ENDORPHINS IN MENTAL HEALTH RESEARCH

ENDORPHINS IN MENTAL HEALTH RESEARCH

Edited by

EARL USDIN, Ph.D.

National Institute of Mental Health, Rockville, Maryland

WILLIAM E. BUNNEY, Jr. M.D.

National Institute of Mental Health, Bethesda, Maryland

and

NATHAN S. KLINE, M.D.

Rockland Research Institute, Orangeburg, New York

1979

Oxford University Press

New York

First published in Great Britain 1979 by
The Macmillan Press Ltd

Printed in Great Britain

Published in the U.S.A. by Oxford University Press, Inc.

Library of Congress Cataloguing in Publication Data

Endorphins in Mental Health Research Conference,
San Juan, P.R., 1977.
Endorphins in mental health research.

Bibliography: p.
Includes index.
1. Endorphins–Congresses. 2. Psychotropic drugs–Congresses. 3. Endorphins–Physiological effect–Congresses. 4. Endorphins–Therapeutic use–Congresses.
I. Usdin, Earl. II. Bunney, William Edward, 1930–
III. Kline, Nathan S. IV. Title.
QP951.E5E52 1977 612′.822 78-13849
ISBN 0-19-520110-8

The members of the Organizing Committee for the Endorphins in Mental Health Research Conference held in Puerto Rico, 10–13 December 1977 were

Floyd Bloom, Salk Institute.
*William E. Bunney, Jr, National Institute of Mental Health.
Avram Goldstein, Stanford University.
John Hughes, Marischal College, Aberdeen (now at Imperial College, London).
Nathan S. Kline, Rockland Research Institute.
Hans Kosterlitz, Marischal College, Aberdeen.
Abel Lajtha, New York State Institute for Neurochemistry and Drug Addiction.
Heinz Lehmann, McGill University.
Candace Pert, National Institute of Mental Health.
Solomon H. Snyder, Johns Hopkins University.
*Earl Usdin, National Institute of Mental Health.

*This book was edited by Drs Usdin and Bunney in their private capacities. No official support or endorsement by the National Institute of Mental Health is intended or should be inferred.

Contents

SECTION ONE: BASIC STUDIES
(B) BIOSYNTHESIS AND DEGRADATION OF ENDORPHINS

SECTION ONE: BASIC STUDIES
(C) FUNCTIONS AND INTERACTIONS OF ENDORPHINS

Foreword

I hope that readers and critics of this volume find it as controversial, interesting and stimulating as I, at least, certainly felt the meeting to be. This meeting on Endorphins in Mental Health Research, held in Puerto Rico in December, 1977 was conceived at the Asilomar meeting on Neuroregulators and Psychiatric Disorders in January 1976, not too long after the first meeting at which the endorphins and the enkephalins raised their heads as fully developed pharmacological entities. (Truly may it be said that a primary outcome of meetings is the begetting of other meetings.) Although there was some doubt as to the need for this meeting when it was originally proposed, by the time it took place, there was little question: the original aim had been an attendance of about 30 or 40, but even with severe restrictions, the organizers had to permit over 150 to attend (including three reporters) and more than 50 papers were given.

Independent of our effort, several psychopharmacologically inclined psychiatrists, led by Nate Kline, arrived at the conclusion that the time was propitious for a meeting on the use of Endorphins in Mental Health, and a request for support was submitted to the Director of the National Institute of Mental Health. Dr Brown agreed that the time was indeed propitious and agreed to give partial support, but he stipulated that the two proposed meetings should be combined.

No attempt has been made in this volume to delete controversy. It is unfortunate that time did not permit inclusion of the discussions at the meeting since, although some of these were almost polemic in nature, they seemed formulated after deep thought by concerned and knowledgeable investigators. Some of these issues have been discussed in the press (see *Medical World News*, January 9, 1978, 86-96).

No conference can work without financial support. I should like to thank most appreciatively the National Institute of Mental Health for providing a large share of such support. In addition, the conference could not have been held without the contribution by the publisher of an advance in lieu of royalties (and for this arrangement, thanks must also be given to the authors). Also, the conference could not have been held if the following companies had not been willing to put their support where their expressed interest was

Endo Laboratories, Inc.
Hoechst-Roussel Pharmaceuticals, Inc.
Hoffman-La Roche, Inc.

ICI Americas, Inc.
Lilly Research Laboratories
Schering Corporation
The Upjohn Company
Wyeth Laboratories

I should like to thank the Council of the American College of Neuropsychopharmacology for allowing us to hold the Endorphins in Mental Health Research Conference in conjunction with their 1977 Annual Meeting. In particular, I thank Dr Morris Lipton, the President, for his invaluable help and cooperation and Dr Alberto DiMascio, the Secretary-Treasurer, and last, but definitely not least, Ms Chris Payne, who did the actual conjunctive cooperation.

Finally, the meeting and the publication could not have succeeded without the help to me of Dr Albert Manian, Mrs Ellen Perella and Mrs Jean Pierce.

Earl Usdin

National Institute of
Mental Health, Rockville,
Maryland

Participants

M. Jules Angst
Psychiatric University Clinic
CH-8029 Zurich 8, Switzerland

Phillip A. Berger
Department of Psychiatry and
Behavioral Sciences
Stanford University Medical School
Stanford, California 94305

Floyd E. Bloom
Salk Institute
P.O. Box 1809
San Diego, California 92112

William D. Brown
Food and Drug Administration
Parklawn Building
Rockville, Maryland 20857

Donald H. Catlin
Department of Pharmacology
UCLA School of Medicine
Los Angeles, California 90024

Steven Childers
Department of Pharmacology and
Experimental Therapeutics
Johns Hopkins University School of Medicine
Baltimore, Maryland 21205

Erminio Costa
NIMH–Saint Elizabeths Hospital
Washington, D.C. 20032

Ian Creese
Department of Pharmacology and
Experimental Therapeutics
Johns Hopkins University School of Medicine
Baltimore, Maryland 21205

Glenn Davis
National Institute of Mental Health
Bethesda, Maryland 20014

H. M. Emrich
Department of Neuropharmacology
Max-Planck Institute for Psychiatry
8 Munich 40, F.R.G.

Frank R. Ervin
Neuropsychiatric Institute, UCLA
Los Angeles, California 90024

Robert C. A. Frederickson
Lilly Research Laboratories
Indianapolis, Indiana 46206

Daniel X. Freedman
Department of Psychiatry
University of Chicago
Chicago, Illinois 60637

Avram Goldstein
Addiction Research Center
Palo Alto, California 94304

Frederick Goodwin
National Institute of Mental Health
Bethesda, Maryland 20014

Lazzlo Graf
Research Institute for
Pharmaceutical Chemistry
Budapest 4, Hungary

Alessandro Guidotti
NIMH–Saint Elizabeths Hospital
Washington, D.C. 20032

Lars-Magnus Gunne
Psychiatric Research Center
University of Uppsala
Ulleraker Hospital
S-750 17 Uppsala, Sweden

Brenton Hanlon
Beckman Instruments, Inc.
Palo Alto, California 94304

Edward Herbert
Department of Chemistry
University of Oregon
Eugene, Oregon 97403

Albert Herz
Max Planck Institute for Psychiatry
8 Munich 40, F.R.G.

John W. Holaday
Walter Reed Army Institute of Research
Washington, D.C. 20013

J. Hong
NIMH–Saint Elizabeths Hospital
Washington, D.C. 20032

Yoshio Hosobuchi
Langley Porter Neuropsychiatric Institute
University of California
San Francisco, California 94143

David Jacobowitz
National Institute of Mental Health
Bethesda, Maryland 20014

Yasuko F. Jacquet
New York State Research Institute for Neurochemistry and Drug Addiction
New York, New York 10035

David Janowsky
Department of Psychiatry
University of California School of Medicine
La Jolla, California 92037

Reese Jones
Langley Porter Neuropsychiatric Institute
University of California
San Francisco, California 94143

Lewis L. Judd
Department of Psychiatry
University of California School of Medicine
La Jolla, California 92037

Roger T. Kelleher
New England Regional Primate Research Center
Southborough, Massachusetts 01772

Werner Klee
National Institute of Mental Health
Bethesda, Maryland 20014

Nathan S. Kline
Rockland Research Center
Orangeburg, New York 10962

Irwin J. Kopin
National Institute of Mental Health
Bethesda, Maryland 20014

Dorothy T. Krieger
Department of Medicine
Mount Sinai Medical Center
New York, New York 10029

William A. Krivoy
NIDA Addiction Research Center
Lexington, Kentucky 40511

Michael J. Kuhar
Department of Pharmacology and Experimental Therapeutics
Johns Hopkins University School of Medicine
Baltimore, Maryland 21205

Fernand Labrie
Laboratory of Molecular Endocrinology
Laval University, Faculty of Medicine
Quebec GIV 4G2, Canada

Abel Lajtha
New York State Research Institute for Neurochemistry and Drug Addiction
Wards Island, New York 10035

David N. Leff
Medical World News
McGraw Hill Publications
New York, New York 10020

Heinz E. Lehmann
Douglas Hospital
Montreal 204, Quebec, Canada

Choh Hao Li
Hormone Research Laboratory
University of California
San Francisco, California 94143

Morris A. Lipton
Department of Psychiatry
University of NC School of Medicine
Chapel Hill, North Carolina 27514

Richard E. Mains
Department of Physiology
University of Colorado Medical Center
Denver, Colorado 80220

Richard J. Miller
Department of Pharmacology
University of Chicago
Chicago, Illinois 60637

Anne Mudge
Physiology Department
Harvard Medical School
Boston, Massachusetts 02114

José M. Musacchio
Department of Pharmacology
New York University Medical Center
New York, New York 10016

Marshall Nirenberg
National Heart and Lung Institute
Bethesda, Maryland 20014

Roberta M. Palmour
Department of Genetics
University of California
Berkeley, California 94720

Jorge Perez-Cruet
Laboratory of Neuropharmacology
Missouri Institute of Psychiatry
St. Louis, Missouri 63139

Agu Pert
National Institute of Mental Health
Bethesda, Maryland 20014

Candace Pert
National Institute of Mental Health
Bethesda, Maryland 20014

Ruth Ann Riese
Beckman Instruments Inc.
Palo Alto, California 94304

R. Schulz
Max Planck Institute for Psychiatry
8 Munich 40, F.R.G.

David S. Segal
Department of Psychiatry
University of California School of Medicine
La Jolla, California 92093

Derek G. Smyth
National Institute for Medical Research
London, NW7, 1AA, U.K.

Sydney Spector
Roche Institute of Molecular Biology
Nutley, New Jersey 07110

Larry Stein
Department of Psychopharmacology
Wyeth Laboratories, Inc.
Philadelphia, Pennsylvania 19101

Hansjörg Teschemacher
Max Planck Institute for Psychiatry
8 Munich 40, F.R.G.

Edward C. Tocus
Food and Drug Administration
Parklawn Building
Rockville, Maryland 20857

Sidney Udenfriend
Roche Institute of Molecular Biology
Nutley, New Jersey 07110

George Uhl
Department of Pharmacology and Experimental Therapeutics
Johns Hopkins University School of Medicine
Baltimore, Maryland 21205

Earl Usdin
National Institute of Mental Health
Parklawn Building
Rockville, Maryland 20857

Barbara Villet
RFD 1
Shushan, New York 12873

Herbert Wagemaker
Department of Psychiatry
Louisville General Hospital
Louisville, Kentucky 40202

Agneta Wahlström
Department of Medicinal Pharmacology
University of Uppsala
S-751 23 Uppsala, Sweden

Stanley J. Watson*
Department of Psychiatry
Stanford University
School of Medicine
Stanford, California 94304

C. David Wise
Wyeth Laboratories
Philadelphia, Pennsylvania 19101

H.-Y. T. Yang
NIMH–Saint Elizabeths Hospital
Washington, D.C. 20032

Walter Zieglgänsberger
Max Planck Institute for Psychiatry
8 Munich 40, F.R.G.

*presented *in absentia.*

Abbreviations

ACTH, adrenocorticotropic hormone (corticotropin)
AIS, abstinence intensity score
Ala, alanine
ANOVA, analysis of variance
Arg, arginine
Asn, asparagine
Asp, aspartic acid
ATP, adenosine triphosphate
BBB, blood/brain barrier
β_c, Beta (camel)
β_h, Beta (human)
β_s, Beta (swine)
Boc, *t*-butyloxycarbonyl
BPRS, Brief Psychiatric Rating Scale
BSA, bovine serum albumin
cAMP, cyclic adenosine monophosphate
CNS, central nervous system
c.p.m., counts per minute
CPRS, Comprehensive Psychopathological Rating Scale
CPZ, chlorpromazine
CRF, corticotropin releasing factor
CSF, cerebrospinal fluid
CTP, cytosine triphosphate
DA, dopamine
DD, differential diagnosis
DDC, diethyldithiocarbamate
DNA, deoxyribonucleic acid
DNP, dinitrophenyl
DOPA, dihydroxyphenylalanine
DOPAC, dihydroxyphenylacetic acid
DSM II, Diagnostic and Statistical Manual of the American Psychiatric Association
DTT, dithiothreitol
ECT, electroconvulsive therapy
EDTA, ethylene diamine tetraacetic acid
EEG, electroencephalogram
EGTA, ethylene glycol *bis*-(β-aminoethyl ether) tetraacetic acid
EKG, electrocardiogram
EMB, explosive motor behavior
EMG, electromyogram
EOG, electrooculogram
e.p.s.p., excitatory postsynaptic potential
EXC, excitement
FDA, (US) Food and Drug Administration
FI, fixed-interval (schedule)
FITC, fluorescein isothiocyanate
FR, fixed-ratio (schedule)
FSH, follicle stimulating hormone
GABA, γ-aminobutyric acid
GH, growth hormone
Glu, glutamic acid
Gly, glycine
GPI, guinea pig ileum
GRN, grandiose expansiveness
GTP, guanosine triphosphate
5-HIAA, 5-hydroxyindoleacetic acid
His, histamine
HOS, hostile belligerence
h.p.l.c. high pressure (or, performance) liquid chromatography
i.c., intracerebral(ly)
Ile, isoleucine
i.m., intramuscular(ly)
IMPS, Inpatient Multidimensional Psychiatric Scale •
IND, Investigational New Drug Application
i.p., intraperitoneal(ly)

IR, inhibitory response
i.v., intravenous(ly)
i.v.t., intraventricular(ly)
Leu, leucine
LH, luteinizing hormone
LHRH, luteinizing hormone releasing hormone
Li, lithium (ion)
LPH, β-lipotropin
LSD, lysergic acid diethylamide
Lys, lysine
MD, manic-depressive psychosis
Me, methyl
mEq, milliequivalents
Met, methionine
MHPG, 3-methoxy-4-hydroxyphenylglycol
MLC, morphine-like compound
MPLM, myenteric plexus-longitudinal muscle
mRNA, messenger RNA
MSH, melanotropin (melanocyte stimulating hormone)
MVD, mouse vas deferens
NA, nucleus accumbens
NE, norepinephrine
NDA, New Drug Application
NIMH, (US) National Institute of Mental Health
Nle, norleucine
NOSIE, Nurses' Observation Scale for Inpatient Evaluation
6-OHDA, 6-hydroxydopamine
PAG, periaqueductal grey
PAR, paranoid projection
PBS, phosphate buffered saline
PCA, perchloracetic acid
PCP, perceptual distortion
Phe, phenylalanine
PIF, prolactin release-inhibiting factor
p.o., per os
POMS, Psychiatric Outpatient Mood Scale
PPi, inorganic phosphate
PRL, prolactin
Pro, proline
REM, rapid eye movement (sleep)
RIA, radioimmunoassay
RNA, ribonucleic acid
s.c., subcutaneous(ly)
s.d., standard deviation
SDS, sodium dodecyl sulfate
s.e.m., standard error of the mean
Ser, serine
SHAS, Subjective High Assessment Scale
SS, stainless steel
TCA, trichloracetic acid
Thr, threonine
t.l.c., thin layer chromatography
tRNA, transfer RNA
Trp, tryptophan
TSH, thyrotropin stimulating hormone
TTX, tetrodotoxin
Tyr, tyramine
UTP, uridine triphosphate
Val, valine
VBS, Verlaufs-Beurteilungs-Skala (Course Assessment Scale)
WAIS, Wechsler Adult Intelligence Scale

Introduction

The recent discovery of opiate receptors in animal and primate brains and the identification of endogenously produced opioid peptides has produced an unparalleled explosion of information in this new field of neuroscience. This book reviews the biosynthesis and degradation of endorphins, their function and interaction with other neurotransmitter and endocrine systems, their localization in brain and peripheral tissue, their structure, new methods for their assay, data related to their clinical importance in man, particularly as related to mental health, and their possible therapeutic use in disease states. Specific issues addressed involve the role of endorphins as neurotransmitters contrasted with their role as endocrine effectors. The regional localization of endorphins may help us to understand their function; thus distribution in the pituitary compared with the brain will be reviewed as well as the distribution of enkephalins within the brain. Other studies review whether the doses of exogenously administered endorphins used in animal and human studies relate to the physiological levels of these substances and their function and whether narcotic antagonists block endorphin function in man and if so, at what doses.

β-Lipotropin
in camel

```
H-Glu-Leu-Thr-Gly-Glu-Arg-Leu-Glu-Gln-Ala-Arg-Gly-Pro-Glu-Ala-Gln-Ala-Glu-Ser-Ala-
                 5                   10                  15                  20

 Ala-Ala-Arg-Ala-Glu-Leu-Glu-Tyr-Gly-Leu-Val-Ala-Glu-Ala-Glu-Ala-Ala-Glu-Lys-Lys-
                 25                  30                  35                  40

 Asp-Ser-Gly-Pro-Tyr-Lys-Met-Glu-His-Phe-Arg-Trp-Gly-Ser-Pro-Pro-Lys-Asp-Lys-Arg-
                 45                  50                  55                  60

 Tyr-Gly-Gly-Phe-Met-Thr-Ser-Glu-Lys-Ser-Gln-Thr-Pro-Leu-Val-Thr-Leu-Phe-Lys-Asn-
                 65                  70                  75                  80
      Met-enkephalin

 Ala-Ile-Ile-Lys-Asn-Ala-His-Lys-Lys-Gly-Gln-OH
                 85                  90
```

β-endorphin

The figure reviews some of the compounds which will be discussed in the following chapters. It has been demonstrated that fragments of β-lipotropin (β-LPH), derived from the pituitary, possess opiate-like activity. These include met-enkephalin, the 61–65 amino acid fragment, and β-endorphin, the C-terminal 31 amino acid fragment of β-LPH.

It should be emphasized that most of our hypotheses concerning the functions of endorphins are derived from many years of investigation of morphine. Morphine was isolated in 1806. The chemical structure was first proven by total synthesis in 1952. Some of the proposed endorphin-mediated behaviors currently under investigation in man include studies of pain, sleep, respiration, sexual activity and endocrine regulation. In addition, a role for endorphins in the symptoms of schizophrenia, catatonia, depression and mania is being intensively studied. Strategies for the study of the function of endorphins in man include single and double-blind, placebo controlled drug trials of β-endorphin, the development of assays for endorphin in the urine, plasma, and CSF, and specific studies attempting to stimulate the release of endorphins by stress, pain, and implanted electrodes in human brain. The most common strategy currently in clinical use and extensively reported in this book involves the use of the specific narcotic antagonists, nalozone and naltrexone, which, theoretically, should displace endogenous endorphins from receptor sites.

The rapid expansion of knowledge in this field has been made possible through the technological development of instruments used in many areas of pharmacology and the existence of well trained pharmacologists, biochemists, neuroendocrinologists, psychiatrists and psychologists. It is my opinion that the excitement in this field has been created by its immediate accessibility, the intriguing and surprising discovery that non-primates and primates produce morphine-like compounds and the large number of basic and clinical investigative corridors that appear to lead from these initial discoveries.

William E. Bunney Jr,
National Institute of
Mental Health, Bethesda, Maryland

Section One
Basic Studies

(A) Localization, Assay and Structure of Endorphins

1
Distribution and pharmacology of the enkephalins

Richard J. Miller, H. Y. Meltzer* and V. S. Fang†
(Departments of Pharmacological and Physiological Sciences, Psychiatry* and Medicine†, University of Chicago)

It is now just over two years since the publication of the structures of two peptides found in the brain which possessed potent opiate agonist activity (Hughes *et al.*, 1975; Simantov and Snyder, 1976). These peptides were named enkephalins and had structures H_2N-Tyr-Gly-Gly-Phe-Met-OH ([Met^5]-enkephalin) and H_2N-Tyr-Gly-Gly-Phe-Leu-OH ([Leu^5]-enkephalin). The structure of [Met^5]-enkephalin is contained in its entirety within the sequence of the hormone β-lipotropin (β-LPH), a 91-amino acid peptide in which [Met^5]-enkephalin constitutes residues 61-65 (Hughes *et al.*, 1975). Moreover, peptides with sequences ranging from β-LPH_{61-65} ([Met^5]. enkephalin) to β-LPH_{61-91} all seem to possess opiate agonist activity (Bradbury *et al.*, 1976*a*; Cox *et al.*, 1976; Lazarus *et al.*, 1976). Several of these related peptides, β-LPH_{61-91} (β-endorphin), β-LPH_{61-76} (α-endorphin) and β-LPH_{61-77} (γ-endorphin) have now been isolated from the brain, pituitary or gastrointestinal tract of several species (Bradbury *et al.*, 1976*b*; Bloom *et al.*, 1978). These observations have stimulated research in many areas of neurobiology and results have been obtained suggesting that the opiate peptides have fundamental roles in many neuronal and endocrine mechanisms.

Owing to their relatively small size and ease of synthesis, the pharmacology of the enkephalins has been intensively investigated and many structural analogues of these peptides have been produced that exhibit a wide spectrum of pharmacological activities (Beddell *et al.*, 1977).

Here we shall discuss the pharmacology of the enkephalins in relation to what is now known about their distribution.

Distribution of the enkephalins studied by radioimmunoassay

Investigation of the distribution of the various opiate peptides has been aided by the development of specific antisera that may be used for both radioimmunoassay (RIA) and immunohistochemistry (Guillemin *et al.*, 1977; Miller *et al.*, 1977*a*; Rossier *et al.*, 1977; Yang *et al.*, 1977). Antisera to both the enkephalin pentapeptides and several of the longer endorphins have been reported. We have determined the distribution of the enkephalins in the CNS and gastrointestinal tract by RIA using these antisera (Kobayashi *et al.*, 1977; Miller *et al.*, 1977*a*). It is important to note that when performing such experiments efficient extraction of the peptides under investigation must be obtained if the data are to be useful in the quantitative sense. Several methods of extraction have been tested. It has been found that extraction of tissue with 0.1 N HCl or 2 N acetic acid leads to high recovery of enkephalins (Miller *et al.*, 1977*a*); 2 N acetic acid also extracts α and β-endorphin efficiently. In the latter case, however, boiling the tissue in acid before homogenization is recommended (Rossier *et al.*, 1977).

After extraction with 0.1 N HCl, the opiate activity found in rat brain can be fractionated by gel filtration. It is clear that some but not all of the opiate activity chromatographs in the same position as authentic [^{3}H] [Met^5] or [Leu^5]-enkephalin on Biogel P-2. Some opiate activity also elutes in the void volume indicating that it has a molecular weight of over 1000. This peak could correspond to opiate peptides such as α or β-endorphin or some other high molecular weight species. Figure 1.1 illustrates this result in the case of rat brain. To monitor opiate activity in each fraction an assay has been

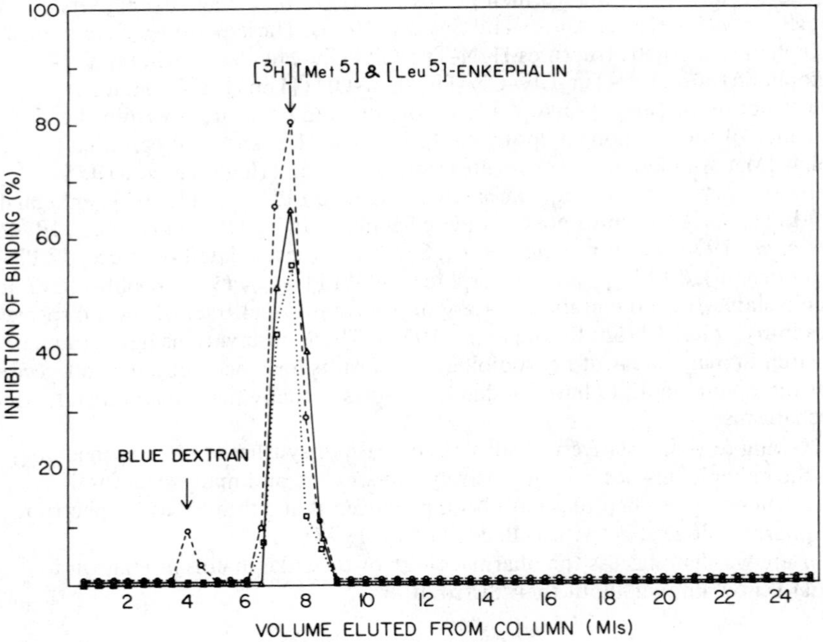

Figure 1.1 Fractionation of 0.1 N HCl extract of whole rat brain on Biogel P-2 column. 0----0, inhibition of opiate receptor binding; □----□, inhibition of [^{125}I] [Leu^5]-enkephalin antibody; △----△, inhibition of binding of [^{125}I] [Met^5]-enkephalin to anti-[Met^5]-enkephalin antibody. (From Miller *et al.*, 1977*a*).

Table 1.1 Regional distribution of brain enkephalin and effects of hypophysectomy (pmol/mg protein)

Rank order	Region	Normal				Hypophysectomized			
		Total	Met	Leu	M/L	Total	Met	Leu	M/L
1	Globus pallidus	35.0	29.5 ± 3.5	5.5 ± 0.10	5.4	36.5	31.5 ± 2.8	5.0 ± 0.35	6.3
2	Central grey	6.5	4.8 ± 0.2	1.7 ± 0.09	2.8	6.6	5.1 ± 0.4	1.5 ± 0.07	3.4
3	Nucleus accumbens	6.3	5.2 ± 0.4	1.1 ± 0.09	4.7	6.5	5.6 ± 0.4	0.91 ± 0.06	6.2
4	Median hypothalamus	5.0	4.4 ± 0.3	0.60 ± 0.07	7.3	4.2	3.7 ± 0.3	0.53 ± 0.01	7.0
5	Amygdala	4.5	3.3 ± 0.3	1.2 ± 0.07	2.8	5.1	3.3 ± 0.2	1.8 ± 0.1	1.8
6	Pons	3.4	2.8 ± 0.4	0.55 ± 0.04	5.1	2.7	2.2 ± 0.4	0.51 ± 0.02	4.3
7	Medulla	3.3	2.6 ± 0.6	0.70 ± 0.06	3.7	2.9	2.2 ± 0.3	0.66 ± 0.08	3.3
8	Caudate/putamen	3.1	2.6 ± 0.4	0.53 ± 0.06	4.9	3.3	2.5 ± 0.2	0.75 ± 0.06	3.3
9	Thalamus	2.6	2.0 ± 0.1	0.64 ± 0.03	3.1	3.0	2.3 ± 0.2	0.66 ± 0.02	3.5
10	Septal area	2.3	2.0 ± 0.3	0.40 ± 0.02	5.0	2.2	1.8 ± 0.2	0.37 ± 0.03	4.9
11	Lateral hypothalamus	2.1	1.9 ± 0.3	0.22 ± 0.02	8.6	1.6	1.4 ± 0.1	0.18 ± 0.01	7.8
12	Midbrain	1.5	1.2 ± 0.1	0.31 ± 0.04	3.9	1.3	1.0 ± 0.1	0.28 ± 0.03	3.6
13	Hippocampus	1.3	1.1 ± 0.08	0.17 ± 0.02	6.5	1.5	1.3 ± 0.10	0.17 ± 0.04	7.7
14	Cerebral cortex	1.3	0.81 ± 0.09	0.44 ± 0.04	1.8	1.4	1.0 ± 0.05	0.37 ± 0.04	2.7
15	Preoptic area	1.1	0.95 ± 0.10	0.11 ± 0.01	8.6	0.9	0.79 ± 0.06	0.10 ± 0.02	7.9
16	Cerebellum	–	0.2 ± 0.03	<0.1	–	–	0.1 ± 0.1	<0.1	–

(From Kobayashi *et al.*, 1977)

developed which utilizes the binding of [^{125}I] [D-Ala^2, D-Leu^5]-enkephalin to opiate receptors in N4TG1 neuroblastoma cells (Miller *et al.*, 1977*a, b*). In the pituitary on the other hand, most of the opiate activity elutes in the void volume and is probably α or β-endorphin. Little opiate material elutes in the region of [Met^5] or [Leu^5]-enkephalin in comparison with the large void volume peak. (Miller *et al.*, 1977*a*).

Table 1.1 illustrates the general distribution of [Met^5] and [Leu^5]-enkephalins in rat brain (Kobayashi *et al.*, 1977). The concentrations reported here are in fair agreement with most other reports. One report gave [Met^5]-enkephalin concentrations that were about twice those reported here (Yang *et al.*, 1977). These authors, however, used microwave irradiation to process tissue before extraction. This method may preserve concentrations of endogenous substances more reliably than conventional methods as it fixes brain tissue more rapidly, destroying the activity of proteases and other potential degradative enzymes. However some problems associated with this method have also been reported (Bloom *et al.*, 1978).

Various points should be noted about the enkephalin distribution in rat brain. Both enkephalins are widely distributed in brain but the distribution is uneven (Hong *et al.*, 1977; Kobayashi *et al.*, 1977; Yang *et al.*, 1977). By far the highest concentrations are in the globus pallidus, which is five times richer in enkephalin than the next richest areas which include the central grey of the mesencephalon, nucleus accumbens, the medial (periventricular) hypothalamus and the amygdala. Concentrations in the caudate/putamen were eleven times lower than in the adjacent globus pallidus. The medial hypothalamus was three times richer in enkephalins than the lateral hypothalamus. Lower enkephalin concentrations were found in the midbrain, hippocampus, cerebral cortex, preoptic area and cerebellum. These data correlate closely with the distribution of enkephalins revealed by immunohistochemistry (see below) and also with the distribution of opiate receptors revealed by autoradiography (Simantov *et al.*, 1977). Opiate receptors are also found in high concentrations in the periaqueductal grey and globus pallidus with low concentrations in the cerebellum. However, there are some differences in distribution. For example, very high concentrations of opiate receptors are found in the caudate/putamen where relatively little enkephalin is found. It is also interesting to compare the distribution of enkephalin with that reported for β-endorphin in the brain. β-endorphin is found in high concentrations in the hypothalamus, as is enkephalin, but is found in extremely small concentrations in the striatum where concentrations of enkephalin are extremely high (Bloom *et al.*, 1978).

The data in table 1.1 also demonstrate that hypophysectomy does not reduce the concentration of [Met^5] or [Leu^5]-enkephalin in any brain area examined. This indicates that the source of enkephalin in the brain cannot be the pituitary. If, in fact, β-LPH and β-endorphin do represent biosynthetic precursors for [Met^5]-enkephalin, then there must be an independent pool of such molecules in the CNS not derived from the pituitary. Such a pool of opiate peptides may not be unlikely in the light of a recent report of another related peptide hormone found in the pituitary (adrenocorticotropin, ACTH) which is also found in the CNS and does not disappear following hypophysectomy (Krieger *et al.*, 1977). These observations are also consistent with another report

Table 1.2 Concentrations of enkephalin in the gastrointestinal tract

[Met⁵]-enkephalin (pmol/g wet weight)

	Guinea pig	Rat
Duodenum	6.2 ± 0.7	1.6 ± 0.2
Jejunum	4.4 ± 0.2	1.1 ± 0.1
Ileum	4.1 ± 0.3	0.81 ± 0.05
Colon	3.3 ± 0.3	0.33 ± 0.01
Cecum	0.7 ± 0.1	0.3 ± 0.01

[Leu⁵]-enkephalin (pmol/g wet weight)

	Guinea pig	Rat
Duodenum	0.55 ± 0.04	0.08 ± 0.01
Jejunum	0.57 ± 0.02	0.09 ± 0.01
Ileum	0.38 ± 0.02	0.1 ± 0.02
Colon	0.67 ± 0.04	0.05 ± 0.01
Cecum	0.1 ± 0.01	0.02 ± 0.003

Results are the mean for three animals.

that the 'total opiate activity' in rat brain extracts is not decreased by hypophysectomy (Cheung and Goldstein, 1976).

Appreciable concentrations of both [Met⁵] and [Leu⁵]-enkephalins are also found in the gastrointestinal tract of human, rat, hamster and guinea pig (Polak *et al.*, 1977; Linnoila *et al.*, 1978). This localization is illustrated in table 1.2 and has been confirmed by immunohistochemistry (see below).

Distribution of enkephalins by immunohistochemistry

The distribution of enkephalins in rat brain was investigated using the same antisera as described above and a modified immunoperoxidase bridge procedure. Rats were perfused through the aorta with 3 per cent paraformaldehyde and 0.5 per cent gluteraldehyde in sodium phosphate buffer. Brains were removed, dissected, dehydrated through alcohol and xylene, and embedded in paraffin; 4 μm sections were cut and stained. Detailed mapping of enkephalin-containing cell bodies and nerve terminals in the CNS has been carried out. Some of the areas in which positive staining of cell bodies and/or nerve terminals has been obtained include in the forebrain: lateral septum, amygdala, hippocampus, globus pallidus, nucleus caudatus and nucleus accumbens; in the midbrain: the nucleus interpeduncularis and periaqueductal grey; and in the lower brainstem: the nucleus parabrachialis, nuclei raphes, locus coeruleus, nucleus tractus soli-

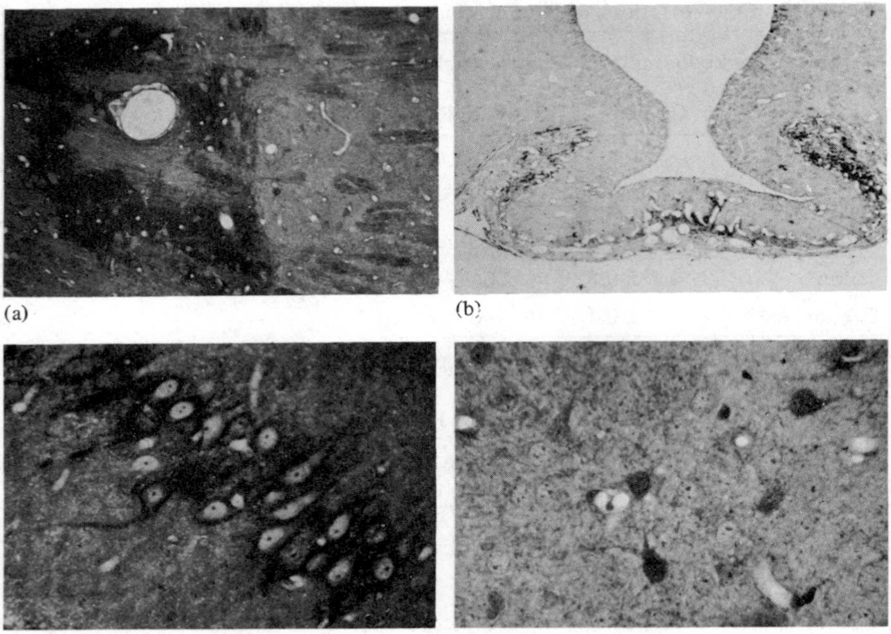

(a) (b) (c) (d)

Figure 1.2 Immunoperoxidase staining of rat brain. Anti-[Leu^5]-enkephalin antibody. (a) Basal ganglia. Note heavy staining in the globus pallidus and relative paucity of staining in the caudate. (b) Median eminence. (c) Hippocampus. (d) Nucleus accumbens. (Sar, Stumpf, Miller, Chang and Cuatrecasas, 1978.)

tarius and formatio reticularis. In the spinal cord staining is also seen, for example in laminae I and II and in the substantia gelatinosa of spinal nerve V. Some examples of this localization are shown in Fig. 1.2.

We have also studied the distribution of [Met^5] and [Leu^5]-enkephalins in the gastrointestinal tract of rat, guinea pig and hamster. In this case, tissue was fixed with either buffered 10 per cent formalin or vapors of diethylpyrocarbonate or *p*-benzoquinone. Immunoperoxidase staining was obtained in nerve fibers all along the gastrointestinal smooth muscle except in the wall of the cecum. Nerve fibers in the guinea pig esophagus and cardia of the stomach were stained with [Met^5] but not [Leu^5]-enkephalin antisera. A network of immunostained fibers was observed in Meissner's plexus of the stomach and small intestine often closely surrounding an unstained cell. Stained nerves were also obtained in the circular muscle layer especially in the colon and rectum (figure 1.3). Staining was not observed in epithelial cells.

Using these antisera, staining is also found in the pituitary gland. In this case anti-[Met^5]-enkephalin antiserum is somewhat more effective than anti-[Leu^5]-enkephalin. Staining is seen in every cell in the intermediate lobe and in scattered cells in the anterior lobe. It is interesting to note that in serial sections those

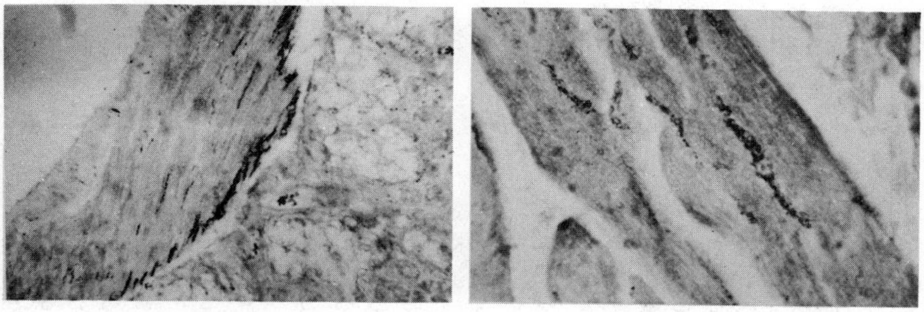

Figure 1.3 Immunoperoxidase staining of guinea pig gastrointestinal tract. (a) Meissner's plexus. Anti-[Leu^5]-enkephalin antiserum. (b) Pylorus of the stomach. Anti-[Met^5]-kephalin antiserum. (Linnoila, DiAugustine, Miller, Chang and Cuatrecasas, 1978.)

cells that stain with anti-enkephalin antisera also stain with antisera to $ACTH_{1-24}$. This observation fits well with data suggesting that opiate peptides and ACTH are both synthesized from a common biosynthetic precursor known as 'Big ACTH' (Mains and Eipper, 1977).

In general the.staining patterns we have obtained are similar to those reported by others (Elde *et al.*, 1976; Hökfelt *et al.*, 1977; Simantov *et al.*, 1977). Some differences are, however, worth mentioning. In contrast to results reported elsewhere (Elde *et al.*, 1976) we have obtained staining of the pituitary gland with our anti-enkephalin antisera. It is not clear whether this is due to cross reactivity of the antisera with β-endorphin, or due to the fact that these antisera are more sensitive than others and are able to detect the low levels of enkephalin found in the pituitary. It is interesting to note that Bloom and colleagues (1978) using the same antisera have compared them with anti-β-endorphin antisera when staining the pituitary. These authors have reported that in fact the anti-[Leu^5]-enkephalin antisera produce a rather different staining pattern from anti-β-endorphin antisera as the anti-[Leu^5]-enkephalin antisera also stain some fiber-like components in the posterior lobe whereas the anti-β-endorphin antisera do not. This suggests that anti-[Leu^5]-enkephalin staining in the pituitary may truly be localizing enkephalin rather than β-endorphin.

Pearse and colleagues (Polak *et al.*, 1977) have also examined the distribution of enkephalin in the gastrointestinal tract. In addition to neuronal elements these authors also detected enkephalin in cells that stained for gastrin as well. We have not detected such cells in the guinea pig gastrointestinal tract, presumably due to interspecies variation.

Pharmacology of the enkephalins

The distribution of the enkephalins as revealed by RIA and immunohistochemistry suggests some possible roles for the enkephalins *in vivo*. Some of these roles are supported by the biological activities of enkephalins and their synthetic analogues as well as by the known pharmacology of opiate agonists. Figure 1.1

Table 1.3 Effect of enkephalin and enkephalin analogues on plasma prolactin levels in male rats

	Plasma prolactin (ng/ml)			
	Pre-injection	10 min	30 min	Opiate receptor affinity (M)
Tyr–Gly–Gly–Phe–Met	13.0 ± 4.5	32.0 ± 10.3	5.7 ± 1.8	2×10^{-8}
Tyr–Gly–Gly–Phe–Leu	11.9 ± 3.4	28.1 ± 5.0	8.0 ± 2.9	1.1×10^{-8}
Tyr–D-Ala–Gly–Phe–D-Leu–HNEt	18.7 ± 10.6	36.1 ± 7.1	29.0 ± 9.4	1×10^{-7}
Tyr–D-Ala–Gly–Phe	10.1 ± 3.9	32.6 ± 4.4	32.4 ± 1.9	7×10^{-8}
Tyr–D-NMeAla–Gly–Phe–D-LeuOMe	6.2 ± 1.0	36.2 ± 3.5	20.5 ± 5.4	9×10^{-8}
Tyr–D-Ala–Gly–Phe–D-Leu	2.2 ± 0.8	41.5 ± 9.5	23.0 ± 4.3	2.6×10^{-9}
Tyr–D-Ala–Gly–*p*ClPhe–D-LeuNHEt	13.4 ± 6.3	62.0 ± 20.6	47.4 ± 14.3	8×10^{-8}
NMeTyr–D-Ala–Gly–Phe–D-MetNH_2	10.4 ± 4.3	30.5 ± 7.2	32.5 ± 6.5	3×10^{-7}
NMeTyr–D-Ala–Gly–Phe–D-LeuNH_2	10.3 ± 5.6	30.7 ± 6.0	29.8 ± 2.8	2×10^{-8}
Tyr–D-Ala–Gly–Phe–Met–Thr	12.4 ± 2.8	34.0 ± 6.9	12.8 ± 5.3	5.6×10^{-9}
Tyr–D-Ala–Gly–*p*ClPhe–D-LeuOMe	10.3 ± 6.0	37.0 ± 7.6	16.0 ± 3.3	2×10^{-9}
Tyr–D-Trp–Gly–Phe–Leu	11.7 ± 2.1	23.4 ± 5.9	14.0 ± 3.2	9×10^{-9}
Tyr–Gly–Gly–TyrOMe–LeuOMe	12.8 ± 2.7	30.9 ± 6.4	12.6 ± 4.7	5×10^{-5}
Tyr–D-Trp–Gly–Phe–D-Leu	15.4 ± 3.5	16.1 ± 3.3	12.4 ± 3.4	8×10^{-6}
Tyr–D-Ala–Gly–Phe–D-Met	12.5 ± 5.2	18.9 ± 5.3	8.6 ± 3.3	1×10^{-8}
Tyr–Gly–Ala–Phe–Leu	21.0 ± 4.9	18.1 ± 2.4	11.3 ± 3.0	8×10^{-6}
Tyr–Gly–Gly–D-Phe–Leu	5.1 ± 2.4	7.4 ± 2.1	3.3 ± 0.9	$> 10^{-4}$
Tyr–D-Ala–Gly–Leu–Leu	11.3 ± 4.5	19.5 ± 6.4	11.5 ± 6.2	$> 10^{-4}$
D-Tyr–D-Ala–Gly–Phe–Leu	19.2 ± 6.0	24.1 ± 5.0	13.0 ± 2.8	3×10^{-4}
D-Ala–Gly–LeuOMe	23.9 ± 4.2	29.8 ± 4.9	26.9 ± 5.0	$> 10^{-4}$
Phe–D-Ala–Gly–Phe–Leu	12.5 ± 5.9	19.4 ± 5.8	7.3 ± 4.2	1×10^{-7}

illustrates the localization of enkephalin in the median eminence of the rat. Such a localization suggests one role for the enkephalins as neuroendocrine modulators. Indeed it has previously been shown that morphine can effect the release of several pituitary hormones, particularly growth hormone (GH) and prolactin (PRL) (Ferland *et al.*, 1976; Kokka *et al.*, 1972). After intraventricular (i.v.t.) injection of enkephalins or their synthetic analogues GH and PRL are released (Cusan *et al.*, 1977; Shaar *et al.*, 1977)–illustrated in table 1.3 for a series of enkephalins. [Met^5] and [Leu^5]-enkephalins increased plasma PRL concentrations at 10 min, but by 30 min levels had returned to normal. Various analogues were also able to increase circulating PRL concentrations. In particular after i.v.t. administration of the analogue H_2N–Tyr–D-Ala–Gly–*p*ClPhe–D-LeuNHEt, plasma PRL levels were still raised after 30 min. As might be expected, analogues with a [D-Ala^2]-substitution which confers metabolic stability on the peptide were most effective in raising PRL levels. Although substitution of a wide range of amino acids in position 2 increases stability, not all such substitutions retain high affinity for the opiate receptor (Miller *et al.*, 1977*c*, 1978; Pert *et al.*, 1977). Thus some substitutions, such as [D-Trp^2], reduce affinity and are less effective in raising PRL. We have also found that some enkephalins are effective in stimulating prolactin secretion when given i.v. Table 1.4 illustrates this result for the analogue [D-Ala^2, D-Leu^5]-enkephalin. The increase in PRL release

Table 1.4 Effect of intravenous enkephalin and naloxone on rat plasma prolactin levels

	Plasma prolactin (ng/ml)		
Treatment	0 min	10 min	30 min
[D-Ala^2, D-Leu^5]	9.0 ± 8.0	25.6 ± 1.3	4.0 ± 3.0
Naloxone + [D-Ala^2, D-Leu^5]	4.0 ± 0.6	3.0 ± 1.0	3.6 ± 3.5

Naloxone, 5 mg/kg (i.v.), or saline (i.v.) was injected 15 min before [D-Ala^2, D-Leu^5], 0.5 mg/kg (i.v.). Results are mean ± s.e.m.

produced by this analogue is reversed by naloxone, indicating that the effect is mediated by the opiate receptor. It has been shown that this enkephalin analogue can produce analgesia after i.v. administration in rats, indicating that it can cross the blood–brain barrier to a certain extent (Wei *et al.*, 1977). This observation, and others indicating that enkephalins do not have a direct PRL-releasing effect on isolated pituitary cells in culture (Rivier *et al.*, 1977), suggests that the effect of intravenous [D-Ala^2 D-Leu^5]-enkephalin is mediated by the hypothalamus. These effects, and those reported by others, together with the localization of the enkephalins in the median eminence, support the notion that these opiate peptides may act as releasing factors *in vivo*.

Enkephalins are also found by RIA and immunohistochemistry in the periaqueductal grey (see above). It is known that electrical stimulation or microinjection of narcotics into this area produces analgesia in animals and man (Mayer and Price, 1976). Thus relocalization of enkephalins supports the hypo-

Table 1.5 Analgesic activity measured by hot plate test

Analogue	ED_{50} μg per mouse i.v.t.
NMe–Tyr–D-Ala–Gly–Phe–D-MetNH_2	0.005
Tyr–D-Ala–Gly–Phe–D-LeuNHEt	0.01
NMeTyr–D-Ala–Gly–Phe–D–Met	0.007
NMeTyr–D-Ala–Gly–Phe–D-MetOMe	0.02
NMeTyr–D-Ala–Gly–Phe–D-LeuNH_2	0.05
Tyr–D-Ala–Gly–Phe–D-LeuO*p*ClPh	0.05
NMeTyr–D-Ala–Gly–Phe–D-LeuOMe	0.05
NMeTyr–D-Ala–Gly–Phe–D-Leu	0.07
Tyr–D-Ala–Gly–*p*ClPhe–D-Leu	0.07
NMeTyr–D-Ala–Gly–Phe–D-MetNHEt	0.07
Tyr–D-Ala–Gly–Phe–D-LeuOMe	0.07
Tyr–D-Ala–Gly–Phe–D-LeuNHEt	0.1
Tyr–D-Ala–Gly–Phe–D-Leu–D-Thr	0.1
Tyr–D-Ala–Gly–Phe–D-Leu–Phe–Gly	0.1
Tyr–D-Ala–Gly–Phe–D-Leu–Thr	0.1
Tyr–D-Ala–Gly–Phe–Met–Thr	0.24
Tyr–D-Ala–Gly–Phe–D-Leu	0.5
Tyr–D-Ala–Gly–Phe–D-Met	0.5
Tyr–D-Ala–Gly–Phe–D-Leu–Thr	0.5
Tyr–D-Ala–Gly–Phe–Thr	0.5
Tyr–D-Ala–Gly–Phe–D-LeuOMe	0.5

thesis that these peptides may also be involved in mediating pain responses and sensations. It is certainly true to say that enkephalins can produce analgesia following i.v.t. and in some cases systemic administration (Belluzzi *et al.*, 1976; Buscher *et al.*, 1976; Miller *et al.*, 1977*a*)–illustrated for a series of enkephalin analogues in table 1.5. It is quite clear that many of these analogues and also β-endorphin produce much more profound analgesia than that reported for [Met^5] and [Leu^5]-enkephalins. The main factor involved here is probably the increased stability of many synthetic enkephalin analogues. However, this is certainly not the only factor. By comparison of table 1.5 with tables 1.6 and 1.7 it can be seen

Table 1.6 Opiate receptor affinity relative to morphine (morphine = 1)

Analogue	Relative affinity
Tyr–D-Ala–Gly–*p*ClPhe–D-Leu	3.5
Tyr–D-Ala–Gly–*p*ClPhe–D-LeuOMe	1.75
Tyr–D-Ala–Gly–Phe–D-Leu	1.34
Tyr–D-Ala–Gly–Phe–Leu	1.09
Tyr–D-Ala–Gly–Phe–Met	0.97
Tyr–D-Ala–Gly–Phe–MetOMe	0.7
Tyr–D-Ala–Gly–Phe–Met–Thr	0.62
Tyr–D-Ala–Gly–Phe–D-Met	0.44
Tyr–D-Ala–Gly–Phe–Leu–Thr	0.44
Tyr–D-Ala–Gly–Phe–Nle	0.4
Tyr–D-Ala–Gly–Phe–LeuOMe	0.4
Tyr–D-Ala–Gly–Phe–D-LeuOMe	0.4

Potency descrepancy bet. analgesia & MVD.

Table 1.7 Potency relative to morphine in the mouse vas deferens assay (morphine = 1)

Analogue	Relative potency
Tyr–D-Ala–Gly–*p*ClPhe–D-Leu	1695
Tyr–D-Ala–Gly–Phe–D-Leu	1227
Tyr–D-Ala–Gly–Phe–Leu–Thr	461
Tyr–D-Ala–Gly–Phe–Leu	267
Tyr–D-Ala–Gly–Phe–Met	229
Tyr–D-Ala–Gly–Phe–Met–Thr	229
NMeTyr–D-Ala–Gly–Phe–D-Leu	229
Tyr–D-Ala–Gly–Phe–D-Met	228
Tyr–D-Ala–Gly–*p*ClPhe–D-LeuOMe	226
Tyr–D-Ala–Gly–Phe–Nle	209
Tyr–D-Ala–Gly–Phe–D-LeuO*p*ClPh	177

Table 1.8 Potency relative to morphine in the guinea pig ileum assay (morphine = 1)

Analogue	Relative potency
Tyr–D-Ala–Gly–Phe–D-LeuOMe	6.04
Tyr–D-Ala–Gly–Phe–D-Leu	1.95
Tyr–D-Ala–Gly–Phe–D-MetOMe	1.76
Tyr–D-Ala–Gly–Phe–MetOMe	1.38
Tyr–D-Ala–Asn–Phe–Leu	1.28
Tyr–D-Ala–Gly–*p*ClPhe–D-Leu	1.0
NMeTyr–Gly–Gly–Phe–Leu	0.93
Tyr–D-Ala–Gly–Phe–D-Met	0.92
Tyr–D-Ala–Gly–Phe–Leu–Thr	0.87
NMeTyr–Gly–Gly–Phe–LeuOMe	0.75
Tyr–D-Ala–Gly–Phe–D-Leu	0.66
Tyr–D-Ala–Gly–Phe–Met–Thr	0.63
NMe_2 Tyr–D-Ala–Gly–Phe–LeuOMe	0.65

Table 1.9 Anti-diarrheal activity

Analogue	ED_{50} mg/kg s.c.
NMeTyr–D-Ala–Gly–Phe–D-LeuNH_2	0.3
NMeTyr–D-Ala–Gly–Phe–D-MetNHEt	0.7
NMeTyr–D-Ala–Gly–Phe–D-MetNH_2	0.8
Tyr–D-Ala–Glu–*p*ClPhe–D-LeuNHEt	1.0
NMeTyr–D-Ala–Gly–Phe–D-Met	2.0
NMeTyr–D-Ala–Gly–Phe–D-MetOMe	2.0
Tyr–D-Ala–Gly–Phe–D-Met	2.0
Tyr–D-Ala–Gly–Phe–D-Leu	3.0
Tyr–D-Ala–Asn–Phe–Leu	3.0
Tyr–D-Ala–Gly–Phe–Thr	3.0
Tyr–Ile–Asn–Met–Leu	8.0

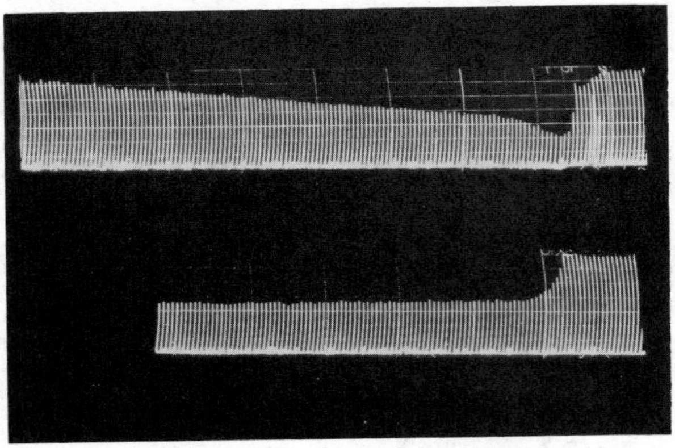

Figure 1.4 Guinea pig ileum traces. Upper trace, effect of [Leu^5]-enkephalin on contractions of the electrically stimulated ileum. Lower trace, effect of [D-Ala^2, D-Leu^5]-enkephalin on the contractions of the electrically stimulated ileum.

that the potencies of various analogues in producing analgesia compared with their relative potencies in one opiate receptor-binding assay or mouse vas deferens bioassays differ considerably. Whether this is due merely to other factors (vas deferens) such as hydrophobicity and access or whether it is due to some receptor heterogeneity is not yet clear (Lord *et al.*, 1977). Such discrepant effects have also been reported by Dutta *et al.* (1977).

As mentioned above, enkephalins are also distributed along the gastrointestinal tracts of several species (Polak *et al.*, 1977). Here again, this distribution suggests an 'in-vivo' role for the enkephalins which ties in with their pharmacology. It is well known that enkephalins and opiate agonists can reduce the magnitude of contractions of the electrically stimulated guinea pig ileum (table 1.8). In addition, opiates and enkephalins have potent anti-diarrheal effects. (figure 1.4, table 1.9; Kosterlitz and Waterfield, 1975). It is likely that under normal conditions enkephalins released from enkephalin-containing nerve terminals in the gastrointestinal tract may control some aspects of gastrointestinal motility. It is interesting to note in passing that neither enkephalin immunoreactivity nor binding of [^{125}I] enkephalins to opiate receptors has been demonstrated in the mouse vas deferens.

It can be seen from this limited discussion that in several cases the distribution of the enkephalins fits in well with their known pharmacology, and the previously observed pharmacology of opiate agonists. Thus localization in the hypothalamus, periaqueductal grey and gut suggests in-vivo roles for enkephalinergic systems as neuroendocrine modulators, mediators of pain responses and modulators of gastrointestinal motility. Other localizations such as the basal ganglia, limbic system and cortex suggest other roles in the control of locomotion and mood for example. However, the possible functions of many other enkephalinergic systems found in the CNS are still quite unknown. The elucidation of these centrally functioning opiate peptides together with the functions of opiate peptides released from the pituitary gland remain subjects for current and future investigation.

ACKNOWLEDGEMENTS

We wish to acknowledge the contributions of our colleagues at the Burroughs-Wellcome laboratories in North Carolina and Beckenham, U.K. and at the University of North Carolina in Chapel Hill and the NIEHS, Research Triangle Park, North Carolina.

REFERENCES

Beddell, C. R., Clark, R. B., Hardy, G. W., Lowe, L. A., Ubatuba, F., Vane, J. R., Wilkinson, S., Miller, R. J., Chang, K-J. and Cuatrecasas, P. (1977). *Proc. R. Soc. B.*, **198** 249–65

Belluzzi, J. D., Grant, N., Garsky, V., Sarantakis, J., Wise, C. D. and Stein, L. (1976). *Nature,* **266** 550–58

Bloom, F. E., Rossier, J., Battenberg, E. L. F., Bayon, A., French, E., Henrikson, S. T., Siggins, G. R., Segal, D., Brown, M., Ling, N. and Guillemin, R. (1978). In *Endorphins*, (ed. E. Costa) Raven Press, New York (in press)

Bradbury, A. F., Smyth, D. G., Snell, C. R., Birdsall, N. J. and Hulme, E. C. (1976*a*). *Nature*, **260**, 793–5

Bradbury, A. F., Feldberg, W. F., Smyth, D. G. and Snell, C. (1976*b*). In *Opiates and Endogenous Opiate Peptides* (ed. H. Kosterlitz), Elsevier/North-Holland, Amsterdam, pp 9–17

Buscher, H., Hill, R., Romer, D., Cardinaux, A., Closse, A., Hauser, D. and Pless, J. (1976). *Nature,* **261**, 423–5

Cheung, A. L. and Goldstein, A. (1976). *Life Sci.,* **19**, 1005–8

Cox, B. M., Goldstein, A. and Li, C. H. (1976). *Proc. natn. Acad. Sci. U.S.A.,* **73**, 1821–3

Cusan, L., Dupont, A., Kledzik, G. S., Labrie, F., Coy, D. H. and Schally, A. V. (1977). *Nature,* **268**, 545–6

Dutta, A. S., Gormley, J. T., Hayward, C. F., Morley, J. S., Shaw, J. J., Stacey, G. J. and Turnbull, M. T. (1977). *Life Sci.,* **21**, 559–62

Elde, R., Hökfelt, T., Johansson, O. and Terenius, L. (1976). *Neuroscience,* **1**, 349–51

Ferland, L., Labrie, F., Coy, D. H., Arimura, A. and Schally, A. W. (1976). *Molec. cell. Endocr.,* **61**, 797–800

Guillemin, R., Ling, N. and Vargo, T. (1977). *Biochem. biophys. Res. Commun.,* 77, 361–6

Hökfelt, T., Elde, R., Johansson, O., Terenius, L. and Stein, L. (1977). *Neurosci. Lett.* **5,** 25–31

Hong, J. S., Yang, H. Y. and Costa, E. (1977). *Brain Res.,* **134**, 383–6

Hughes, J., Smith, T. W., Kosterlitz, H. W., Fothergill, L. H., Morgan, B. A. and Morris, H. (1975). *Nature,* **255**, 577–9

Kokka, W., Garcia, J. F. and Elliot, H. W. (1972). *Endocrinology,* **90**, 735–43

Kosterlitz, H. W. and Waterfield, A. A. (1975). *A. Rev. Pharmac.,* **15**, 29–47

Kobayashi, R., Palkovits, M., Miller, R., Chang, K.-J. and Cuatrecasas, P. (1977). *Life Sci.* **22,** 527–30

Krieger, D. T., Liotta, A. and Brownstein, M. (1977). *Proc. natn. Acad. Sci. U.S.A.,* **74**, 648–52

Lazarus, L., Ling, N. E. and Guillemin, R. (1976). *Proc. natn. Acad. Sci. U.S.A.,* **73**, 1145–8

Linnoilla, I., DiAugustine, R., Miller, R. J., Chang, K.-J. and Cuatrecasas, P. (1978). *Neuroscience* (in press)

Lord, J. A. H., Waterfield, A. A., Kosterlitz, H. and Hughes, J. (1977). *Nature,* **267**, 495–9

Mains, R. and Eipper, B. (1977). *Proc. natn. Acad. Sci. U.S.A.,* **74**, 3014–5

Mayer, D. J. and Price, D. D. (1976). *Pain,* **2**, 379–404

Miller, R. J., Chang, K.-J., Cooper, B. and Cuatrecasas, P. (1977*a*). *J. biol. Chem.,* **253,** 531–8

Miller, R. J., Chang, K.-J., Leighton, H. J. and Cuatrecasas, P. (1977*b*). *Life Sci.*, **22,** 378–89

Miller, R. J., Chang, K.-J., Cuatrecasas, P. and Wilkinson, S. (1977*c*). *Biochem. biophys. Res. Commun.,* **74**, 1311–8

Miller, R. J., Chang, K.-J., Cuatrecasas, P., Wilkinson, S., Lowe, L., Beddell, C. and Follenjant, R. (1978). In *Centrally Acting Peptides* (ed. J. Hughes) Macmillan, London

Pert, C. B., Pert, A., Chang, K.-J. and Fong, B. T. W. (1976). *Science*, **194**, 330–2
Polak, J. M., Sullivan, S., Bloom, S., Faler, R. and Pearse, A. G. E. (1977). *Lancet*, x, 972–4
Rivier, C., Vale, W., Ling, N., Brown, M. and Guillemin, R. (1977). *Endocrinology*, **100**, 238–41
Rossier, J., Bayon, A., Vargo, T., Ling, N., Guillemin, R. and Bloom, F. E. (1977). *Life Sci.*, **21**, 847–51
Sar, M., Stumpf, W., Miller, R. J., Chang, K.-J. and Cuatrecasas, P. (1978). *J. comp. Neurol.*, (in press)
Shaar, C. J., Frederickson, R. C. A., Diminjer, N. B. and Jackson, L. (1977). *Life Sci.*, **21**, 853–60
Simantov, R. and Snyder, S. H. (1976). *Proc. natn. Acad. Sci. U.S.A.*, **73**, 2515–9
Simantov, R., Kuhar, M., Uhl, G. and Snyder, S. H. (1977). *Proc. natn. Acad. Sci. U.S.A.*, **76**, 2167–71
Yang, H. Y., Hong, J. and Costa, E. (1977). *Neuropharmacology*, **16**, 303–7
Wei, E. T., Tseng, L. F., Loh, H. H. and Li, C. H. (1977). *Life Sci.*, **21**, 321–8

2

β-Endorphin: cellular localization, electrophysiological and behavioral effects

F. E. Bloom, J. Rossier, E. L. F. Battenberg, A. Bayon, E. French, S. J. Henriksen, G. R. Siggins, N. Ling*, and R. Guillemin*
(The A. V. Davis Center for Behavioral Neurobiology and The Neuroendocrinology Laboratory* of the Salk Institute, La Jolla, California

Tremendous excitement has been generated by the isolation, purification, and subsequent synthesis of the opioid peptides. Our collaborative efforts have been directed at the questions of where β-endorphin is stored in brain and pituitary, how such structures are related to those storing the enkephalins and possibly other biogenic substances, and the functions of these peptides expressed through their electrophysiological properties. Although none of these questions is yet completely answered, sufficient data have been accumulated (Bloom *et al.*, 1976, 1977*a, b*; Guillemin *et al.*, 1977*a, b, c*; Rossier *et al.*, 1977*a, b, c*; Nicoll *et al.*, 1977; Henriksen *et al.*, 1977; French *et al.*, 1977) to enable us to give this overview and progress report.

REGIONAL IMMUNOASSAY OF BRAIN AND PITUITARY β-ENDORPHIN

The naturally occurring opioid peptides all share common N-terminal amino acid sequences with C-terminal fragments of β-lipotropin (LPH). These common sequences have led to two sorts of conjecture: the endorphins may represent prohormone forms of the enkephalins, or conversely that the enkephalins may merely be breakdown products of the endorphins (see Goldstein, 1976).

To attack this problem we have developed specific antisera which can distinguish the enkephalin pentapeptides from α-and β-endorphin. As described in more detail elsewhere (Guillemin *et al.*, 1977*b*; Rossier *et al.*, 1977*a, c*) our radioimmunoassays (RIA) for α or β-endorphin show no cross reactivity to β or α-endorphin respectively, and neither assay reads either enkephalin.

Endorphin and enkephalin immunoassayable material in rat pituitary

As already reported (Bloom *et al.*, 1977*a*), in rat pituitary as well as in mouse, kitten, pig, and frog pituitary, immunocytochemical and RIA studies indicate that α and β-endorphin are found in every cell of the intermediate lobe, and in isolated cells—corresponding to those reactive to antisera against adrenocortico-

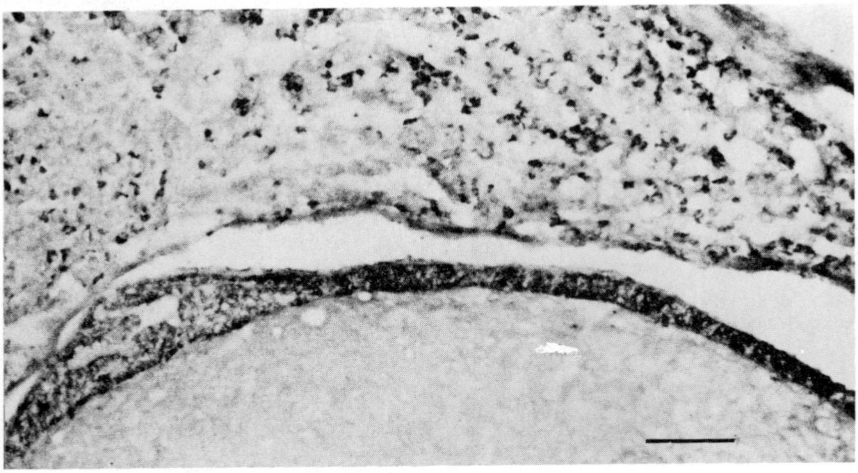

Figure 2.1 Localization of β-endorphin in the kitten pituitary. Immunoperoxidase staining with RB100–10/76, as described in Bloom *et al.* (1977*a*) (Calibration bar = 50 μm).

tropin (ACTH)—in the adenohypophysis (figure 2.1); neither α nor β-endorphin is detected in the neurohypophysis. Material immunoreactive in enkephalin RIA is restricted to the neuro-intermediate lobe (see Rossier *et al.*, 1977*c*).

The relationships between β-endorphin and enkephalin levels in brain and pituitary were evaluated by RIA after long-term hypophysectomy and adrenalectomy (Rossier *et al.*, 1977*c*). Neither treatment altered significantly the amount of brain β-endorphin-like immunoreactive substance attributable to authentic β-endorphin. After adrenalectomy, both β-endorphin and enkephalin showed corresponding fivefold increases in the adenohypophysis. These data indicate that the brain content of β-endorphin is not dependent upon the presence of pituitary β-endorphin.

Characterization of β-endorphin-like immunoreactive substances

The RIA used for measurements of β-endorphin is specific for the Leu^{14}–His^{27} segment of the molecule (Guillemin *et al.*, 1977*b*). This antiserum binds, in an equimolar ratio, β-LPH and 31 000 dalton prohormone (31 K precursor) which has been isolated from pituitary tumor cells and found to contain both ACTH and β-LPH (Mains *et al.*, 1977). Therefore, we separated the immunoreactive β-endorphin-like components by gel filtration. Brain extracts were passed through a Biogel P60 column and eluted with 4 M guanidine. Consistently, two peaks of immunoreactivity were resolved with the β-endorphin RIA. One peak coincides precisely with the location of radiolabeled synthetic β-endorphin, while the other peak (amounting to 37 per cent of the total β-endorphin-like immunoreactive substance) was eluted in a broad zone of larger molecular weight (10 000–30 000 daltons) which did not coincide closely with the elution pattern of either β-LPH or the 31 000 dalton prohormone. Moreover, the β-endorphin-like immunoreactive substance corresponding to labeled β-endorphin (63 per cent of the total immunoreactive material) was clearly separable from the enkephalin peak detected by the RIA for enkephalin (figure 2.2).

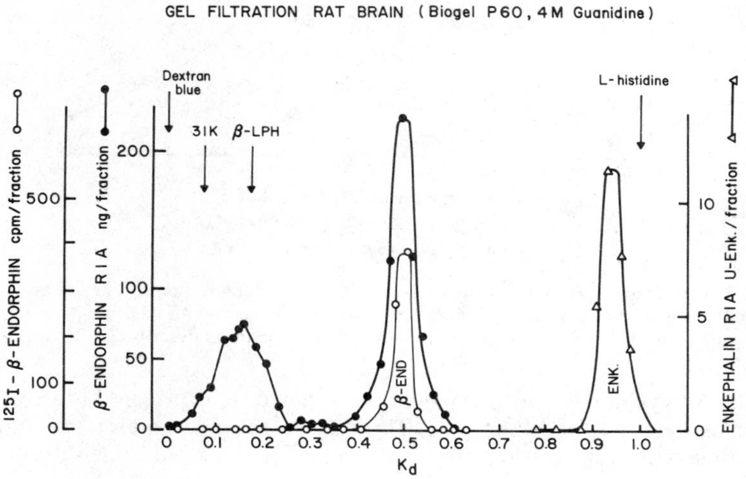

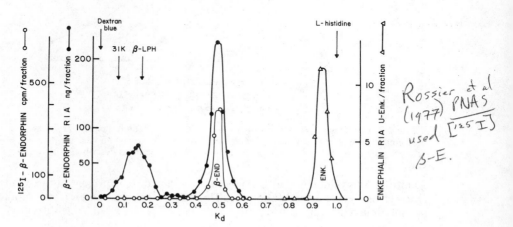

Figure 2.2 Gel filtration of rat brain extract. Two rats were killed by microwaves and their brains homogenized in 1 N acetic acid. After centrifugation, the supernatant was applied to a Biogel P60 column and eluted with 4 M guanidine. To express the results K_d values were calculated. β-endorphin (●●) and enkephalin (△△) immunoreactivity were assayed by RIA. In another run [^{125}I] β-endorphin was applied to the column and the radioactivity was monitored (○○). The elution peak of 31K prohormone and of β-LPH is also indicated by amount (see Rossier, *et al.*, 1977*c* for details).

Rossier et al (1977) PNAS used [125I] β-E.

Striatum and cerebral, cerebellar and hippocampal cortices all show significant amounts of the larger molecular weight substances (see Rossier *et al.*, 1977*c*). In hypothalamus, septum, pons, medulla and mesencephalon, the fraction of total β-endorphin-like immunoreactive substances attributable to the larger molecular weight substances was much less. The material which is present in brain extracts from the non-cortical regions is therefore most likely identical to β-endorphin. However, values obtained with β-endorphin RIA in extracts of striatal and cortical regions appear to be due to an as yet uncharacterized cross-reacting larger molecule, which may or may not be either β-LPH (Krieger *et al.*, 1977) or the 31K common precursor of β-LPH and ACTH (Mains *et al.*, 1977). Furthermore, by immunocytochemistry, under certain conditions some of our β-endorphin antisera (RB100-10/76 and RB263-11/76) stain myelinated fibers; this is especially pronounced in cortical regions (cerebral, hippocampal and cerebellar cortex). By RIA the degree of cross-reactivity with purified myelin basic protein (MW 18 500) was determined to be 0.001 per cent on a molar basis (figure 2.3). Large

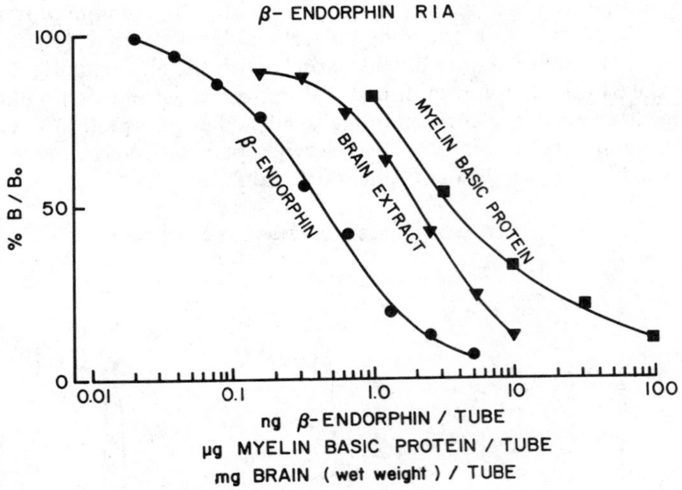

Figure 2.3 Cross-reactivity of serum RB100–10/76 with myelin basic protein. RIAs were performed as described in Guillemin *et al.* (1977*b*). Pure ovine myelin basic protein was a generous gift of Dr J. Villarreal. Rat brain extract was prepared as described in Rossier *et al.* (1977*a*).

quantities of myelin basic protein would be expected to be present in the brain extracts assayed here for β-endorphin. This molecule could, therefore, be another possible source for the cross-reacting larger molecule separated by gel-filtration.

Regional separation of β-endorphin and enkephalin

When extracts of all brain regions are corrected for RIA values due to the uncharacterized high molecular weight material, significant amounts of β-endorphin were found within whole brain and in hypothalamus and midbrain. However, no material attributable to the specific β-endorphin component could be found in extracts of the enkephalin-rich neostriatum (caudate–globus pallidus–putamen)

Table 2.1 Distribution of opioid peptide in the diencephalon

	Weight (mg tissue)	β-endorphin (ng/g)	Enkephalin (U/g)	Ratio β-endorphin (col.1) / Enkephalin (col.2)
Thalamus	55	329 ± 19	36 ± 5	9.1
Dorsal preoptic	35	742 ± 156	140 ± 22	5.2
Ventral preoptic	57	987 ± 127	260 ± 31	3.8
Hypothalamus	31	217 ± 32	134 ± 17	1.6

Means ± s.e.m. are for 12 rat brains dissected into quadrants of the diencephalon as described elsewhere (Rossier *et al.*, 1977*c*).

or of the cerebral, cerebellar or hippocampal cortices. These latter regions all contain significant amounts of enkephalin according to others and as confirmed by our enkephalin RIA here. When the same regions are assayed for β-endorphin and enkephalin, there is clearcut independent variation from region to region of the two classes of opioid peptides. Furthermore, when the diencephalon was dissected in accordance with the distribution of immunocytochemically detected β-endorphin neurons and fibers (see below), the ratio between β-endorphin and enkephalin values was found to vary from 1.6 in hypothalamus to 9.1 in periaqueductal thalamus (table 2.1). In addition, globus pallidus and caudate nucleus which contain large numbers of immunocytochemically detected enkephalin fibers (Elde *et al.*, 1976; Simantov *et al.*, 1977; Watson *et al.*, 1977) contain virtually no β-endorphin. Thus, these data strongly suggest that β-endorphin and enkephalin are found in the brain within different neuronal systems.

Tissue extraction and fixation procedures

Obviously, the methods for stabilizing brain peptides after death and extracting them for RIA are critical in their quantification (also see Cheung *et al.*, 1977; Yang *et al.*, 1977). In our RIAs, we evaluated various methods of tissue stabilization and extraction. As others have already shown (see Hambrook *et al.*, 1976; Miller *et al.*, 1977) the enkephalins are quite unstable in tissue homogenates or in plasma; in contrast, β-endorphin appears to be very stable in rat plasma, with no significant degradation in serum diluted 1:10 over 30 min at 37 °C (Rossier *et al.*, 1977*a*). Similarly, in a freely moving rhesus monkey, CSF sampled repeatedly *in vivo* after i.v.t. injection of β-endorphin showed a slow disappearance rate of about 50 per cent/hour (Ommaya, Bloom, Rossier and Guillemin, unpublished; figure 2.4). However, when exposed to brain homogenates, β-endorphin disappears

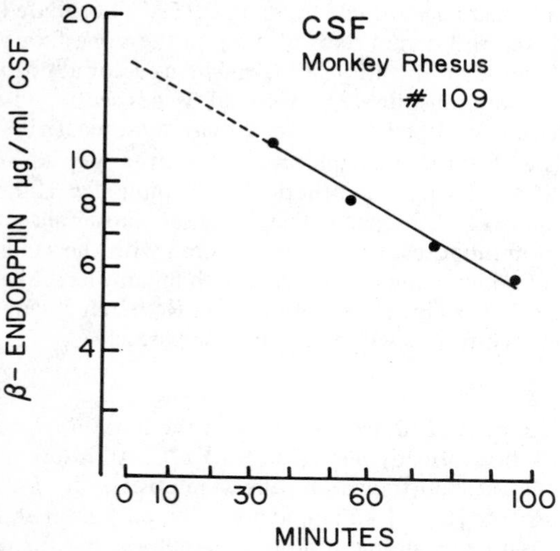

Figure 2.4 Degradation of β-endorphin in CSF. 100 μg of β-endorphin were injected in the CSF of a living rhesus monkey. At various times, aliquots of the CSF were taken out, heated to 95 °C for 2 min and assayed for β-endorphin. The primate model for long-term study of i.v.t. administered drugs developed by Wood *et al.* (1977), was used.

much more rapidly, showing a half-life of around 4 min when 1 μg of synthetic peptide is exposed to 40 mg brain homogenate at 37 °C. Disappearance of β-endorphin was accompanied by simultaneous appearance of α-endorphin (Rossier *et al.*, 1977a).

After comparing several methods of peptidase inactivation, we find that boiling the intact tissue is the best procedure for the β-endorphin RIA. Compared with the values obtained with decapitation and no boiling, heat inactivation of peptidases can be seen as an absolute prerequisite for β-endorphin assays: β-endorphin values were ten times lower when the samples were not boiled. This striking difference is not found for enkephalin, whose values decrease only by half without boiling. Also interesting is that with boiling, α-endorphin immunoreactivity was below the sensitivity of the assay. This may indicate that α-endorphin is not a primary compound in the rat brain and arises mainly from the degradation of β-endorphin after tissue disruption (see Rossier *et al.*, 1977*a*).

IMMUNOCYTOCHEMICAL STUDIES

Immunocytochemical results with anti-enkephalin sera have been reported by several laboratories (Elde *et al.*, 1976; Hökfelt *et al.*, 1977; Sar *et al.*, 1977; Watson *et al.*, 1977; Simantov *et al.*, 1977). With the availability of anti-β-endorphin sera showing significant immunoreactivity in RIAs, we evaluated several sera and several methodological modifications. Of the six anti-endorphin sera available to us, we found good immunoreactivity in pituitary, brain and intestine with two, (RB100:10/76 and RB263 11/76); other sera showed reactivity in RIA, but were weak or negative in immunocytochemical staining. Of various fixative procedures, we routinely find that a 5 min perfusion with ice-cold 4 or 5 per cent depolymerized paraformaldehyde in 0.15 M phosphate buffer, followed by a 3-hour immersion of 3–5 mm slabs of brain in the same fixative gave optimal results. Higher or lower concentrations of formaldehyde or addition of 1% or more glutaraldehyde were unsuitable, as were all tissues sectioned after embedding in paraffin. In each case described below, positive immunoreactivity was established by absorption tests with synthetic β-endorphin and other peptides (see Guillemin *et al.*, 1977*a*): addition of 1 μg of synthetic β-endorphin (RB 100, diluted 1/500 or 1/1000), for 24 hours at 5 °C blocked all staining seen in serial sections of a brain which showed good immunoreactivity when reacted with the same sera unblocked. A limited number of comparisons were made with an anti-leu-enkephalin serum provided by Dr R. J. Miller (Burroughs-Wellcome, Research Triangle, North Carolina). More detailed results will be reported separately.

Staining patterns

In rat, frog, pig and mouse pituitary, results with the immunoperoxidase method were comparable to those already described for FITC. All intermediate lobe cells and the adenohypophyseal corticotroph cells were positive for β-endorphin (figure 2.1). With the Miller anti-[Leu^5]-enkephalin we saw only faint staining of some corticotroph cells, minimal staining of intermediate lobe, but distinct fiber-like staining within the neurohypophysis (to be published).

In brain, the β-endorphin-reactive tissue elements were found to be much more restricted than those reacting to enkephalin antisera. Two groups of β-endorphin-

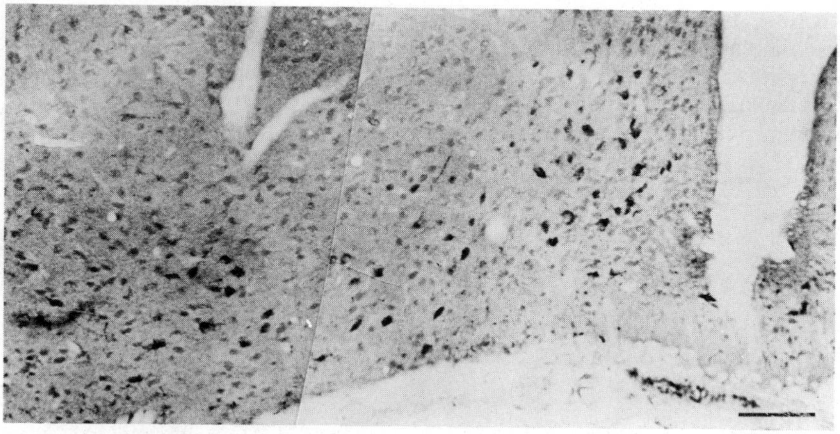

Figure 2.5 Localization of β-endorphin in the rat basal hypothalamus. Immunoperoxidase staining with RB100–10/76; calibration bar = 25 μm.

reactive neurons have been seen (figure 2.5). Both are located within the basal hypothalamus, one being within and dorso-lateral to the arcuate nucleus in its middle to posterior third, while the other is somewhat more anterior and quite lateral in the basal hypothalamus. Some β-endorphin-reactive cells form a continuous line across the floor of the third ventricle.

Large, long and thick varicose processes can be seen within these nuclei and can be followed in serial sections within the diencephalon and midbrain. These varicose fibers are mostly confined to midline structures near the ventricular surfaces, with a few exceptions.

Fibers are most dense in the anterior hypothalamic area, especially at the level of the decussation of the anterior commissure, and within the stria terminalis, and somewhat less dense in the lateral septum and nucleus accumbens. Within the hypothalamus proper, the paraventricular, supraoptic and suprachiasmatic nuclei show moderately heavy innervation, as does the lateral hypothalamic portion of the anterior hypothalamus and median eminence. Midline structures within the thalamic and pontine periaqueductal grey show consistent innervation, especially the anterior paraventricular nucleus (figure 2.6) and the dorsal raphe and locus coeruleus, at which point the fibers disappear laterally. Caudal to the locus coeruleus, fibers reactive with anti-β-endorphin are extremely scarce.

Positive reactivity was also seen when serum RB 263 was purified by affinity chromatography in which the gel was conjugated with synthetic β-endorphin, (1.7 mg β-endorphin per ml Sepharose). This product gave a lower titer in RIA than RB 100, but showed good affinity for β-endorphin. When used for immunocytochemical studies, this serum product gave all the results described above, but also revealed a profuse staining of myelinated axons which were especially prominent in pre-pyriform and rhinencephalic cortex, hippocampus and limbic cortex, and within the cingulate gyrus and cerebellum. This reactivity was totally abolished by preincubation of the sera with β-endorphin; when the serum was preincubated with well-purified myelin basic protein, only the myelinated fiber reactivity was abolished leaving a staining pattern identical to that seen with

RB 100. These observations, coupled with the results of the immunoassays on material separated by gel-filtration suggest that some common reactive component exists between the immunogen segment of β-endorphin and myelin basic protein. This unexpected common sequence and cross-reactivity could cause confusion in mapping and assays. Surprisingly, not all myelinated tracts exhibit the reactivity

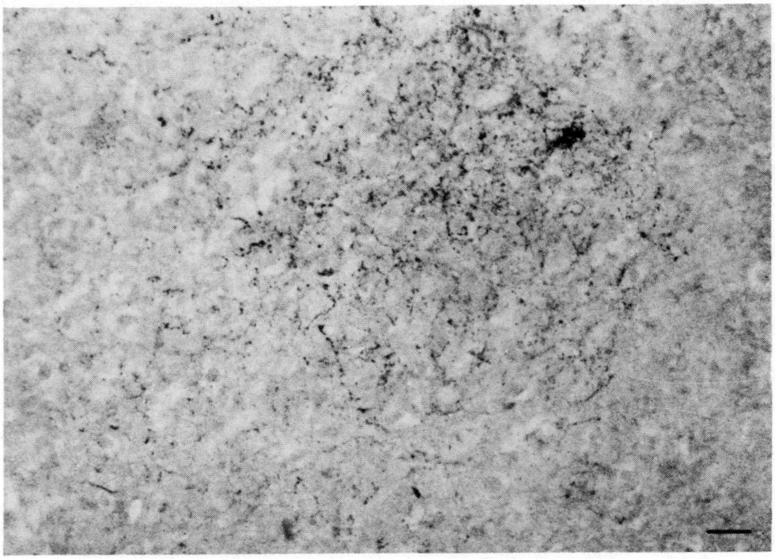

Figure 2.6 Localization of β-endorphin in the rat paraventricular nucleus. As in figure 5; calibration bar = 10 μm.

to β-endorphin sera, but mainly those myelinated fibers in the limbic cortical regions. When tested in higher concentrations, especially in brains of immature animals, RB 100 can also show some myelinated fiber staining. Nevertheless, despite the apparent regional selectivity of the myelin cross reactivity, we assume that this has no functional significance except as it may need to be reckoned with in accurate assays of β-endorphin.

In comparison with the reported distribution and appearance of enkephalin-reactive neuronal processes, it seems clear that different sets of target areas, with some overlap, and different sets of nerve cells are involved. Hökfelt *et al.* (1977) report that enkephalin-containing neurons are mainly short interneurons present in discrete regions throughout the CNS. In contrast β-endorphin-reactive cells are restricted to the basal hypothalamus and long processes from these cells are restricted mainly within midline fields near the ventricular surfaces.

ELECTROPHYSIOLOGY

Single unit studies

We have recently reported the results of surveying the responsivity of neurons in various portions of the rat brain to iontophoretic applications of the enkephalins and endorphins (Nicoll *et al.*, 1977). In cerebral cortex, brainstem (especially lateral reticular nucleus), caudate nucleus and thalamus, most responsive cells were inhibited by opiates and by each of the peptides. In contrast, pyramidal cells in the hippocampus were exclusively excited by opiates and by the peptides. A lower degree of responsivity, with mixed inhibitions and excitations, was exhibited by cerebellar Purkinje cells. In each region tested, both excitatory and inhibitory effects could be antagonized by iontophoretic or by parenterally injected naloxone.

More recent studies (French *et al.*, 1977) have focused on the unexpected excitation seen in hippocampus. In view of the known cholinergic excitatory input to hippocampus from septum, we evaluated effects of the peptides and acetylcholine in the presence of naloxone and cholinergic antagonists. However, cholinergic antagonists had no effect on opioid peptide excitations, and conversely naloxone had no effect on acetylcholine excitations.

EEG Studies

Opiate alkaloids alter spontaneous electroencephalographic (EEG) patterns when administered systemically to man or animals (Teitelbaum *et al.*, 1976); enkephalins do so when given i.c. (Urca *et al.*, 1977). At high systemic doses of these agents, or when placed at certain intracerebral sites, these agents can precipitate epileptiform activity. We have recently observed (Henriksen *et al.*, 1977) that endorphins are also powerful epileptigenic agents when administered i.v.t. to rats, and can produce these EEG effects at molar doses far less than comparable doses of the opiate alkaloids. In our experience, β-endorphin is the most potent and long-lasting epileptogenic agent. [Met^5]-enkephalin produces similar electroencephalographic alterations only at much higher molar doses and then only for short periods. However, the difference in apparent potency of [Met^5]-enkephalin compared with β-endorphin could merely reflect relative peptidase degradation. Given the apparently different distributions of β-endorphin and the enkephalins discussed earlier, the determination of the primary site(s) of action of these peptides for this effect becomes critical.

In rats implanted with chronic cortical as well as subcortical electrode arrays, epileptiform discharges appear within 90–120 s after infusion of β-endorphin. The emergent epileptiform discharges are often preceded by increased exploratory behavior and vigorous sniffing. During the initial ictal episode rats appear alerted but motionless and can exhibit occasional olfactory and gustatory stereotypies. Frequently at the end of the initial episode the animal will exhibit a series of wet-dog shakes (see Bloom *et al.*, 1976). Depending on the dose, multiple ictal episodes can be observed, all of which are followed by a prolonged period of interictal spiking lasting up to 4 hours at the higher dose ranges. Of particular interest to us has been the fact that at low doses (0.5–1.0 ng) the only overt behavioral effect seems to be the precipitation of these seizures. They appear to be the lower threshold effect of β-endorphin and can occur in rats devoid of any other behavioral signs or analgesia.

Although electroencephalographic seizures are precipitated by β-endorphin, we have never observed a behavioral convulsion following either acute or chronic administration. The seizural activity seems to be primarily restricted to limbic structures and appears not to extend into motor systems. Repeated injections of β-endorphin result in an attenuation of the epileptic response, suggesting the development of tolerance. At higher doses of β-endorphin, when rigidity is marked, EEGs show cortical synchrony and slow wave activity as well as the interictal spikes. This synchronous activity can be desynchronized by minimally-arousing stimuli of any modality, but is not affected by nociceptive stimuli.

The entire electrographic response can be either reversed or blocked by administering the specific opiate antagonist naloxone (2-5 mg/kg i.p.) before or after the emergence of the discharges. Intravenous injection of β-endorphin (human or porcine) in amounts up to 25 mg/kg produces no overt EEG changes in our rats.

We previously postulated (Bloom *et al.*, 1976) that the potent behavioral changes (see Segal, this volume) induced by β-endorphin in rats might make these peptides potential etiologic factors in some mental illnesses. We further suggested that if this view were valid, opiate antagonists might offer some therapeutic benefit. Although Gunne *et al.* (1977) reported that 0.4 mg naloxone reduced auditory hallucination intensity in four out of six chronic schizophrenics, others (Davis *et al.*, 1977; Volavka *et al.*, 1977) as well as ourselves (Janowsky *et al.*, 1977*a, b*) using two to threefold higher doses and double blind protocols have been unable to repeat these positive results with naloxone. However on the basis of our behavioral, EEG and unit recording observations, these doses of naloxone may still be too low to reverse the central effects of endorphins (see Janowsky, this volume). Furthermore, in the subclassification of opiate receptors proposed by Martin and associates (Martin *et al.*, 1976; also see Lord *et al.*, 1977), some opiate agonist actions may require 3-6 times more naloxone for reversal. Most recently, Kline *et al.* (1977) have observed immediate short term improvement in psychotically depressed patients and longer latency, longer duration improvements in some chronic schizophrenics after i.v. infusion of β-endorphin (total dose 3-9 mg per 6 hours). These preliminary clinical results, which would suggest that peripheral endorphin has positive therapeutic benefits, are difficult to reconcile with animal studies indicating minimal transient central effects of the peptide only with extremely high doses peripherally.

It remains unclear from these results where and how blood-borne endorphin can produce behavioral improvement in man. Our initial RIAs for endorphins in human plasma and CSF reveal extremely low levels. How could the peripheral peptides produce presumptive central actions? We have recently reported (Guillemin *et al.*, 1977*c*; Rossier *et al.*, 1977*b*) that every stress known to release ACTH into rat blood also releases β-endorphin concomitantly and in approximately equimolar amounts. This concomitant release is probably explained by the common cellular storage and synthesis of the two peptide hormones, possibly as a result of their synthesis within the same prohormones (Mains *et al.*, 1977). It should be realized that the blood levels which would be achieved by doses of β-endorphin reported (Tseng *et al.*, 1976) to produce analgesia in mice after i.v. injection would be several orders of magnitude greater than the peak level reached in our rats under acute painful stress. Such astronomical levels are unlikely to be achieved physiologically in blood, and if necessary for analgesia, suggest that the pituitary endorphin does not mediate stress analgesia. Even the much lower i.v. doses of β-endorphin reported to produce analgesia in cats (Feldberg and Smyth, 1977) would still be at least two orders of magnitude greater than the physiological endorphin range in the rat (1-10 ng/ml) (Guillemin *et al.*, 1977*c*; Rossier *et al.*, 1977*b*). Nevertheless, the present data are insufficient to reach definite conclusions, and considerable degrees of species-related specificity must be sought and documented. Thus we find (Foote, Henriksen, and Bloom; unpublished) that the squirrel monkey is much less sensitive to i.v.t. administered β-endorphin when evaluated for analgesia and EEG changes, but is quite sensitive to the depression of respiratory activity. More work is clearly needed for this important question to be answered. Since peripheral target tissues respond to ACTH with secretory products which in turn produce feedback regulation of ACTH release, we have wondered whether there exist similar feedback regulated peripheral targets for endorphin. Such targets might include cells adjacent to the endorphin-rich cells of the gastrointestinal tract or the circumventricular organs found deep within the recesses of the brain (such as the pineal, median eminence, sub-commissural and subfornical organs) which are on the blood side of the blood-brain barrier. If any of the latter cells were responsive to endorphin levels in the blood, their innervation might conceivably signal higher centers neuronally. This is the route through which angiotensin (Fitzsimons, 1975) and neurotoxic amino acids (Olney, 1977) would appear to work, and may be the route by which blood-borne endorphins cause release of adenohypophyseal hormones (Rivier *et al.*, 1977).

SUMMARY

Using antisera specific for β-endorphin, cells containing this peptide have been identified in adenohypophysis, neural lobe of the pituitary and within the tubero-basal hypothalamus. The sera used in RIA for β-endorphin quantitation support the cytochemical observations that the hypothalamus and diencephalon are richest in β-endorphin, while areas reported by others and confirmed by us as rich in enkephalins (such as globus pallidus, caudate nucleus, and substantia gelatinosa) are devoid of detectable β-endorphin. We conclude that β-endorphin-rich cells exist in the brain separately from those reactive to anti-enkephalin sera, and that the brain endorphin and enkephalin systems are each separate from the endorphin-rich cells of the pituitary. Electrophysiological studies with single cells and EEG recordings indicate that in rat, epileptiform discharges within the limbic system represent a lower threshold response than analgesia, but the site and synaptic mechanism of the effect are not yet known. The physiological range of variation for plasma β-endorphin in the rat is several orders of magnitude lower than that reported to be required for i.v. endorphin to produce analgesia. To determine whether blood-borne β-endorphin or opiate antagonists may be helpful in the therapy of mental illness will require significant extensions of these experimental observations.

ACKNOWLEDGEMENTS

This work was supported by grants from The William Randolph Hearst Foundation, National Institute of Drug Abuse (DA 01785), National Institute of Child Health and Human Development (HD 09690) and National Institute of

Arthritis, Metabolic and Digestive Diseases (AM 18811). We thank Dr J. Gupta of Endo for naloxone.

REFERENCES

Bloom, F., Battenberg, E., Rossier, J., Ling, N., Leppaluoto, J., Vargo, T. M. and Guillemin, R. (1977*a*). *Life Sci.*, **20**, 43–8

Bloom, F. E., Rossier, J., Battenberg, E. L. F., Bayon, A., French, E., Henricksen, S., Siggins, G. R., Segal, D., Browne, R., Ling, N. and Guillemin, R. (1977*b*). *Endorphins*, (ed. E. Costa) Raven Press, New York, in press.

Bloom, F. E., Segal, D., Ling, N., and Guillemin, R. (1976). *Science*, **194**, 630–2

Cheung, A. L., Stavinhoa, W. B., and Goldstein, A. (1977). *Life Sci.*, **20**, 1285–90

Davis, G. C., Bunney, W. E., Jr., de Fraites, E. G., Kleinman, J. E., Van Kammen, D. P., Post, R. M. and Wyatt, R. J. (1977). *Science*, **197**, 74–7

Elde, R., Hökfelt, T., Johansson, O. and Terenius, L. (1976). *Neuroscience*, **1**, 349–51

Feldberg, W. J. and Smyth, D. G. (1977). *J. Physiol., Lond.*, **265**, 25P–27P

Fitzsimons, J. T. (1975). *Prog. Brain Res.*, **42**, 215–33

French, E. D., Siggins, G. R., Henriksen, S. J. and Ling, N. (1977). *Neurosci. Abstr.*, **3**, 291

Goldstein, A. (1976). *Science*, **193**, 1081–6

Guillemin, R., Bloom, F. E., Rossier, J., Minick, S., Henriksen, S., Burgus, R. and Ling, N. (1977a). In *Sixth International Conference on Endocrinology*, (ed. I. McIntyre) Elsevier, North Holland, Amsterdam, in press.

Guillemin, R., Ling, N. and Vargo, T. M. (1977b). *Biochem. biophys. Res. Commun.*, 77, 361–6

Guillemin, R., Vargo, T., Rossier, J., Minick, S., Ling, N., Rivier, C., Vale, W. and Bloom, F. (1977c). *Science*, **197**, 1368–9

Gunne, L. M., Lindstrom, L. and Terenius, L. (1977). *J. Neural Transmission*, **40**, 13–19

Henriksen, S. J., Bloom, F. E., Ling, N. and Guillemin, R. (1977). *Neurosci. Abstr.*, **3**, 293

Hambrook, J. M., Morgan, B. A., Rance, M. J. and Smith, C. F. C. (1976). *Nature*, **262**, 782–3

Hökfelt, T., Elde, R., Johansson, O., Terenius, L. and Stein, L. (1977). *Neurosci. Lett.*, **5**, 25–31

Janowsky, D. S., Segal, D. S., Abrams, A., Bloom, F. and Guillemin, R. (1977a). *Psychopharmacology*, **53**, 295–7

Janowsky, D. S., Segal, D. S., Bloom, F., Abrams, A. and Guillemin, R. (1977b). *Am. J. Psychiat.*, **134**, 926–7

Kline, N. S., Li, C. H., Lehmann, H. E., Lajtha, A., Laski, E. and Cooper, T. (1977). *Archs gen. Psychiat.*, **34**, 1111–3

Krieger, D. T., Liotta, A., Suda, T., Palkovits, M. and Brownstein, M. J. (1977). *Biochem. biophys. Res. Commun.*, **76**, 930–6

Lord, J. A. H., Waterfield, A. A., Hughes, J. and Kosterlitz, H. W. (1977). *Nature*, **267** 495–9

Mains, R., Eipper, E. and Ling, N. (1977). *Proc. natn. Acad. Sci. U.S.A.*, **74**, 3014–8

Martin, W. R., Eades, C. G., Thompson, J. A., Huppler, R. E. and Gilbert, P. E. (1976). *J. Pharmac. exp. Ther.*, **197**, 517–32

Miller, R. J., Chang, K. J. and Cuatrecasas, P. (1977). *Biochem. biophys. Res. Commun.*, **74**, 1311–7

Nicoll, R. A., Siggins, G. R., Ling, N., Bloom, F. E. and Guillemin, R. (1977). *Proc. natn. Acad. Sci. U.S.A.*, 74, 2584–8

Olney, J. W., Rhee, V. and DeGubareff, T. (1977). *Brain Res.*, **120**, 151–7

Rivier, C., Vale, W., Ling, N., Brown, M. and Guillemin, R. (1977). *Endocrinology*, **100**, 238–41

Rossier, J., Bayon, A., Vargo, T., Ling, N., Guillemin, R. and Bloom, F. (1977*a*). *Life Sci.*, **21**, 847–52

Rossier, J., French, E., Rivier, C., Ling, N., Guillemin, R. and Bloom, F. (1977*b*). *Nature*, **270**, 618–20

Rossier, J., Vargo, T. M., Minick, S., Ling, N., Bloom, F. and Guillemin, R. (1977*c*). *Proc. natn. Acad. Sci. U.S.A.*, **74**, 5162–5

Sar, M., Stumpf, W. E., Miller, R. J., Chang, K. J. and Cuatrecasas, P. (1977). *Neurosci. Abstr.* **3**, 301
Simantov, R., Kuhar, M. J., Uhl, G. R. and Snyder, S. H. (1977). *Proc. natn. Acad. Sci. U.S.A.*, **74**, 2167–71
Teitelbaum, H., Blosser, J. and Catravas, G. (1976). *Nature*, **260**, 158–9
Tseng, L.-F., Loh, H. H. and Li, C. H. (1976). *Nature*, **263**, 239–40
Urca, G., Frenk, H. and Liebeskind, J. (1977). *Science*, **197**, 83–6
Volavka, J., Mallya, A., Baig, S., and Perez-Cruet, J. (1977). *Science*, **196**, 1227–8
Watson, S. J., Akil, H., Sullivan, S. and Barchas, J. D. (1977). *Life Sci.*, **21**, 733–8
Wood, J. H., Poplack, D. G., Bleyer, W. A. and Ommaya, A. K. (1977). *Science*, **195**, 499–501
Yang, H. Y., Hong, J. S. and Costa, E. (1977). *Neuropharmacology*, **16**, 303–7

3

Immunohistochemical and biochemical studies of the enkephalins, β-endorphin, and related peptides

Stanley J. Watson, Huda Akil, and Jack D. Barchas
(Nancy Pritzker Laboratory of Behavioral Neurochemistry, Department of Psychiatry and Behavioral Sciences, Stanford University School of Medicine, Stanford, California)

There are several hypotheses concerning the relationships between the various endorphins and enkephalins (Hughes *et al.*, 1975; Li and Chung, 1976; Guillemin *et al.*, 1976; Bradbury *et al.*, 1976). Such hypotheses include the possibility that β-endorphin or a similar pituitary peptide is primarily a precursor of met-enkephalin (Cox *et al.*, 1975), that met-enkephalin and other peptides such as α and γ-endorphin are breakdown products of β-endorphin (Austen *et al.*, 1977), or that the enkephalins and β-endorphin constitute two distinct endogenous opioid systems (Watson *et al.*, 1977*a, b, c*; Akil *et al.*, 1978; Bloom *et al.*, 1977*b*). Furthermore, because of the history of their discovery, the enkephalins have been primarily associated with the brain (Hughes *et al.*, 1975; Simantov and Snyder, 1976), while α, β, and γ-endorphin have been primarily linked to the intermediate and anterior lobes of the pituitary (Cox *et al.*, 1975; Guillemin *et al.*, 1976; Li and Chung, 1976; Bloom *et al.*, 1977*a*; Bradbury *et al.*, 1976; Graf *et al.*, 1976; Teschemacher, 1975), and particularly to β-lipotropin (β-LPH) their putative prohormone (Moon *et al.*, 1973; Pelletier *et al.*, 1977). Elucidation of the relationships between these endogenous opioid peptides is a crucial first step towards a better understanding of their biosynthetic and degradative pathways, and as a prerequisite for the study of their physiological functions.

In this chapter, we have used anatomical, immunological, and biochemical approaches, coupled with some lesion and pharmacological studies in order to investigate the relationships between met-enkephalin, leu-enkephalin, β-endorphin, and β-LPH in mammalian brain. Further, because of the recently discovered relationship between β-LPH (and β-endorphin) and adrenocorticotropin (ACTH) in mouse pituitary cell cultures (Mains *et al.*, 1977), we have attempted an immunocytochemical characterization of ACTH in brain—particularly in relation to β-LPH and β-endorphin.

Finally, because of the close anatomical association of the two enkephalins, we have attempted to examine potential differences in their interaction with post-synaptic sites, that is, with the putative opiate receptors.

GENERAL METHODS

Antibodies to the peptides

The antisera used in these studies were obtained from a variety of sources. Met and leu-enkephalin antisera were produced in this laboratory. They were obtained from animals immunized against a BSA–glutaraldehyde–enkephalin complex (Sullivan *et al.*, 1977). Antisera against human β-LPH were obtained from Dr C. H. Li (Hormone Research Laboratory, University of California, San Francisco) (Rao and Li, 1977). This antibody was produced against extracted β-LPH which was injected uncomplexed into rabbit. Rabbit antisera against the C-fragment of β-LPH was prepared against β-endorphin$_{1-9}$ complexed to BSA by a carbodiimide linkage by R. Mains and B. Eipper. They also immunized rabbits with AtT-20/D-16v mouse pituitary tumor (Eipper *et al.,* 1976). Anti-ACTH immunoglobulin was harvested from this complex antiserum using synthetic ACTH$_{1-24}$ attached to an affinity column.

Since the antibodies were utilized for both RIA and immunocytochemistry, their specificity had to be characterized with two sets of criteria in mind. For RIA, cross-reactivity is defined as the ability of other substances to compete against the binding of the primary labeled immunogen. Small degrees of cross-reactivity, possible due to multiple populations of antibodies are thus detected and quantified. Immunocytochemical studies depend on the type of specificity necessary for RIA as well as the assumption that only one type of antibody in the antiserum is producing the anatomical demonstration. For example, the met-enkephalin antiserum used in the following studies for RIA has been characterized for the competition of other substances against met-enkephalin binding. In the immunocytochemical studies, the met-enkephalin antiserum has been further characterized by the demonstration that, of the substances tried, only met-enkephalin could block antibody binding to the anatomical structures. Table 3.1 shows the peptides used in blocking experiments in immunocytochemical studies with these five antibodies. Each antibody was blocked only by the peptide against which it was raised. In the case of leu-enkephalin antibody, there is less than 10 per cent cross-reactivity with met-enkephalin. However, the antiserum seems to have at least two main antibody populations, one of which (<10 per cent) recognizes met and leu-enkephalin, and one which recognizes leu-enkephalin only. The leu-enkephalin antiserum is incubated with 10 μM met-enkephalin and still demonstrates enkephalin-positive cells, whereas the addition of 1 μM leu-enkephalin was sufficient to completely block activity. The β-LPH antiserum is <1 per cent cross-reactive with β-endorphin. Again, β-endorphin at 10 μM does not block that antiserum, whereas 5 nM β-LPH will completely block the activity. Neither ACTH or met- or leu-enkephalin exhibits significant cross-reactivity. The β-endorphin$_{1-9}$ antiserum is not cross-reactive with met- or leu-enkephalin or ACTH. However, it is 100 per cent cross-reactive with β-LPH.

Table 3.1 Summary of antisera and cross-reactivity

Antisera and titer	Cross-reactivity
Met-enkephalin (1/200) (our laboratory)	Not blocked by leu-enkephalin, β-endorphin β-LPH, ACTH, β-MSH (0.5% cross–reactive with leu-enkephalin by RIA)
Leu-enkephalin (1/200) (our laboratory)	Not blocked by met-enkephalin, β-LPH, β-endorphin, ACTH, β-MSH (< 1% cross reactive with met-enkephalin by RIA)
β-LPH (1/800) (C. H. Li)	Not blocked by met-enkephalin, β-endorphin leu-enkepahlin, ACTH, β-MSH (< 10% cross–reactive with β-endorphin by RIA)
β-END (1/800) (Mains and Eipper)	Not blocked by met-enkephalin, leu-enkephalin, ACTH, β-MSH (100% cross–reactive with β-LPH)
ACTH (1/1500) (Mains and Eipper)	Not blocked by β-endorphin, β-LPH, met-enkephalin, leu-enkephalin, β-MSH

Extraction of enkephalins and β-LPH

Since some experiments required the simultaneous measurement of β-LPH and the endogenous opioids, we have devised a technique for their extraction from the same brain tissue. Of paramount importance was avoiding the possibility of breakdown of larger peptides into enkephalins, or of enkephalins into smaller fragments. The following technique was therefore adopted

(1) Tissue is dissected, frozen immediately on dry ice, and homogenized in 5 volumes of ice-cold 0.4 N perchloric acid (PCA).

(2) The homogenate is centrifuged at 40 000 *g* for 20 min. Under these conditions, the supernatant contains the enkephalins, while the pellet contains at least 85–90 per cent of the β-LPH.

(3) The enkephalin-containing supernatant is carefully decanted, its pH adjusted to 7.4 with KOH. The white precipitate is spun down and discarded. This second supernatant can now be either assayed directly in the enkephalin RIA or can be further purified and concentrated using biobeads and/or an anion exchange column (AG1–X2). The details of this purification have been reported elsewhere (Akil *et al.*, 1978).

(4) The β-LPH-containing pellet (from step 2) is resuspended by homogenization in 5 volumes of ice-cold, double -distilled H_2O.

(5) This homogenate is centrifuged again at 40 000 *g* for 20 min. Under these conditions, β-LPH is in the supernatant.

(6) The β-LPH-containing supernatant is then adjusted for pH with KOH and assayed directly in the RIA or applied to a 1 × 12-cm Sephadex G10 column, run in acetic acid. The β-LPH-containing fraction is then concentrated by evaporation and assayed.

This procedure yields good recovery of the enkephalins (90 per cent) and β-LPH (65–75 per cent), as monitored with both unlabeled and labeled peptides.

There is no evidence of enzymatic breakdown after the homogenization in PCA. Rat whole brain, pituitary, or brain parts as small as 10 mg of tissue have been extracted in this way.

Measurement by binding and RIA

The opiate receptor assay was used not only for measuring levels of endogenous opioids, but for more detailed studies of the kinetics of leu-enkephalin and met-enkephalin binding in various regions of rat brain.

The preparation of crude homogenates was modified from the standard procedure of Pasternak *et al.* (1976) to include three washes of the pellet in 50 nM Tris HCl buffer (pH 7.7 at 25 °C). The homogenate was incubated at room temperature for 1 hour between this second and third wash—a procedure which appeared to enhance enkephalin binding. Appropriate concentrations of labeled ligands ([^{3}H] naloxone, New England Nuclear; [^{3}H] leu-enkephalin, Amersham/Searle; [^{3}H] met-enkephalin, New England Nuclear) were added to aliquots of the binding preparations, and the assays were carried out at 0–20 °C for 90–180 min. Rapid filtration under vacuum on glass fiber filters (GF/B Whatman) was used to separate bound from free ligand. The extent of enkephalin breakdown in drug incubation with tissue preparations from various brain regions was monitored by centrifugation of the samples and application of aliquots of the supernatant to a t.l.c. system (*n*-butanol: pyridine: acetone: H_2O; 15:10:3:12). The behavior of the [^{3}H] labeled compounds (labeled on the tyrosine) was compared to that of tyrosine, enkephalins, and the peptide fragments of enkephalin containing tyrosine. This permitted an estimation of relative breakdown of the two enkephalins in different brain regions.

Radioimmunoassay for the enkephalins are carried out in Tris HCl buffer (0.2 M, pH 7.3) and bound and free ligands are separated by ammonium sulfate precipitation. The immunogens were obtained by coupling leu or met-enkephalin to BSA by glutaraldehyde or carbodiimide conjugation. The procedure of coupling and characterization has been described elsewhere (Akil *et al.*, 1978; Sullivan *et al.*, in press). The met-enkephalin antiserum exhibits high specificity, with no cross reactivity with β-endorphin or β-LPH at 1 μM, and less than 0.5 per cent cross reactivity with leu-enkephalin.

β-LPH radioimmunoassay uses an antiserum obtained from Dr C. H. Li (University of California, San Francisco) (Rao and Li, 1977). The assay is carried out at a dilution of 1/20 000 in sodium phosphate buffer (pH 7.5). Bound and free β-LPH are separated with charcoal absorption. The assay is sensitive to less than 5 fmol β-LPH. In our hands, it exhibits less than 1 per cent cross-reactivity with β-endorphin and no cross-reactivity to α and γ-endorphin, met or leu-enkephalin, β-MSH, or ACTH.

Immunocytochemistry

Tissue is prepared for immunocytochemistry according to Hökfelt *et al.* (1977) and Watson *et al.* (1977). Briefly, adult, male, Sprague-Dawley rats were perfused via the aorta with 4 per cent formaldehyde–0.1 M phosphate buffer at 4 °C for 30 min at 130 mmHg pressure. The brain is removed, blocked, and placed in cold perfusate for 2 hours. It is then removed into 5 per cent sucrose PBS buffer at

4 °C overnight, and then frozen with liquid nitrogen, sectioned in a cryostat at –20 °C and kept at –20 °C until used. The various rabbit antisera are diluted with 0.3 per cent Triton–PBS and incubated with the section for 1 hour at 37°C and then at 4 °C for 16–48 hours. The sections are washed, then incubated with FITC-conjugated goat anti-rabbit IgG (1/80-Cappel Labs, Cochranville, Pennsylvania) for 1 hour at 37 °C. They are rewashed, covered with a coverslip and viewed with a Leitz Orthoplan microscope.

RESULTS

Enkephalin system

Using anti-enkephalin antisera, several groups have studied the distribution of enkephalin-like immunoreactivity in rat brain (Watson *et al.*, 1977; Hökfelt *et al.*, 1977; Elde *et al.*, 1976; Simantov *et al.*, 1977). The results of these investigations are remarkably consistent. They have shown the enkephalin system to be composed of many local cell groups throughout the brainstem. The existence of met and leu-enkephalin raises the question of whether these two peptides are found in the same or different neuronal pools. To carry out such anatomical studies, it is necessary to have a specific antiserum against each of the two enkephalins which is not cross-reactive with the other enkephalin. Although this ideal has not been reached, good met-enkephalin antiserum and fair leu-enkephalin antiserum have been produced in this laboratory (table 3.1).

We have studied enkephalin distribution using serial sections through the rat brain. The sections were incubated with met-enkephalin antiserum plus 10 μM leu-enkephalin peptide (even though this antibody does not show detectable cross-reactivity to leu-enkephalin) or leu-enkephalin antiserum with 10 μM met-enkephalin peptide. These sections showed almost identical patterns of the distribution of met and leu-enkephalin. Studies are in progress using both met and leu-enkephalin antisera sequentially on the same section through the lateral septal nucleus. Preliminary results using the controls as outlined below for multiple antigen studies, show that both antisera demonstrate the same cells and fibers. One interpretation of these results is that the antisera were cross-reacting with the 'other' enkephalin, even though 10 μM of that peptide was present. Another likely interpretation appears to be that met and leu-enkephalin come from the same neuronal pool and coexist in the same cells. If this were the case, differences between their functions would not be due to the cell of origin. Rather, differential roles of the two enkephalins might be due to differences in storage, release, or postsynaptic events. In the next section, we describe some experiments aimed at uncovering potentially different binding sites available to the two pentapeptides.

Kinetic properties of met and leu-enkephalin binding in various brain regions

We reasoned that if the two enkephalins can bind somewhat different subpopulations of opiate receptors, they would exhibit differential binding patterns and relationships in various brain regions. The properties of opiate receptors in various brain regions were therefore examined by dissecting the following areas: cortex, striatum, hippocampus and septum, hypothalamus, midbrain and medulla–pons.

Parts from 25 animals were pooled for each experiment. The tissue was prepared for radioreceptor binding as described above. [^{3}H] naloxone, [^{3}H] leu-enkephalin and [^{3}H] met-enkephalin binding was examined in the same tissue under the same conditions for a range of concentrations from 0.25 to 64 nM. The study was carried out in duplicate and the whole experiment was repeated twice. Scatchard analysis for each ligand in each brain region generally revealed two components of binding for all ligands; a high-afinity-low-capacity component, and a lower-affinity/higher-capacity component. In general, a given ligand such as leu-enkephalin exhibited similar K_d values in various brain regions, but significantly different numbers of binding sites. In our hands, and throughout all brain regions, the V_{max} for leu-enkephalin binding was significantly lower than that for met-enkephalin binding. Furthermore, the ratio of the binding sites varied significantly from one region to the other. For example, in cortex [^{3}H] leu-enkephalin V_{max} was 4.7 pmol/g, and [^{3}H] met-enkephalin V_{max} was 9.7 pmol/g, a leu/met ratio of 49 per cent. On the other hand, in striatum V_{max} for leu-enkephalin was 8.4 pmol/g, V_{max} for met-enkephalin was 11.9 pmol/g, with a ratio of 70%. Those two ratios were found to be significantly different ($P < 0.01$). In general, the number of [^{3}H] met-enkephalin sites compared closely with [^{3}H] naloxone sites in most regions.

The differential number of binding sites for met and leu-enkephalin in various regions cannot be attributed to differential breakdown of these two substances in the assay. Careful studies measuring breakdown by t.l.c. as described above did not reveal any such differential degradation of the two enkephalins. Nor can the differential ratios be attributed to errors of estimating concentrations or specific activity of the labeled ligands, since these would be constant across all regions.

These studies suggest that leu and met-enkepahlin may have access to somewhat different populations of opiate receptors. This may prove to be an important postsynaptic mechanism of distinguishing between these two opioid peptides which seem to be contained within the same neurons.

β-LPH/β-endorphin system

When Hughes *et al.* (1975) first published their sequences of met and leu-enkephalin they pointed out that the sequence of met-enkephalin could be found in β-LPH at position 61–65. Relatively soon after, the C-fragment of β-LPH (also called β-endorphin) was shown to have opiate-like activity (Li and Chung, 1976; Bradbury *et al.*, 1976). There has been much speculation about the biosynthesis of met-enkephalin from β-LPH through β-endorphin. We were interested in the possibility that β-LPH and β-endorphin might exist in brain. Using the β-LPH and β-endorphin antisera mentioned above and in table 3.1, we have mapped these peptides in rat brain (Watson *et al.*, 1977*a*, *c*; Akil *et al.*, 1978). The distribution of β-LPH-like immunoreactivity and β-endorphin-like immunoreactivity (Bloom *et al.*, 1977*b*) are apparently identical. In a study outlined below, we were able to show that they are found within the same hypothalamic cells and fibers throughout the brain.

The β LPH/β-endorphin system has only one major group of cells in the brain–in the region of the arcuate nucleus and lateral to it. From this cell group, fibers project to many structures throughout the brainstem. When the distribution of the enkephalin-positive cells is compared to the cells of β-LPH/β-endorphin system, there is no detectable overlap. Although both systems have fibers in the hypothalamus, thalamus, and midbrain, there are areas where one system has fibers and the other does not. For example, there are enkephalin fibers and cells in spinal cord and striatum, whereas there were no detectable cells or fibers of β-endorphin or β-LPH. It seemed possible that the two opiate peptide systems (enkephalin and endorphin) are anatomically and biochemically separate. In order further to evaluate this hypothesis, we carried out the following lesion study.

Effect of lesions on β-LPH and met-enkephalin

We reasoned that if β-LPH was primarily the precursor for met-enkephalin, or if met-enkephalin was a breakdown product of β-LPH/β-endorphin, then lesions which alter the larger peptides should secondarily alter met-enkephalin. If, on the other hand, the β-LPH/β-endorphin system is independent of the met-enkephalin system, then it is theoretically possible to perform lesion studies which differentially alter the levels of the peptides in question. We therefore placed lesions in two areas: the basal hypothalamus, which was chosen because it contained what appeared to be the sole β-LPH/β-endorphin cell group; and the ventral central grey region, which contains β-LPH-positive terminals, and met-enkephalin terminals and cell bodies.

Fifteen male, Sprague-Dawley rats were assigned to three groups: a sham operated control, a ventral central grey-lesioned group, and a posteromedial hypothalamus-lesioned group. The lesions were all unilateral. In the case of the hypothalamus, four small lesions were placed in an array to destroy completely the β-LPH-positive cell system. In a parallel group of animals, periaqueductal central grey and hypothalamic lesions were performed and their sites were verified histologically and by immunocytochemistry.

Ten days after surgery, the animals were killed, and the brains extracted. The cerebellum, cortex, septal area and hippocampus—all areas containing relatively low levels of endogenous opioids—were dissected away. The remaining brainstem was divided into two regions—a posterior area including the medulla-pons, the central grey and surrounding tectum and tegmentum with the colliculi, and an anterior region containing the thalamus, subthalamus, hypothalamus and striatum. The parts were immediately frozen on dry ice and β-LPH and met-enkephalin were extracted as described above. The β-LPH and met-enkephalin RIAs were used to measure the levels of the peptides.

Table 3.2 summarizes the results obtained. It should be noted that, since the lesions were unilateral, a drop to 50 per cent of control levels represents a complete loss of activity on one side, if one assumes the systems to be uncrossed. However, since the lesioned sites were near the midline, it is possible that, in some cases, the lesion was not confined to one side of the brain. The β-LPH levels reported in this paper should be considered relative rather than absolute, since the antibody was directed against human and not rat β-LPH. Preliminary evidence suggests lower affinity of the antibody to the rat peptide, which would lead us to underestimate the levels.

As can be seen from the table, the lesions produced a different pattern of effects on β-LPH and met-enkephalin levels. Thus, hypothalamic lesions produced a consistent decrease in levels of β-LPH throughout both regions, with the values dropping to below 50 per cent of controls. This is consistent with the notion that

Table 3.2 Effect of unilateral lesions on met-enkephalin and β-LPH in two regions

	Hypothalamus Met-enkephalin*	β-LPH†
Posterior region	Controls = 1110 ± 193 Lesioned = 890 ± 230 %C = 80%	Controls = 5.0 ± 0.4 Lesioned = 2.3 ± 0.8 %C = 45%
	Not significant	$P < 0.02$
Anterior region	Controls = 1431 ± 85 Lesioned = 1159 ± 165 %C = Not significant	Controls = 2.5 ± 0.4 Lesioned < 1.2 %C < 50%
	Central grey Met-enkephalin	β-LPH
Posterior region	Controls = 1110 ± 193 Lesioned = 457 ± 81 %C = 41%	Controls = 5.0 ± 0.4 Lesioned = 3.5 ± 0.4 %C = 70%
	$P < 0.01$	$P < 0.025$
Anterior region	Controls = 1431 ± 85 Lesioned = 758 ± 112 %C = 53%	Controls = 2.50 ± 0.4 Lesioned = 2.45 ± 0.2 %C = 98%
	$P < 0.01$	Not significant

*Enkephalin given in pmol/g tissue; †β-LPH given in pmol/g equivalent

we have destroyed the major cell group of β-LPH/β-endorphin on one side and totally eradicated β-LPH immunoreactivity (verified in similar animals by immunohistochemistry). These same hypothalamic lesions had considerably less effect on met-enkephalin levels in the same tissue, since both the anterior and posterior regions exhibited a non-significant drop (to 80 per cent of controls) in met-enkephalin levels.

Central grey lesions, on the other hand, produced the opposite pattern (table 3.2). The had more effect on met-enkephalin levels ($P < 0.01$) than they did on β-LPH. While the posterior region, which contained the lesioned area, exhibited a significant decrease in β-LPH, the levels in the anterior region remained completely unaltered.

It therefore appears that hypothalamic lesions can eradicate β-LPH immunoreactivity with little change in met-enkephalin, while central grey lesions can dramatically alter met-enkephalin with little change in β-LPH in more anterior sites. These findings tend to support the notion of two separable opioid systems. They further argue against the possibility that met-enkephalin is merely the result of breakdown of β-LPH/β-endorphin.

ACTH, β-LPH, and β-endorphin

β-LPH has been localized in the pituitary within the corticotrophs of the anterior lobe and all the cells of the intermediate lobe (Moon *et al.*, 1973). Electron microscopic studies have demonstrated the presence of ACTH-like and β-LPH-like immunoreactivity (ACTH-LI and β-LPH-LI) in the same granule of pituitary cells (Pelletier *et al.*, 1977). Bloom *et al.* (1977*a*) have shown that β-endorphin-like immunoreactivity (β-endorphin-LI) is found in the same pituitary cell population as β-LPH-LI and ACTH-LI. In another study, that group has shown parallel plasma levels of ACTH-LI and β-endorphin-LI after physiological stress (Guillemin *et al.*, 1977). The biochemical relationship between β-LPH, β-endorphin, and ACTH has been strengthened by studies in a mouse pituitary tumor cell line (AtT-20/DV16) by Mains, Eipper, and Ling (1977). They have shown that there is a 31 000 dalton precursor protein which contains ACTH and β-LPH (and therefore β-MSH, β-endorphin, and met-enkephalin).

Recently, both β-LPH-LI and ACTH-LI have been shown in brain by RIA (Krieger *et al.*, 1977a, b; Akil *et al.*, 1978) and by immunocytochemistry (Watson *et al.*, 1977c; Watson *et al.*, 1978). Using immunocytochemistry β-endorphin-LI as well has been demonstrated in rat brain (Bloom *et al.*, 1977; Watson *et al.*, 1977*a*). These three immunoreactivities (β-LPH, β-endorphin, and ACTH) have strikingly similar distributions. All three have one major cell group in the region of the arcuate nucleus (and a few cells slightly lateral) and project throughout the brainstem in a very similar pattern. Because of this similar anatomical pattern in brain and their identical cells of origin in pituitary, we undertook a study to determine whether all three peptides were located in the same hypothalamic cells.

Procedure for detecting multiple antigens by immunocytochemistry

For multiple antigen studies carried out in the same section, the sections were obtained from colchicine-pretreated rats and then prepared as described in the Immunocytochemistry section, photographed, coverslips were removed and the slides washed. They were soaked overnight in 6 M guanidine HCl, re-covered, and viewed the next day. Guanidine was used so that most antigen-antibody bonds would be dissociated. All slides had a modest level of specific fluorescence remaining. Specific areas were exposed to ultraviolet light until all fluorescence was extinguished. They were then re-photographed, the coverslip removed, washed, and incubated with goat anti-rabbit IgC (without FITC). The goat anti-rabbit IgG was used to block any remaining bound rabbit IgG so that subsequent FITC-goat anti-rabbit could not bind in an anatomically specific fashion. The second primary antibody (for example anti-β-endorphin) was then started in an overnight incubation and the entire process was repeated. In a few slides a third primary antibody (anti-β-LPH) was studied on the same sections.

The sections studied were taken from the arcuate region of the hypothalamus so that the β-LPH, β-endorphin, and ACTH-positive cell groups could be compared. In those coronal sections it was also possible to study fibers from hypothalamus, thalamus, and amygdala.

Several control conditions are necessary in this type of study

(1) Excess authentic peptide was shown to block the appropriate antiserum (figure 3.2 c, d). Other peptides were shown not to interfere with the specific demonstrations.

(2) Although guanidine seemed to dissociate some of the antigen–antibody bonds, it was necessary to show that the demonstration of the second (or third)

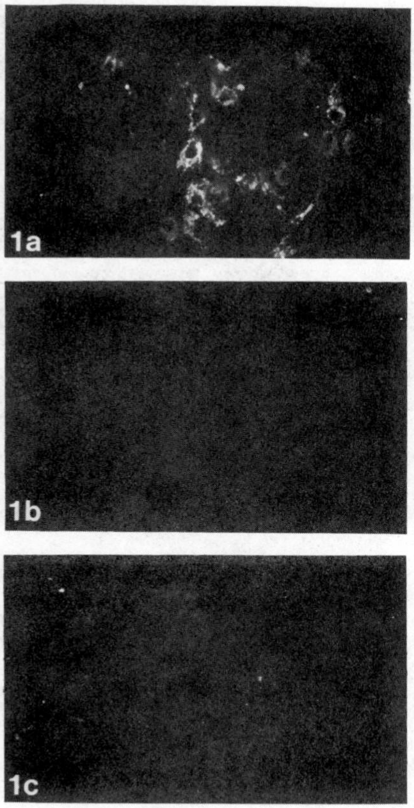

Figure 3.1 Control series demonstrating that FITC-goat-anti-rabbit IgG does not rebind to the section in an anatomically specific fashion. (a) ACTH-positive cells in the arcuate region of rat hypothalamus, pretreated with colchicine. (50 μg i.v.t. at 48 h) ×280. (b) The same area as in (a) after a 16-h exposure to 6 M guanidine HCl and unfiltered ultraviolet for 30 min. Note the complete absence of fluorescence. ×280. (c) The same area after (b) and after incubation with goat-anti-rabbit IgG (1/50) for 1 h at 37°C, wash and exposure to FITC-goat-anti-rabbit IgG (1/80, 1 h at 37°C). Note the absence of specific fluorescence. ×280.

peptide was not simply a rebinding of the FITC-goat anti-rabbit IgG to the remaining primary antibody. After guanidine treatment, some sections were incubated with FITC-goat anti-rabbit alone to show that there was no specific binding (figure 3.1a, b, c).

(3) Sections were prepared in which the second primary antiserum (for example, anti-β-endorphin) was blocked by the appropriate peptide (β-endorphin).

(4) It was shown that after guanidine treatment, all three peptides could be visualized, depending upon specific antiserum (figures 3.2b, d; 3.3c; 3,4c; 3.5b, c).

(5) Antisera to other peptides, such as the enkephalins, were shown to bind to completely different structures on the same sections.

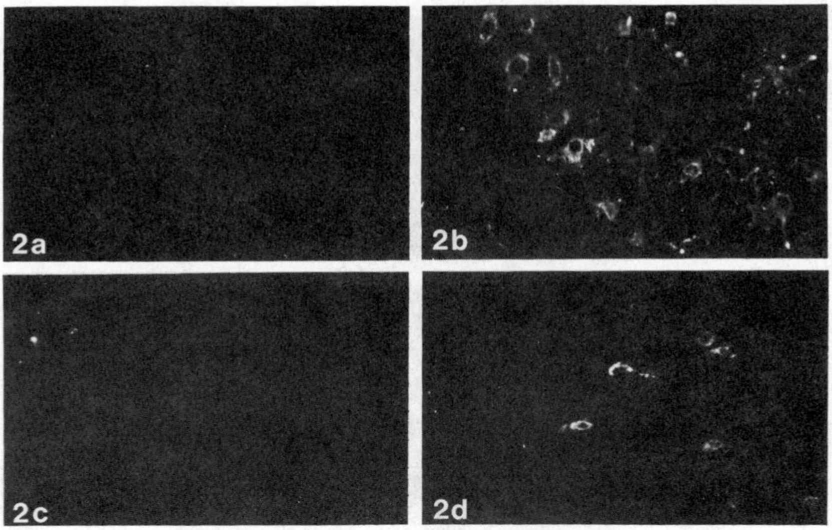

Figure 3.2 Two control series demonstrating that 6 M guanidine HCl does not substantially interfere with visualization of β-endorphin (a, b) or ACTH (c, d) and that ACTH peptide blocks ACTH antiserum (c, d). (a) Blocked ACTH antiserum followed by β-endorphin antiserum. 100 μM $ACTH_{1-24}$ blocked the ACTH antiserum used in this hypothalamic section. ×280. (b) After (a) was photographed, it was incubated in guanidine HCl, exposed to ultraviolet, incubated in goat anti-rabbit IgG, finally β-endorphin antiserum and then FITC-goat anit-rabbit. Note the β-endorphin positive cells. ×280. (c) Blocked ACTH antiserum followed by unblocked ACTH antiserum. A control using 100 μM $ACTH_{1-24}$ in ACTH antiserum was produced. Note the absence of specific fluorescence. ×280. (d) The section was reincubated in unblocked anti-ACTH antiserum. Several ACTH-positive cells are now clearly visible. ×280.

These controls were carried out and showed that the binding seen with all three antisera was only blocked by the appropriate peptide (Figure 3.2), that re-binding of FITC-goat-anti-rabbit was not seen (figure 3.1), and that guanidine did not obviously harm the peptides (figures 3.3, 3.4, 3.5).

The results of this study are best seen in figures 3.3, 3.4, and 3.5. ACTH-positive cells in the arcuate region are also demonstrated by anti-β-endorphin antiserum (figure 3.3). When the section is incubated with anti-β-endorphin first and then anti-ACTH, as the second main antibody, the same hypothalamic fibers are seen with both antisera (figure 3.4). Finally, when the entire procedure is run on the same section using all three anti-sera sequentially, the same cells are demonstrated each time (figure 3.5). It seems reasonable to conclude that the immunoreactivity detected by these three antisera is present in one general set of cells and fibers in brain. One interpretation of these results is that all three antibodies were recognizing a single protein (31000 dalton precursor?) (Mains *et al.*, 1977) at three separate antigenic sites. It is also possible that these antisera were demonstrating the presence of three distinct peptides β-LPH, β-endorphin, and ACTH. More biochemical work is necessary before this question can be resolved.

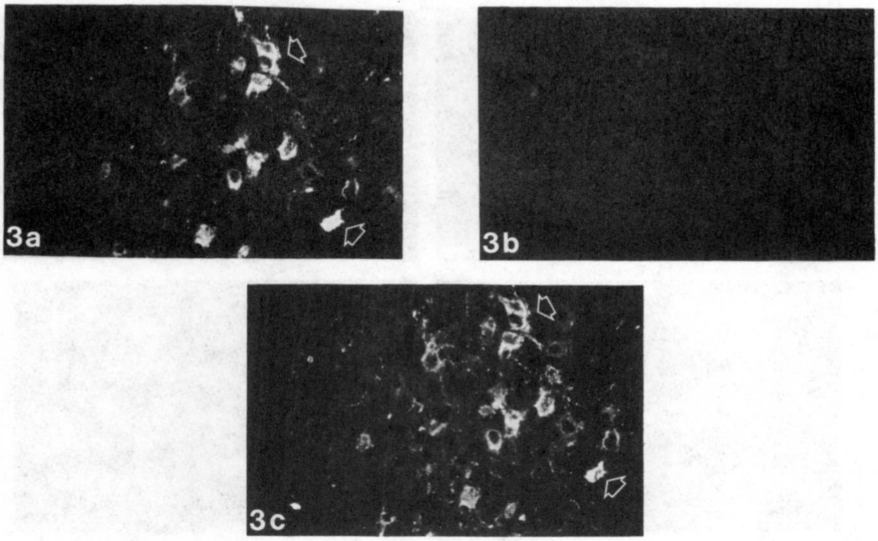

Figure 3.3 An experimental series showing ACTH-positive cells (a) in the accurate region of colchicine-pretreated rat, the loss of activity (b) after guanidine and ultraviolet treatment and the revisualization of the same cells (c) after exposure to the anti-β-endorphin.

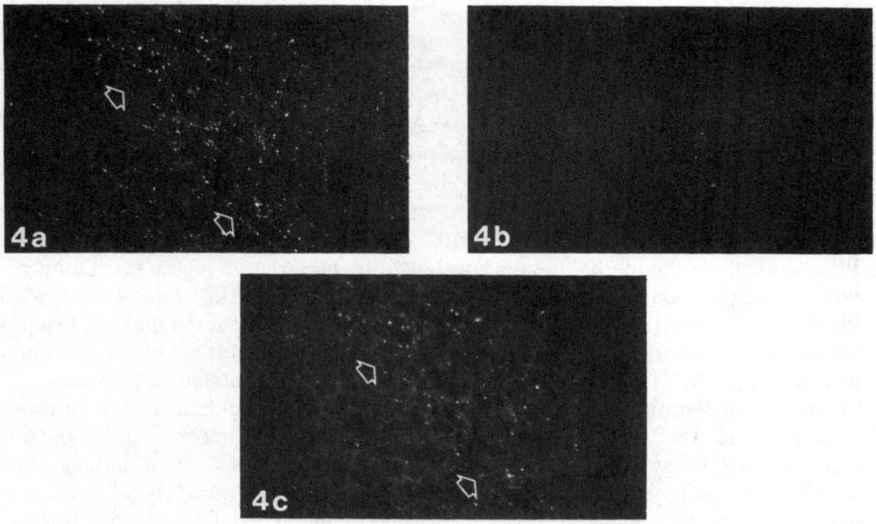

Figure 3.4 An experimental series showing β-endorphin-positive fibers (a) in the dorsomedial hypothalamus of a colchicine-pretreated rat, the loss of activity (b) after guanidine and ultraviolet treatment and the revisualization of the same fibers (c) after exposure to ACTH antiserum.

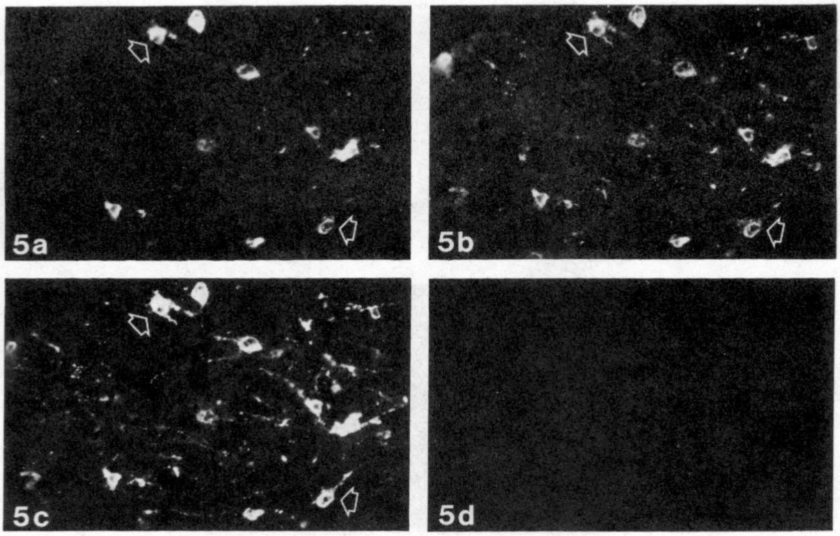

Figure 3.5 An experimental series showing ACTH-positive hypothalamic cells (a), and the disappearance of fluorescence in the section after guanidine and ultraviolet (d). The same cells are visible after exposure to anti-β-endorphin (b). They can be visualized again after a second treatment with guanidine, ultraviolet and exposure to anti-β-LPH (c). These cells are demonstrated by all three antisera. Between each treatment the area was treated with guanidine HCl and ultraviolet resulting in a complete loss of specific activity—as in (d). Parallel peptide-blocked controls were uniformly negative. Colchicine-pretreated adult rat (50 μg i.v.t. at 48 h). ×280.

CONCLUSIONS AND DISCUSSION

The present immunocytochemical–biochemical studies suggest the existence of two distinct systems of endogenous opioids in rat brain: an enkephalin-containing system with multiple groups of cell bodies distributed throughout the CNS predominantly with short projections (Watson *et al.*, 1977*b*; Elde *et al.*, 1976; Hökfelt *et al.*, 1977; Simantov *et al.*, 1977), and a β-endorphin system with one major group of cells in the medial-basal hypothalamus (periarcuate region) and longer projections (Watson *et al.*, 1977*a, c*; Bloom *et al.*, 1977*b*; Akil *et al.*, 1978). Within the enkephalin system met and leu-enkephalin cannot be distinguished using highly specific antisera. The β-endorphin system also contains β-LPH-like immunoreactivity and ACTH-like immunoreactivity within the same neuron. Specific lesions can differentially alter the levels of β-LPH and met-enkephalin in various brain regions, as a function of lesion site. Although the pituitary contains the β-endorphin-ACTH system, it is not clear whether it contains an enkephalin system.

Although we have shown that β-endorphin and β-LPH are not merely precursors of enkephalin, they may be critical in the enkephalin synthetic pathway. If this were the case, one would expect them to have a relatively short life in the enkephalin neurons, since they have not been visualized in these neurons, and exist in very low concentrations in some enkephalin-rich areas such as the striatum. The opposite hypothesis—that enkephalin is merely a breakdown product of the C-fragment of β-LPH—appears somewhat less likely. Using many extraction procedures which attempt to halt enzymatic breakdown, the levels of enkephalin in brain appear at least an order of magnitude higher than those of β-endorphin or β-LPH. There are many areas which are rich in one substance and relatively poor in the other. Finally, the existence of specific neurons with immunoreactivity to one opioid peptide and not to the other argues in favor of two distinct systems.

The existence of this two-part opioid system in the brain raises several critical questions concerning their function, regulation, and interactions. If, in fact, each of these systems contains two active peptides within its neurons (met-enkephalin and leu-enkephalin in one, β-endorphin and ACTH in the other), questions of the nature of their function, of their storage, release, postsynaptic effects and regulations become more complex than in the case of classically characterized neurotransmitter systems. The met and leu-enkephalin binding studies reported in this paper, along with evidence from other laboratories (Martin *et al.*, 1976; Lord *et al.*, 1976; Akil *et al.*, 1978) suggests that the differentiations between the enkephalins may be, in part, postsynaptic. The notion of multiple opiate receptors extends further to distinguish between enkephalin effects and β-endorphin-like effects (Lord *et al.*, 1976). Finally, the potential role of brain ACTH, and its possible interactions with β-endorphin remain totally obscure.

Thus, studies of both pre and postsynaptic characteristics of each of the active peptides, within each of the two opioid systems are crucial to an understanding of their physiological functions.

ACKNOWLEDGEMENTS

We wish to thank Dr C. H. Li for generously providing β-LPH and the β-LPH antiserum. We also wish to thank Drs Mains and Eipper for generously providing the anti-ACTH and anti-β-endorphin antisera. S.J.W. is the recipient of MH 11028 and a Bank of America Giannini Foundation Postdoctoral Fellowship. H.A. is the recipient of Sloan Foundation Fellowship in Neurophysiology, BR 16091. J.D.B. holds Research Scientist Development Award, MH 24161. Various aspects of the work were supported by NIDA grants, DA 1522 and DA 01207, and by NIMH Program-Project grant, MH 23861.

REFERENCES

Akil, H., Watson, S. J., Berger, P. A. and Barchas, J. D. (1978). In *The Endorphins: Advances in Biochemical Psychopharmacology*, **18**, Raven Press, New York

Austen, B. M., Smyth, D. G. and Snell, C. R. (1977). *Nature*, **269**, 619–21

Bloom, F., Battenberg, E., Rossier, J., Ling, N., Leppaluoto, J., Vargo, T. M. and Guillemin, R. (1977*a*). *Life Sci.*, **20**, 43–8

Bloom, F., Rossier, J., Battenberg, E., Vargo, T., Minick, S., Ling, N. and Guillemin, R. (1977*b*). Presentation at the Annual Meeting of the Society for Neuroscience, Anaheim, California

Bradbury, A. F., Feldberg, W. F., Smyth, D. G. and Snell, C. R. (1976). *Opiates and Endogenous Opioid Peptides*, (ed. H. W. Kosterlitz) Elsevier/North-Holland, Amsterdam, pp.9–17

Cox, B. M., Opheim, K. E., Teschemacher, H. and Goldstein, A. (1975). *Life Sci.*, **16**, 1777–82

Eipper, B. A., Mains, R. E. and Guenzi, D. (1976). *J. biol. Chem.*, **251**, 4121–6

Elde, R., Hökfelt, T., Johannsson, O. and Terenius, L. (1976). *Neuroscience*, **1**, 349–51

Graf, L., Ronal, A. Z., Bajusz, S., Csek, G. and Seze'kely, J. T. (1976). *FEBS Lett.*, **64**, 181–4

Guillemin, R., Ling, N. and Burgus, R. (1976). *C. r. hebd. Séanc. Acad. Sci. Paris, Ser. D.*, **282**, 783–5

Guillemin, R., Vargo, T., Rossier, J., Minick, S., Ling, N., Rivier, C., Vale, W. and Bloom, F. (1977). *Science*, **197**, 1367–9

Hökfelt, T., Elde, R., Johansson, O., Terenius, L. and Stein, L. (1977). *Neurosci. Lett.*, **5**, 25–31

Hughes, J., Smith, T. W., Kosterlitz, H. W., Fothergill, L. A., Morgan, B. A. and Morris, H. R. (1975). *Nature*, **258**, 577–9

Krieger, D. T., Liotta, A. and Brownstein, M. J. (1977*a*). *Proc. natn. Acad. Sci. U.S.A.*, **74**, 648–52.

Krieger, D. T., Liotta, A., Suda, T., Palkovits, M. and Brownstein, M. J. (1977). *Biochem. biophys. Res. Commun.*, **73**, 930–6

Li, H. L. and Chung, D. (1976). *Proc. natn. Acad. Sci. U.S.A.*, **73**, 1145–8

Lord, J. A. H., Waterfield, A. A., Hughes, J., and Kosterlitz, H. W. (1976). In *Opiates and Endogenous Opioid Peptides*, (ed. H. W. Kosterlitz) Elsevier/North Holland, Amsterdam, pp. 275–80

Mains, R. E., Eipper, B. A. and Ling, N. (1977). *Proc. natn. Acad. Sci. U.S.A.*, **74**, 3014–8

Martin, W. R., Eades, G. G., Thompson, J. A., Huppler, R. E. and Gilbert, P. E. (1976). *J. Pharmac. exp. Ther.*, **197**, 518–32

Moon, H. D., Li, C. H. and Jennings, B. M. (1973). *Anat. Rec.*, **175**, 524–38

Pasternak, G. W., Simantov, R. and Snyder S. H. (1976). *Molec. Pharmac.*, **12**, 504–13

Pelletier, G., Leclerc, R., Labrie, F., Cote, J., Chretien, M. and Les, M. (1977). *Endocrinology*, **100**, 770–6

Rao, A. J. and Li, C. H. (1977). *Int. J. Peptide Protein*, **10**, 169

Simantov, R., Kuhar, M. J., Uhl, G. R. and Snyder, S. H. (1977). *Proc. natn. Acad. Sci. U.S.A.*, **74**, 2167–71

Simantov, R. and Snyder, S. H. (1976). *Life Sci.*, **18**, 781–8

Sullivan, S., Akil, H., Watson, S. J. and Barchas, J. D. *Commun. Psychopharm.*, **1**, 605–10

Teschemacher, H., Opheim, K. E., Cox, B. M. and Goldstein, A. (1975). *Life Sci.*, **16**, 1771–6

Watson, S. J., Akil, H. and Barchas, J. D. (1977*a*). Presentation (*Annual Meeting of the Society for Neuroscience*, Anaheim, California

Watson, S. J., Akil, H., Sullivan, S. O. and Barchas, J. D. (1977*b*). *Life Sci.*, **25**, 733–8

Watson, S. J., Barchas, J. D. and Li, C. H. (1977*c*). *Proc. natn. Acad. Sci. U.S.A.*, **74**, 5155–8

Watson, S. J., Richard, C. W. and Barchas, J. D. (1978). *Science*, (in press)

4

Effects of opiates and opioid peptides on motor behaviors: sites and mechanisms of action

Agu Pert, Louise A. DeWald, Helen Liao and Carlos Sivit (Section on Biochemistry and Pharmacology, Biological Psychiatry Branch, National Institute of Mental Health, Bethesda, Maryland)

In addition to their analgesic effects, opiates have profound effects on motor behaviors. This is not surprising since extrapyramidal as well as mesolimbic structures which have been shown to have important functions in regulating motor activity (Costall *et al.*, 1977; Kelly *et al.*, 1975) are among the highest in opiate receptor concentration (Atweh and Kuhar, 1977; Hiller *et al.*, 1973; Kuhar *et al.*, 1973), enkephalin content (Hong *et al.*, 1977) and enkephalinergic terminals (Elde *et al.*, 1976; Simantov *et al.*, 1977).

Small doses of morphine produce increases in spontaneous locomotor activity (Babbini and Davis, 1972), while large doses cause an initial depression and catatonia which is followed by motor excitation (Babbini and Davis, 1972; Costall and Naylor, 1973). These psychomotor, as well as catatonic, effects of opiate agonists have generally been ascribed to their actions on various components of the nigrostriatal dopamine system, especially the striatum (Kuschinsky, 1976; Lal, 1976).

The purpose of these studies was to analyze further the mechanisms and sites of action of opiate alkaloids and opioid peptides in modulating motor behaviors.

Effects of morphine and opioid peptides on locomotor activity following intraventricular injections

Thirty-one male Sprague-Dawley rats (300–350 g) were stereotactically implanted with chronic indwelling cannulae guides constructed from 22-gauge stainless steel tubing. The tips of these guide cannulae were aimed for an area 1.5 mm dorsal to the ventricular system (AP 3.0; LAT 0.0, DV +2.0; König and Klippel, 1965). Injections were made through 27-gauge injectors which protruded 1.5 mm past the guide cannulae. One week following surgery, the rats were divided into four groups and injected with either 25 μg morphine sulfate (n = 8), 25 μg β-endorphin (n = 8),

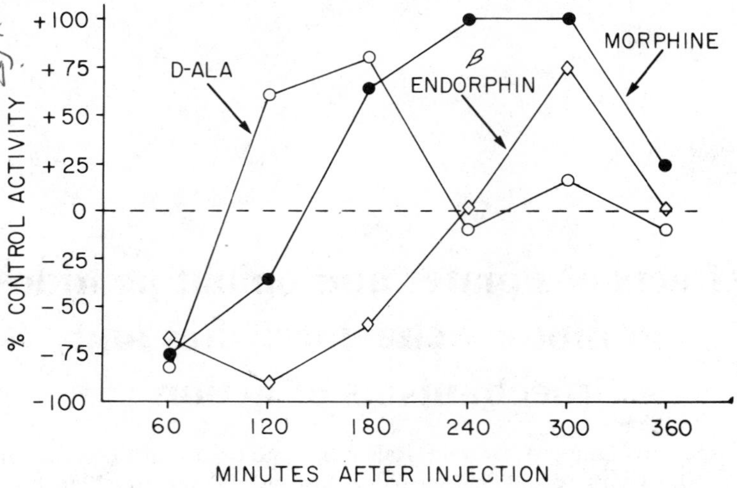

Figure 4.1 Biphasic effects of morphine, β-endorphin and [D-Ala^2, Met^5]-enkephalinamide on spontaneous horizontal locomotor activity following intraventricular injections (25 μg).

25 μg [D-Ala^2, Met^5-enkephalinamide (Pert *et al.*, 1976) ($n = 8$) or 5 μl sterile H_2O ($n = 7$). All drugs were dissolved in sterile water and injected in a volume of 5 μl at a rate of 1 μl per 15 s. Immediately after injections the animals were placed in clear Plexiglas chambers (23 × 23 × 15 cm) which were mounted in Motron activity meters (Model 40Fc). Horizontal and vertical activity were monitored in 60 min segments for 6 h.

Figure 4.1 illustrates the biphasic effects of morphine, [D-Ala^2, Met^5]-enkephalinamide and β-endorphin on locomotor activity. All three compounds produced an initial depression of activity which was followed by motor excitation. No qualitative differences were noted in the actions of these three compounds. [D-Ala^2, Met^5]-enkephalinamide produced the shortest depressive phase, while β-endorphin exhibited the longest.

Increased locomotor activity following injections of morphine and [D-Ala^2, Met^5]-enkephalinamide into the forebrain

The biphasic effects of opiates on locomotor activity suggested that the two behavioral components (depression and activation) may be mediated through different neural structures. An attempt was made to localize these two actions by assessing the effects of morphine on locomotion following injections into specific brain sites. Since the nucleus accumbens in the limbic forebrain contains a relatively high concentration of opiate receptors and enkephalin terminals (Elde *et al.*, 1976) and has been implicated in locomotor behavior (Kelly *et al.*, 1975; Jackson *et al.*, 1977), it is conceivable that some of the locomotor effects of opiates could be mediated through this structure.

Thirty-five male Sprague-Dawley rats, anesthetized with sodium pentobarbitone, were implanted stereotactically with bilateral intracerebral cannulae guides constructed from 23-gauge hypodermic tubing. The guide cannulae tips were aimed for a region 2 mm dorsal to the n. accumbens (AP 9.4, LAT 1.5, DV 2.0). Drugs were injected into the n. accumbens through 30-gauge injectors which protruded 2 mm past the guide tips. Drug and control solutions were administered in a volume of 1 μl and a rate of 1 μl per 30 s. One group of 10 animals was injected bilaterally in the n. accumbens with 5 μg morphine sulfate (that is, a 10 μg total dose), 10 μg apomorphine and 1 μl of water (the drug vehicle). All animals received both drugs and the vehicle in a counterbalanced order 7 days apart. Another group of animals ($n = 9$) was injected in the n. accumbens with both 10 μg [D-Ala^2, Met^5]-enkephalinamide and 1 μl of water in a counterbalanced order as above. Immediately after injections the animals were placed in the Motron motility meters. Horizontal and vertical activity was monitored in 30-min segments for 6 h. Animals in these studies were always injected at 1000 h and removed from the apparatus at 1600 h.

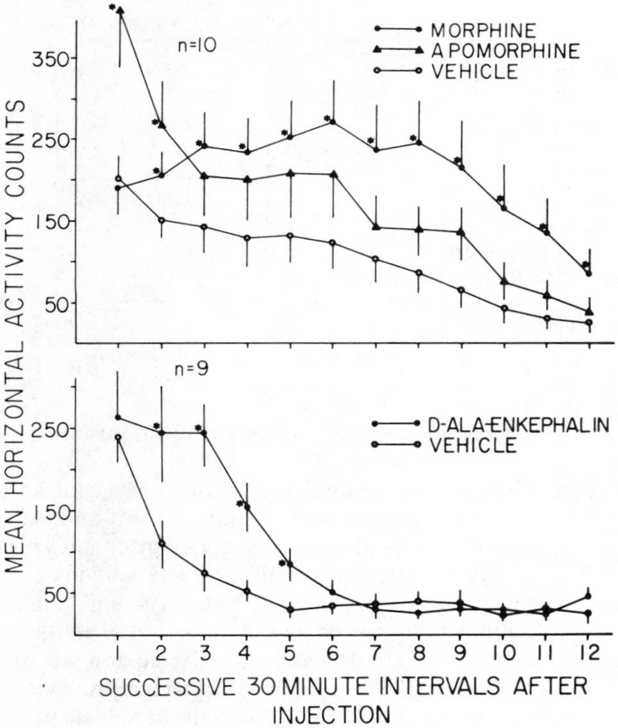

Figure 4.2 Time course of horizontal hypermotility after bilateral injections of (top) vehicle alone (○), morphine 5 μg (●), apomorphine 10 μg (▲) or (bottom) [D-Ala^2, Met^5]-enkephalinamide 10 μg (●) into the nucleus accumbens. Repeated measures analyses of variance revealed a significant drug effect for both groups of rats. Vertical lines indicate s.e.m. Similar results were obtained for vertical activity. $*P < 0.05$ for comparisons between effects produced by the drugs and the vehicle at each time point. (Pert and Sivit, 1977; by courtesy of *Nature*).

Figure 4.2 illustrates the effects of apomorphine, morphine and [D-Ala^2, Met^5]-enkephalinamide on motor activity following injection into the nucleus accumbens. Apomorphine produced an immediate increase in both horizontal and vertical spontaneous activity after injections into the n. accumbens. This effect was dissipated rapidly over 1 h and was no longer detectable 90 min after injection. Morphine, however, induced a more gradual increase in activity which reached asymptotic levels in approximately 3 h and was still present 5.5–6 h after injection. The excitatory effect of [D-Ala^2, Met^5]-enkephalinamide also had a gradual onset but was not as persistent as that of morphine.

Interestingly, the hyperactivity induced by morphine was antagonized by naloxone but not by haloperidol, while the hyperactivity induced by apomorphine was antagonized by haloperidol and not by naloxone (Pert and Sivit, 1977).

Table 4.1 Coordinates for intracerebral morphine injections

Structure	Coordinates			
	AP	LAT	DV	*n*
Caudate nucleus	7.5	2.5	1.0	9
Lateral hypothalamus	4.5	1.5	−3.0	10
Ventral thalamus	4.5	2.0	−0.4	8
Amygdala	4.2	3.4	−3.4	8
Dorsal hippocampus	3.8	2.2	2.0	8
Substantia nigra	2.2	1.8	−2.2	8
Ventral tegmentum	1.8	0	−2.5	10
Periaqueductal grey matter	0.6	0.5	−0.5	9
Mesencephalic reticular formation	0.6	2.0	−1.5	10

(König and Klippel, 1965.)

Effects of morphine on locomotor activity following injections into other brain regions

Eighty male Sprague-Dawley rats were implanted with 23-gauge intracerebral cannulae guides in the brain regions indicated in table 4.1. All cannulae were bilateral with the exception of the periaqueductal grey matter and ventral tegmentum. One week after surgery the bilaterally implanted rats were injected bilaterally with either 5 μg morphine sulfate or 1 μl of sterile water. The unilaterally implanted rats were injected with either 10 μg morphine sulfate or 1 μl of sterile water. Morphine sulfate was dissolved in 1 μl sterile water and injected at a rate of 1 μl per 30 s. Injections were made through 30-gauge injectors which protruded 2 mm past the guide tips. All animals received both morphine and the vehicle in a randomized order at least 7 days apart. Immediately after injections the animals were placed in the Motron activity meters. Horizontal and vertical activity was monitored in 30-min segments for 2 h.

Table 4.2 illustrates the effects of morphine on spontaneous locomotor activity following injections into various brain sites. The most profound effect of morphine on locomotor activity was seen following injections into the periaqueductal grey

Table 4.2 Effects of morphine on spontaneous vertical and horizontal locomotor behavior following intracerebral injections

Structure	Min after injection							
	0–30		30–60		60–90		90–120	
	H	V	H	V	H	V	H	V
Caudate nucleus	0	0	0	0	0	0	0	0
Lateral hypothalamus	0	0	0	↓	0	↓	0	0
Ventral thalamus	↓	↓	↓	↓	0	0	0	0
Amygdala	0	0	0	0	0	0	0	0
Dorsal hippocampus	↓	↓	↓	↓	0	↓	0	0
Substantia nigra	↑	↓	↑	↓	0	↓	↑	0
Ventral tegmentum	0	0	0	0	0	0	0	0
Periaqueductal grey matter	↓↓	↓↓	↓↓	↓↓	0	0	0	0
Mesencephalic reticular formation	0	0	0	0	0	↓	0	0

↓, Moderate depressant effects; ↓↓, intense depressant effects; ↑, moderate excitatory effects; 0, No significant effect; H, Horizontal activity; V, Vertical activity.

matter. Unilateral injections of 10 μg into this region produced an immediate and pronounced depression of both vertical and horizontal motor activity which persisted for 60 min. Two of the nine rats exhibited spontaneous hyper-reactivity which has been described previously by Jacquet and Lajtha (1974). This effect is apparently non-specific since we were unable to antagonize it with naloxone (5 mg/kg i.p.). Furthermore, hyper-reactivity following injections of morphine into the PAG is elicited equally well by both (+) and (–)-morphine (Jacquet *et al.*, 1977) and is not found following injections of other opiate alkaloids or opioid peptides (Jacquet and Lajtha, 1974; Pert, unpublished observations). Bouts of hyper-reactivity alternated with periods of depressed motility and catatonia. Data from these two rats were not included in the analysis. Bilateral injections into the caudate nucleus, amygdala and the mesencephalic reticular formation, as well as unilateral injections into the ventral tegmentum proved to be relatively ineffective in modifying spontaneous motor output. Injections into the dorsal hippocampus, and into the ventral thalamus were, however, effective in depressing both horizontal and vertical activity for 30–90 min. Injections into the lateral hypothalamus and the mesencephalic reticular formation produced a slight depression of the vertical motor component which became significant only 30–60 min after application. Bilateral injections of morphine into the substantia nigra produced a complex reaction. Vertical activity decreased while horizontal locomotor activity increased. The increased horizontal motor activity was also accompanied by stereotypic lateral head movements. These movements appeared to contribute to the increase in horizontal motor activity.

Catatonic effects of opiates following intraventricular injections

Successively higher doses of opiate agonists induce a catatonic-like state that is characterized by muscular rigidity (Wand *et al.*, 1973; Costall and Naylor, 1973). Opiate-induced catatonia can be differentiated from neuroleptic-induced catalepsy

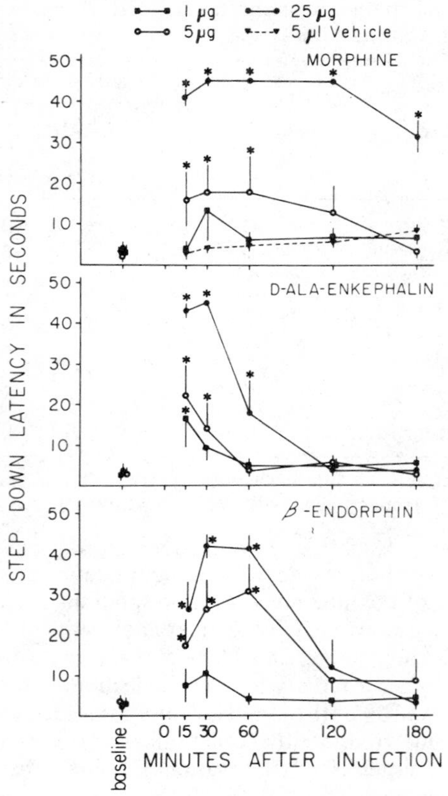

Figure 4.3 Catatonic effects of morphine, β-endorphin and [D-Ala^2, Met^5]-enkephalinamide following i.v.t. injections.

in that the opiate catatonic effect is also accompanied by loss of the righting reflex, muscular rigidity and inhibition of nociceptive reactions while the cataleptic state induced by neuroleptics is not. Segal *et al.* (1977) have recently extended this differentiation to β-endorphin.

The purpose of this study was to compare and contrast the catatonic effects of morphine, β-endorphin and [D-Ala^2, Met^5]-enkephalinamide following i.v.t. injections.

Seventy-seven male Sprague-Dawley rats were prepared with ventricular cannulae as before. After recovery they were injected with 1, 5 or 25 μg of morphine, [D-Ala^2, Met^5]-enkephalinamide or 5 μl of sterile water. Three groups of animals were also pretreated with 2 mg/kg of nalozone i.p. immediately before i.v.t. injections of 25 μg of morphine, [D-Ala^2, Met^5]-enkephalinamide or β-endorphin. Catatonia was assessed 15, 30, 60, 120 or 180 min after an i.v.t. injection. An objective measure of catatonia was obtained by simply placing the animal's front paws on a horizontal wooden bar 10 cm high and measuring the amount of time that it took the rat to step down. An arbitrary limit of 45 s was imposed on each trial.

Injections of 25 μg of either morphine, β-endorphin or [D-Ala[2], Met[5]]-enkephalinamide into the ventricles produced a significant catatonic reaction that was characterized by muscular rigidity (figure 4.3). Similar findings have been reported by Segal *et al.* (1977) and Jacquet and Marks (1976) for β-endorphin after injections into either the ventricles or the periaqueductal grey matter. The catatonic effects of morphine were still seen in some animals even 3 h after injection. The catatonic effects of [D-Ala[2], Met[5]]-enkephalinamide and β-endorphin, on the other hand, persisted for only 1 h. Lower doses of the three compounds had lesser effects. No qualitative differences were noted in the catatonia induced by each compound.

Catatonic sites of action

To ascertain whether the catatonic effects of opiates have specific neural foci, some of the animals that had been used previously to identify the neural substrates that mediate the locomotor effects of morphine were again injected with either morphine (5 μg bilaterally or 10 μg unilaterally) or 1 μl of saline as above. All animals received both saline and morphine in a randomized order 7 days apart. They were tested for catatonia 15 and 30 min after injection.

While a modest but significant catatonic effect was elicited after injections of morphine into the hippocampus, the most pronounced catatonia was obtained after injections into the PAG. Two of the eight rats, however, again exhibited spontaneous hyper-reactivity alternating with catatonia, following unilateral injections of 10 μg of morphine. Injections into other structures were relatively ineffective in modifying step-down latencies.

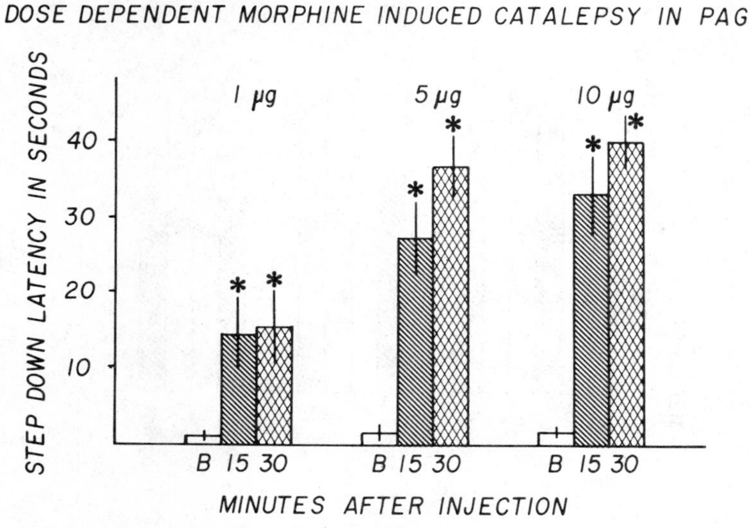

Figure 4.4 Catatonic effects of 1 μg (n = 5), 5 μg (n = 6) and 10 μg (n = 7) of morphine following injections into the periaqueductal grey matter of the mesencephalon. Baseline measures (B) were always taken 30 min before the morphine injections. Two animals in the 10 μg group were not included in the analysis since they exhibited hyperexcitability along with catatonia.

Sharpe *et al.* (1974) have reported that the hyper-reactivity elicited by injections of morphine into the PAG is dose dependent—only relatively high (and presumably toxic) doses produce this response. It was of interest to ascertain whether catatonia could be observed following injections of morphine into the PAG without the confounding hyper-reactivity, by using lower doses of morphine.

For this, 17 male Sprague-Dawley rats were prepared with unilateral PAG cannulae as above. The animals were divided into three groups and injected with either 1, 5 or 10 μg of morphine. Figure 4.4 illustrates the dose-dependent catatonic effect of morphine following PAG injections. Although hyper-reactivity accompanied catatonia in two of the rats injected with 10 μg of morphine, none of the animals injected with the lower doses demonstrated this reaction. Even 1 μg of morphine was clearly sufficient to induce a significant catatonic response.

Effect of naloxone on spontaneous motor activity

If enkephalin does play a part in modulating motor behaviors, and if these systems are tonically active, it should be possible to modify motor activity with specific opiate antagonists.

Sixty male Sprague-Dawley rats (350–400 g) were tested for 30 min in the Motron activity apparatus. On the basis of their performance during this session, they were divided into six matched groups. Five days later they were injected with either 0.1, 0.5, 1.5 or 10 mg/kg of naloxone or 1 ml/kg saline i.p. Fifteen minutes

Naloxone 5 mg/kg ip
↓ locomotor activity.

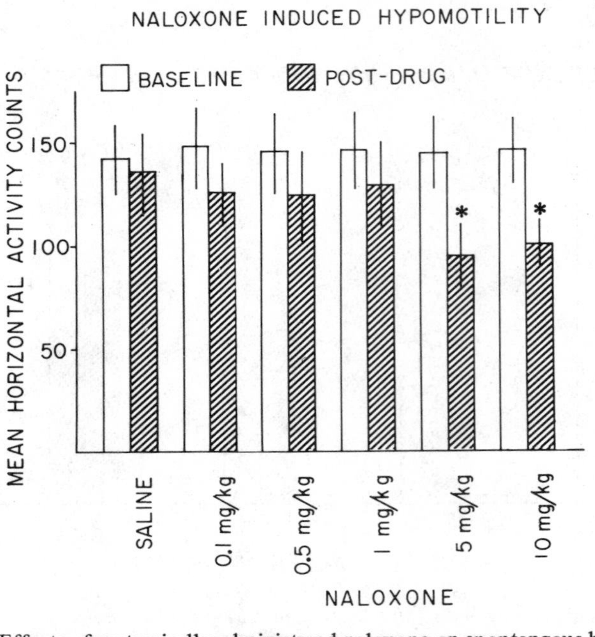

Figure 4.5 Effects of systemically administered naloxone on spontaneous horizontal locomotor activity. $*P < 0.05$ for comparisons of post-drug performance with baseline performance.

after the injection the animals were placed in the activity apparatus for a second 30 min session. Figure 4.5 illustrates the effects of naloxone on horizontal motor activity. Although the lower doses of naloxone were not effective in modifying spontaneous locomotor activity, the highest doses (5 and 10 mg/kg) clearly depressed this behavior.

Effects of opiates on the nigrostriatal system

Opiates exert profound effects on the nigrostriatal dopamine system. Increased dopamine synthesis is indicated by the ability of opiate agonists to increase the conversion of radioactive tyrosine into dopamine in the striata of rodents (Clouet and Ratner, 1970; Costa *et al.*, 1973; Loh *et al.*, 1973). Opiates have also been found to raise the dopamine utilization in whole brain (Gunne *et al.*, 1969) or striata of rats (Kuschinsky and Hornykiewicz, 1972) and mice (Kuschinsky and Hornykiewicz, 1974). It is not clear, however, whether these effects of opiates are due to their direct action on nigrostriatal dopaminergic neurons or on neurons which are associated with the nigrostriatal dopamine pathways.

In the next series of studies we utilized the rotational model first introduced by Andén *et al.* (1966) and extended by Ungerstedt (1971) to examine the effects of morphine on nigrostriatal activity. Essentially this model is based on the principle that animals will rotate away from the striatum with the preponderance of dopaminergic activity. A dopaminergic imbalance is usually created by unilaterally lesioning the substantia nigra either electrolytically or by injections of 6-hydroxydopamine (6-OHDA). Such lesions result in the degeneration of ascending dopaminergic neurons in the nigrostriatal pathway and the development of dopamine receptor supersensitivity in the corresponding striatum (Creese *et al.*, 1977).

Dopaminergic drugs which enhance dopaminergic activity by releasing dopamine from terminals (amphetamine) induce rotational behavior ipsilateral to the lesion while dopaminergic agonists which act postsynaptically (apomorphine) induce rotational behavior which is contralateral to the lesion, presumably due to their actions on the striatum which has developed supersensitive dopamine receptors. These differential effects are most clearly seen after 6-OHDA lesions (Iwamoto *et al.*, 1976*a*; Costall *et al.*, 1976).

Effects of morphine on rotational behavior following unilateral 6-OHDA lesions to substantia nigra

Twenty-eight male Sprague-Dawley rats (200–250 g) were injected unilaterally in the substantia nigra (AP 2.2, LAT 1.8, DV −2.2) with 9 μg of 6-OHDA dissolved in a solution of sterile saline containing 0.2 mg/ml of ascorbic acid. The injection volume was 3 μl and the injection rate was 1 μl per 30 s. Approximately 2 weeks following lesioning, the rats were injected with either 1 mg/kg apomorphine or 2.5 mg/kg *d*-amphetamine intraperitoneally. All rats received both drugs in a randomized order, 3 days apart. Rotational behavior was assessed 15 min after injection by placing the animal in a clear Plexiglas cylinder (28 cm in diameter and 27 cm high) and recording the direction and number of rotations made in 5 min.

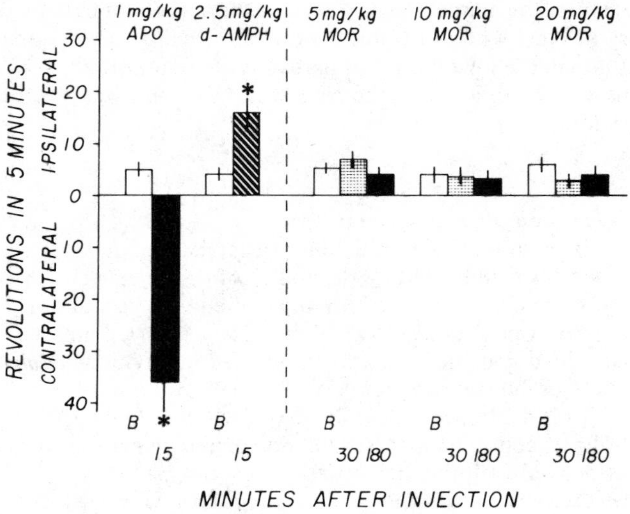

Figure 4.6 Effects of apomorphine (APO), amphetamine (*d*-AMPH) and morphine (MOR) on rotational behavior in rats lesioned unilaterally with 6-OHDA in the substantia nigra. $*P < 0.05$ for comparisons of post-drug performance with pre-drug baseline. B, baseline rotational levels.

Only rats that demonstrated a clear differential response to apomorphine and amphetamine (contralateral rotations to apomorphine and ipsilateral rotations to amphetamine) were selected for use in the subsequent study aimed at evaluating the acute effects of morphine on rotational behavior. Fourteen rats met this criterion. Approximately 3 weeks after the 6-OHDA lesions, morphine administration was initiated. All rats in this series received injections of 5, 10 and 20 mg/kg morphine i.p. in a randomized order, 5 days apart. Each animal was tested 30 min and 180 min after injection.

The results of this study appear in figure 4.6. Apomorphine induced rotations contralateral to the lesion with a mean of 7.2 per min while amphetamine produced rotations in the opposite direction with a mean of 3.1 per min. Morphine was found to be completely ineffective in inducing rotational behavior at any of the doses tested.

acute

The lack of effect of morphine was surprising since Iwamoto *et al.* (1976*b*) have recently reported that opiate agonists induce ipsilateral rotations in rats that have unilateral substantia nigra lesions. Fuxe and Ungerstedt (1970) have also reported morphine-induced asymmetry to the operated side in animals with unilateral lesions in the substantia nigra. Von Voigtlander and Moore (1973), on the other hand, failed to observe any effect of morphine on rotational behavior following 6-OHDA lesions to the striatum in mice.

Since a variety of brain regions outside the extrapyramidal system appear to mediate the motor depressant effects of opiates, it is possible that the actions of systemically administered morphine in these areas may inhibit the expression of rotational behavior in certain situations. Since animals become tolerant rapidly to the motor depressant effects of morphine (Babbini and Davis, 1972) but not the excitatory actions, it is possible that the effects of morphine on rotational behavior could be unmasked after chronic administration.

The 14 rats used in the previous study were divided into two groups of 7 animals each. One group was injected with saline every day for 10 days and the other group was injected with 10 mg/kg morphine sulfate. All animals were tested for rotational behavior 60 min before the injection and 30 min after the injection. On day 11 all rats were injected with saline.

Chronic administration of morphine was found to produce rotations ipsilateral to the lesion. Furthermore, the rotational behavior clearly increased in intensity over time. An abrupt change to saline on day 11 in animals that had been treated with morphine eliminated this behavior (figure 4.7).

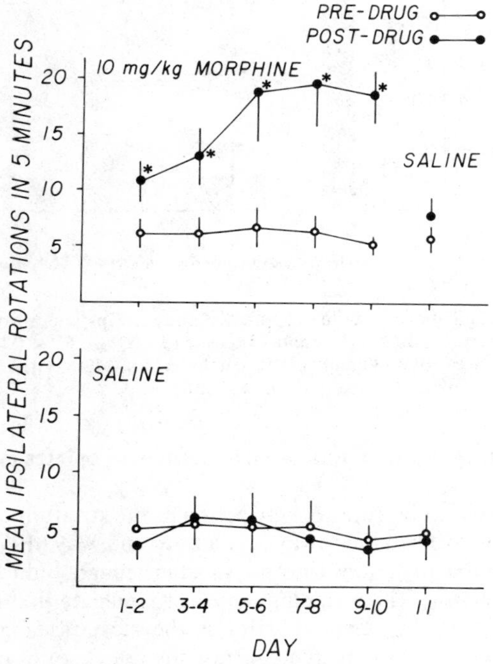

Figure 4.7 Effects of chronic intraperitoneal morphine (10 mg/kg) on rotational behavior following 6-OHDA lesions to substantia nigra. Animals in both groups were injected with saline on day 11. $*P < 0.05$ for comparisons of post-drug performance with pre-drug performance. $n = 7$ in each group.

Although chronically administered morphine was found to induce ipsilateral rotations in animals lesioned unilaterally in the substantia nigra, is this effect pharmacologically specific and is it determined through activation of the dopamine system? To answer these questions, rats from the previous study that had received chronic morphine received injections of morphine together with naloxone and haloperidol. All animals were injected with morphine 20 min before testing and haloperidol (0.5 mg/kg i.p.) 15 min before testing or naloxone (5 mg/kg i.p.)

or saline 25 min before testing. All three drug combinations were administered to all animals in a randomized order 5 days apart.

Both haloperidol and naloxone effectively inhibited the ipsilateral rotations induced by morphine (figure 4.8).

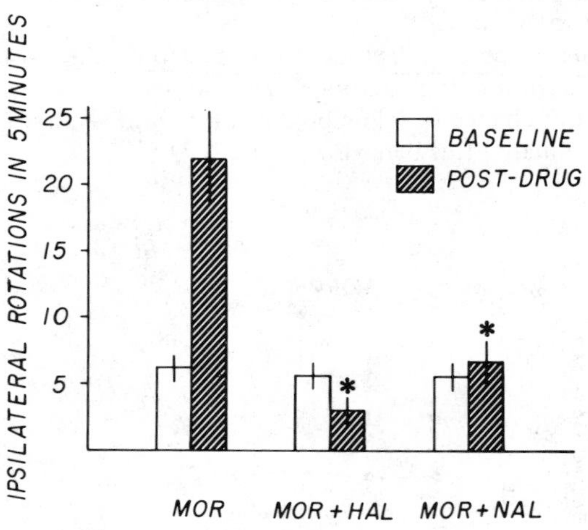

Figure 4.8 The antagonism of morphine (10 mg/kg)-induced ipsilateral rotations in 6–OHDA lesioned rats by haloperidol (0.5 mg/kg) and naloxone (5 mg/kg). $*P < 0.05$ for comparisons of post-drug performances following morphine + haloperidol (MOR + HAL) and morphine + naloxone (MOR + NAL) against morphine alone (MOR).

Rotational behavior induced by unilateral injections of opiates into the substantia nigra

Do opiates induce ipsilateral rotations by acting in the striatum or by activating the dopaminergic nigrostriatal pathways? Iwamoto and Way (1977) have recently reported that morphine injections into the substantia nigra induce rotations contralateral to the injection. These findings appear to indicate that morphine activates the nigrostriatal pathways by a direct action in the substantia nigra. The purpose. of the next study was to compare and contrast the effects of morphine, β-endorphin and [D-Ala^2, Met^5]-enkephalinamide on rotational behavior after direct injections into the substantia nigra.

Twenty-five male Sprague-Dawley rats were implanted with bilateral cannula guides situated 2 mm above the substantia nigra (AP 2.2, LAT 1.8, DV −2.2). After recovery the animals were divided into three groups. One was injected unilaterally in the substantia nigra with 1, 5, and 10 μg of morphine sulfate or 1 μl of sterile water. The other two groups were injected with identical quantities of β-endorphin or [D-Ala^2, Met^5]-enkephalinamide. All drugs were dissolved in sterile water and injected in a volume of 1 μl. All animals in a given group were injected with all doses of the drug and the vehicle in a randomized order 5 days apart. The animals were tested for rotational behavior for 3 min at 30, 60, 120 and 180 min after injection.

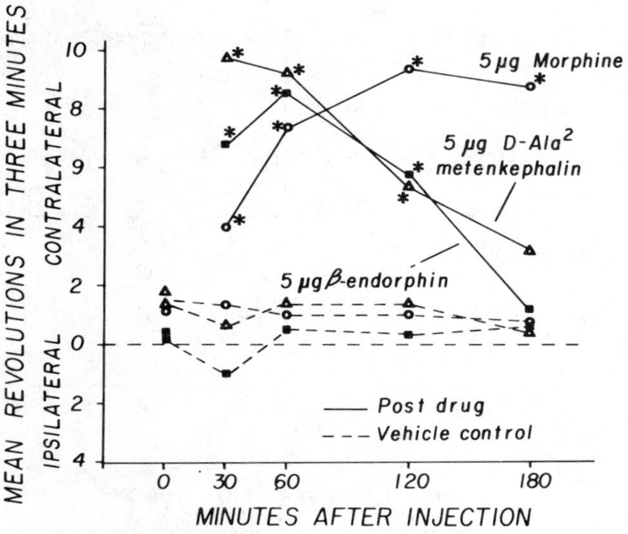

Figure 4.9 Effects of 5 μg of morphine, β-endorphin, and [D-Ala^2, Met^5]-enkephalinamide on rotational behavior following unilateral intranigral injections. $^*P < 0.05$ for comparisons of drug-induced behavior with the vehicle baseline.

Figure 4.9 illustrates the effects of unilateral intranigral injections of 5 μg of β-endorphin, morphine and [D-Ala^2, Met^5]-enkephalinamide on rotational behavior. All three compounds were found to induce rotations contralateral to the injection. The effects of β-endorphin and [D-Ala^2, Met^5]-enkephalinamide decreased over the observation period while the effects of morphine were actually enhanced. In subsequent experiments we found that pretreatment with 5 mg/kg of naloxone antagonizes the effects of all three opiate agonists following injections into the substantia nigra.

Although unilateral injections of opiates into the substantia nigra were found to produce rotational behavior, it is possible that other structures of the extrapyramidal system are also involved in mediating the effects of morphine in the 6-OHDA lesioned animals above. To test this possibility two groups of rats ($n = 5$ each) were prepared with chronic indwelling cannula guides in either the caudate nucleus (AP 7.5, LAT 2.5, DV 1.0) or the globus pallidus (AP 6.0, LAT 2.5, DV 0). After recovery, each rat was injected unilaterally with 5 μg of morphine through 30-gauge injectors which protruded 2 mm below the guide cannulae. The animals were tested for rotational behavior 30 and 60 min after injection as before.

To ascertain whether chronic pretreatment with morphine enhances the response, the same animals were tested again with 5 μg of morphine following treatment with 10 mg/kg of morphine i.p. for 10 days.

Figure 4.10 illustrates the effects of unilateral injections of morphine into the caudate nucleus and the globus pallidus in drug-naive rats and in the same animals following chronic systemic treatment with morphine. Morphine failed to elicit rotational behavior after unilateral injections into these two structures under either condition.

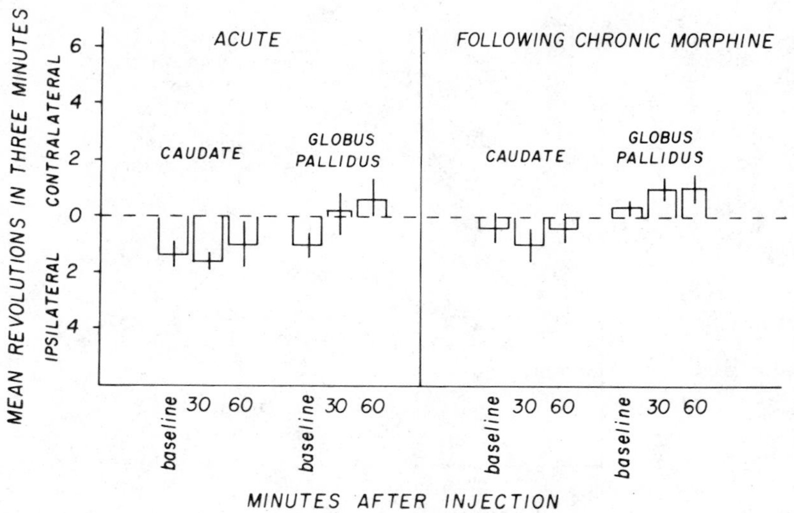

Figure 4.10 Effects of unilateral injections of 5 μg of morphine into the caudate nucleus and globus pallidus of drug-naive rats and the same rats following chronic treatment with systemic morphine. No significant rotational response was seen in either case following unilateral morphine.

DISCUSSION

These studies indicate that the complex effects of opiates on motor behaviors have specific neural substrates or foci. Most significantly, the differential effects of opiates on locomotor activity appear to be mediated through entirely different neural circuits and structures. Thus, the excitatory effects of opiates appear to be mediated through the mesolimbic component of the dopamine system, as well as the substantia nigra, while the depressant effects appear to be determined by the actions of opiates in the periaqueductal grey matter, hippocampus, ventral thalamus, and to some extent, the lateral hypothalamus.

Both opiates (Babbini and Davis, 1972; Oka and Hosoya, 1976) and various catecholaminergic agonists (Maj *et al.*, 1972; Thornburg and Moore, 1973; Greyer *et al.*, 1972) have been reported to increase spontaneous locomotor activity in rodents after systemic injections. The nucleus accumbens, a terminal region for the mesolimbic dopamine pathways originating from area A10, has been implicated as a principal focus for the excitatory actions of amphetamine (Kelly *et al.*, 1975) and apomorphine (Jackson *et al.*, 1975; Grabowska and Andén, 1976). These compounds affect activity by either increasing the availability of dopamine at the synapse, or by a direct action on dopamine receptors, as dopamine receptor blockers antagonize their excitatory actions. Our findings (Pert and Sivit, 1977) indicate that, at least in the rat forebrain, opiates produce excitatory effects that are dissociated from direct dopaminergic actions. It is possible that parallel neurohumoral systems exist in the forebrain to regulate motility–one encoded by dopamine and the other by enkephalin.

On the other hand, the excitatory effects of opiates on horizontal motor activity which were seen following bilateral injections into the substantia nigra do appear to be determined by a direct or indirect activation of the ascending dopaminergic nigrostriatal neurons. This assumption is supported by the finding that haloperidol was able to block morphine-induced rotational behavior in rats that had been lesioned unilaterally in the substantia nigra with 6-OHDA. The effects of opiates at the level of the substantia nigra, however, may contribute differently to their overall excitatory actions since hyperactivity induced by injections into this structure was also accompanied by stereotypy.

A number of investigators (Kuschinsky, 1976; Lal, 1976) have postulated that the cataleptic and psychomotor effects of opiates are determined by their actions in the striatum. This assumption is not supported by the present finding. Bilateral injections of morphine into the caudate nucleus did not alter motor activity or induce catatonia and unilateral injections did not produce rotational behavior.

The most critical focus for the motor depressant and catatonic effects of opiates appears to be the periaqueductal grey matter which has also been identified as one of the principal regions mediating the analgesic effects of opiates (Pert and Yaksh, 1974; Jacquet and Lajtha, 1974; Herz *et al.*, 1970). It is not entirely clear, however, how the actions of opiates in this brain region are ultimately translated into depression of locomotor activity and catatonia. The effects of opiates here do appear to be independent of the catecholamines since injections of chlorpromazine into the PAG do not elicit catalepsy. Interestingly however, injections of chlorpromazine into the caudate nucleus do produce catalepsy (Pert, unpublished observation). Thus, it appears that the catatonic actions of morphine are not determined by a blockade of dopaminergic transmission. In fact, it is possible to separate neuroanatomically the cataleptic effects of dopamine-blocking agents from the catatonic effects of opiates.

Injections of morphine into the ventral thalamus and hippocampus also depressed motor acitivty. It is interesting that the ventral thalamic nuclei receive inputs from the globus pallidus, cerebellum and motor cortex, and project in turn to the motor cortex. Although neither opiate receptors nor enkephalinergic terminals are strikingly abundant in this region, it is still possible that enkephalinergic neurons, strategically located, serve to modulate motor effects relayed through these nuclei. Although the hippocampus is not classically a motor region, lesions in this area have been reported to modify motor activity (Douglas, 1967; Kimble, 1968). It is not clear at this point, however, what aspects of motor behavior are regulated by enkephalin in the hippocampus.

One of the most interesting findings to emerge from this series of studies is the depressant effect of naloxone on motor activity. This appears to reinforce the notion that endogenous enkephalinergic systems do, in fact, have a role in modulating motor behavior. The systems that are tonically active, however, appear to be the ones that mediate the excitatory effects of opiates since only depression of motor behavior was observed following the administration of this opiate antagonist.

Our findings regarding the actions of opiates on the nigrostriatal system confirm and extend the recent findings of Iwamoto *et al.* (1976*a, b*) and Iwamoto and Way (1977). Using the rotational model, opiates were clearly found to increase the activity of the ascending dopaminergic nigrostriatal system. Interestingly, no tolerance appeared to develop to this effect; chronic administration of morphine produced a progressively greater response. We have suggested that the increasing effects of morphine in the 6-OHDA lesioned rats was due to the development of tolerance to the motor-depressant actions which presumably mask the appearance of rotational behavior. It is, of course, possible that the progressively increasing response to morphine in this model represents adaptive changes directly in the substantia nigra in response to chronic receptor occupation. This remains to be tested.

Although opiates appear to increase ascending nigrostriatal dopaminergic transmission by increasing the activity of dopaminergic cells in the zona compacta of the substantia nigra (Iwatsubo and Clouet, 1976; Nowycky, 1976), it is still not clear whether this is a direct action on the zona compacta neurons or whether it is an indirect effect through some other system in the substantia nigra. The effects on rotational behavior seen following systemic administration of morphine to lesioned animals or direct injections into the substantia nigra could be exerted by an inhibitory action of morphine on neurons which are inhibitory to zona compacta cells. In this respect, it is interesting to note that we have also seen contralateral rotational behavior following unilateral injections of a local anesthetic into the substantia nigra.

Considering the close association of enkephalinergic neurons and opiate receptors with the motor system and the profound effects of opiate alkaloids and opioid peptides on motor behavior, it is clear that enkephalinergic neuronal systems play an important part in modulating motor output. It remains to be determined, however, what are the precise functional roles of the enkephalinergic systems in this behavior and in what circumstances the enkephalinergic systems are called into play.

Since the enkephalinergic systems do appear to have a critical role in modulating motor activity, it is quite possible that dysfunctions in these systems may underlie or contribute to the etiology of some psychomotor disturbances in man.

REFERENCES

Andén, N. E., Dahlstrom, A., Fuxe, K. and Larson, K. (1966). *Acta pharmac. Tox.*, **24**, 263–74

Atweh, S. F. and Kuhar, M. J. (1977). *Brain Res.*, **129**, 1–12

Babbini, M. and Davis, W. M. (1972). *Br. J. Pharmac.*, **46** 213–24

Clouet, D. H. and Ratner, M. (1970). *Science*, **168**, 854–6

Costa, E., Carenzi, A., Guidotti, A. and Revvecta, A. (1973). In *Frontiers in Catecholamine Research*, (eds E. Usdin and S. H. Snyder) Pergamon Press, New York

Costall, B., Marsden, C. D., Naylor, R. J. and Pycock, C. J. (1976). *Brain Res.*, **118**, 87–113

Costall, B., Marsden, C. D., Naylor, R. J. and Pycock, C. J. (1977). *Brain Res.*, **123**, 89–111

Costall, B. and Naylor, R. J. (1973). *Arzneim.-Forsch. (Drug Res.)*, **23**, 674–83

Creese, I., Burt, D. R. and Snyder, S. H. (1977). *Science*, **197**, 596–9

Douglas, R. J. (1974). In *The hippocampus*, (eds R. L. Isaacson and K. H. Pibram) Plenum Press, New York

Elde, R., Hökfelt, T., Johansson, O. and Terenius, L. (1976). *Neuroscience*, **1**, 349–511

Fuxe, K. and Ungerstedt, U. (1970). In *Amphetamine and Related Compounds*, (eds E. Costa and S. Garattini) Raven Press, New York

Geyer, M. A., Segal, D. S. and Mandell, A. J. (1972). *Physiol. Behav.*, **8**, 653–8

Grabowska, M. and Andén, N. E. (1976). *J. Neur. Trans.*, **38**, 1–8

Gunne, L. M., Jonsson, J. and Fuxe, K. (1969). *Eur. J. Pharmac.*, **5**, 338–42

Herz, A., Albus, K., Metys, T., Schubert, P. and Teschemacher, H. J. (1970). *Neuropharmacology,* **9**, 539–51
Hiller, J. M., Pearson, J. and Simon, E. J. (1973). *Res. Commun. Chem. Pathol. Pharmac.*, **6**, 1052–61
Hong, J. S., Yang, H. Y. T., Fratta, W. and Costa, E. (1977). *Brain Res.*, **134**, 383–6
Iwamoto, E. T., Loh, H. H. and Way, E. L. (1976*a*) *Eur. J. Pharmac.*, **37**, 339–56
Iwamoto, E. T., Loh, H. H. and Way, E. L. (1976*b*). *J. Pharmac. exp. Ther.*, **197**, 503–16.
Iwamoto, E. T. and Way, E. L. (1977). *J. Pharmac. exp. Ther.*, **203**, 347–59
Iwatsubo, K. and Clouet, D. H. (1976). *Pharmacologist,* **18**, 178
Jackson, D. M., Andén, N. E., and Dahlstrom, A. (1975). *Psychopharmacologia*, **45**, 139–49
Jacquet, Y. F., Klee, W. A., Rice, K. C., Iijima, I. and Minamikawa, J. (1977). *Science,* 198, 842–5
Jacquet, Y. and Lajtha, A. (1974). *Science*, **185**, 1055–7
Jacquet, Y. F. and Marks, N. (1976). *Science,* **194**, 632–5
Kelly, P. H., Seviour, P. W. and Iversen, S. D. (1975). *Brain Res.*, **94**, 507–22
Kimble, D. P. (1968). *Psychol. Bull.*, **70**, 285–95
König, J. F. R. and Klippel, R. A. (1963). *The Rat Brain.* Krieger, New York
Kuhar, M. J., Pert, C. B. and Snyder, S. H. (1974). *Nature,* **245**, 447–50
Kuschinsky, K. (1976). *Arzneim.-Forsch. (Drug Res.)* **26**, 563–7
Kuschinsky, K. and Hornykiewicz, O. (1972). *Eur. J. Pharmac.*, **19**, 119–22
Kuschinsky, K. and Hornykiewicz, O. (1974). *Eur. J. Pharmac.*, **26**, 41–50
Lal, H. (1976). *Life Sci.*, **17**, 483–96
Loh, H. H., Hitzemann, R. J. and Way, E. L. (1973). *Life Sci.*, **12**, 33–41
Maj, J., Grabowska, M. and Gajda, L. (1972). *Eur. J. Pharmac.*, **17**, 208–14
Nakamura, K., Kuntzman, R., Maggio, A. and Conney, A. H. (1973). *Neuropharmacology*, **12**, 1153–60
Nowycky, M. C. (1976). Ph. D. thesis, Yale University
Oka, T. and Hosoya, E. (1976). *Psychopharmacologia*, **47**, 243–8
Pert, A. and Sivit, C. (1977). *Nature,* **265**, 645–7
Pert, A. and Yaksh, T. (1974). *Brain Res.*, **80**, 135–40
Pert, C. B., Pert, A., Change, J. -K. and Fong, B. T. W. (1976). *Science,* **194**, 330–32
Segal, D. S., Browne, R. G., Bloom, F., Ling, N. and Guillemin, R. (1977). *Science,* **198**, 411–14
Sharpe, L. G., Garnett, J. E. and Cicero, T. J. (1974). *J. behav. Biol.*, **11**, 303–13
Simantov, R., Kuhar, M. J., Uhl, G. R. and Snyder, S. H. (1977). *Proc. natn. Acad. Sci. U.S.A.*, **74**, 2167–71
Thornburg, J. E. and Moore, K. E. (1973). *Neuropharmacology,* **12**, 853–66
Ungerstedt, U. (1971). *Acta physiol. scand.*, **82** (suppl. 367), 69–93
Von Voigtlander, P. F. and Moore, K. E. (1973). *Neuropharmacology,* **12**, 451–62
Wand, P., Kuschinsky, K. and Sontag, K. H. (1973). *Eur. J. Pharmac.*, **24**, 189–93

MFB (LH) has LE axons, but not cell bodies.

5
Mapping of leu-enkephalin-containing axons and cell bodies of the rat forebrain

David M. Jacobowitz, Michael A. Silver and William G. Soden
(Laboratory of Clinical Science, National Institute of Mental Health, Bethesda, Maryland)

The suggestion that the enkephalin peptides represent natural ligands for the opiate receptors (Hughes *et al.*, 1975) has resulted in several recent reports on the distribution of the enkephalin pentapeptides by immunohistochemical methods (Elde *et al.*, 1976, Hökfelt *et al.*, 1977, Simantov *et al.*, 1977; Watson *et al.*, 1977; Sar and Stumpf, 1977; Uhl *et al.*, in this volume). These studies have focused attention on small varicose endings reminiscent of catecholamine-containing terminals. Furthermore, cell bodies were observed to contain the immunoreactive peptides following treatment with colchicine (Hökfelt *et al.*, 1977).

There is currently only one report of a possible long axonal enkephalin pathway which appears to emanate from the nucleus amygdaloideus centralis and courses through the stria terminalis to terminate in the red nucleus of the stria terminalis (Uhl *et al.* in this volume). In this laboratory preliminary immunofluorescent observations of the localization of leu-enkephalin-containing nerves revealed that, in addition to abundant fine varicose fibers, there is a population of larger axonal-like processes present throughout the forebrain. The mapping of the distribution of these axonal-like processes, in addition to perikarya of the forebrain, comprises most of this communication.

MATERIALS AND METHODS

The antibody for leu-enkephalin was generously provided by Dr Richard Miller. The preparation and characterization of the antibody has been described (Miller *et al.*., 1978). Preliminary results on the distribution of axons and cell bodies as revealed with indirect fluorescence immunohistochemistry (Coons, 1958) is presented in this communication. Details for the specific procedure for leu-enkephalin immunofluorescence have been described by Elde *et al.* (1976). The method as presently used, with minor modifications, is as follows. Male Sprague-Dawley rats (200–400 g) were perfused through the ascending aorta with 60 ml of cold buffer followed by 350 ml of ice-cold 4 per cent paraformaldehyde in 0.1 M phosphate buffer (pH 7.3–7.4). A hemostat was used to clamp off the descending aorta. Preparation of the buffer has been described (Laties *et al.*, 1967). The brains were placed in a brain slicer (Jacobowitz, 1974) and 3-mm slices were fixed (4 °C) for 90 min and washed in 5 per cent sucrose in 0.1 M phosphate buffer (24 h at 4 °C). The tissue slices were frozen on a chuck and 20 μm sections were cut in a cryostat.

The slides were dipped briefly into phosphate-buffered saline (PBS) and incubated in a humidity box for 30 min at 37 °C with either leu-enkephalin antiserum (0.1 per cent Triton-X-100 in PBS) or preimmune serum diluted 1/100 which served as the control. The slides were washed 3 times, 5 min each, in 0.2 per cent Triton-X-100 in PBS (4 °C) and then incubated as above with fluorescein-labeled rabbit antiserum (Cappel, Downington, Pennsylvania) to goat IgG (0.04 mg/ml) diluted 1/60 with PBS containing 0.1 per cent Triton-X-100. The slides were washed as above with a fourth wash in PBS. The slides were mounted in glycerin–PBS (3:1). Sections were examined under a Leitz Orthoplan microscope equipped with a Ploem illuminator.

RESULTS

Mapping axonal pathways

The telencephalon and diencephalon were studied for fluorescence localization of enkephalin-like immunoreactivity. As described previously (Elde *et al.*, 1976;

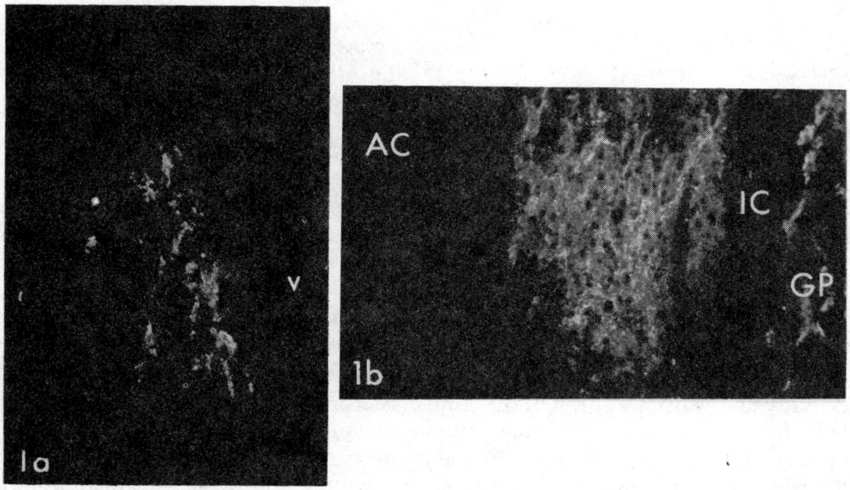

Figure 5.1 a, Lateral septal area, shows dense varicose plexus of enkephalin nerves; v, lateral ventricle (approximate level A7100) × 130. b, Nucleus interstitialis stria terminalis. Varicosities are seen between the anterior commissure (AC) and the internal capsule (IC); GP, globus pallidus (level of A6860) × 75.

Hökfelt *et al.*, 1977; Simantov *et al.*, 1977; Watson *et al.*, 1977), enkephalin was observed primarily in small varicose nerve-like processes (figure 5.1). However, there were axon-like processes that could be followed for a considerable distance, they were traced from the lateral hypothalamus to the level of the nucleus accumbens (figure 5.2). These large axonal processes were mapped. Pairs of

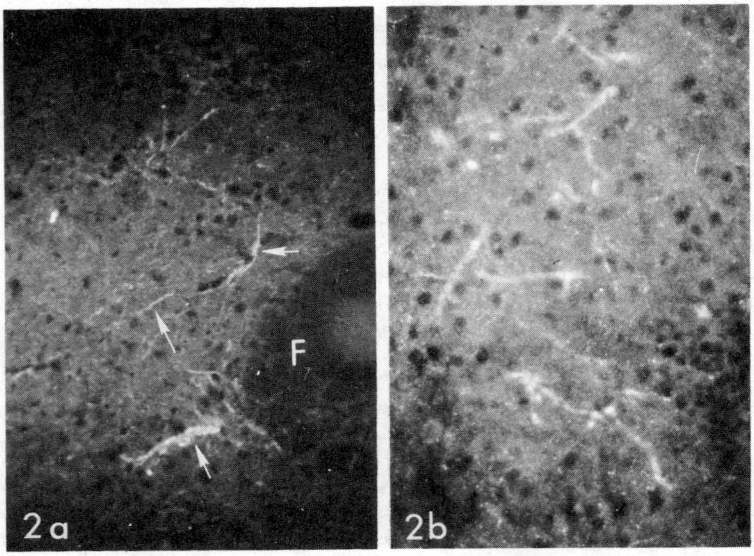

Figure 5.2 a, Lateral hypothalamus; large axonal processes (arrows) lateral to the fornix (F); (level of A4700) × 130. b, Enkephalin-containing processes in the tractus septohypothalamicus medial to the nucleus accumbens (level of A9400) × 210.

sections were used, one for immunofluorescence examination, the other was stained with 0.1 per cent Thionin. Drawings of the sections were made from projected stained slides. The precise localization of the axons were superimposed on these drawings. The results were finally plotted on drawings prepared from the atlases of the rat brain (König and Klippel, 1963; Jacobowitz and Palkovits, 1974).

Figures 5.3–5.6 are mappings of what we interpret to be axonal pathways of leu-enkephalin-containing nerves. The direction of these axons cannot be interpreted until lesion studies are performed. A major movement of axons is observed in the supraoptic commisure (CSDV, Maynert's commissure, figures 5.3b–d) which can be followed rostrally and medially through the median forebrain bundle and dorsally and ventrally through the fornix. A crossover tract seems to occur at the basal hypothalamus via the supraoptic commissure and ventral to the ventromedial nucleus (figures 5.3a–c). At the point of separation of the optic tract from the proximity of the internal capsule, large axon-like processes are apparent in the ansa lenticularis (figures 5.3a, 5.4a–d). Some of these axons seem to course medially through the ventral aspect of the internal capsule and laterally just ventral to the globus pallidus and caudate/putamen. There is a long axonal bundle in the stria terminalis just medial to the internal capsule (figure 5.5d).

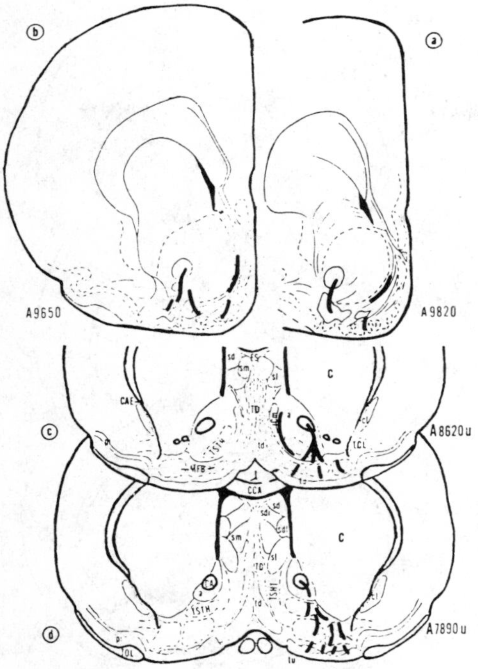

Figure 5.3 Schematic of preterminal enkephalin-containing axons. Frontal sections are numbered in the lower right corner with coordinates anterior to the frontal zero plane of the König and Klippel (1963) stereotaxic atlas and catecholaminergic atlas of Jacobowitz and Palkovits (1974). The axonal processes are shown as heavy lines. For abbreviations refer to the above atlases.

At the level of the anterior commissure (figure 5.5c) axons are observed in the stria terminalis and the nucleus interstitialis stria terminalis. There appears to be a large formation of axons just ventral to the rostral globus pallidus within the median forebrain bundle-preoptic lateralis region. Whether this projection emanates from the globus pallidus can only be conjecture. This formation extends rostrally and ventrally to the anterior commissure (pars posterior, figures 5.5a–b) within the dorsal aspect of the median forebrain bundle. A projection appears to course through the tractus diagonalis and the tractus septohypothalamicus (figures 5.5a and 5.6). Fibers enter the anterior commissure to cross the midline (figure 5.5c); at a more rostral level it would seem that axons emanate from the anterior commisssure to proceed ventrally towards the olfactory tubercle (figures 5.6a–d and figure 5.7).

Mapping cell bodies

Enkephalin-containing cell bodies are normally very sparse throughout the brain. Only after colchicine treatment (Hökfelt *et al.*, 1977) are numerous immunofluorescent cell bodies observed. In this study, a similar neurotoxic reagent,

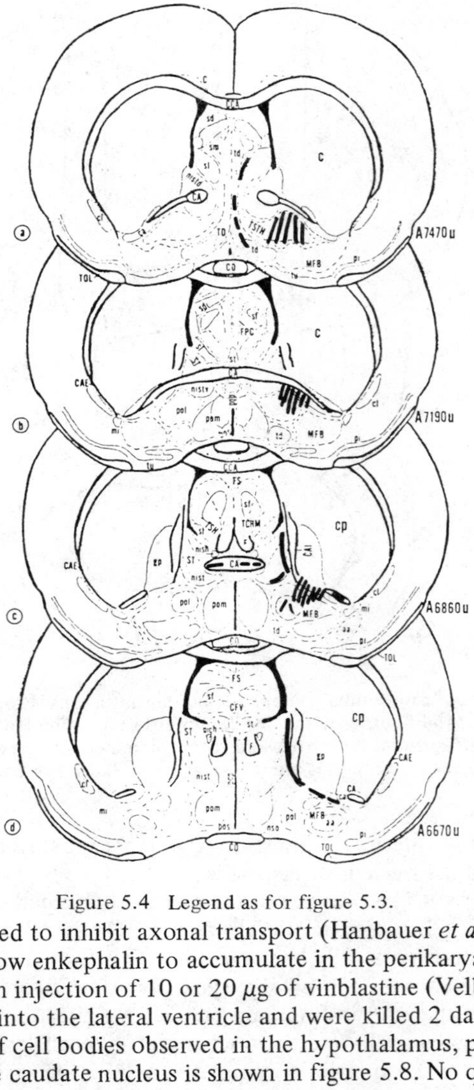

Figure 5.4 Legend as for figure 5.3.

vinblastine, was used to inhibit axonal transport (Hanbauer *et al.*, 1974; Palkovits *et al.*, 1974) to allow enkephalin to accumulate in the perikarya.

Rats received an injection of 10 or 20 μg of vinblastine (Velban, Lilly) (1 μg/μl in saline) into the lateral ventricle and were killed 2 days after the injection. A mapping of cell bodies observed in the hypothalamus, preoptic area, septal area and the caudate nucleus is shown in figure 5.8. No quantitative or semiquantitative significance is intended in these maps. Numerous somata are observed in the hypothalamus (dorsomedialis, paraventricularis, periventricularis, ventromedialis and arcuate nuclei) (figures 5.8e–i), preoptic area (figures 5.8c–d), red nucleus of the stria terminalis (figures 5.8b–d and 5.9), septal area (dorsal, medial, intermediate nuclei and tractus septohypothalamicus) (figures 5.8a–c), nucleus accumbens (figure 5.8a) and the medial caudate nucleus (figures 5.8a–d). Since the lateral extent of the penetration of vinblastine is unknown, this mapping is preliminary. Of particular interest was the presence of a large cluster of cell bodies in the nucleus ventromedialis, pars lateralis (figures 5.8i).

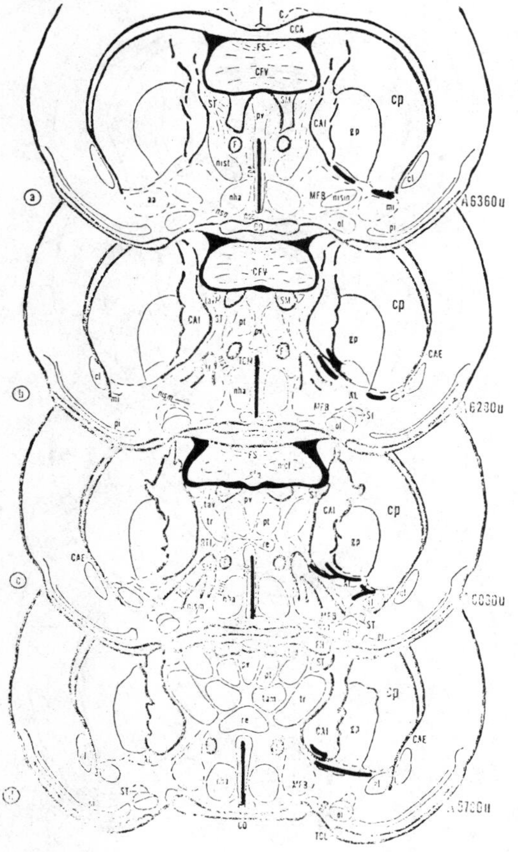

Figure 5.5 Legend as for figure 5.3.

Other interesting features were brought to light by vinblastine treatment. Normally, fine discrete varicose processes are seen in the external (palisade) layer of the median eminence (figure 5.10a). After vinblastine treatment, an additional fiber system was apparent throughout the internal layer of the median eminence (figure 5.10b). These fibers contain enlarged processes with distorted and swollen varicosities suggestive of early stages of degeneration.

The caudate nucleus usually contains small to moderate numbers of varicose fibers. After vinblastine an abundant number of axonal-like processes were seen in the dorsomedial region of the caudate nucleus within the internal capsule myelinated bundles (figures 5.8a, b, d).

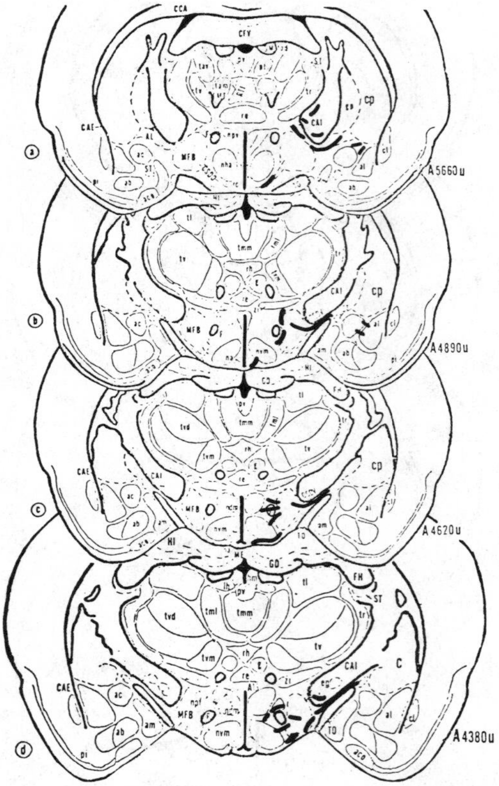

Figure 5.6 Legend as for figure 5.3.

DISCUSSION

The present mapping of possible long axonal enkephalinergic pathways is of significance for further work that will use this knowledge for the experimental manipulations required for stimulation or ablation studies for example. There is a major movement of axons within the ansa lenticularis, an area which contains noradrenergic axons (Jacobowitz, 1973; 1975). It would be of interest to ascertain whether enkephalin is also contained within certain aminergic nerves.

More rostrally, a large area of axons is seen just ventral to the globus pallidus which is the region within the brain richest in enkephalin (Elde *et al.*, 1976; Hong *et al.*, 1977). This proximity to the globus pallidus suggests that the latter

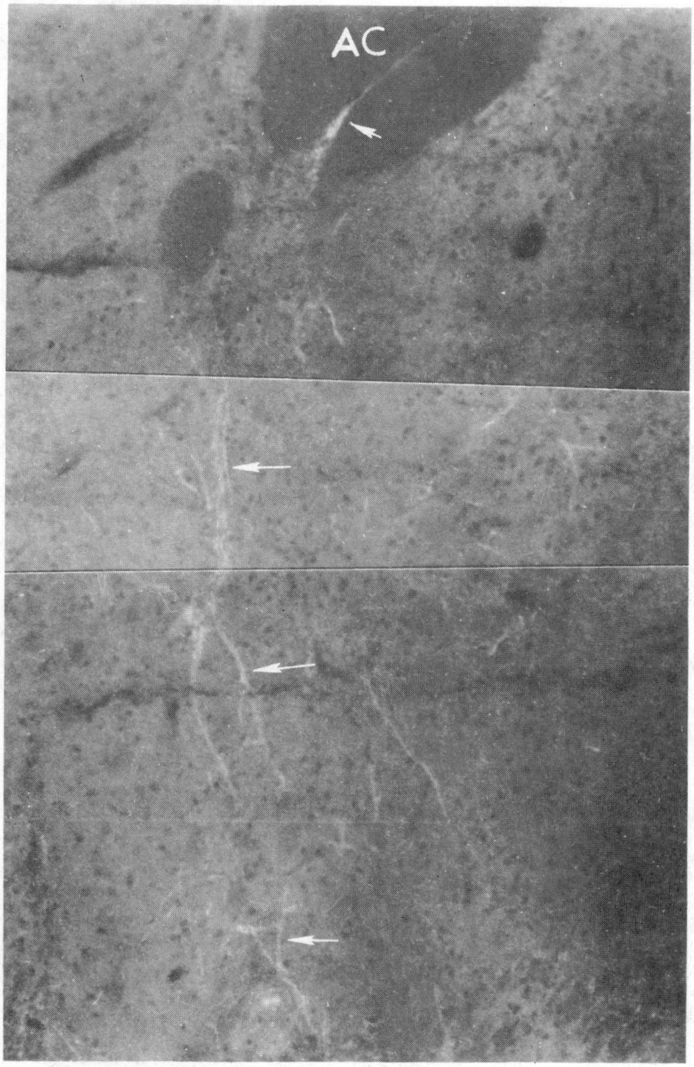

Figure 5.7 Montage of enkephalinergic axons (arrows) which appear to emanate from the anterior commissure (AC) and course ventrally through the nucleus accumbens towards the olfactory tubercle; (level of A8600) × 130

area may be the source of this large projection. Because of the density of fluorescent processes within the globus pallidus, cell bodies were difficult to detect. Such a population of perikarya could account for this rostral projection which appears

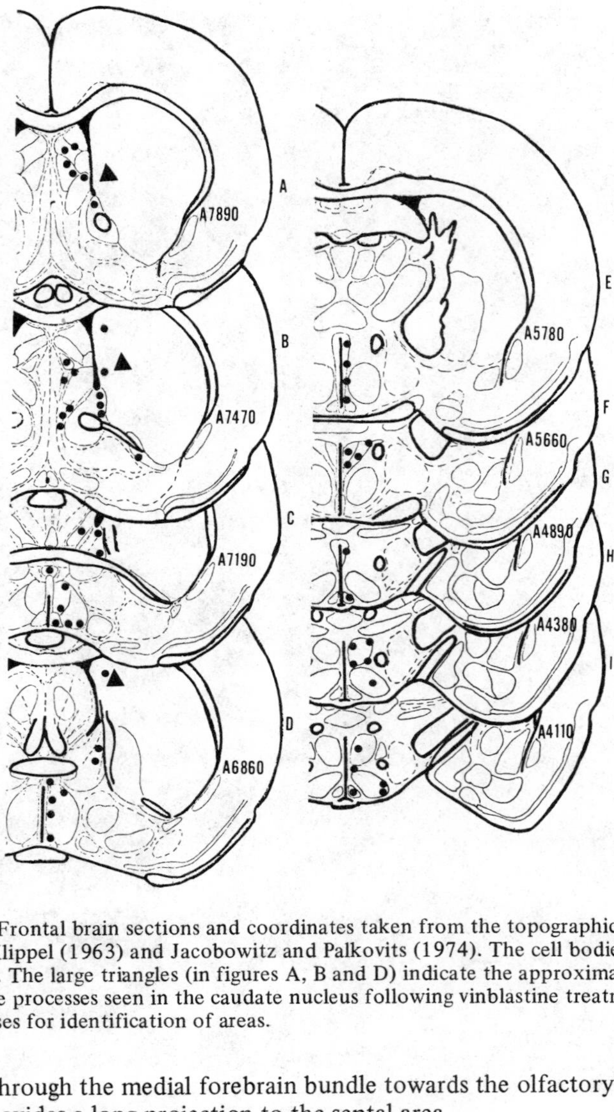

Figure 5.8 Frontal brain sections and coordinates taken from the topographic atlases of König and Klippel (1963) and Jacobowitz and Palkovits (1974). The cell bodies are plotted as filled circles. The large triangles (in figures A, B and D) indicate the approximate position of the axon-like processes seen in the caudate nucleus following vinblastine treatment. See original atlases for identification of areas.

to course through the medial forebrain bundle towards the olfactory tubercle and possibly provides a long projection to the septal area.

The widespread population of enkephalinergic cell bodies in the hypothalamus, preoptic and septal areas is consistent with the interpretation that enkephalin is generally contained within interneurons.

A large cluster of cell bodies was found in the lateral part of the ventromedial nuclues which is the 'satiety center'. Stimulation of this area results in reduced eating. In this regard it is interesting that morphine addicts show a marked reduction in appetite (Goodman and Gilman, 1970).

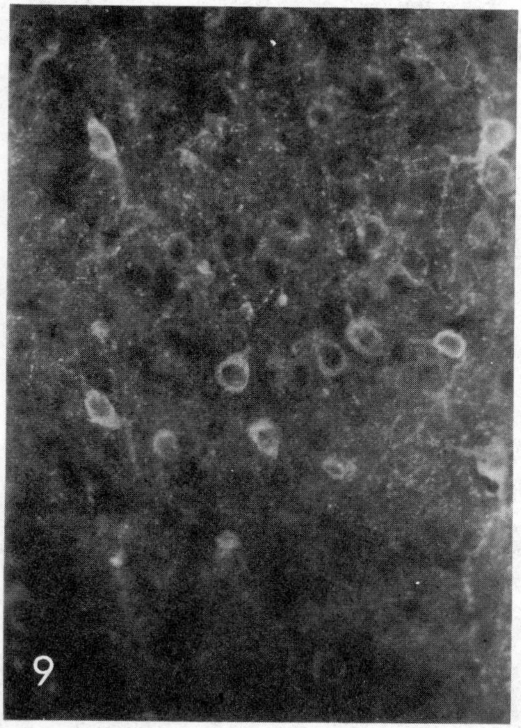

Figure 5.9 Enkephalin-containing perikarya following vinblastine treatment (20 μg, 2 days); nucleus interstitialis stria terminalis, dorsal (level of A7000) × 345.

The median eminence is a major center for neuroendocrine activity in the brain. The significance of the dense population of enkephalin varicosities in the external layer of the median eminence is currently unknown. This localization seems to be identical to that of the tuberoinfundibular dopaminergic neurons. After vinblastine treatment another system of enkephalin processes was observed in the zona interna of the median eminence. This region also contains noradrenergic nerves (Fuxe and Hökfelt, 1969), and peptidergic neurons such as vasopressin, oxytocin and neurophysin (see review by Zimmerman, 1976). A possible enkephalin-aminergic, or other hormonal interaction at the median eminence level, needs to be elucidated.

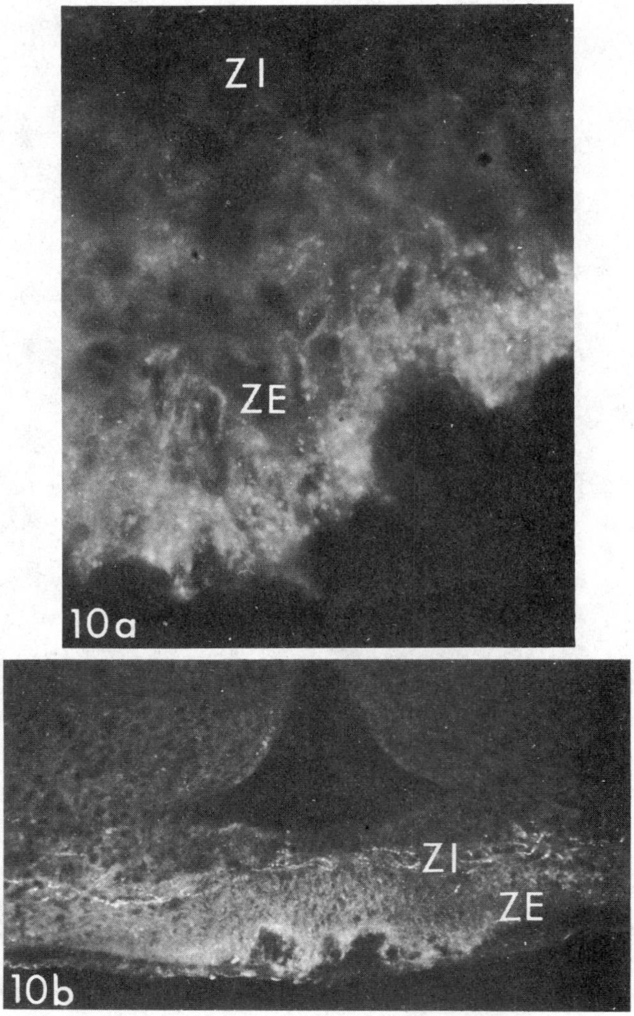

Figure 5.10 Median Eminence. a, Fine varicose terminals are noted in the zona externa (ZE) × 640; b, Vinblastine-treated rat (10 μg, 1 day). Note enlarged axonal processes in the zona interna (ZI) × 100.

ACKNOWLEDGEMENT

The authors are indebted to Dr Richard Miller for generously contributing the enkephalin antibody used in this study.

REFERENCES

Coons, A. H. (1958). In *General Cytochemical Methods*, (ed. J. F. Danielli) Academic Press, New York

Elde, R., Hökfelt, T., Johansson, O. and Terenius, L. (1976). *Neuroscience*, **1**, 349–51

Fuxe, K. and Hökfelt, T. (1969). In *Frontiers in Neuroendocrinology*, (eds. W. F. Ganong and L. Martini) Oxford University Press, Oxford

Goodman, L. S., and Gilman, A. (eds), (1970. *The Pharmacological Basis of Therapeutics*, The Macmillan Company, New York

Hanbauer, I., Kopin, I. J. and Jacobowitz, D. M. (1974). In *Proceedings of the Wenner-Gren Symposium on Dynamics of Degeneration and Growth in Neurons*, (eds K. Fuxe, L. Olson and Y. Zutterman), Pergamon Press, Oxford

Hökfelt, T., Ljungdahl, Å., Terenius, L., Elde, R. and Nilson, G. (1977). *Proc. natn. Acad. Sci. U.S.A.*, **74**, 3081–5

Hong, J. S., Yang, H.-Y. T. and Costa, E. (1977). *Neuropharmacology*, **16**, 451–3

Hughes, J., Smith, T. W., Kosterlitz, H. W., Fothergill, L. A., Morgan, B. A. and Morris, H. R. (1975). *Nature*, **258**, 577–9

Jacobowitz, D. (1973). In *Frontiers in Catecholamine Research*, (eds E. Usdin and S. Snyder), Pergamon Press, Oxford

Jacobowitz, D. M. (1975). In *Anatomical Neuroendocrinology*, (eds W. E. Stumpf and L. D. Grant), Karger, Basel

Jacobowitz, D. M. (1974). *Brain Res.*, **80**, 111–5

Jacobowitz, D. M. and Palkovits, M. (1974). *J. comp. Neurol.*, **157**, 13–28

König, J. F. R. and Klippel, R. A. (1963). *The Rat Brain: A Stereotaxic Atlas of the Forebrain and Lower Parts of the Brain Stem*, Williams and Wilkins, Baltimore

Laties, A. M., Lund, R. and Jacobowitz, D. (1967). *J. Histochem. Cytochem.*, **15**, 535–41

Miller, R. J., Chang, K. J., Cooper, B. and Cuatrecasas, P. (1978). *J. biol. Chem.*, **253,** 531–8

Palkovits, M., Richardson, J. S. and Jacobowitz, D. M. (1974). *Brain Res.*, **81**, 183–8

Sar, M., Stumpf, W. E., Miller, R. J., Chang, K. J. and Cuatrecasas, P. (1977). *Society for Neuroscience, (Abstracts)*, **III**, 1977).

Simantov, R. Kuhar, M. J., Uhl, G. R., Snyder, S. H. (1977). *Proc. natn. Acad. Sci. U.S.A.*, **74**, 2167–71

Watson, S. J., Akil, H., Sullivan, S. and Barchas, J. D. (1977). *Life Sci.*, **22**, 733–8

Zimmerman, E. A. (1976). In *Frontiers in Neuroendocrinology* (eds L. Martini and W. F. Ganong), Raven Press, New York

See also BR 166 75-94, 1979.

6
Histochemical localization of the enkephalins

George Uhl, Michael J. Kuhar, Robert R. Goodman and Solomon H. Snyder
Departments of Pharmacology and Experimental Therapeutics and
Psychiatry and the Behavioral Sciences
The Johns Hopkins University School of Medicine, Baltimore, Maryland

The opiate-like pentapeptides methionine-enkephalin and leucine-enkephalin (Hughes, 1975; Hughes *et al.*, 1975; Simantov and Snyder, 1976) are found in the mammalian brain. In biochemical studies, their regional localization resembles that of opiate receptor binding (Hughes, 1975; Simantov *et al.*, 1976*a*; Pasternak *et al.*, 1975) and in subcellular fractionation studies, they are localized to the synaptosomal fractions that contain nerve terminals (Simantov *et al.*, 1976*b*). Electrophysiologic studies indicate that the enkephalins can have potent effects on neuronal firing rates (Zieglgänsberger *et al.*, 1976; Duggan *et al.*, 1976; Frederickson and Norris, 1976; Bradley *et al.*, 1976; Young *et al.*, 1977; Nicoll *et al.*, 1977). Taken together, these findings suggest that the enkephalins may be neurotransmitters or neuromodulators in the mammalian brain.

Because antisera highly specific to the enkephalins can be obtained, enkephalin-containing cells can be localized by immunohistochemical techniques. Initial studies reported the presence of enkephalin-containing fibers and terminals in anatomical areas shown to have opiate receptors by autoradiographic techniques (Elde *et al.*, 1976; Simantov *et al.*, 1977; Watson *et al.*, 1977). Subsequent studies, utilizing the intraventricular injection of colchicine, revealed the location of several groups of enkephalin-containing cell bodies throughout the brain (Hökfelt *et al.*, 1977*a*; Hökfelt *et al.*, 1977*b*; Uhl *et al.*, 1978*a,b*). This report contains information on the localization of enkephalin-containing neurons in various parts of the brain and discusses some of their implications.

METHODS

Specific antisera directed against met and leu-enkephalin were raised in rabbits following a series of injections of enkephalin-hemocyanin conjugates linked with glutaraldehyde as described elsewhere (Childers *et al.*, 1978). Radioimmunoassay revealed negligible cross-reactivity with a variety of peptides including α and β-

endorphins. Further, each enkephalin antiserum has more than 200-fold greater affinity for the enkephalin pentapeptide against which it was directed than for the other pentapeptide.

Normal Sprague-Dawley male rats (100 g) were used for initial studies. For improved visualization of enkephalin-containing cell bodies, 50 μg of colchicine in 25 μl of 0.9 per cent saline was injected into the lateral ventricle 2 days before the rats were killed (Uhl *et al.*, 1977).

In some animals, electrolytic lesions of the amygdala or knife cuts of the stria terminalis were made as previously described (Uhl *et al.*, 1978*c*). Animals were perfused with a buffered depolymerized paraformaldehyde solution, brains were soaked, frozen and sectioned on a cryostat, and sections were processed for immunohistochemical staining by the indirect technique of Coons and co-workers (1958) as described previously (Uhl *et al.*, 1977). Adjacent sections stained with antiserum previously incubated overnight at 4 °C with 1 M enkephalin served as controls for non-specific fluorescence.

RESULTS

Specificity of immunohistochemical fluorescence

Specific enkephalin-like immunofluorescence observed in these studies was eliminated by preadsorption of serum with the peptide against which the serum was directed. For example, the very intense staining in the globus pallidus was nearly eliminated by the preadsorption treatment (figure 6.1a and b). This specific fluorescence is distributed unevenly through the brain, and is localized to neuronal perikarya and to structures resembling fibers and terminal varicosities.

Mapping studies in the brainstem

In the spinal cord, immunofluorescent fibers and terminals were observed to be highly concentrated in the substantia gelatinosa, though densities were also found in other areas such as the ventral horn and the white matter adjacent to the substantia gelatinosa (figures 6.1c and d). At the junction of the medulla oblongata and the spinal cord, the substantia gelatinosa of the spinal trigeminal nucleus shows a dense fiber and terminal fluorescent pattern. Further, the substantia gelatinosa possesses enkephalin-containing cell bodies which are concentrated in the dorsal and ventral portions and tend to be localized in the more medial aspect of the substantia gelatinosa (figure 6.2). The nucleus commissuralis displayed a fiber and terminal fluorescence pattern similar in intensity to that of the substantia gelatinosa. Lower levels of fluorescent fibers were observed through several aspects of the reticular formation (figure 6.2).

At the level of the nucleus raphe magnus, the most dense fiber and terminal fluorescence occurs in the nucleus of the solitary tract, with less fluorescence over the tract itself. The greatest density of cells in this area occurs just outside the borders of nucleus raphe magnus, in the region overlying the dorsal border of the pyramids.

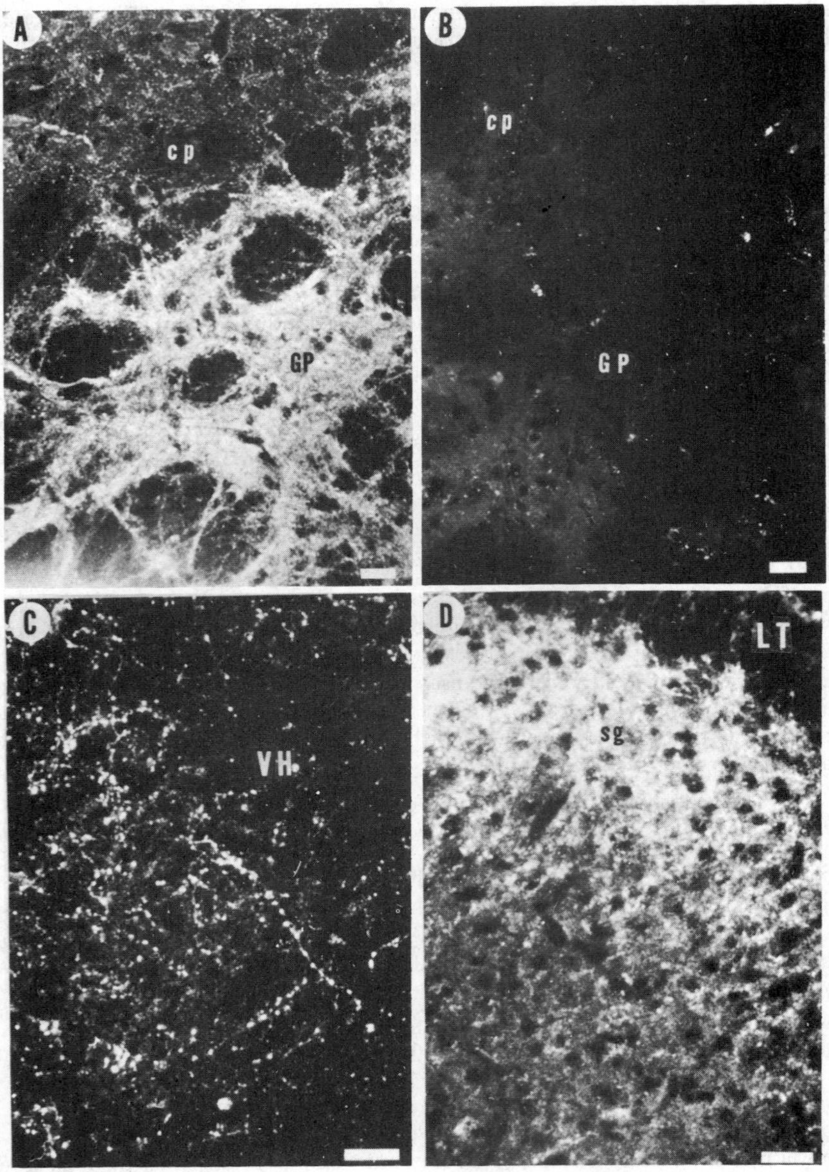

Figure 6.1 Immunofluorescence micrographs of (A and B) the globus pallidus (GP) and nucleus caudatus/putamen (cp) and of the cervical spinal cord showing (C) the ventral horn (VH) and (D) Lissauer's Tract (LT) and substantia gelatinosa (sg). Micrographs A and B were taken from serial sections, but the primary serum used for staining in B was previously adsorbed overnight with 1 mM leu-enkephalin to establish a control. All sections were stained with rabbit antiserum against leu-enkephalin. Bars, 25 μm. From Simantov *et al.* (1977).

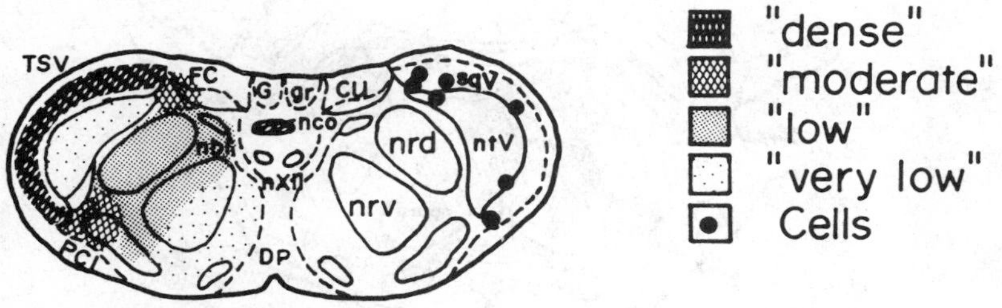

Figure 6.2 Enkephalin immunofluorescence at the decussation of the pyramids. cu, cuneate nucleus; DP, decussation of the pyramids; FC, cuneate fasciculus; G, gracile fasciculus; gr, gracile nucleus; nbi, basilar internal nucleus of Cajal; nco, nucleus commissuralis; nrd, dorsal medullary reticular nucleus; nrv, ventral medullary reticular nucleus; ntv, nucleus of the spinal tract of the trigeminal; nXII, hypoglossal nucleus; PCI, inferior cerebellar peduncle; rl, lateral reticular nucleus; sgV, substantia gelatinosa of the trigeminal; TSV, spinal tract of the trigeminal.

These groups of cells are continuous with a few cells contained within the raphe magnus nucleus itself. Many of the cells lying dorsal and lateral to the raphe magnus appear to be bipolar or fusiform in shape. This contrasts with the classical description of larger, multipolar raphe magnus cells of the cat (Pierce *et al.*, 1960). Cell bodies are also observed in the medial vestibular nucleus and the dorsal cochlear nucleus (figure 6.3). Again, varying densities of fibers and terminals were observed in the reticular formation. The facial nucleus, in the ventral portion of the medulla, displays a prominent network of fibers and terminals (figure 6.3).

At the level of the locus coeruleus, the densest fiber, terminal and cell body fluorescence is found in the medial aspect of the dorsal tegmental nucleus of Gudden. Fluorescent fibers, terminals and cells are apparent in the parabrachial nuclei. Terminals and fibers appear again to be distributed somewhat unevenly through the reticular formation (figure 6.4).

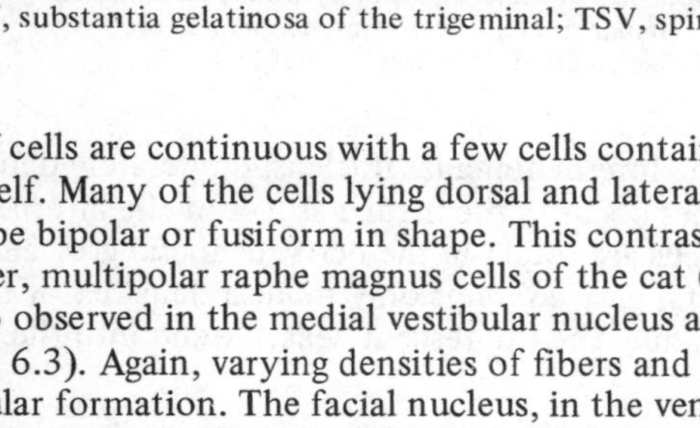

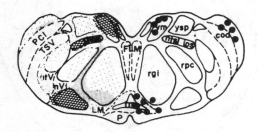

Figure 6.3 Enkephalin immunofluorescence at the level of the raphe magnus. cod, dorsal cochlear nucleus; FLM, medial longitudinal fasciculus; LM, medial lemniscus; nts, nucleus of the solitary tract; ntV, nucleus of the spinal tract of the trigeminal; nVII, nucleus of the facial nerve; P, pyramid; PCI, inferior cerebellar peduncle; ps, parasolitary nucleus; rgi, gigantocellular reticular nucleus; rm, nucleus raphe magnus; rpc, parvocellular reticular nucleus; TSV, spinal tract of the trigeminal; vm, medial vestibular nucleus; vsp, spinal vestibular nucleus. See figure 6.2 for key.

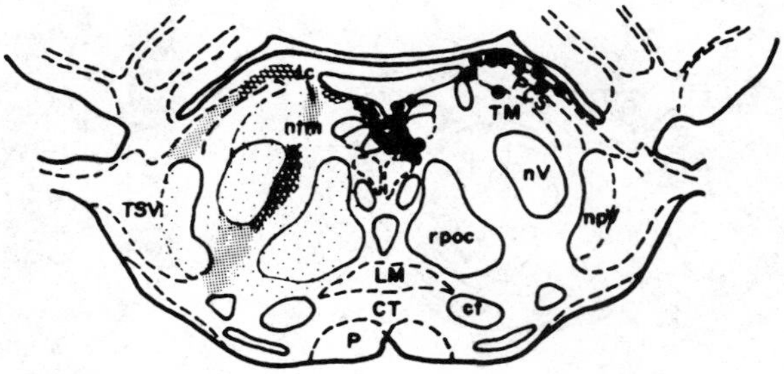

Figure 6.4 Enkephalin immunofluorescence at the level of the exit of the trigeminal. CT, trapezoid body; ct, nucleus of the trapezoid body; lc, locus coeruleus; LM, medial lemniscus; npV, main nucleus of the trigeminal; ntm, nucleus of the mesencephalic tract of the trigeminal; nV, motor nucleus of the trigeminal; P, pyramid; PCS, superior cerebellar peduncle; rpoc, caudal pontine reticular nucleus; TM, mesencephalic tract of the trigeminal; TSV, spinal tract of the trigeminal. See figure 6.2 for key.

At the level of the interpeduncular nucleus, moderately dense fiber fluorescence and cell bodies occur in the medial aspect of the interpeduncular nucleus. Other fluorescent cells are found in the periaqueductal grey and in areas lateral to it. The periaqueductal grey contains only modest densities of fiber and terminal fluorescence, which, like the fluorescent cells, extend into the lateral midbrain (figure 6.5).

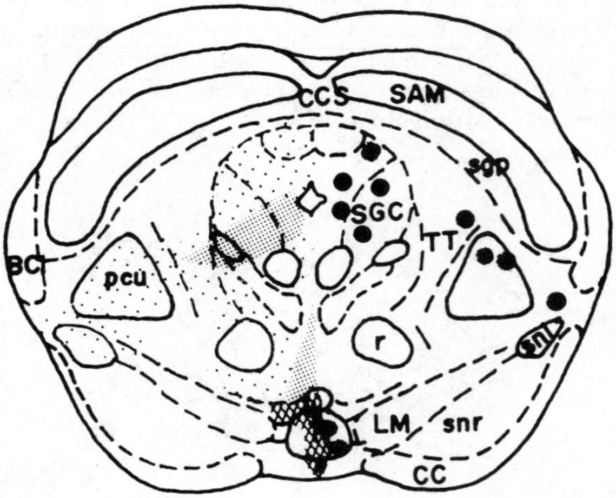

Figure 6.5 Enkephalin immunofluorescence at the level of the interpeduncular nucleus. BCI, brachium of the inferior colliculus; CC, cerebral peduncle; CCS, commissure of the superior colliculus; ipn, interpeduncular nucleus; LM, medial lemniscus; nIII, occulomotor nucleus; ncu, cuneiform nucleus; r, red nucleus; SAM, superior colliculus; SGC, central grey; sgp, deep grey of the superior colliculus; snl, lateral substantia nigra; snr, reticulata of the substantia nigra; TT, tectospinal tract.

Delineation of enkephalin-containing pathways

We have observed enkephalin-containing cell bodies and fibers in more rostral areas such as the central nucleus of the amygdala, the interstitial nucleus of the stria terminalis, the medial and lateral preoptic areas and the lateral septal nucleus. Many hypothalamic nuclei also have enkephalin-containing neurons. More dimly fluorescent perikarya are observed in the central caudate/putamen. To elucidate the various projections of such cell groups, several lesion studies have been undertaken. Because of the high concentration of enkephalin-immunoreactive cells in the central nucleus of the amygdala and fibers in the stria terminalis, experiments were designed to test the hypothesis that there was an enkephalin-containing amygdalo-fugal pathway. Lesions were placed in the central nucleus of the amygdala in some rats, and the stria terminalis pathway was sectioned in other animals (figure 6.6). When these animals were prepared for histochemistry, it was found that lesions in the central nucleus of the amygdala resulted, 10 days later, in a loss of fiber fluorescence in the ventrolateral stria terminalis (figure 6.7a compared with b). Lesions placed near the central nucleus, but which did not impinge upon it, did not alter the fluorescence in the stria terminalis (figure 6.7c). In the animals where the stria terminalis was sectioned 3 days before killing, there appears to be an accumulation of fluorescent material in fibers in areas posterior to the lesion (figure 6.7d). Anterior portions of the stria terminalis showed a depletion of fluorescence, though noticeably less fluorescence was lost than after central amygdala lesion. These data suggest the existence of an amygdalo-fugal enkephalin-containing pathway schematically shown in figure 6.8. Further evidence for the existence of such a pathway is the finding that the enkephalin-containing fibers are found in the lateral and ventral part of the stria terminalis, which is known to contain fibers rising from the central nucleus of the amygdala (DeOlmos, 1972).

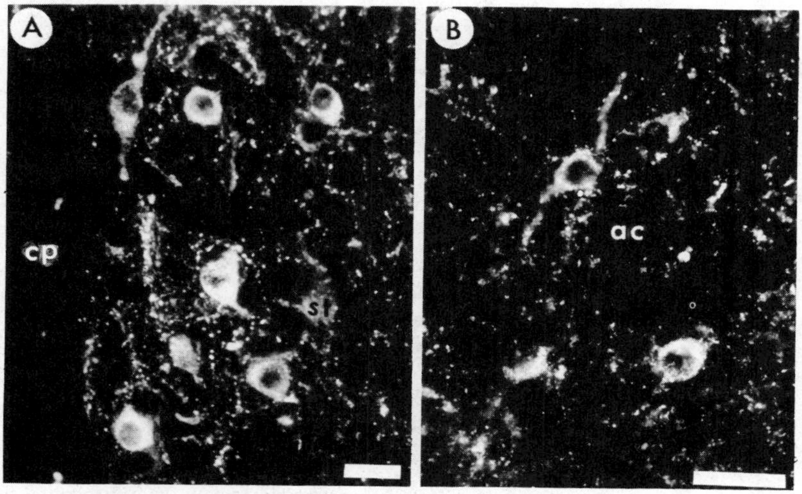

Figure 6.6 Photomicrographs of immunofluorescence in colchicine-pretreated rats. A, Enkephalin fluorescence in the interstitial nucleus of the stria terminalis (st) and the caudate/putamen (cp). B, Enkephalin fluorescence in the central (ac) amygdaloid nucleus. Bars, 25 μm. (From Uhl *et al.*, 1978c).

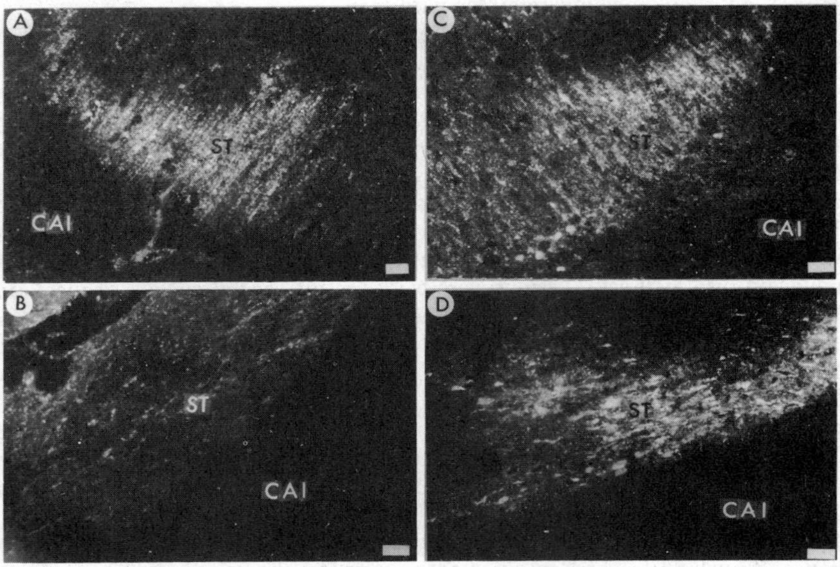

Figure 6.7 Photomicrographs of enkephalin immunofluorescence in the ventrolateral stria terminalis (ST) and internal capsule (CAI). A, Normal; B, Ipsilateral to electrolytic lesion destroying the central amygdala; C, Ipsilateral to electrolytic lesion sparing the central amygdala; D, Ipsilateral and posterior to knife cut of the stria terminalis; B and C, 10 d survival time; D, 2 d survival time. Bars, 25 μm. (From Uhl *et al.*, 1978c).

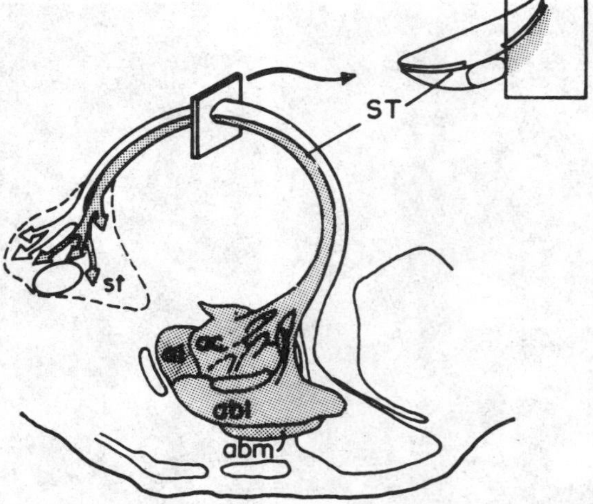

Figure 6.8 Origin, course and termination of fibers running through the centrolateral stria terminalis as determined by classical degeneration methods. Fibers arising from the central (ac), lateral (al), basolateral (abl) and basomedial (abm) amygdaloid nuclei pass through the ventrolateral stria terminalis (ST) and end in the interstitial nucleus of the stria terminalis (st). From the work of DeOlmos (1972).

Cuello and co-workers (1978) have reported evidence for the existence of another enkephalin-containing tract. Knife cuts separating the globus pallidus from the caudate/putamen, as well as other lateral and anterior structures, resulted in an almost total loss of enkephalin fluorescence in the globus pallidus. These results suggest the existence of an enkephalin-containing system afferent to the globus pallidus. But there is some concern that such knife cuts might also sever penetrating vascular branches supplying the globus pallidus. The location of cell bodies whose fibers pass to the globus is also not clear in this study. Accordingly, we have examined residual enkephalin fluorescence after injection of kainic acid into the head of the caudate/putamen. Intrastriatal injections of kainate results in a dramatic loss of neurons whose cell bodies are in the striatum, while processes and terminals of cell bodies that lie outside the caudate/putamen are apparently spared (Schwarcz and Coyle, 1977; Coyle *et al.*, 1978). In animals killed 48 hours after 2 $\mu g/\mu l$ injections of kainic acid into the head of the caudate/putamen, neuronal cell loss is evident on the injected side at the level of the nucleus accumbens. At the level of the globus pallidus, however, neuronal loss is not evident in either the caudate/putamen or the globus pallidus. Nevertheless, we have observed substantial depletion of enkephalin fluorescence in restricted portions of the globus pallidus following kainate; these preliminary studies suggest a pathway from cells in the head of the caudate/putamen to terminal fields in lateral aspects of the globus. Further studies are obviously necessary to determine whether other parts of the caudate/putamen or other brain regions contribute to the dense fluorescence which remains in the medial portions of the globus pallidus.

DISCUSSION

The observations reported here are in general agreement with those of Hökfelt and co-workers (Elde *et al.*, 1976; Hökfelt *et al.*, 1977*a* and *b*). However, there are some discrepancies. Whereas we have observed substantial numbers of cells in the inferior colliculus, Hökfelt *et al.* (1977*a*) report cells localized to the superior colliculus but not the inferior colliculus. We have also observed concentrations of cells in the dorsal tegmental nucleus of Gudden and the interpeduncular nucleus, areas in which Hökfelt *et al.* (1977*a*) did not report any cells.

As noted in earlier studies, our more detailed explanation of brainstem enkephalin underscores the similarities in distribution of peptide-containing fibers and terminals and opiate receptors (Simantov *et al.*, 1977; Atweh and Kuhar, 1977*a* and *b*; Atweh and Kuhar, 1977*c*). For example, the substantia gelatinosa zones of the spinal cord and nucleus of the spinal tract of the trigeminal are enriched in both receptor and peptide. The interstitial nucleus of stria terminalis has been reported to be enriched in both receptor (Atweh and Kuhar, 1977*c*) and enkephalin (Elde *et al.*, 1976; Simantov *et al.*, 1977). Similarly, the interpeduncular nucleus is markedly enriched in receptors. Within the nucleus, densities of receptor and peptide are restricted to similar zones in dorsal and medial portions of the nucleus (Simantov *et al.*, 1977). On the other hand, varying concentrations of enkephalin-containing fibers were observed throughout the reticular formation whereas the receptor concentration was not especially striking. This finding might be rationalized since certain densities of enkephalin-reactive fibers might possess receptors at their terminal fields only and not along the total length of the axon.

It is also conceivable that some of the autoradiographically determined opiate receptors are for other opioid peptides in other neuronal systems, such as β-endorphin (Bradbury *et al.*, 1976). However, immunohistochemical studies of the distribution of β-endorphin reveal a much more restricted distribution, with a marked localization of cell bodies to the hypothalamus. Fibers and terminals of these cells do not seem to extend to the brainstem nor are substantial densities of such fibers or terminals observed in the brainstem.

Opiates and opioid peptides are well known for their analgesic properties. These drugs or peptides could interact with the endogenous systems thought to be involved in the integration of nociceptive stimuli that are found in the following areas: substantia gelatinosa of the spinal cord, substantia gelatinosa of the spinal trigeminal nerve, nucleus raphe magnus and periaqueductal grey. The precise nature of function of these endogenous peptide-containing neurons in the regulation of nociceptive stimuli is an exciting frontier.

Enkephalin-containing neurons are found in areas associated with other sensory functions. Several structures possibly related to auditory function are enriched in enkephalin-containing elements especially cell bodies. These include the dorsal cochlear nucleus, the medial geniculate body, the paraolivary nucleus, the area between the superior olive and the trapezoid body, the lateral lemniscus and inferior colliculus. Opiates are also known to influence numerous visceral functions such as nausea and vomiting. The enkephalin-containing neurons within the nuclei associated with the vagus nerve are possibly the systems related to these functions.

ACKNOWLEDGEMENT

This research was supported by USPHS Grant DA 00266 and M. J. K. is the recipient of RSDA Type II, MH 00053. G. U. is supported by USPHS Training Grant 5 TO1 GM 01183-13.

REFERENCES

Atweh, S. F. and Kuhar, M. J. (1977*a*). *Brain Res.*, **124**, 53–68

Atweh, S. F. and Kuhar, M. J. (1977*b*). *Brain Res.*, **129**, 1–12

Atweh, S. F. and Kuhar, M. J. (1977*c*). *Brain Res.*, **134**, 393–405

Bradbury, A., Smyth, D., Snell, C., Birdsall, N. and Hulme, E. (1976). *Nature*, **260**, 793–5

Bradley, P. B., Briggs, I., Gayton, R. J. and Lambert, L. A. (1976). *Nature*, **261**, 425–6

Childers, S., Schwarcz, R., Coyle, J. T. and Snyder, S. H. (1978). In *Endorphins*, (eds. E. Costa and M. Trabucci) Raven Press, New York, in press

Coons, A. H. (1958). In *General Cytochemical Methods,* (ed. J. F. Danielli) Academic Press, New York

Cox, B. and Goldstein, A. L. C. (1976). *Proc. natn. Acad. Sci. U.S.A.*, **73**, 1821–3

Coyle, J. T., Molliver, M. E. and Kuhar, M. J. (1978). *J. comp. Neurol.*, (in press)

Cuello, C. and Iversen, L. (1978). In *Endorphins*, (eds. E. Costa and M. Trabucci) Raven Press, New York, in press

DeOlmos, J. (1972). In *Neurobiology of the Amygdala,* (ed. B. Eleftheriou) Plenum Press, New York, pp. 145–204

Duggan, A. W., Hall, J. G., Headley, P. M. (1976). *Nature*, **264**, 456–8

Elde, R., Hökfelt, T., Johansson, O. and Terenius, L. (1976). *Neuroscience*, **1**, 349–55

Frederickson, R. C. and Norris, F. H. (1976). *Science,* **194**, 440–2

Hökfelt, T., Elde, R., Johansson, O. C., Terenius, L. and Stein, L. (1977*a*). *Neurosci Lett.*, **5**, 25–31

Hökfelt, T., Ljungdahl, A., Terenius, L., Elde, R. and Nilsson, G. (1977*b*). *Proc. natn. Acad. Sci. U.S.A.*, **74**, 3081–5

Hughes, J. (1975). *Brain Res.*, **88**, 295–308

Hughes, J., Smith, T. W., Kosterlitz, H. W., Fothergill, L. A., Morgan, B. A. and Morris, H. R. (1975). *Nature*, **258**, 577–9

Nicoll, R., Siggins, G., Ling, N., Bloom, F. and Guillemin, R. (1977). *Proc. natn. Acad. Sci. U.S.A.*, **74**, 2584–8

Pasternak, G. W., Goodman, R. and Snyder, S. H. (1975). *Life Sci.*, **16**, 1765–9

Pierce, E., Brodal, A. and Walberg, F. (1960). *J. comp. Neurol.*, **114**, 116–88

Schwarcz, R. and Coyle, J. T. (1977). *Brain Res.*, **127**, 235–49

Simantov, R., Kuhar, M. J., Pasternak, G. W. and Snyder, S. H. (1976*a*). *Brain Res.*, **106**, 189–97

Simantov, R., Kuhar, M. J., Uhl, G. R. and Snyder, S. H. (1977). *Proc. natn. Acad. Sci, U.S.A.*, **74**, 2167–71

Simantov, R., Snowman, A. M. and Snyder, S. H. (1976*b*). *Brain Res.*, **107**, 650–7

Simantov, R. and Snyder, S. H. (1976). *Proc. natn. Acad. Sci. U.S.A.*, **73**, 2515–9

Uhl, G. R., Goodman, R. R., Kuhar, M. J. and Snyder, S. H. (1978*a*). In *Endorphins*, (eds. E. Costa and M. Trabucci) Raven Press, New York, in press

Uhl, G. R., Goodman, R. R., Kuhar, M. J. and Snyder, S. H. (1978*b*). *Brain Res.*, (in press)

Uhl, G. R., Kuhar, M. J. and Snyder, S. H. (1977). *Proc. natn. Acad. Sci. U.S.A.*, **74**, 4059–63

Uhl, G. R., Kuhar, M. J. and Snyder, S. H. (1978*c*). *Brain Res.*, in press 149 223-228, 1978

Watson, S. J., Akil, H., Sullivan, S. and Barchas, J. D. (1977). *Life Sci.*, **21**, 733–8

Young, W. S., Bird, S. J. and Kuhar, M. J. (1977). *Brain Res.*, **129**, 366–70

Zieglgänsberger, W., Fry, J. P., Herz, A., Moroden, L. and Wunsch E. (1976). *Brain Res.*, **115**. 160–4

7

Isolation and characterization of endogenous [α]-n-acyl derivatives of the C and C′ of lph

D. G. Smyth and Siraik Zakarian (National Institute for Medical Research, Mill Hill, London)

Studies of pituitary peptides, carried out 3 years ago, revealed that the constituent fragments of lipotropin (LPH) have an independent existence in the pituitary gland (Bradbury *et al.*, 1975). A second series of peptides was found in similar quantity (table 7.1) and it was proposed that these were derived from a prohormone to adrenocorticotropin (ACTH). It is now clear that the two groups of peptides account for the major part of a single chain 31K precursor which is the common prohormone of LPH and ACTH (Mains, Eipper and Ling, 1977). Thus it is to be expected that the elaboration of ACTH and of α-melanocyte stimulating hormone (α-MSH) which represents the N-terminal region of ACTH, would be accompanied by the release of LPH and its fragments. Since the N-terminal residue of α-MSH is acetylated (Harris and Roos, 1957), it would seem possible that the N-terminal residues of the LPH fragments formed simultaneously might also undergo acetylation and be retained in the pituitary gland.

Table 7.1 Yields of peptides isolated from porcine pituitary (~ 1200 glands, 500 g)

No met-E or leu-E in pituitary

Pro-β-MSH			pro-ACTH		
Residues	Fragment	Yield (μmol)	Residues	Fragment	Yield (μmol)
1–91	β-lipotropin	6.3	1–19	Peptide I	6.8
1–58	γ-lipotropin	8.1	22–40	Peptide II	6.8
1–38	N-fragment	7.2	1–40	I - - - II	2.1
41–58	β-MSH	10.5	43–82	ACTH	15.0
61–87	C′-fragment	5.0	61–82	CLIP	1.1
61–91	C-fragment	9.1			

We report here the isolation and identification of a naturally occurring acyl form of LPH C-fragment (residues 61–91, also known as β-endorphin). We report also the corresponding derivative of LPH C′-fragment (residues 61–87). Both peptides are present in substantial quantity in porcine pituitary and further evidence indicates that they occur in brain.

N-ACYL PEPTIDES IN PITUITARY

The procedure previously employed for the isolation of peptides from porcine pituitary (Bradbury *et al.*, 1976; Smyth *et al.*, 1978) was slightly modified. Before ion exchange chromatography on CM-Sephadex C25, the mixture of peptides was neutralized and insoluble peptides were removed by centrifugation. This step eliminates most of the ACTH which has a limited solubility and which previously had interfered with the resolution of basic peptides during chromatography. Using the modified procedure, the resolution of C-fragment from residual ACTH on SP-Sephadex C25 was complete (figure 7.1) and emerging with less retention that ACTH was a new peptide (I) which was subsequently isolated by gel filtration on Sephadex G50 in 50 per cent acetic acid. Its composition was identical with that of C-fragment (table 7.2). In the corresponding stage of isolation of the C′-fragment,

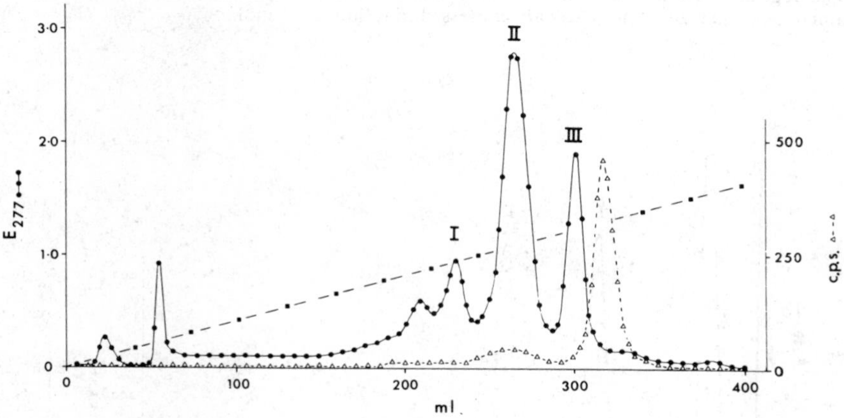

Figure 7.1 Chromatography of N-acyl C-fragment (I), ACTH (II) and C-fragment (III) on SP–Sephadex C25. (60 × 0.9 cm) with a gradient from 0.02M to 0.5M NaCl at pH 7.0.

again a more basic peptide was observed which exhibited less retention than C′-fragment (figure 7.2) while possessing the same composition. Radiolabeled C and C′-fragments added to the pituitary homogenate were isolated in a single form only. The derivatives of the C and C′ fragments therefore do not appear to be artifacts produced during isolation.

The differences between the less basic forms of C and C′-fragments and their normal counterparts were localized at the N-termini of the respective peptides. Digestion of the C or C′-fragment derivatives by trypsin and aminopeptidase M

Table 7.2 Amino acid composition of N-acyl C-fragment (LPH_{61-91}) and N-acyl C′fragment (LPH_{61-87}).

	N-acyl C-fragment	Theory	N-acyl C′-fragment	Theory
Asp	2.1	2	1.9	2
Thr	2.8	3	3.0	3
Ser	2.0	2	2.0	2
Glu	3.0	3	2.1	2
Pro	1.4	1	0.9	1
Gly	2.9	3	2.1	2
Ala	1.9	2	1.9	2
Val	1.2	2	1.3	2
Met	0.7	1	0.9	1
Ile	0.3	1	0.3	1
Leu	1.9	2	1.9	2
Tyr	1.0	1	1.0	1
Phe	1.9	2	1.8	2
Lys	4.9	5	3.2	3
His	0.8	1	0.9	1
Arg	–	–	–	–

The peptides were hydrolyzed in 6 N HCl at 110 °C for 16 h and analyzed on a Beckman 120 C amino acid analyzer. The values are expressed in residues per mol.

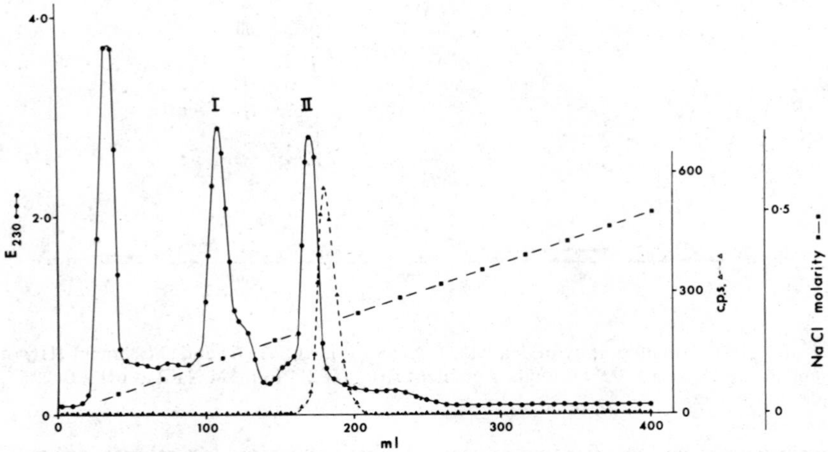

Figure 7.2 Chromatography of N-acyl C′-fragment (I) and C′-fragment (II) on SP–Sephadex C25 (60 × 0.9 cm) with a gradient from 0.02M to 0.5M NaCl at pH 7.0.

released the expected amino acids except for tyrosine, and the yield of glycine which follows the N-terminal tyrosine in sequence was low (table 7.3). These data suggest that the differences between the less basic peptides and their parent peptides reside in a modification at the N-terminal tyrosine.

Table 7.3 Amino acids released by enzymic digestion of C′-fragment and N-acyl C′-fragment.

	N-acyl C′-fragment	C′-fragment
Asp	–	–
Thr	2.0	2.0
Ser + Asn	4.3	4.2
Glu	0.9	0.9
Pro	–	–
Gly	0.4	2.1
Ala	1.8	2.1
Val	1.9	1.9
Met	1.0	0.8
Ile	1.1	1.1
Leu	2.3	2.0
Tyr	<0.1	0.9
Phe	2.1	1.8

Digestions of peptide (20 nmol) with trypsin (0.2 nmol) and aminopeptidase M (0.4 nmol) were carried out at pH 8.0, 37 °C for 16 h with a trypsin: peptide ratio of 1:50 and aminopeptidase M: peptide ratio of 1:20 (w/w) and analysis was performed on a Beckman 120 C analyzer.

The differing chromatographic properties of the pairs of related peptides seem to be due to the presence of an acyl substituent attached to the terminal NH_2 group. The less basic form of C-fragment (20 nmol) was digested with chymotrypsin (1:10, pH 5, 5 h, 37 °C) which cleaved the peptide chain on the carboxyl side of the N-terminal tyrosine at position 1 and the phenylalanine at position 4. Neither the released tyrosine nor the tetrapeptide was retained by a column of Dowex 50 X 2 (5 × 0.9 cm) in the H^+ form and the products were shown to be present in the H_2O eluate by acid hydrolysis, consistent with the absence of a free α-amino group in the acyl peptide. Corresponding results were obtained with the less basic form of C′-fragment while control experiments with 'normal' C and C′-fragments showed, as expected, that tyrosine and the tetrapeptide were retained on the Dowex column.

The identification of the two derivatives as N-acyl forms of the C and C′-fragments rests on their chromatographic properties, their compositions given by acid and enzymic hydrolysis, and on the isolation of the acylated forms of the N-terminal tyrosine residues. In current experiments the nature of the acyl substituent is being examined. The amounts of C-fragment and N-acyl C-fragment obtained from 1200 pig pituitaries (approximately 500 g) were 9.3 μmol and 3.2 μmol, respectively; and the amounts of C′-fragment and N-acyl C′-fragment were 5.0 μmol and 4.8 μmol. Thus the ratio of C-fragment to acyl C-fragment in porcine pituitary was approximately 3:1 and the ratio for C′-fragment to acyl C′-fragment about 1:1.

∴ don't know ID of acyl group

While α-MSH is present in pituitary, this acetylated peptide occurs also in brain (Rudman *et al.*, 1973). It was therefore of interest to investigate whether the N-acyl forms of C- and C′-fragments occur in brain as well as in pituitary.

N-ACYL PEPTIDES IN BRAIN

To detect the lower concentrations of C and C′-fragments expected in brain, the peptides in brain homogenates were fractionated by gel filtration on a column of Sephadex G75 in a dissociating solvent and the resolved peptides were located by immunoassay. Figure 7.3 shows the resolution of a standard mixture containing pmol quantities of radiolabeled LPH, C-fragment and met-enkephalin on the G75 column. Ion exchange chromatography on columns of SP Sephadex C25 was subsequently carried out to separate peptides with different charge.

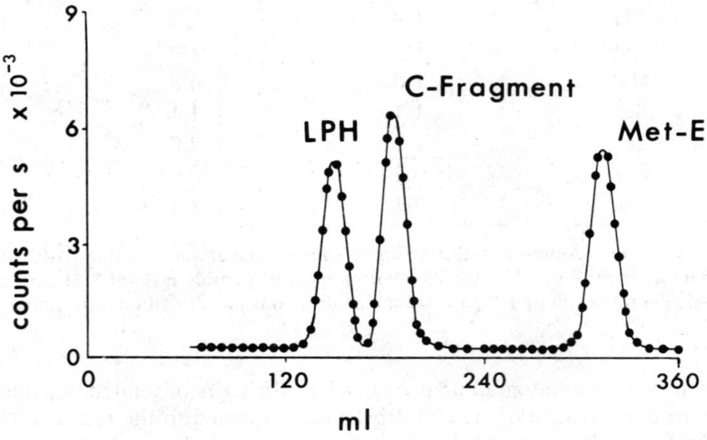

Figure 7.3 Gel filtration of [^{125}I] LPH, C-fragment and met-enkephalin on Sephadex G75 (70 × 2.5 cm) in 50 per cent acetic acid.

Antibody against C-fragment was prepared by coupling natural porcine C-fragment to bovine γ-globulin and rabbits were immunized by multisite injection in complete Freunds adjuvant, followed by booster injections at intervals for 3 months with incomplete Freunds adjuvant. Immunoassay was carried out for C-fragment reactivity using displacement of [^{125}I] C-fragment by the method of Rees *et al.* (1971). Antibody against leu-enkephalin, which cross-reacts about 20 per cent with met-enkephalin, was obtained from Miles Laboratories, Stoke Poges, UK and immunoassay with this antibody was performed according to the method of Weissman *et al.* (1976).

The specificity of the c-fragment antiserum was determined against standard solutions of porcine C-fragment, C′-fragment, LPH and met-enkephalin. The specificity to the acyl peptides was also examined. At a dilution of 1/16,000 the antibody was capable of measuring as little as 0.05 to 0.1 pmol of C-fragment. Its affinity for C′fragment was approximately one-quarter and its affinity for porcine LPH one-sixth that of C-fragment (figure 7.4); met-enkephalin did not react. Each of the acyl peptides was immunologically indistinguishable from its parent peptide (figure 7.5), in agreement with the COOH-terminal specificity of the antibody

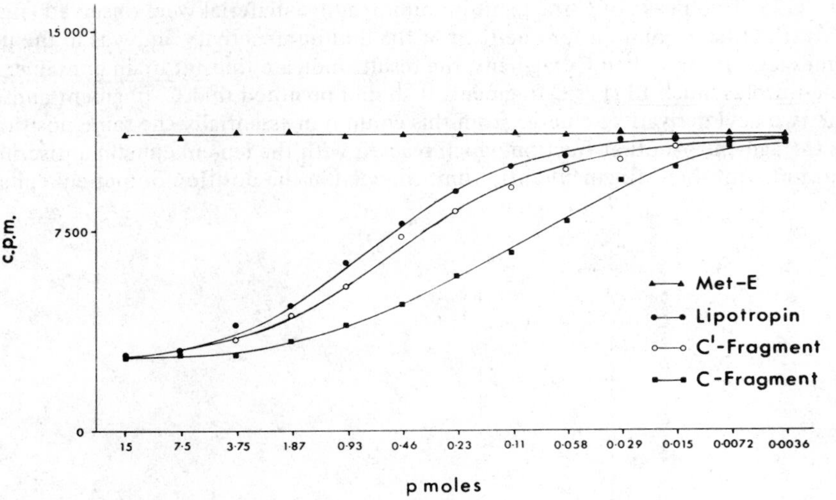

Figure 7.4 Radioimmunoassay standard curves for C-fragment, C′-fragment, LPH and met-enkephalin.

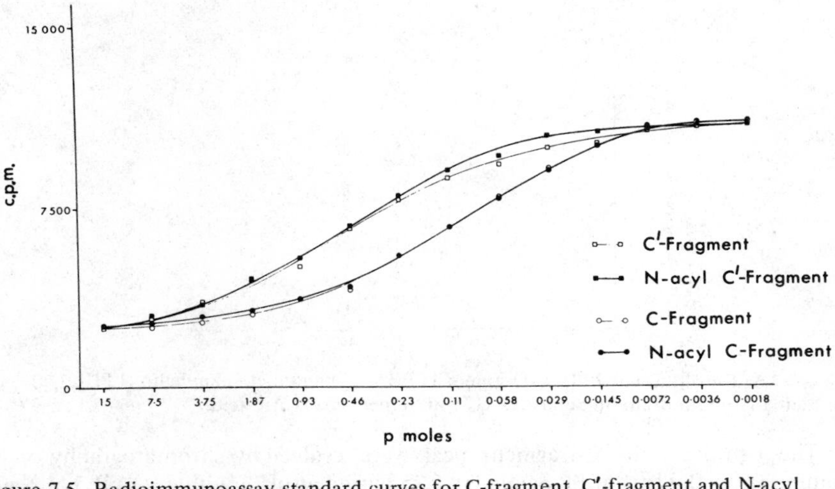

Figure 7.5 Radioimmunoassay standard curves for C-fragment, C′-fragment and N-acyl derivatives.

Rats (inbred, August strain) were killed by stunning and decapitation and the brains, less cerebellum, were removed within 30 s. Homogenization of the brains from two rats was at 4 °C for 1 min in acid acetone (acetone, hydrochloric acid, water; 40:1:5) and after centrifugation the supernatants were concentrated *in vacuo* to remove acetone and lyophilized. The residues were taken up in 50 per cent acetic acid and gel filtration was performed on a column (70 × 2.5 cm) of Sephadex G75. Two peaks of C-fragment immunoreactive material were observed (figure 7.6): the first accounted for one-fifth of the immunoreactivity and was in the posi-times less strongly than C-fragment, the results indicate that rat brain contains one-third as much LPH as C-fragment. It should be noted that C′-fragment and the two acyl derivatives emerge from this column in essentially the same position as C-fragment. Another fraction which reacted with the leu-enkephalin antiserum but not with the C-fragment antiserum, emerged in the position of met-enkephalin.

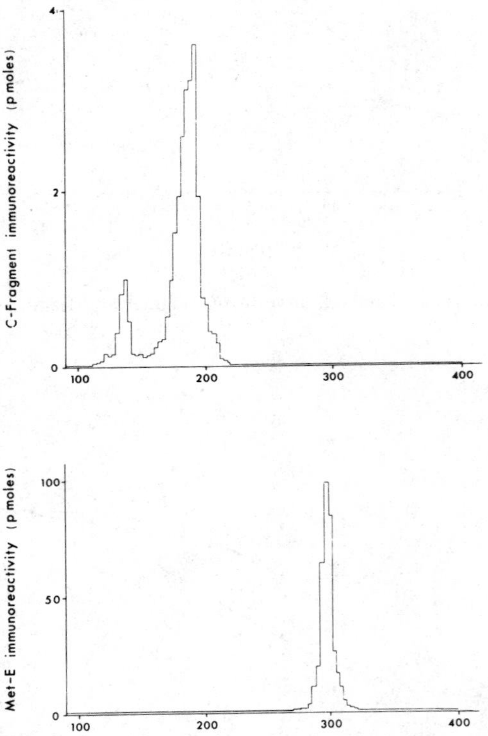

Figure 7.6 Resolution of LPH, C-fragment (LPH_{61-91}) and met-enkephalin (LPH_{61-65}) extracted from rat brain on Sephadex G75 in 50 per cent acetic acid.

The peptides in the 'C-fragment' peak were resolved by chromatography on a column (60 × 0.9 cm) of SP-Sephadex C25 eluted at pH 7 with a 0 to 0.5 M NaCl gradient. Four peaks of C-fragment immunoreactive material were seen, corresponding to the elution positions of N-acyl C′-fragment, C′-fragment, N-acyl C-fragment and C-fragment. Although the recovery of immunoreactivity was less than quantitative on this column, it could be seen that the amounts of the four peptides were in the proportion 1:4:2:10, as assessed by C-fragment immunoreactivity. However, C′-fragment and its acyl derivative are detected four times less sensitively than C-fragment and the results suggest that in this series C′-fragment is the predominant peptide in brain. (rat) except for ME.

The immunoreactive peptides emerging from the Sephadex G75 column in the met-enkephalin position were fractionated on a column (30 × 0.9 cm) of SP-Sephadex C25 eluted at pH 4 with a 0 to 0.5 M NaCl gradient (figure 7.7). Two principal peaks of immunoreactive peptides were obtained, the first emerging without retention, accounted for <20 per cent of the immunoreactivity, the second emerging in

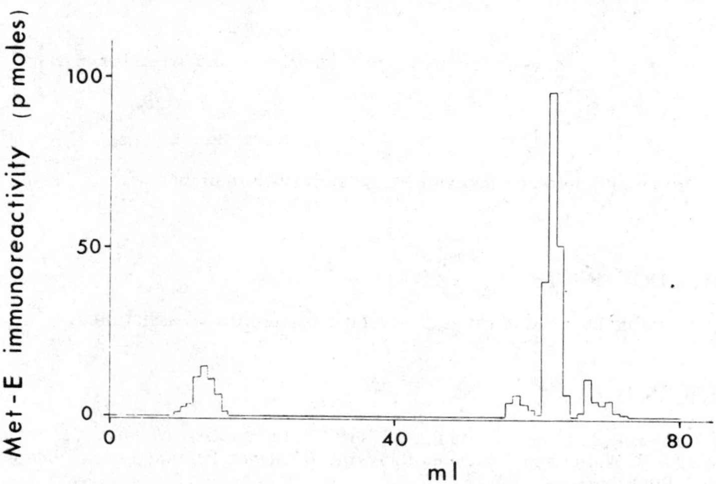

Figure 7.7 Chromatography on SP-Sephadex C25 of met-enkephalin extracted from rat brain.

the position of met-enkephalin. This is consistent with the interpretation that the first peptide lacks basic amino groups and might be an acyl form of met-enkephalin. The sensitivity of the antiserum to the N-acyl pentapeptide is not known but from other specificity data the acyl peptide would be expected to react less strongly than met-enkephalin (Weissman *et al.*, 1976) and the amounts present could be greater than indicated in the figure. A provisional estimate of the amounts of the 'opiate' peptides in rat brain indiates that the LPH content is in the region of 7 pmol/g brain, C-fragment 17 pmol/g, C′fragment 27 pmol/g and met-enkephalin 670 pmol/g. The N-acyl derivatives appear to be present in amounts less than the parent peptides.

The finding that several of the peptide fragments derived from the 31K prohormone can exist as N-acyl derivatives (figure 7.8) suggests a possible control mechanism for the release of one biological activity without concomitant release of a different activity associated with another region. Thus cells that produce α-MSH would at the same time acetylate the C-fragment, eliminating its opiate activity. Conversely, cells producing C-fragment in its basic form would not produce α-MSH. In this way the two peptides could be released independently to act as neurotransmitters.

In summary, N-acyl forms of lipotropin C and C′-fragments were isolated from porcine pituitary and identified; the acyl peptides were present in substantial quantity. Evidence has been obtained that similar N-acyl derivatives occur in brain. The N-acylation reaction offers a possible mechanism for the independent release of multiple biological activities from the 31K ACTH-LPH prohormone.

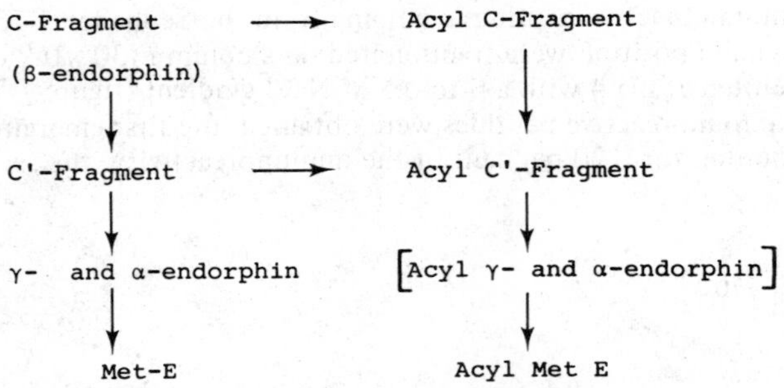

Figure 7.8 Proposed opioid peptides and N-acyl derivatives in brain.

ACKNOWLEDGEMENTS

The authors thank D. E. Massey and N. Clark for technical assistance.

REFERENCES

Bradbury, A. F., Smyth, D. G. and Snell, C. R. (1975). In *Peptides: chemistry, structure and biology,* (eds R. Walter and J. Meienhofer) *Proc. 4th Amer. Peptide Symp., Michigan,* Ann Arbor Sci. Publishers, pp. 609–15

Bradbury, A. F., Smyth, D. G. and Snell, C. R. (1976). In *Polypeptide Hormones: molecular and cellular aspects.* (eds R. Porter and D. W. Fitzsimons) Ciba Foundation Symp. 41 (new series), Amsterdam, Elsevier/Excerpta Medica/North Holland, pp. 61–75

Harris, J. I. and Lerner, A. B. (1957). *Nature,* **179**, 1346–7

Mains, R. E., Eipper, B. A. and Ling, N. (1977). *Proc. natn. Acad. Sci. U.S.A.*, **74**, 3014–18.

Rees, L. H., Cook, D. M., Kendall, J. W., Allen, C. F., Kramer, R. M., Ratcliffe, J. G. and Knight, R. A. (1971). *Endocrinology*, **89**, 254–61

Rudman, D., Del Rio, A. E., Hollins, B. M., Houser, D. H., Keeling, M. E., Sutin, J., Scott, J. W., Sears, R. A. and Rosenberg, M. Z. (1973). *Endocrinology,* **92**, 372–9

Smyth, D. G., Snell, C. R. and Massey, D. E. (1978). *Biochem. J.* (in press)

Weissman, B. A., Gershon, H. and Pert, C. B. (1976). *FEBS Lett.*, **70**, 245–8

cold-water swims & forced running ↓ [³H]-D-Ala²-Met⁵-Enk amide binding
∴ endorphins are occupying OR's.
heat stress no effect on " "
sleep deprivation ↑ " "
sleep dep effect doesn't make sense, Should be a stress, yet seemingly doesn't release endorphins to occupy OR's

8

Behavioral manipulation of rats causes alterations in opiate receptor occupancy

Candace B. Pert and Donald L. Bowie (Section on Biochemistry and Pharmacology, Biological Psychiatry Branch, National Institute of Mental Health, Bethesda, Maryland)

The notion that about half of the opiate receptors of rat brain are associated with endogenous ligand even after extensive washing of brain membranes at 0 °C explains a number of observations: if brain membranes are subjected to a preliminary incubation at 37 °C, subsequent binding of [^{3}H] opiates is approximately doubled, the assumption being that the endogenous ligand, by dissociating much more rapidly at the higher incubation temperature, makes additional opiate receptor sites available for binding (Pasternak *et al.,* 1975*a*, *b*). If sodium chloride is included in the preincubation medium—even at 0 °C—the subsequent binding of [^{3}H] opiates is similarly increased (Simantov *et al.,* 1976). The agonist dihydromorphine, has been shown to dissociate from opiate receptors about three times more rapidly in the presence of sodium ion at 0 °C (Pert and Snyder, 1974), and the assumption is that sodium ion also speeds up the dissociation of the endogenous opiate agonist. In other experiments, membrane preparations from rats injected with low doses of opiate antagonists or high doses of opiate agonists show almost twice as much [^{3}H] opiate binding after extensive washing at 0 °C than saline-injected controls. If the assay is conducted in the presence of sodium, however, the control membrane preparations become elevated to the level of the membranes from opiate-injected rats so that a significant difference between the two is no longer apparent (Pert and Snyder, 1976). These findings can be explained if the opiate alkaloids displace some of the endogenous ligand from opiate receptors *in vivo* and the remaining endogenous ligand (except in the presence of sodium ion) dissociates much more slowly from opiate receptors during membrane preparation than the opiate alkaloids.

We now report some of the characteristics of the binding of [^{3}H] [D-Ala^2, Met^5]-enkephalinamide to rat brain membranes. This enkephalin analogue retains 50 per cent of its affinity for opiate receptors while entirely losing its susceptibility to enzymatic degradation by dilute brain membrane preparations (Pert *et al.*, 1976). Using the [^{3}H] [D-Ala^2] analogue as a prototype endogenous peptide ligand, we observe that the ion dependence of its dissociation from opiate receptors is identical to that expected of the endogenous ligand as ascertained from preincubation experiments. Furthermore, we demonstrate that it is possible to alter receptor occupancy by submitting rats to behavioral manipulation immediately before decapitation.

METHODS

See figure and table legends.

RESULTS

The association of the [^{3}H] [D-Ala^2] analogue is shown in figure 8.1. At both temperatures, the active opiate levorphanol displaces about 80 per cent of the total binding while dextrorphan, its pharmacologically inert enantiomer, is without effect at the same concentration (1×10^{-6} M). This suggests that 80 per cent

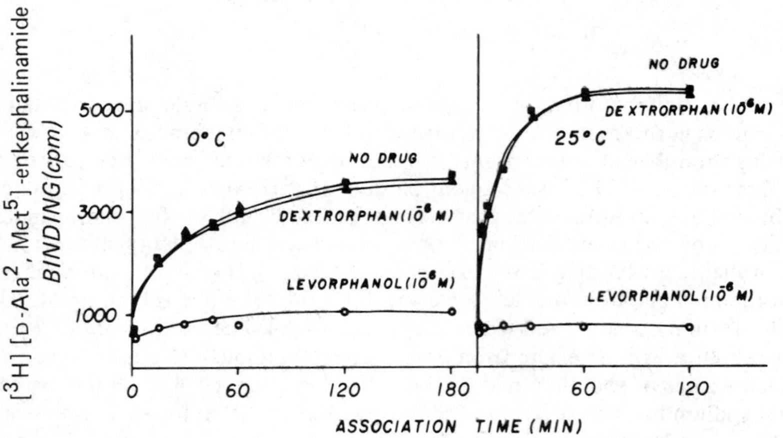

Figure 8.1 Association of [^{3}H] [D-Ala^2, Met^5]-enkephalinamide. Two rats were decapitated; the cerebellum was removed and the brain homogenized in 100 vol of cold (4 °C) Tris buffer (Trizma Preset Crystals, pH 7.0 at 25 °C) with a Polytron at setting 5 for 15 s. The crude homogenate was centrifuged at 12 000 *g* for 15 min; the supernatant was discarded. The pellet was again suspended in 100 vol of cold buffer and centrifuged again at 12 000 *g* for 15 min. The pellet was resuspended in 20 ml of cold buffer, vortexed (approximately 10 s) and polytroned briefly. 100 μl each of homogenate was added to duplicate samples using 10 $\times$ 75 mm glass test tubes, at appropriate temperatures, containing the following: 50 000 c.p.m. of the [^{3}H] [D-Ala^2]-analogue (New England Nuclear, 47 Ci/mmol), sufficient buffer for a 500 μl assay. At each subsequent time point (abscissa), duplicate samples were vortexed briefly, then filtered through Whatman GF/B filters under reduced pressure and washed with two 7 ml portions of cold buffer in a cycle less than 10 s in duration. Each filter was placed in a vial with 10 ml scintillation fluid (Aquasol, New England Nuclear) and counted in a Beckman LS-230 Scintillation Counter at an efficiency of 40%. Duplicate control samples containing 10^{-6} M levorphanol (○) and 10^{-6} M dextrorphan (▲) were also filtered at each time point.

of the binding is stereospecific and pharmacologically relevant. In all subsequent experiments, levorphanol (1×10^{-6} M) was used as a 'blank' value which was subtracted from the binding which occurred without the presence of a cold drug to obtain 'specific binding.' At 0 °C, the [^{3}H] [D-Ala^2] analogue equilibrates very slowly, requiring about 2 h. Binding at 25 °C occurs more rapidly, reaching an equilibrium which is about 30 per cent higher at 1 h. The calculated k_1 at 0°C and 25°C are respectively 2.4×10^7/M min and 9.6×10^7/M min.

The effects of manganese ion and sodium ion on [^{3}H] [D-Ala^2, Met^5]-enkephalinamide binding are shown in table 8.1. At 25 °C, manganese ion enhances receptor binding with as little as 0.5 mM manganese chloride, an effect previously

Table 8.1 Effect of ions on the binding of [^{3}H] [D-Ala^2, Met^5]-enkephalinamide

[Mn^{2+}] (mM)	Binding (c.p.m.) 0 °C	Binding (c.p.m.) 25 °C	[Na^+] (mM)	Binding (c.p.m.) 25 °C	[$Na^+ + Mn^{2+}$] (mM)	Binding (c.p.m.) 25 °C
0	727	742	1	743	1 + 3	1245
0.1	–	800	5	820	5 + 3	1097
0.5	593	1632	20	841	20 + 3	1066
1	634	1123	100	461	100 + 3	828
3	547	1144				
5	462	1109				
10	328	1038				

The opiate receptor homogenate was prepared as described in figure 8.1. 100 μl of the homogenate was added to an assay mixture containing 5 000 c.p.m., 0.24 mM [^{3}H] [D-Ala^2, Met^5]-enkephalinamide concentrated ion to give the indicated final concentraction, and sufficient buffer for a 500 μl assay. Incubation was carried out at 25 °C for 60 min or 0 °C for 120 min. Samples were counted as described in figure 8.1.

reported for opiate alkaloid agonists (Pasternak *et al.*, 1975*b*). Sodium chloride which reduces binding of the analogue at 100 mM appears to be less inhibitory compared to its effects on alkaloid agonists (Pert and Snyder, 1974; Simon *et al.*, 1973), while manganese ion appears to be able to 'counteract' the inhibitory effect of sodium ion. Strangely, when the assay is conducted at 0°C, manganese has a marked inhibitory effect on binding.

Figure 8.2 shows the effects of added ions on the dissociation rate of [^{3}H] [D-Ala^2] analogue. At 25 °C manganese ions slow the rate of dissociation of the analogue from the receptors by about twofold, whereas sodium ions cause a threefold increase in the dissociation rate. Manganese and sodium ions added together appear to 'counteract each other' and restore the dissociation rate to that which occurs when no ions are added. The effects of the ions on dissociation rate are sufficient to account for their effects on specific binding. At 0 °C, the half-lives of [^{3}H] [D-Ala^2] dissociation from opiate receptors are 26 min (in the presence of NaCl) and 64 min when no ions are added (data not shown). Curiously, at 0 °C manganese decreases receptor binding by about 50 per cent, just as previously reported for opiate alkaloid agonists (Pasternak *et al.*, 1975*b*), and at 0 °C the half-life of manganese dissociation is decreased to 50 min.

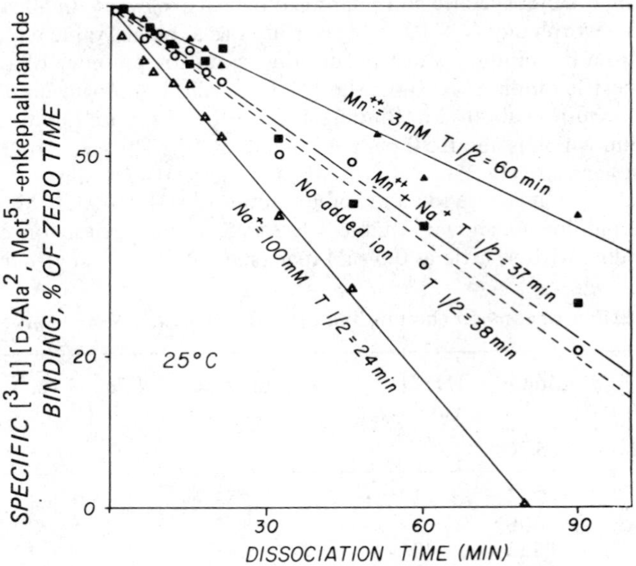

Figure 8.2 Dissociation of endogenous ligand at 25 °C. The homogenate was prepared as in figure 8.1 up to the point of the second suspension. The pellets were resuspended (100 vol) in cold buffer containing 100 mM NaCl. The suspension was homogenized briefly and allowed to incubate for 1 h at 0 °C. At 1 h the homogenate was centrifuged at 12 000 *g* for 15 min. The pellet was resuspended in exactly 100 vol of cold buffer containing 50 000 c.p.m. [^{3}H] [D-Ala^2, Met^5]-enkephalinamide/ml and 3 mM $MnCl_2$. The homogenate was then allowed to incubate for 2 h at 25 °C. At this time 30 ml was aliquoted into 4 tubes and centrifuged at 12 000 *g* for 15 min. The pellets were resuspended in 30 ml buffer at 25 °C and poured into Erlenmeyer flasks containing enough concentrated ions and cold [D-Ala^2, Met^5]-enkephalinamide to give a final resuspension of the following: (1) no ions (○); (2) 3 mM $MnCl_2$ (▲) + 10^{-7} M cold [D-Ala^2, Met^5]-enkephalinamide; (3) 100 mM NaCl (△) + 10^{-7} M cold [D-Ala^2, Met^5]-enkephalinamide; and (4) 3 mM $MnCl_2$ + 100 mM NaCl (♦) + 10^{-7} M cold [D-Ala^2, Met^5]-enkephalinamide. Two ml of each homogenate was filtered per time point in alternating cycles. For the zero time point, the 30 ml was added to the flask containing the ions and cold [D-Ala^2, Met^5]-enkephalinamide, swirled briefly and 2 × 2 ml filtered immediately. Samples were then prepared for counting as described in figure 8.1.

From experiments shown in figure 8.3 and table 8.2, the ion dependence of the dissociation of the endogenous ligand from opiate receptors can be indirectly surmised. Membranes were washed once and then allowed to dissociate in various ionic media for 0, 30 or 60 min. They were then centrifuged, resuspended in a buffer containing no added ions and incubated with [^{3}H] [D-Ala^2] for exactly 30 min at 0 °C (figure 8.3). Inclusion of sodium in the preincubation medium resulted in a time-dependent increase in the sites available for binding, consistent with an increased dissociation rate of the endogenous ligand from the membrane receptors. On the other hand, manganese reduced the number of sites available for binding, presumably by slowing the dissociation rate of the endogenous ligand from the membrane receptors. Inclusion of both sodium and manganese gave intermediate binding which is consistent with the counteractive effect seen on

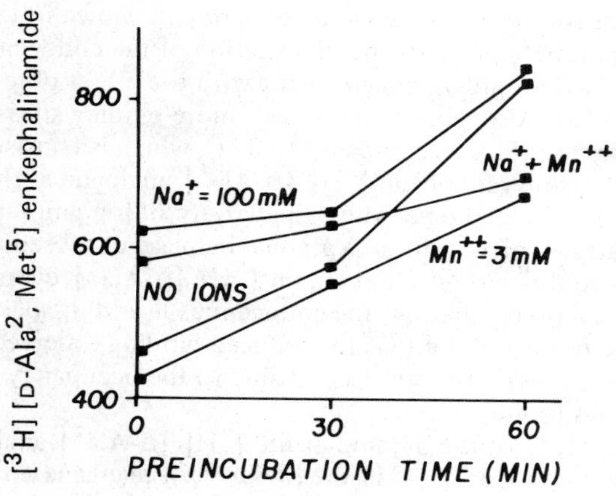

Figure 8.3 Ion dependence of dissociation of endogenous ligand(s) from brain membranes. Preincubation time course and ion effect on the stereospecific binding of [^{3}H] [D-Ala^2, Met^5]-enkephalinamide. Two rat brain homogenates were prepared as described in figure 8.1 and 4 × 30 ml portions were submitted to the final centrifugation. The pellets were resuspended in 100 vol cold buffer containing either 3 mM $MnCl_2$, 100 mM NaCl, no ions, or 3 mM $MnCl_2$ and 100 mM NaCl together, and were allowed to incubate at 25 °C for the indicated time, centrifuged at 12 000 *g* for 10 min and then resuspended in 2.7 ml cold buffer. Homogenates from each time point were then assayed immediately as in figure 8.1 for exactly 30 min at 0 °C. Levorphanol (10^{-6} M) controls were assayed with each ionic condition.

Table 8.2 Binding of [^{3}H] [D-Ala^2, Met^5]-enkephalinamide after preincubation under various conditions

Preincubation conditions	Binding (c.p.m.)
1 h	
0 °C	
No ion	710
3 mM $MnCl_2$	919
100 nM NaCl	1779
Na + Mn	1885
25 °C	
No ion	1177
3 mM $MnCl_2$	977
100 mM NaCl	1527
Na + Mn	1290

Brain homogenates were preincubated as in figure 8.3 at 0 and 25 °C for 1 h with either NaCl (100 mM), no added ions, $MnCl_2$ (3 mM) or NaCl + $MnCl_2$. The homogenates were each centrifuged at 12 000 *g* for 15 min, resuspended in 10 ml cold buffer and assayed as in figure 8.1 for 60 min.

[^{3}H] [D-Ala^2] dissociation. In a separate experiment shown in table 8.2, it is apparent that manganese prevents the dissociation of the endogenous ligand at 25 °C but not at 0 °C, a finding in agreement with the effect observed on [^{3}H] [D-Ala^2] dissociation. Also, about 40 per cent more binding sites become available after preincubation at 25 °C as compared to 0 °C, which is consistent with the two-fold greater dissociation rate of the [^{3}H] [D-Ala^2] analogue at the higher temperature in the absence of added ions. Thus, the pattern of ion and temperature effects during preincubation which result in a gradual increase in subsequent binding is strikingly similar to the pattern observed on [^{3}H] [D-Ala^2] dissociation. This suggests that during preincubation, the endogenous ligand dissociates slowly from membrane opiate receptors and that the reduced binding observed after minimal dissociation has been permitted to occur is due to the occupancy of opiate receptors by endogenous ligand.

A Scatchard analysis of the binding of the [^{3}H] [D-Ala^2] analogue to non-preincubated membranes at 25 °C in the presence of manganese ion is shown in figure 8.4. Binding can be resolved into a high (2.7×10^{-10}) affinity and low

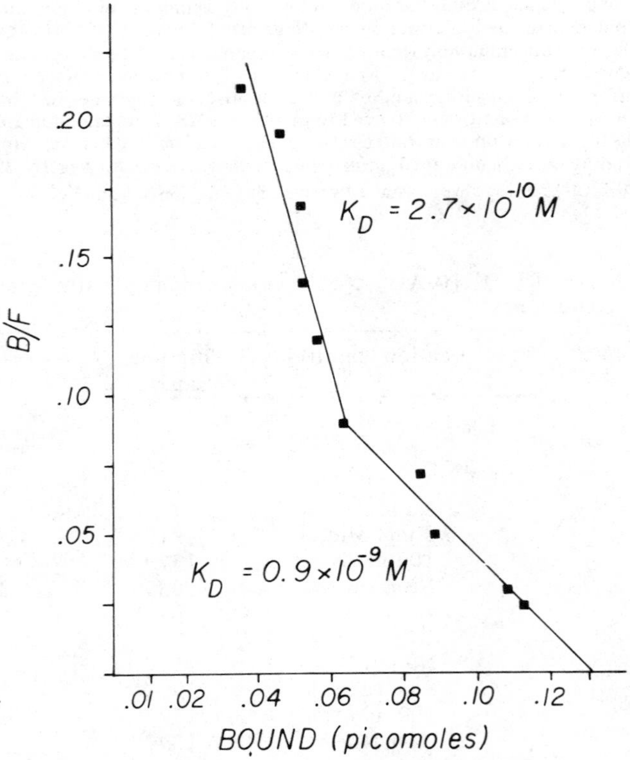

Figure 8.4 Scatchard analysis of the saturable binding of [^{3}H] [D-Ala^2, Met^5]-enkephalinamide. The opiate assay was performed as in figure 8.1 except the amounts of [^{3}H] [D-Ala^2, Met^5]-enkephalinamide varied between 5 000 c.p.m. (0.24 nM) and 200 000 c.p.m. (9.6 nM) and Mn^{2+} (3 mM) was included. The samples were incubated at 25°C for 60 min, then filtered and counted as described in figure 8.1.

(0.9×10^{-9}) affinity component. Calculation of the dissociation constant using the appropriate k_1 and k_{-1} determined by direct measurement 1.2×10^{-10} M, a value in close agreement with the high affinity site as determined by Scatchard analysis.

Presumably, the amount of binding detectable in brain homogenates maintained at 0 °C is inversely proportional to the level of opiate receptor occupancy in the animal at the moment of death—or at least homogenization. Since the brain is originally homogenized in a large volume (100 vol) and the supernatant fluid containing released endorphins is rapidly removed, it seems unlikely that increased association of receptors with endorphins could occur after homogenization. Opiate receptor ligand probably begins to dissociate from the moment of homogenization. The dissociation rate at 0 °C, however, is fairly slow, so that perhaps half of the receptor-bound ligand is lost by the time the assay is complete, assuming identical dissociation rates for [D-Ala^2, Met^5]-enkephalinamide and the actual endogenous ligand. Conceivably, the true endogenous ligand may dissociate even more slowly so that very little receptor-bound ligand is lost. In order to ascertain whether significant alterations in opiate receptor occupancy occur at decapitation or in the minutes between decapitation and homogenization, three groups of six rats each were compared. One group was decapitated, dissected and homogenized immediately, one was decapitated and the head allowed to remain at room temperature for 1 hour before removal of the brain and the third was decapitated after spending 1 hour under sodium pentobarbitone anesthesia (50 mg/kg). There was no significant difference in the binding of the [^{3}H] [D-Ala^2] analogue among these three groups, the values being respectively 1096 ± 156 c.p.m., 1083 ± 140 c.p.m. and 1301 ± 151 c.p.m. This experiment suggests that apparent opiate receptor occupancy as measured by binding of the [^{3}H] [D-Ala^2] analogue is related to conditions in the animals' brain at the last moment before decapitation.

In order to investigate the possibility that profound stress alters opiate receptor occupancy, rats were forced to swim in an ice-water bath for 5 min. After this, they were removed and allowed to recuperate in an individual cage for various times before decapitation. The control group was merely placed in the empty ice bucket for 5 min. The results of this experiment are shown in figure 8.5. There is no difference between [^{3}H] [D-Ala^2] binding in the individually assayed brains of the control group, the rats killed immediately after the ice-water swim and the rats allowed to recover for 5 min. However, after 15 and 20 min of recovery from the ice-water swim, [^{3}H] [D-Ala^2] binding in rat brains was reduced by about 40 per cent. By 45 min, binding had returned to control levels. To ascertain that diminished binding in the stressed group was really due to increased receptor occupancy by endogenous ligand, individual homogenates from the stressed and control rats were preincubated at 0 °C with and without added sodium ions and at 25 °C with and without added manganese ions (table 8.3). Inclusion of 100 mM sodium chloride in the preincubation media raised the binding in the homogenates of the stressed animals' brains to control levels. Preincubation at 25 °C also reversed the reduction in binding in the homogenates from stressed animals. However, by including manganese ion in the preincubation medium at 25 °C, the difference between the stressed and control animals is preserved. These results are consistent with the notion that sodium ion and increased preincubation temperature both accelerate the dissociation of endogenous ligand from the membrane receptors, while manganese ion somehow stabilizes the ligand–receptor complex.

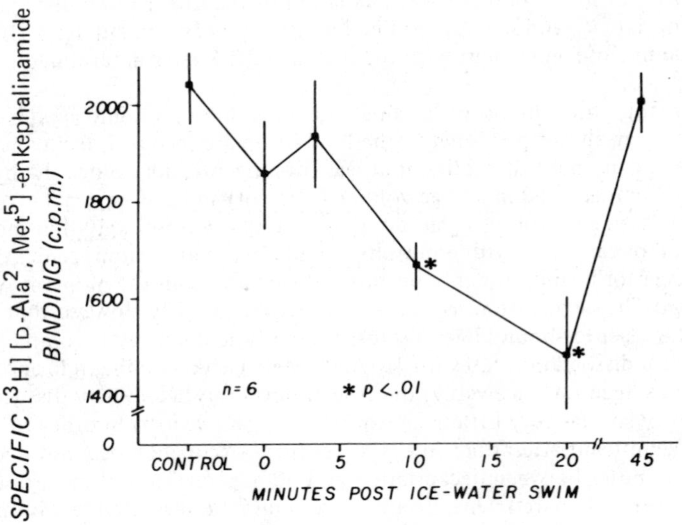

Figure 8.5 Assay of cold-stressed rats for stereospecific [^{3}H] [D-Ala^2, Met^5]-enkephalinamide binding. Rats were placed in a bucket containing ice water (4 °C) for 5 min and allowed to swim freely. At the end of the swim period they were placed in a plastic cage containing pine chips for the indicated time to recover. Control rats were placed in an empty bucket for 5 min and then placed in a cage for the indicated recovery period. n = 6 for all groups. At the end of this period, the rats were decapitated in a counterbalanced order and the brains (minus the cerebellum) were frozen in dry ice. The brains were weighed and then individually assayed for displacement of [^{3}H] [D-Ala^2, Met^5]-enkephalinamide for 60 min at 0 °C as described in figure 8.1.

The apparent increased opiate receptor occupancy is due either to an increased release of enkephalin or endorphin on to opiate receptors or else a slowing of their dissociation rate from receptors. In either case, such an enhanced opiate receptor occupancy must surely alter the psychological state of the rats into something which might be most aptly designated 'relief euphoria.' In any case, as shown in table 8.4, heat stress is unable to alter opiate receptor occupancy either immediately or after a 10 min recovery.

As shown in table 8.5, brains of rats who are deprived of sleep for 24 h by confinement in a slowly rotating drum (Stefurak *et al.*, 1977) bind about 25 per cent more [^{3}H] [D-Ala^2] analogue than controls. Apparently, opiate receptor occupancy is reduced during sleep deprivation so that it might be surmised that sleep either releases endorphins and/or enkephalins or results in their slower dissociation from receptors.

The effect of mild exercise was examined (figure 8.6) by forcing rats to run in an activity wheel for 15 min. Their brains showed a decrease in [^{3}H] [D-Ala^2] binding immediately after the cessation of running. Binding levels returned to control values rapidly, within 5 to 10 min. The pool of receptor-associated endorphin is presumably the pool of the greatest functional significance. Cessation of running must therefore be correlated in rats with a euphoric feeling induced by increased opiate receptor occupancy.

Table 8.3 Stress-induced alterations in opiate receptor occupancy are modified by ionic conditions

Preincubation	Binding (c.p.m.)		% Change
	Control	Stressed	
0 °C			
No ion added	1136 ± 142	593 ± 201*	–48
100 mM NaCl	1351 ± 398	1355 ± 606	0
25 °C			
No ion added	1483 ± 191	1307 ± 205	0
3 mM $MnCl_2$	1303 ± 150	948 ± 122*	–27

*$P < 0.01$

Four rats were subjected to cold stress as described in figure 8.5 and allowed to recover for 20 min. The brains (minus the cerebellum) of control and stressed rats were obtained in a counter-balanced fashion and frozen in dry ice. After weighing, the brains were homogenized in 100 vol cold buffer and two 12 ml aliquots of the homogenate of each rat were preincubated at 0 °C ±100 mM NaCl and two aliquots were preincubated at 25 °C ± 3 mM $Mncl_2$ for 60 min. The homogenate was centrifuged at 12 000 *g* for 10 min and resuspended in 800 μl cold Tris buffer. 100 μl aliquots of each homogenate were assayed in duplicate with 50 000 c.p.m. at 0 °C for 60 min. Control values of duplicate 10^{-6} M levorphanol were also assayed with each preincubation ionic condition. Samples were filtered and counted as in figure 8.1.

Table 8.4 Heat stress does not affect opiate receptor occupancy

	[^{3}H] [D-Ala^2, Met^5]-enkephalinamide binding (c.p.m.)
Control	1455 ± 144
Immediately after heating (5 min at 70 °C)	1598 ± 105
After 10 min recovery	1501 ± 36

Rats (n = 6) were placed in an oven set at 70 °C in a cage containing saw chips for 5 min. One group was allowed to recover in a cage from the heat for 10 min at room temperature. Control rats were placed in a cold oven for 5 min and then in the cage for 10 min. The brains were removed and assayed at 0 °C for 60 min as described in figure 8.1.

Table 8.5 Sleep deprivation reduces opiate receptor occupancy

	[^{3}H] [D-Ala^2, Met^5]-enkephalinamide
Control	1172 ± 73
Sleep deprived (24 h)	1446 ± 99*

Six rats sleep-deprived by the method of Stefurak *et al.* (1977) were killed alternately with six control rats maintained for 24 h with access to the same amount of food and water. Individual rat brains were assayed as in figure 8.5 (Mendleson, Gillin, Wyatt and Pert, unpublished).

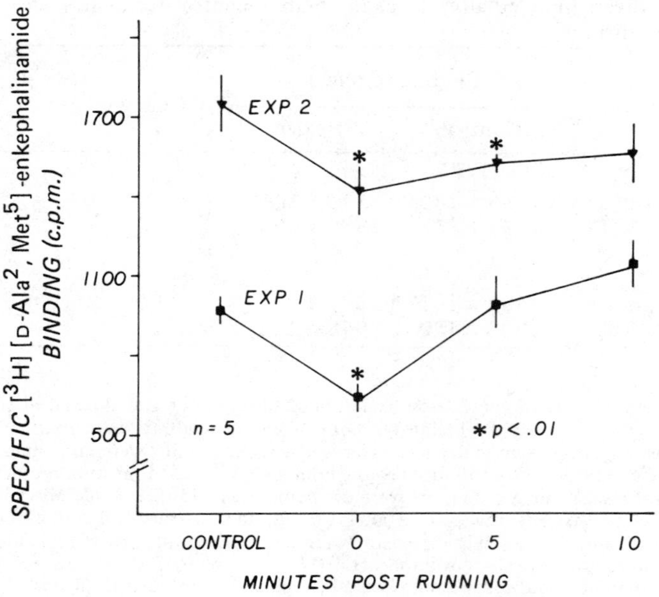

Figure 8.6 Effect of exercise on stereospecific [^{3}H] [D-Ala^2, Met^5]-enkephalinamide binding. Each rat was placed in a rotating drum that was coupled to a laboratory stirrer motor (T-Line Model 106, Talboys Engineering, Emerson, New Jersey) and was forced to run for 15 min at 40–50 r.p.m. At the end of the forced run they were sacrificed or allowed to recover in a plastic cage containing pine chips for the indicated time. The brains (minus the cerebellum) were removed in a counterbalanced order, frozen in dry ice and subsequently assayed individually for 60 min at 0 °C for displacement of stereospecific [^{3}H] [D-Ala^2, Met^5]-enkephalinamide binding as described in figure 8.1.

DISCUSSION

We have demonstrated that the binding of [^{3}H] [D-Ala^2, Met^5]-enkephalinamide to rat brain membranes is susceptible to modification by the inclusion of sodium or manganese ion in the incubation medium. These effects, moreover, were due to effects on receptor dissociation. Association rates were not affected by ionic manipulations (data not shown).

We tested the assumption that reduced binding seen in homogenates that have been thoroughly washed but maintained at 0 °C is due to the 'clogging' of opiate receptors with endogenous ligand so that the radiolabeled ligand cannot gain access. The reduced binding can be reversed in a time-dependent fashion by inclusion of sodium ion at 0 °C or by increasing the temperature to 25 °C. At 25 °C, manganese ion is able to prolong the reduced binding. This pattern of ion and temperature susceptibility is identical to the pattern of effects on the dissociation rate of a [^{3}H] peptide agonist, [^{3}H] [D-Ala^2, Met^5]-enkephalinamide.

By rapidly homogenizing brains in a large volume of ice-cold buffer, preparing well-washed membranes and carrying out the assay at 0 °C, endogenous ligand associated with opiate receptors at the time of the animals' death can be estimated.

We have shown that cold stress and exercise both increase opiate receptor occupancy. Sleep deprivation diminishes opiate receptor occupancy by endogenous ligand.

Apparent receptor heterogeneity may result from differential occupancy

In these experiments, there appears to be an overall average of 50 per cent occupancy of opiate receptors in rat brain. This level is altered by various physiological states. Presumably there is a very wide range of differing receptor occupancies in various brain areas mediating differing behaviors. A cluster of receptors on a given neuron which is 90 per cent occupied by endorphins (and hence 90 per cent in the agonist conformation) would be expected to respond very differently to the application of a mixed agonist–antagonist than would another neuron which is only 10 per cent occupied (90 per cent in the antagonist conformation). Thus, differing occupancy by endogenous ligands would be expected to produce an apparent receptor heterogeneity. Presumably the endogenous ligands, like [D-Ala^2, Met^5]-enkephalinamide, have a very slow dissociation rate relative to the dissociation rates of the alkaloid agonists and antagonists. Thus, when receptor dissociation is the rate-limiting step the alkaloids would be expected to compete much less efficiently with endogenous ligands and this is, in fact, what is seen in competitive binding studies (Lord *et al.*, 1977).

Opiate receptor occupancy and chronic opiate administration

It is worth speculating about the mechanism of the development of tolerance and physical dependence in the light of the new way that we must envisage opiate receptors. The opiate receptors on each neuron must be differentially associated with endogenous ligand so that they have an accustomed neurophysiological 'set point' determined by the proportion of opiate receptors occupied and hence held in the agonist conformation. It seems reasonable to assume, as proposed originally by Kosterlitz and Hughes (1975), that endogenous ligand synthesis and release must gradually slow down in response to repeated flooding of the brain with opiates.

If the proportion of receptors in the agonist conformation (the homeostatic 'set point') is to remain constant, the inevitable consequence of diminished endorphin/enkephalin release is that opiate alkaloids will gradually replace endorphins on the receptor. Since opiate alkaloids have a much faster dissociation rate than endorphins, their ability to 'hold' the receptor in the agonist state is greatly reduced. Thus, larger and larger doses of morphine would be required to achieve the same degree of transformation into the agonist state since less slowly dissociating endorphin would be present to 'lend a hand'. This would account for tolerance.

Withdrawal signs would become apparent when the 'set point' is exceeded by conversion into the antagonist conformation due to morphine's dissociation from the receptors, the abstinence syndrome becoming more pronounced with time as morphine's contribution to receptor occupancy increased. Smaller doses of antagonist would be expected to precipitate withdrawal as tolerance progressed, since morphine would be expected to be more readily displaced than endorphin. Experimental support for this speculation is lacking (Pert and Snyder, 1976), but it may be necessary to use other methods (radioimmunoassay?) which discriminate between opiate and endorphin-occupied receptors.

REFERENCES

Kosterlitz, H. W. and Hughes, J. (1975). In *The Opiate Narcotics,* (ed. A. Goldstein) Pergamon Press, New York pp. 245–50
Lord, J. A. H., Waterfield, A. A., Hughes, J. and Kosterlitz, H. W. (1977). *Nature,* **267**, 445–9
Pasternak, G. W., Wilson, R. H. and Snyder, S. H. (1975*a*). *Molec. Pharmac.,* **11**, 340–51
Pasternak, G. W., Snowman, A. M. and Snyder, S. H. (1975*b*). *Molec. Pharmac.,* **11**, 735–44
Pert, C. B. and Snyder, S. H. (1974). *Molec. Pharmac.,* **10**, 868–79
Pert, C. B. and Snyder, S. H. (1976). *Biochem. Pharmac.,* **25**, 847–53
Pert, C. B., Pert, A., Chang, J–K. and Fong, B. T. W. (1976). *Science,* **194**, 330–2
Simantov, R., Snowman, A. M. and Snyder, S. H. (1976). *Molec. Pharmac.,* **12**, 977–86
Simon, E. J., Hiller, J. M. and Edelman, I. (1973). *Proc. natn. Acad. Sci. U.S.A.,* **70**, 1947–9
Stefurak, S. J., Stefurak, M. L., Mendelson, W. B., Gillin, J. C. and Wyatt, R. J. (1977). *Pharmac. Biochem. Behav.,* **6**, 137–9

9

Participation of [Met^5]-enkephalin in the action of antipsychotic drugs

J. S. Hong, H.-Y. T. Yang, J. C. Gillin*, W. Fratta and E. Costa,
(Laboratory of Preclinical Pharmacology and
*Laboratory of Clinical Psychopharmacology,
National Institute of Mental Health,
Saint Elizabeths Hospital
Washington, DC 20032, U.S.A.)

Several lines of indirect investigation indicate that the two polypeptides, [Leu^5] and [Met^5]-enkephalin which are stored in brain neurons and function as endogenous ligands for opiate receptors may be operative in a number of brain functions including regulation of extrapyramidal motility, reward seeking behavior and responsiveness to aversive stimuli. This notion is consistent with the high content of [Met^5]-enkephalin in striatum, nucleus accumbens, amygdala and nucleus interpeduncularis (Hong *et al.*, 1977*b*). In rats, the intraventricular injection of β-endorphin, like that of morphine, decreases spontaneous motor activity, elicits muscular rigidity (Bloom *et al.*, 1977) and reduces the acetylcholine metabolism in hippocampus via a regulation of the trans-synaptic activation taking place in septum (Moroni *et al.*, 1977*a, b*). Belluzzi and Stein (1977) reported that the pattern of [Met^5] and [Leu^5]-enkephalin self-administration in rats is consistent with the hypothesis that [Leu^5] and [Met^5]-enkephalin mediate the drive-reducing reward function. Thus, they propose a model in which drive-inducing and drive-reducing reward function are mediated by norepinephrine and [Met^5]-enkephalin, respectively. Furthermore, recent reports concerning clinical experiments with naloxone (Gunne *et al.*, 1977; Davis *et al.*, 1977; Janowsky *et al.*, 1977) and β-endorphin (Kline *et al.*, 1977) on mental patients encourage the working hypothesis that an abnormality in the function of endogenous opiate peptides may be operative in psychosis.

In an attempt to contribute additional evidence on the possible roles of [Met^5] and [Leu^5]-enkephalin in psychosis, we studied the effects of chronic administration of psychotropic agents on the [Met^5]-enkephalin content in striatum and in several other brain regions. Chronic administration of cataleptogenic antischizophrenic drugs endowed with dopamine (DA) receptor blocking activity selectively increase the [Met^5]-enkephalin content of striatum and nucleus accumbens which are innervated by DA terminals. In addition, chronic administration of lithium (Li) or reserpine or brain hemitransection also increases the [Met^5]-enkephalin content of rat striatum. Since the characteristics of the action of antischizophrenics on striatal [Met^5]-enkephalin content differ from those of Li, on the basis of such circumstantial evidence we have proposed as a working hypothesis that despite the apparent similarity, the mechanism whereby striatal [Met^5]-enkephalin is increased by reserpine, antischizophrenics and brain hemisection differs from the increase caused by Li.

ROLE OF MONOAMINERGIC NEURONS IN THE REGULATION OF STRIATAL MET-ENKEPHALIN CONTENT

Striatal [Met^5]-enkephalin content after hemitransection

To explore whether striatal [Met^5]-enkephalin neurons are regulated trans-synaptically by dopaminergic axon terminals, we have determined the striatal [Met^5]-enkephalin content following the interruption of dopaminergic transmission by a unilateral brain hemitransection. The procedure for hemitransection has been described previously (Hong *et al.*, 1977*c*). Seven days after hemitransection, striatal [Met^5]-enkephalin content of the hemitransected side tends to be higher than that of the contralateral intact side but this difference was not statistically significant. However, 30 days after the hemitransection, the [Met^5]-enkephalin content of the hemitransected side is about 70 per cent higher than the contralateral side (figure 9.1); the [Met^5]-enkephalin content of the latter was always equal to that of unoperated control rats.

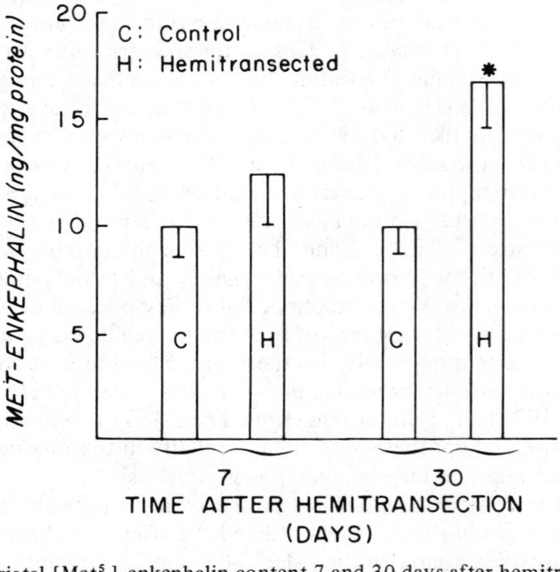

Figure 9.1 Striatal [Met^5]-enkephalin content 7 and 30 days after hemitransection (AP 4380 μM according to König and Klippel (1967)). [Met^5]-enkephalin was determined by the radioimmunoassay method described previously by Yang *et al.* (1977).

Striatal [Met^5]-enkephalin content after chronic treatment with reserpine
Since striatum receives monoaminergic fibers which originate from the cell bodies located in mesencephalon and rhombencephalon, in order to ascertain whether the increase of striatal [Met^5]-enkephalin elicited by hemitransection was due to a monoaminergic denervation of this brain structure, we have studied whether reserpine, one of the major tranquilizers used in the past to deplete serotonin and catecholamine content from axon terminals, like hemitransection, increased striatal [Met^5]-enkephalin content. Chronic treatment with reserpine (0.5 mg/kg day, i.p) for 10 days doubled the striatal [Met^5]-enkephalin content (table 9.1).

Table 9.1 Effect of chronic administration of reserpine (0.5 mg/kg day, i.p.) on striatal [Met^5]-enkephalin

Treatment	Period of treatment (day)	[Met^5]-enkephalin (ng/mg protein)
Saline	1	10 ± 0.8
Saline	10	10 ± 1.0
Reserpine	1	9.5 ± 1.0
Reserpine	10	20 ± 2.5*

Reserpine was given at the rate of 0.5 mg/kg day, i.p.
*$P < 0.001$ compared with saline-treated rats. $N = 6$–10.

The striatal [Met^5]-enkephalin content remained unchanged in rats killed 3 hours after a single injection of reserpine (0.5 mg/kg i.p.), suggesting that the action of reserpine on striatal [Met^5]-enkephalin content occurred after a certain time delay.

STRIATAL [MET^5]-ENKEPHALIN CONTENT FOLLOWING CHRONIC TREATMENT WITH HALOPERIDOL

Dose response
Haloperidol, a DA receptor blocker, was used to disclose whether catecholamines or serotonin are involved in reserpine induced increase of striatal [Met^5]-enkephalin content. A single dose of haloperidol (2 mg/kg) failed to change the [Met^5]-enkephalin content of rat hypothalamus and striatum, whereas a chronic administration of haloperidol (2 mg/kg daily i.p., for 3 weeks) doubled the [Met^5]-enkephalin content of rat striatum (table 9.2). In the same brain, the [Met^5]-enkephalin content of hypothalamus, medulla oblongata, septum and pituitary remained unchanged.

Successive experiments have shown that the increase in striatal [Met^5]-enkephalin content is proportional to the dose of haloperidol. A dose close to an average clinical dose (0.1 mg/kg i.p.) given daily for 3 weeks appears to be greater

Table 9.2 Graded increase of striatal [Met^5]-enkephalin after chronic administration of various doses of haloperidol for 3 weeks

Dose (mg/kg day)	[Met^5]-enkephalin (ng/mg protein)	% of control
0	10 ± 1.2	
0.1	13.5 ± 1.5	135
0.25	14.5 ± 1.5	145
0.5	16 ± 2.0	160
1.0	20 ± 3.5	200
2.0	20 ± 4.0	200

Each value is the mean ± s.e.m. of at least six determinations.
All the values are significantly different from the value of saline-treated controls ($P < 0.05$).

than the threshold dose necessary to elicit a significant accumulation of [Met^5]-enkephalin in striatum. A maximal accumulation of striatal [Met^5]-enkephalin was obtained after a daily dose of 1 mg/kg (table 9.2).

Time Course

Rats received 1 mg/kg of haloperidol i.p. for various periods so we could study whether the duration of the treatment influenced the extent of the increase in striatal [Met^5]-enkephalin content. The striatal [Met^5]-enkephalin content gradually increased from 10 ng/mg protein (0 day) to 14 ng/mg (1 week), 18 ng/mg protein (2 weeks) and 20 ng/mg protein (3 weeks) (table 9.3). In other experiments, we studied how long the increase of striatal [Met^5]-enkephalin persisted when haloperidol treatment was discontinued. Rats were killed at various

Table 9.3 Time course of the increase in striatal [Met^5]-enkephalin following chronic administration of haloperidol

Period of treatment (day)	[Met^5]-enkephalin (ng/mg protein)	% of control	P
Saline	10 ± 1.2		
1	9.5 ± 1.0	95	>0.05
7	14 ± 1.8	140	<0.05
14	18 ± 2.2	180	<0.001
21	20 ± 2.5	200	<0.001

Each value is the mean ± s.e.m. of at least six determinations. Day 1 represents animals killed 1 hour after receiving one injection of haloperidol (1 mg/kg). Haloperidol was given at the rate of 1 mg/kg day times after the termination of a 3-week administration daily of 2 mg/kg i.p. of haloperidol to evaluate how long the increase in striatal [Met^5]-enkephalin persisted. Striatal [Met^5]-enkephalin was still maximally elevated 2 days after withdrawal; it was still increased 1 week after withdrawal, but was back to control level 2 weeks after haloperidol withdrawal.

Location of [Met^5]-enkephalin increase

We also examined whether chronic administration of haloperidol would affect the [Met^5]-enkephalin content of other brain regions. As shown in figure 9.2, after 3 weeks of haloperidol (2 mg/kg day) treatment, the [Met^5]-enkephalin content was elevated not only in the nucleus caudatus and globus pallidus but also in the nucleus accumbens. However, such treatment failed to alter the [Met^5]-enkephalin content in other brain areas studied.

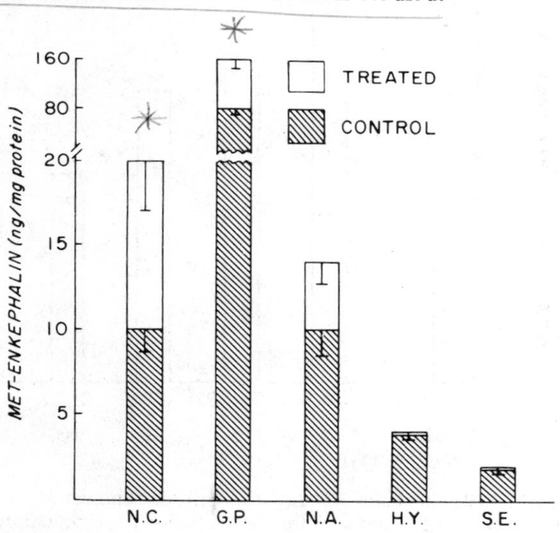

Figure 9.2 [Met^5]-enkephalin content of various brain regions after daily injection of haloperidol (2 mg/kg day) for 3 weeks. N.C., nucleus caudatus; G.P., globus pallidus; N.A., nucleus accumbens; H.Y., hypothalamus; S.E., septum.
The [Met^5]-enkephalin content of haloperidol-treated rats is significantly different from that of saline-treated controls in N.C., G.P. and N.A. ($P < 0.05$) but not in H.Y. and S.E. ($P > 0.05$). $N = 6$–10.

EFFECTS OF CATALEPTOGENIC AND NON-CATALEPTOGENIC ANTISCHIZOPHRENIC DRUGS

A great number of antischizophrenic drugs impair extrapyramidal function (Snyder *et al.*, 1974*a, b*) and this is related to their ability to block striatal DA receptors (Creese *et al.*, 1976). Because chlorpromazine, haloperidol and pimozide impair extrapyramidal function they are termed cataleptogenic (Creese *et al.*, 1976); in contrast, clozapine, although it blocks DA receptors, fails to cause extrapyramidal side-effects (DeMaio, 1972). This drug and thioridazine are two anti-schizophrenics which are devoid of extrapyramidal activity; for this reason they are at present termed non-cataleptogenics. The reason for the difference in the extra-pyramidal liability between clozapine and other cataleptogenic antipsychotics may be found in the ability of clozapine to block the function of cholinergic muscarinic receptors (Snyder *et al.*, 1974*b*; Racagni *et al.*, 1976).

An increase of striatal [Met^5]-enkephalin content was also observed after 2 weeks of daily administration of pimozide (1.5 mg/kg day, i.p.) or chlorpromazine (6.0 mg/kg day, i.p.), two cataleptogenic antischizophrenic drugs. A similar treatment with the non-cataleptogenic antischizophrenic drug, clozapine (10 mg/kg day, i.p.) failed to change the striatal [Met^5]-enkephalin content (figure 9.3).

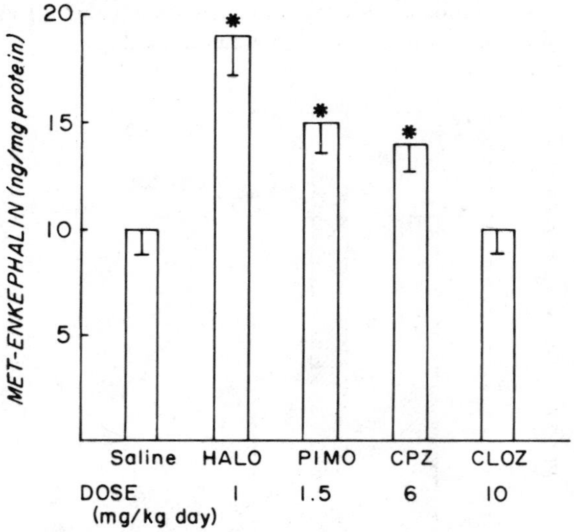

Figure 9.3 Striatal [Met^5]-enkephalin content after chronic administration of various antipsychotics for 14 days. HALO, haloperidol; PIMO, pimozide; CPZ, chlorpromazine; CLOZ, clozapine.
All the drugs were given i.p. *Results were significantly different from the saline-treated animals ($P < 0.05$).

EFFECT OF CHRONIC ADMINISTRATION OF LiCl ON STRIATAL [MET^5]-ENKEPHALIN CONTENT

Lithium has been used successfully in treating manic depressive patients (Schou, 1976; Bunney, 1976). To examine whether brain [Met^5]-enkephalin content could be affected by Li treatment, we have administered Li i.p. (5 mEq/kg) and measured striatal [Met^5]-enkephalin content at various times thereafter. [Met^5]-enkephalin content remained unchanged in rats killed 1 day after receiving a single injection of Li (5 mEq/kg i.p.). However, seven daily injections of this dose of Li elevated striatal [Met^5]-enkephalin content dramatically (figure 9.4). Various amounts of Li were injected chronically, seven daily doses as low as 1 mEq/kg

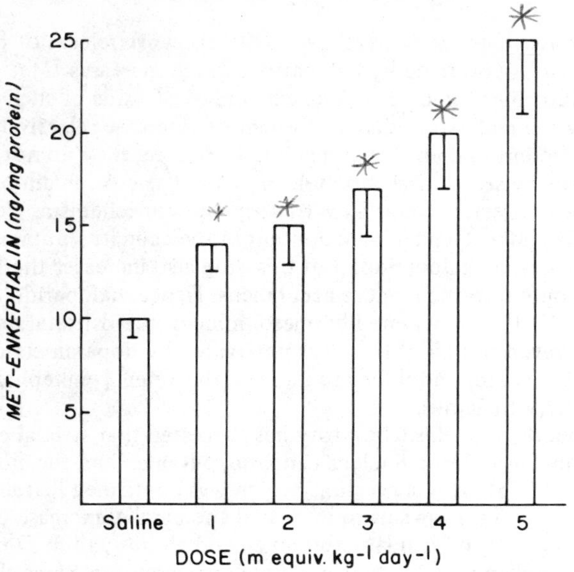

Figure 9.4 A graded increase of striatal [Met^5]-enkephalin after chronic administration of various doses of LiCl for 7 days. All the values are significantly different from saline-treated controls ($P < 0.05$). $N = 6–10$.

already increased striatal [Met^5]-enkephalin content. The time course of the increase in striatal [Met^5]-enkephalin content elicited by Li was characterized by a 2 or 3-day delay in the onset and by habituation occurring after 1 week or 10 days of treatment.

SPECULATIONS AND CONCLUSIONS

Three DA receptor blockers, haloperidol, chlorpromazine and pimozide, which relieve some symptoms of schizophrenia in man and cause catalepsy in animals and extrapyramidal side-effects in man (Snyder *et al.*, 1974*b*) can elevate the [Met^5]-enkephalin content of striatum when given chronically. Haloperidol was studied in greater detail and it was found to increase striatal [Met^5]-enkephalin content by 40 per cent after a 3-week treatment at a dosage of 0.1 mg/kg day i.p. (table 9.2). This haloperidol dose is comparable to that used clinically (Usdin and Efron, 1972). Higher doses of haloperidol cause a greater increase of striatal [Met^5]-enkephalin. Peak effects (100 per cent increase) are obtained with 1 mg/kg day for 3 weeks. Although our results suggest that striatal [Met^5]-enkephalin content may be elevated in patients treated with haloperidol, they fail to indicate whether the concentration of [Met^5]-enkephalin available at the synaptic cleft is increased or decreased in haloperidol treated patients. Recent reports indicate that the content of two molecular forms of 'endorphin' may be elevated in spinal fluid of schizophrenic patients before they receive any antischizophrenic medication (Terenius *et al.*, 1976); considering this report and our finding that haloperidol increases [Met^5]-enkephalin content, it would be tempting to speculate that a defect associated with psychosis is the excessive release of [Met^5]-enkephalin; this is corrected by haloperidol which increases [Met^5]-enkephalin content by favoring storage. However, the practical value of such speculation is decreased by the realization that antipsychotics increase selectively the [Met^5]-enkephalin content of some brain regions. Therefore, they do not act on some general regulatory step in the metabolism of [Met^5]-enkephalin but their effect appears to be indirect; perhaps via a trans-synaptic mechanism. We found that not only is the [Met^5]-enkephalin content in the caudatus/putamen or in globus pallidus increased by haloperidol, but this drug also increases the [Met^5]-enkephalin content in the nucleus accumbens. Hence, haloperidol seems to act on structures that are innervated by mesolimbic or nigrostriatal dopaminergic neurons. However, not all of the areas innervated by dopaminergic neurons are affected because haloperidol fails to increase the [Met^5]-enkephalin content in septum and hypothalamus.

Previous work from this laboratory has suggested that striatal enkephalinergic neurons are intrinsic to the nucleus caudatus/putamen and the globus pallidus (Hong *et al.*, 1977*a*). This suggestion, which was confirmed histologically by Hökfelt *et al.* (1977), allows us to infer that the parallel increase of [Met^5]-enkephalin found in the caudatus/putamen and globus pallidus reflects an increase in the [Met^5]-enkephalin content in striatal interneurons. Since the antipsychotic agent preferentially increases the [Met^5]-enkephalin in the nucleus accumbens and striatum, it may be inferred that in these structures a blockade of DA receptors regulates [Met^5]-enkephalin production or storage, perhaps trans-synaptically. This possibility is supported by the similar increase in striatum [Met^5]-enkephalin content caused by reserphine injections and brain hemitransection, both procedures, like haloperiodol, block dopaminergic transmission.

When the action of cataleptogenic DA receptor blockers on striatal [Met^5]-enkephalin content is considered in contrast to the ineffectiveness of clozapine, a non-cataleptogenic DA receptor blocker, it appears that there is a correlation between the potency of these drugs to cause DA receptor supersensitivity in animals (Gnegy *et al.*, 1977*a, b*) or extrapyramidal side-effects including tardive dyskinesia in man (Sayers *et al.*, 1975) and their ability to elevate striatal [Met^5]-enkephalin content (see figure 9.3). Clozapine fails to increase DA receptor supersensitivity and [Met^5]-enkephalin in striatum, whereas haloperidol, pimozide and chlorpromazine can elicit both effects. The inability of clozapine to raise striatal [Met^5]-enkephalin suggests that we should now test whether the increase in striatal [Met^5]-enkephalin elicited by antipsychotics requires a trans-synaptic mechanism involving a cholinergic interneuron. In some way this increase of striatal [Met^5]-enkephalin content is reminiscent of the DA receptor supersensitivity following chronic haloperidol as described by Sayers *et al.* (1975), Gnegy *et al.* (1977*a, b*) and Costa (1977). Also, this supersensitivity appears after 2 weeks of chronic administration of cataleptogenic antipsychotics but not after chronic treatment with clozapine.

Therapy with Li not only alleviates the symptoms of mania but it prevents the recurrence of the manic depressive symptomatology; many molecular mechanisms regulating neuronal function are affected by this drug but none has been shown to be crucial in explaining the therapeutic actions of Li. Is the increase in striatal [Met^5]-enkephalin caused by Li relevant to its antimanic action? At present, a stumbling block to an affirmative answer is our lack of understanding of the mechanisms involved in the increase of striatal [Met^5]-enkephalin by haloperidol and Li. Indeed, if the mechanisms were similar it would be difficult to explain how Li and haloperidol act by a similar mechanism despite the different profiles of their clinical indications. A daily injection of Li for 7 days with a dose as low as 1 mEq/kg day, increases by 40 per cent the striatal [Met^5]-enkephalin content. The extent of this increase is greater when the dose of Li is increased. However, an important difference between Li and haloperidol was revealed by the studies of the time course of the action on striatal [Met^5]-enkephalin. This study revealed that there was a 2 to 3-day lag before the elevation of striatal [Met^5]-enkephalin was observed (data not shown). More important, the effect of haloperidol lasted after it had stopped being administered. Even 1 week after haloperidol withdrawal, the [Met^5]-enkephalin striatal content was still elevated. In contrast, the increase in striatal [Met^5]-enkephalin caused by Li was evident during the first week of treatment. When Li treatment was continued for 2 weeks, the increase in striatal [Met^5]-enkephalin vanished during the second week. Both haloperidol and Li increase striatal [Met^5]-enkephalin after a time lag; a few days for Li, about 1 week for haloperidol. In both cases, one can relate this characteristic time lag to their respective therapeutic actions. An important difference is the persistence of the striatal [Met^5]-enkephalin increase in the case of haloperidol and the temporary character of the response to Li. This difference might suggest that the molecular mechanism involved in the increase of [Met^5]-enkephalin by Li is different from that caused by haloperidol. It has been reported that Li administration inhibits DA synthesis in striatum (Friedman and Gershon, 1973) which, in turn, might interrupt dopaminergic transmission. Since a haloperidol-induced increase of striatal [Met^5]-enkephalin is probably a result of a dopaminergic blockade, it seemed logical to speculate that the effect of Li on striatal [Met^5]-enkephalin content may also be mediated through a dopaminergic mechanism. However, if this were the case, it would be difficult to explain the discrepancy between the time courses of the increase in striatal [Met^5]-enkephalin caused by haloperidol and by Li. We could speculate that haloperidol may change a rate-limiting step in the regulation of striatal [Met^5]-enkephalin, perhaps by inducing a rate-limiting enzyme which acts trans-synaptically while the effect of Li on striatal [Met^5]-enkephalin may reflect a compensatory change; perhaps a decrease in the release rate of [Met^5]-enkephalin.

SUMMARY

This study demonstrates that chronic administration of antipsychotics, reserpine and Li elevates [Met^5]-enkephalin content in striatum and nucleus accumbens. However, the underlying mechanism for raising the [Met^5]-enkephalin content is not known. We are now studying the effects of these drugs on the release and biosynthesis of [Met^5]-enkephalin to determine whether the increased [Met^5]-enkephalin is a result of a reduction in its release or of an increase in its biosynthesis.

REFERENCES

Belluzzi, J. and Stein, L. (1977). *Nature* **266**, 556–8

Bloom, F., Segal, D., Ling, N. and Guillemin, R. (1976). *Science,* **194**, 630–2

Bunney, W. E., Jr (1976). *Neurosci. Res. Prog. Bull,* **14**, 124–31

Costa, E., Gnegy, M. E. and Uzunov, P. (1977). *Naunyn Schmiedeberg's Archs Pharmac.,* **297**, 547–8

Creese, I., Burt, D. R. and Snyder, H. (1976). *Science,* **192**, 481–3

Davis, G. C., Bunney, W. E., Jr., Defraites, E. G., Kleinman, J. E., van Kammen, D. P., Post, R. M. and Wyatt, R. J. (1977). *Science,* **197**, 74–7

DeMaio, D. (1972). *Arzneimittel-Forsch,* **22**, 919–21

Friedman, E. and Gershon, S. (1973). *Nature,* **243**, 520–1

Gnegy, M. E., Lucchelli, A. and Costa, E. (1977*a*). *Naunyn Schmiedeberg's Archs Pharmac.* **202**, 558–64

Gnegy, M. E., Uzunov, P. and Costa, E. (1977*b*). *J. Pharmac. exp. Ther.* (in press)

Gunne, L.-M., Lindstrom, L. and Terenius, L. (1977). *J. Neural Transmission,* **40**, 13–9

Hökfelt, T., Elde, R., Johansson, O., Terenius, L. and Stein, L. (1977). *Neurosci. Lett.* **5**, 25–31

Hong, J. S., Yang, H.-Y. T. and Costa, E. (1977*a*). *Neuropharmacology,* **16**, 451–3

Hong, J. S., Yang, H.-Y. T., Fratta, W. and Costa, E. (1977*b*). *Brain Res.,* **134**, 383–6

Hong, J. S., Yang, H.-Y. T., Racagni, G. and Costa, E. (1977*c*). *Brain Res.,* **122**, 541–4

Janowsky, D. S., Segal, D. S., Abrams, A., Bloom, F. and Guillemin, R. (1977). *Psychopharmacology,* **53**, 295–7

Kline, N. S., Li, C. H., Lehmann, H. E., Lajtha, A., Laski, E. and Cooper, T. (1977). *Archs gen. Psychiat.,* **34**, 1111–4

König, J. F. R. and Klippel, R. A. (1967). *The Rat Brain,* Krieger, Huntington, New York

Moroni, F., Cheney, D. L. and Costa, E. (1977*a*). *Nature,* **267**, 267–8

Moroni, F., Cheney, D. L. and Costa, E. (1977*b*). *Naunyn Schmiedeberg's Archs Pharmac.,* **299**, 149–53

Racagni, G., Cheney, D. L., Zsilla, G. and Costa, E. (1976). *Neuropharmacology,* **15**, 723–36

Sayers, A. C., Burki, H. R., Ruch, W. and Asper, H. (1975). *Psychopharmacologia, (Berl),* **41**, 97–104

Schou, M. (1976). *Neurosci. Res. Prog. Bull.,* **14**, 117–31

Snyder, S. H., Banerjee, S. P., Yamamura, H. I. and Greenberg, D. (1974*a*). *Science,* **184**, 1243–53

Snyder, S., Greenberg, D. and Yamamura, H. I. (1974*b*). *Archs gen. Psychiat.,* **31**, 58–61

Terenius, L., Wahlström, A., Lindstrom, L. and Widerlov, E. (1976). *Neurosci. Lett.,* **3**, 157–62

Usdin, E. and Efron, D. H. (1972). *Psychotropic Drugs and Related Compounds,* Department of Health Education and Welfare Publication, Washington, DC

Yang, H.-Y. T., Hong, J. S. and Costa, E. (1977). *Neuropharmacology,* **16**, 303–7

10
Brain endorphin levels increase after long-term chlorpromazine treatment

C. David Wise* and Larry Stein (Wyeth Laboratories, PO Box 8299, Philadelphia, Pennsylvania 19101, U.S.A.)

Observations in animals (Bloom *et al.*, 1976; Jacquet and Marks, 1976) and man (Terenius *et al.*, 1976; Gunne *et al.*, 1977; Kline *et al.*, in press) suggest the possible involvement of brain endorphins in mental illness. Terenius *et al.* (1976) reported that four chronic schizophrenics exhibited elevated levels of endorphins in their cerebrospinal fluid during 'a symptom-rich' phase of their disease. In two of these patients, whose condition improved during neuroleptic therapy, there was a return to low endorphin level (Gunne *et al.*, 1977). These findings are consistent with the idea that some psychotic symptoms might be caused by excessive endorphin activity. We report here raised endorphin levels in brains of rats after long-term administration of the antipsychotic agent chlorpromazine (CPZ), but not after the structurally-related antidepressant imipramine. This raises the possibility that the therapeutic action of antipsychotics may be associated with changes in endorphin activity.

Endogenous endorphins in rat brain extracts were assayed by competition for opiate receptor binding (Pert and Snyder, 1974; Simantov *et al.*, 1976). Endorphin was extracted from whole rat brain (minus cerebellum) by the procedure of Simantov *et al.* (1976). Non-specific binding was defined as the amount of isotope bound in the presence of 1 μM of non-radioactive morphine or levallorphan. Stereospecific binding was calculated by subtracting the value for non-specific binding from the total amount of isotope bound in the absence of cold morphine or levallorphan, or in the presence of dextrallorphan (1 μM). One unit of endorphin activity was defined as that amount of extract which yielded 50% inhibition of $[^3H]$-morphine binding as determined by log–probit analysis.

Chlorpromazine, imipramine and apomorphine were administered to different groups of rats in their powdered diet for 4 weeks. Increasing drug doses were given to achieve the final levels shown in table 10.1. The rats were killed by immersion

*Present address: Laboratory of Clinical Psychopharmacology, Division of Special Mental Health Research, National Institute of Mental Health, William A. White Building, Saint Elizabeth's Hospital, Washington, DC.

in carbon dioxide, decapitated, and their brains immediately removed for endorphin extraction.

Only CPZ treatment produced a statistically significant increase in brain endorphin content (table 10.1). Specificity of effect of CPZ is suggested by the observation that imipramine, a structurally-related antidepressant, produced no such increase. If CPZ elevated brain endorphins by blockade of dopamine receptors (the currently favored explanation of its antipsychotic action (Van Rossum, 1966; Snyder, 1976), then apomorphine, which stimulates dopamine receptors, might lower endorphin levels. However, the apomorphine treatments had no measurable effect on brain endorphins (table 10.1).

Table 10.1 Effect of long-term administration of chlorpromazine, apomorphine and imipramine on endorphin levels in rat brain

Treatment	Final dose (mg/kg, p.o.)	No. of animals	Mean endorphin concentration (units/g wet tissue) ± s.e.m.	Percentage increase
No drug control	–	19	5.9 ± 0.35	–
Apomorphine	10	8	6.0 ± 0.47	1.6
Imipramine	20	10	6.6 ± 0.38	11.8
Chlorpromazine	20	19	7.6 ± 0.62*	28.8

Rats were administered drugs in their diet over a period of 4 weeks. The whole brain (minus cerebellum) was then extracted and assayed in an opiate binding assay. One unit of endorphin is defined as that amount of material that yields 50 per cent receptor occupancy in the opiate binding assay.

*Differs from no drug at $P < 0.05$

It is possible that the presence of CPZ in the extract interfered with the binding assay (Clay and Brougham, 1975; Creese *et al.*, 1976), and thus caused a spuriously elevated estimate of endorphin content. To evaluate this possibility, large single doses of CPZ, imipramine, or apomorphine were injected i.p. in different groups of rats in a short-term experiment. The animals were killed and their brains removed for analysis 1 hour later, when peak brain levels of CPZ are reached (Gothelf and Karczmar, 1963). No drug-induced changes in opiate receptor binding activity were obtained in the short-term experiment (table 10.2). We also observed that long-term administration of CPZ had no significant effect on opiate receptor density or affinity (Wise and Stein, unpublished).

Thus, we find that long-term (but not short-term) administration of CPZ significantly raises the brain concentration of endorphins. Long-term administration of CPZ similarly is required for effective antischizophrenic activity (Casey *et al.*, 1960). Raised brain levels of other neurotransmitters, such as dopamine, serotonin and acetylcholine, usually are associated with a reduction in the activity of dopaminergic, serotonergic, and cholinergic neurons (Rommelspacher and

Table 10.2 Effect of single doses of chlorpromazine, apomorphine and imipramine on endorphin levels in rat brain

Treatment	Dose (mg/kg, i.p.)	No. of animals	Mean endorphin concentration (units/g wet tissue) ± s.e.m.
Saline control	–	7	5.4 ± 0.70
Apomorphine	10	7	6.4 ± 0.93
Imipramine	20	8	5.8 ± 0.76
Chlorpromazine	20	8	5.5 ± 1.26

Rats received a single i.p. dose of drug and were killed 1 hour later. The endorphin in whole brain (minus cerebellum) was extracted and assayed in an opiate binding assay ([^{3}H]-etorphine was used as the ligand). One unit of endorphin is defined as that amount of material that yields 50 per cent receptor occupancy in the opiate binding assay.

Kuhar, 1974; Roth *et al.*, 1973; Wang and Aghajanian, 1977). By analogy, increased brain levels of endorphin might reflect a reduced activity of endorphin neurons. If so, it would appear that long-term administration of CPZ somehow lowers the activity of endorphin neurons.

The present observation of CPZ-induced increases in brain levels of endorphin may appear at first inconsistent with the earlier report (Terenius *et al.*, 1976) of neuroleptic-induced decreases in CSF endorphin. However, if long-term CPZ treatment reduces endorphin activity as we suggest, the neuronal stores (and hence, brain levels) of endorphin could increase while that released into CSF could decrease.

ACKNOWLEDGEMENT

We thank B. A. Brehmeyer, W. J. Carmint and N. S. Buonato for technical assistance.

REFERENCES

Bloom, F., Segal, D., Ling, N. and Guillemin, R. (1976). *Science,* **194**, 630–2
Casey, J. F., Bennett, I. F., Lindley, C. J., Hollister, L. E., Gordon, M. H. and Springer, N. N. (1960). *Archs gen. Psychiat.,* **2**, 210–20
Clay, G. A. and Brougham, L. R. (1975). *Biochem. Pharmac.,* **24**, 1363–7
Creese, I., Feinburg, A. P. and Snyder, S. (1976). *Eur. J. Pharmac.,* **36**, 231–5
Gothelf, B., and Karczmar, A. G. (1963). *Int. J. Neuropharmac.,* **2**, 39–49
Gunne, L.-M., Lindstrom, L. and Terenius, L. (1977). *J. Neural Transmission,* **40**, 13–22
Jacquet, Y. F. and Marks, N. (1976). *Science,* **194**, 632–5
Kline, N. S., Li, C. H., Lehman, H. E., Lajtha, A., Laski, E. and Cooper, T. *Archs gen. Psychiat.* (in press)
Pert, C. and Snyder, S. H. (1974). *Molec. Pharmac.,* **10**, 868–79
Rommelspacher, H. and Kuhar, M. J. (1974). *Brain Res.,* **81**, 243–51
Roth, R. H., Walters, J. T. and Aghajanian, G. K. (1973). In *Frontiers of Catecholamine Research* (eds E. Usdin and S. H. Snyder), Pergamon Press, Oxford
Simantov, R., Kuhar, M. J., Pasternak, G. W. and Snyder, S. H. (1976). *Brain Res.,* **106**, 189–97

Snyder, S. H. (1976). *Am. J. Psychiat.*, **133**, 197–202
Terenius, L., Wahlström, A., Lindstrom, L. and Widerlov, E. (1976). *Neurosci. Lett.*, **3**, 157–62
Van Rossum, J. M. (1966). *Archs int. Pharmacodyn.*, **160**, 492–4
Wang, R. V. and Aghajanian, G. K. (1977). *Brain Res.*, **132**, 186–93

11
A re-evaluation of the opioid peptides present in the central nervous system utilizing microfluorometry

Sidney Udenfriend, Menachem Rubinstein and Stanley Stein
(Roche Institute of Molecular Biology, Nutley, New Jersey 07110, U.S.A.)

The recent emergence of a physiology of analgesia and behavior is based on the demonstration of a morphine receptor (Goldstein *et al.*, 1971) followed by the isolation and characterization of peptides with opioid or behavioral activity, that is, enkephalins (Hughes *et al.*, 1975) and β-endorphin (Li and Chung, 1976). The precursor relationship of β-lipotropin (β-LPH) to the opioid peptides was then realized. Since then, other congeners of enkephalin and endorphin have been reported in tissues.

The presence of so many clearly related compounds in tissue extracts makes it necessary for chemical corroboration of findings obtained by bioassay and immunoassay procedures. What is needed is the introduction of biochemistry. For this purpose specific and sensitive chemical procedures for assaying each of the many congeners are required. Before enkephalin was found, our laboratory had developed specific fluorometric assays for peptides, with a sensitivity in the picomole range, and applied them to various aspects of peptide chemistry, including the assay of oxytocin and vasopressin in the pituitary (Gruber *et al.*, 1976) and of carnosine (β-alanyl histidine) in the olfactory bulb (Wideman *et al.*, 1978). More recently we have applied such methods to the opioid peptides in various tissues for two purposes: to initiate studies on the biosynthesis of these peptides and, to develop specific methods for each of the peptides and use them in pharmacologic studies.

Our studies turned first to the rat since this laboratory animal has been used traditionally for experimental studies on analgesia and behavior. Also, the biochemistry of peptides can only be elucidated in small laboratory animals. To carry out such studies with relatively few animals requires analytical procedures which are 100 to 1000 times more sensitive than those traditionally used in peptide chemistry. The reagent, fluorescamine, possesses such sensitivity. Fluorometric assay, together with a receptor binding assay, utilizing neuroblastoma–glioma hybrid cells, has been used in our laboratory for the isolation and characterization of the opioid peptides in rat tissues and in re-evaluating findings from other laboratories.

PROCEDURES

The reagent fluorescamine is a non-fluorescent substance which reacts almost instantaneously with primary amines to yield highly fluorescent products. Excess reagent rapidly decomposes to yield non-fluorescent products. Since amino acids, peptides, and proteins are primary amines they too yield intense fluorescence. Instrumentation has been devised to use fluorescamine for monitoring chromatographic columns during protein and peptide fractionation (Böhlen *et al.*, 1975) and for amino acid assay (Stein *et al.*, 1973). The sensitivity of both systems is in the picomole range.

The instrument used for chromatographic separation of peptides utilizes a stream sampling valve that directs a preset percentage of a column effluent to the fluorometric detection system, while the remainder proceeds to a fraction collector. An aliquot of each fraction collected from the chromatographic column is then assayed for opiate-like activity. The procedure that we developed for bioassay (Gerber *et al.*, 1978) utilizes neuroblastoma–glioma cells (Klee and Nirenberg, 1974) in a competitive binding assay with [^{3}H] [Tyr, Leu^5]-enkephalin as the displaced ligand. This radioreceptor assay permits the monitoring of a complete chromatographic run (as many as 60 fractions) in a day. Less than 0.5 pmol of enkephalins or endorphins can be measured. Similar quantities of β-LPH and other opiate-related proteins can be assayed after digestion with trypsin. The final stages of identification and isolation are carried out with high performance liquid chromatography (h.p.l.c.) columns having efficiencies of about 3000 theoretical plates (Rubinstein *et al.*, 1977*a*).

PEPTIDE AND PROTEIN STANDARDS

It is important to re-emphasize the necessity of establishing the purity and homogeneity of a peptide before experimental use. Detection of peptides by conventional means requires relatively large amounts. Many peptides are expensive or difficult to obtain in quantity. As a result many investigators do not check their purity. With the fluorescamine systems we have been able to check for purity using as little as 50 pmol so that the procedure is essentially non-destructive. In our experience, essentially all commercially obtained peptides must be repurified. Some (figure 11.1) contain relatively large amounts of contaminants. Use of these impure preparations in the development of bioassays or immunoassays could lead to erroneous results.

PEPTIDES IN THE RAT PITUITARY GLAND

As stated above, the rat was selected for this study because most previous experimental studies on analgesia and behavior have been done on this animal and also because only in such small laboratory animals can carefully controlled

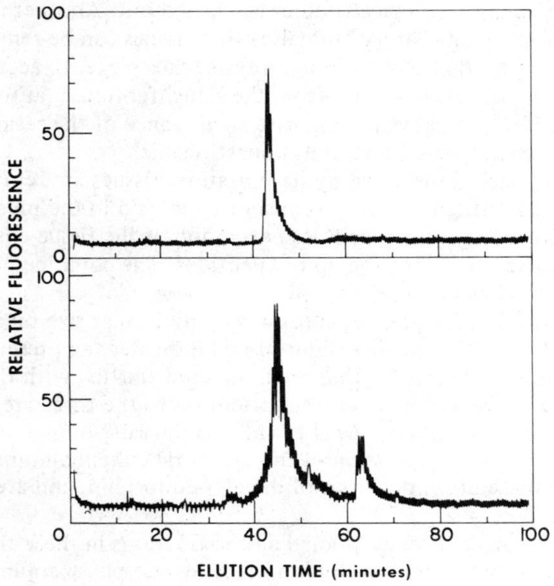

Figure 11.1. Comparison by h.p.l.c. of two preparations of β-LPH. Bottom panel, commercial source; top panel, from C. H. Li.

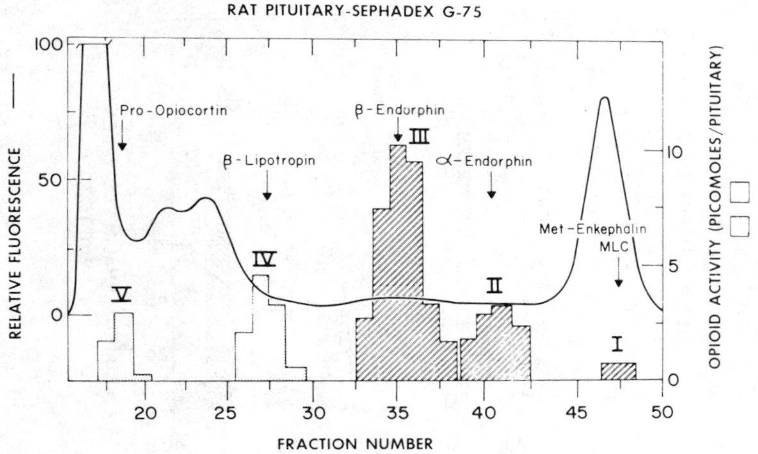

Figure 11.2. Chromatography of a rat pituitary extract on Sephadex G-75. Aliquots of fractions in the high molecular weight region of the chromatogram (> 4000 daltons) were digested with trypsin prior to the radioreceptor assay. Activity units have been converted into picomoles for each opioid peptide.

biochemical and pharmacological studies be carried out. Another reason for using individual small laboratory animals is that tissues can be removed and worked up so rapidly that little or no autolysis takes place. In accumulating large amounts of tissue, particularly that from the slaughter-house, autolysis is inevitable. The quantitative and even qualitative significance of the residual peptides isolated from such autolyzed material is questionable.

In our studies each rat is killed by decapitation, tissues are removed within 15 s and frozen. The tissue is then homogenized in acid in the presence of protease inhibitors and centrifuged. Re-extraction of the tissue ensures essentially quantitative recovery of all of the opioid peptides. The combined extracts are then subjected to chromatography.

The initial chromatographic separation is by molecular size on a Sephadex G-75 column. The elution profile (figure 11.2) indicates the presence of five distinct areas of opioid activity, that are numbered starting with the smallest (last to be eluted). We will first turn our attention to the three areas representing substances below 4000 daltons. Area I, which is the salt volume of the column, corresponds to the elution position of the synthetic enkephalin marker. Area II corresponds to the elution positions of α and γ-endorphin, and area III to that of β-endorphin.

For further identification we pooled all the fractions in these three areas and subjected the material to analysis by h.p.l.c. A reverse-phase column was precalibrated with the synthetic endorphins and enkephalins (figure 11.3A). Chromatography of the pooled low molecular weight extract of rat pituitaries revealed the presence of six opioid substances. As shown in figure 11.3B the first peak of

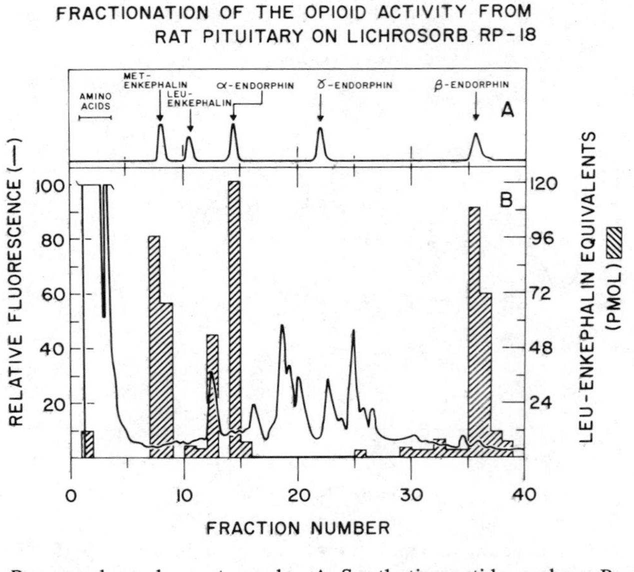

Figure 11.3. Reverse-phase chromatography. A, Synthetic peptide markers; B, pooled and concentrated fractions corresponding to the low molecular weight region of the Sephadex G-75 chromatogram in figure 11.2.

opioid activity is at the position of the free amino acids and does not correspond to any of the peptide markers. Dr Spector in our department, tested this substance in a morphine radioimmunoassay and found it to cross-react with antibody to morphine. This pituitary substance is apparently the non-peptide morphine-like compound, which he first discovered in 1975 (Ginzler *et al.*, 1976). Spector's results are presented in chapter 53.

The second peak on the reverse-phase column (figure 11.3B) corresponds to the [Met^5]-enkephalin marker. Rechromatography on both Sephadex G-10 and h.p.l.c. confirmed the presence of [Met^5]-enkephalin in the rat pituitary. Negligible activity is present at the position of the [Leu^5]-enkephalin marker. The third peak of activity does not correspond to any of the markers which were used and is still unidentified. The fourth peak corresponds to α-endorphin; there is no activity at the γ-endorphin position.

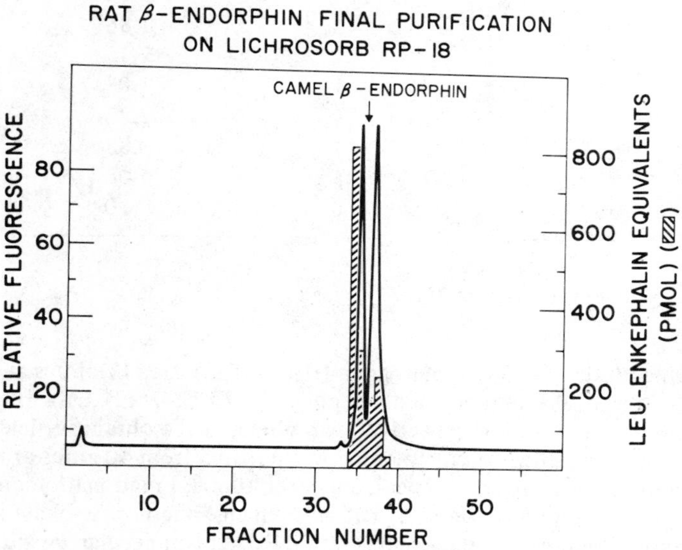

Figure 11.4. Final purification step of rat β-endorphin on an h.p.l.c. reverse-phase column. Fractions 34 and 35 were combined and used for the characterization of rat β-endorphin.

The fifth and largest of the low molecular weight opioid substances was eluted at the position of the β-endorphin marker. To obtain enough of this material for isolation, 200 frozen rat pituitaries (commercial) were used. Following chromatography on Sephadex G-75 the area corresponding to β-endorphin was collected and subjected to two steps of h.p.l.c. The peak of activity on the final h.p.l.c. (figure 11.4) was collected (about 6 nmol) and an aliquot subjected to amino acid assay. As shown in table 11.1 rat β-endorphin is identical in composition to β-endorphin from the camel, sheep and other animals. Identity with camel β-endorphin was also shown by comparing tryptic fragments of the two on h.p.l.c. (Rubinstein *et al.*, 1977*b*).

Table 11.1 Amino acid composition of camel and rat β-endorphins

Amino Acid	Camel*	Rat†
Asx	2	2.11
Thr	3	3.01
Ser	2	1.58
Glx	3	3.08
Pro	1	1.28
Gly	3	2.81
Ala	2	2.13
Cys	0	0
Val	1	1.18
Met	1	0.94
Ile	2	1.86
Leu	2	2.15
Tyr	1	1.08
Phe	2	2.22
His	1	0.88
Lys	5	5.06
Arg	0	0

*Li and Chung (1976).
†Rubinstein *et al.* (1977*b*).

Returning to the G-75 chromatogram (figure 11.2), area IV elutes at the position of the β-LPH marker (kindly supplied by Dr C. H. Li). On h.p.l.c. of this area one peak of biological activity was obtained. To obtain sufficient pure material for characterization the peptide was purified from 40 anterior pituitaries which we obtained from rats immediately after killing. Fractionation on a Sephadex G-75 column followed by cation exchange and reverse-phase h.p.l.c. yielded about 2 nmol of homogeneous rat β-LPH. The molecular weight, obtained on a Biogel column, was found to be the same as that of β-LPH from other species (about 12 000). The amino acid compositions of some β-LPH are shown in table 11.2. Similarities are seen, particularly with respect to the basic amino acids, but each β-LPH is distinct. This contrasts with the close interspecies homology of the β-endorphins.

In our initial studies we noticed only four areas of opioid activity on Sephadex G-75 columns. Only a small amount of β-LPH activity was observed and no activity was seen in the area corresponding to the largest proteins. However, when aliquots from the collected fractions were treated with trypsin before performing the radioreceptor assay the activity of the β-LPH peak was markedly increased and a fifth area of activity was revealed which was eluted just after the void volume (figure 11.2). When the high molecular weight region (area V) was rechromatographed no activity appeared in the β-LPH region nor in any other region. This showed that the activity in area V is not an artifact resulting from

Table 11.2 Amino acid composition of various β-lipotropins*

Amino Acid	Sheep	Human	Rat
Asx	2	10	7
Thr	4	4	4
Ser	5	4	4
Glx	12	13	12
Pro	5	7	10
Gly	8	12	8
Ala	13	8	4
Cys	0	0	0
Val	2	2	4
Met	2	2	2
Ile	2	1	2
Leu	6	7	7
Tyr	3	3	3
Phe	3	3	4
His	2	2	3
Lys	10	10	12
Arg	5	6	5
Trp	1	1	–

*From Rubinstein *et al.* (1977*a*).

contamination with the smaller peptides. From its position on Sephadex G-75 as well as on Biogel P-30 the large opioid protein was found to have a molecular weight of approximately 30 000. This value assumes that the molecule is linear. However, the molecular weight can be as high as 70 000 if it is globular. An extract containing the large opioid protein was digested with trypsin and the fragments were resolved by h.p.l.c. The only biologically active substance generated was the nonapeptide β-LPH_{61-69}. This is the same peptide as that formed when β-LPH or the endorphins are treated with trypsin. There was no trace of the corresponding leucine nonapeptide that could represent a corresponding congener of [Leu^5]-enkephalin. This establishes that the pituitary contains within it a precursor of the opiate peptides much larger than β-LPH. Initial reports concerning this large precursor were presented at the Fifth American Peptide Symposium (Udenfriend, 1977) and in two subsequent reports (Rubinstein *et al.*, 1977*a*, and 1978).

Utilizing cultured pituitary cells and radiolabeled amino acids, Mains *et al.* (1977) also obtained evidence of a protein of about 31 000 daltons which reacts with antibodies to both ACTH and β-endorphin. A similar 31 000 dalton protein which cross-reacts with antibodies to ACTH was reported by Roberts and Herbert (1977). We have also shown that the partially purified rat protein interacts with antibody to ACTH. The name pro-opiocortin has been suggested (Rubinstein *et al.*, 1978) to indicate the precursor relationship to both ACTH and opioid peptides.

Table 11.3 Endogenous opiates in rat pituitary

	pmol per pituitary		
	A	B	C
Pro-opiocortin	18		
β-LPH	17		+
β-Endorphin	33	740	13
γ-Endorphin	<0.1		
α-Endorphin	11		
[Met^{5}]-enkephalin	3		
Morphine-like compound	0.1–4?		

A, Determined on duplicate sets of four pooled glands by radioreceptor assay after column chromatography. B, From Guillemin *et al.* (1977). C, C. H. Li (personal communication).

The amounts of each of the above opioid substances present in whole rat pituitaries is shown in table 11.3. It should be noted that the values are presented in molar units rather than units of mass. This is to make apparent the quantitative interrelationships among these congeners which, because of the great differences in mass, are otherwise obscured. As an example, 500 ng of enkephalin represents 1 nmol whereas 500 ng of pro-opiocortin is less than 0.02 nmol. Investigations on the biosynthesis and metabolism of peptides, as well as their comparative pharmacology, can only be interpreted when molar units are used; reporting values in arbitrary units is even more confusing.

To our knowledge there has been little quantitative data on the opioid peptides in the pituitary. In recent publications from Guillemin's laboratory it was reported that rat pituitaries contain 2.6 μg (740 pmol) of β-endorphin per gland (Guillemin *et al.*, 1977; Rossier *et al.*, 1977). This was based on a radioimmunoassay. It should be noted (table 11.3) that our values for β-endorphin are much lower as are those found by C. H. Li (personal communication).

PEPTIDES IN THE CAMEL PITUITARY

A key contribution to the opioid peptide field was the isolation of β-endorphin from camel pituitaries by Li and Chung (1976). Selection of the camel for investigation was unusual but quite fortunate since in all other species β-LPH had been the congener isolated. The absence of β-LPH led to the isolation of the chromatographically similar congener, β-endorphin.

When the analgesic activity of β-endorphin was reported, the unusually large amounts in the camel pituitary suggested that this animal was also unusual with respect to its response to pain. What made us question the chemical findings in the camel pituitary were observations made by us on rat pituitaries. We observed that β-LPH and pro-opiocortin were major components of pituitaries which we rapidly dissected out and extracted. However, when we purchased rat pituitaries which were frozen and thawed the pro-opiocortin was essentially absent, β-LPH

Table 11.4 Endogenous opiates in camel pituitary (nmol per pituitary)

	A	B	C
Pro-opiocortin	20	24	
β-LPH	23	20	+
β-Endorphin	<0.5	11	0.03
γ-Endorphin	9	7	
α-Endorphin	9	7	
[Met^5]-enkephalin	2	4	
Morphine-like compound	+	+	

A and B, Determined on individual glands by radioreceptor assay after column chromatography. C, C. H. Li (personal communication).

was markedly diminished and β-endorphin and the smaller congeners were correspondingly increased. These are the changes one would expect if autolysis had occurred and they made us think of the findings in the camel. Were the very low β-LPH and high β-endorphin levels typical of the camel or were they the result of autolysis which arose during collection of the 1000 glands that were used? We discussed this with C. H. Li and decided to investigate this jointly with him using individual camel pituitaries which were rapidly removed, frozen and lyophilized. In our laboratories, using chemical and bioassay methods, and individual glands we found that fresh camel pituitaries, like pituitaries of other species contain large amounts of β-LPH as well as pro-opiocortin; β-endorphin values are lower and in some instances barely detectable (table 11.4). C. H. Li (personal communication) has found similar low levels of β-endorphin in fresh camel pituitaries using immunoassay. It would appear therefore, that the unusually large amounts of β-endorphin and small amounts of β-LPH originally found in camel pituitaries is an index of autolysis after collection and is not indicative of an unusual opioid physiology of the species.

It should be noted that all studies which are carried out on large numbers of glands collected at the slaughterhouse are subject to errors arising from autolysis. Since most of the peptide hormones which we recognize today were isolated from tissues which were obtained from such collections they too are suspect and require re-evaluation.

HUMAN SPINAL FLUID

Spinal fluid has been investigated by several laboratories and although opioid activity has been detected by most of them there is some dispute as to its nature. Wahlström *et al.* (1976) have presented evidence for two substances which can be separated by chromatography; one of these they tentatively identify as [Met^5]-enkephalin. With our procedures, utilizing from 5 to 8.5 ml samples of human spinal fluid, only one peak of opioid activity was observed on h.p.l.c. This peak did not coincide with [Met^5]-enkephalin, but eluted with amino acids. Aliquots were given to Dr Spector who identified it as non-peptide morphine-like material, which reacts with antibody to morphine. If [Met^5]-enkephalin or any of the other opioid peptides are present in human spinal fluid they must be there in amounts below 0.1 pmol/ml.

As for [Met^5]-enkephalin, it would be surprising to find any in spinal fluid since the pentapeptide is rapidly degraded by peptidases in this fluid. When [^{3}H] [Tyr, Leu^5]-enkephalin was added to human spinal fluid at 37 °C [^{3}H]-tyrosine was quantitatively liberated within 1 hour. It is our firm belief that the dispute over the identity of the opioid activity in human spinal fluid is a result of the failure to take into account the non-peptide opiate (Ginzler *et al.*, 1976; Blume *et al.*, 1977).

THE ENKEPHALINS IN BRAIN

The original purification and characterization of [Met^5] and [Leu^5]-enkephalins by Hughes *et al.* (1975) was an elegant piece of work. Others corroborated their identification. We have been able to assay the enkephalins in guinea pig striatum after separating them by h.p.l.c. We find approximately 150 pmol of [Met^5]-enkephalin per striatum and about 30 pmol of [Leu^5]-enkephalin. With tissues from six animals we were able to purify sufficient striatal [Met^5]-enkephalin to identify it by amino acid analysis. The quantities of striatal [Leu^5]-enkephalin in the guinea pig are, however, quite small and confirmatory chemical identification of this peptide will require larger amounts of tissue.

BIOCHEMICAL CONSIDERATIONS

With the finding of pro-opiocortin it becomes apparent that the biosyntheses of ACTH and opioid peptides are intimately connected. It remains to be seen whether pro-opiocortin is the original ribosomal product or whether a still larger protein is the product of gene expression. As shown in figure 11.5 there is apparently a cleavage which separates the ACTH activity from the opioid activity of the pro-opiocortin. Following this there are successive cleavages to yield several products which interact with opiate receptors.

The significance of the different endorphins must be considered. The presence of large amounts of α and γ-endorphin in fresh pituitaries may have some significance physiologically as well as biochemically. They deserve as much study as does β-endorphin. The nature and specificity of the peptidases involved at each step are of great interest. Also of interest are the residual peptides which have no opioid or ACTH activity. One such fragment is β-MSH. Are the other fragments without activity? Even if they are, some of them might serve as specific markers for following the metabolism of the overall pathway.

Finally, because we are dealing here with a series of congeners, each possessing significant homology with its precursors, it will be very difficult to achieve absolute specificity for any one of them with radioimmunoassay or bioassay of crude tissue extracts. A combination of reliable chromatography plus immunoassay or bioassay are the minimal requirements for specific estimation of each of these congeners.

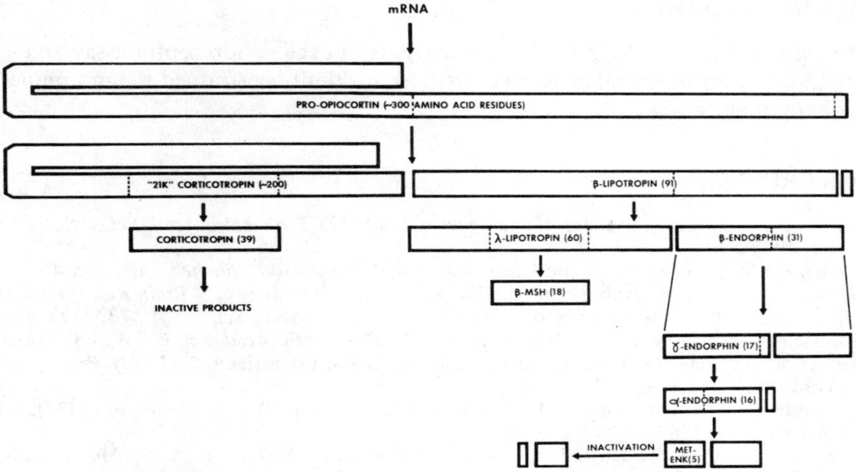

Figure 11.5. Interrelationships between pro-opiocortin and peptides arising from it.

PHYSIOLOGICAL CONSIDERATIONS

The question remains as to which of the congeners is released by the pituitary gland. Reports by Guillemin *et al.* (1977) and by Krieger *et al.* (in press) suggest that ACTH and opiate peptides are released into the blood in equal amounts. The most obvious explanation is that pro-opiocortin is delivered to the secretory granules and before or coincident with release the active peptides are generated by proteolysis. Alternatively, pro-opiocortin itself may be the substance released. That this may be the case is our finding (tables 11.3 and 11.4) that pro-opiocortin is a major component of both rat and camel pituitaries. Thus intact pro-opiocortin may actually represent the product released by the pituitary in response to stress. Once released it would be cleaved by enzymes in the blood into ACTH and perhaps a number of opiate peptides, each with a specific function. Since pro-opiocortin has a molecular weight of at least 30 000 and the sum of ACTH and β-endorphin is only 8000 there is even the possibility that it contains within it sequences of other biologically active peptides. Pro-opiocortin thus represents a duplex, or perhaps multiplex, hormone which ensures the simultaneous presence at certain receptor sites of two or more chemical agents that the body has elaborated to cope with stress. It is even possible that the overall behavioral effects of pro-opiocortin differ from those of its individual components. This would be true if the effects of endorphins are influenced by ACTH and vice versa. Should pro-opiocortin prove to contain within itself even additional components as active as ACTH and endorphin then its effects *in vivo* would very well differ from those of any of its individual components. Isolation of pro-opiocortin is essential for elucidating the significance of the endorphins as well as of ACTH and may provide us with a greater understanding of the physiology of stress and behavior.

ACKNOWLEDGMENTS

We wish to thank Ms L. D. Gerber for carrying out the radioreceptor assay and Mr L. Brink for technical assistance. Dr J. Shorr kindly performed the morphine radioimmunoassays.

REFERENCES

Blume, A. J., Shorr, J., Finberg, J. and Spector, S. (1977). *Proc. natn. Acad. Sci. U.S.A.*, **74**, 4927–31

Böhlen, P., Stein, S., Stone, J. and Udenfriend, S. (1975). *Analyt. Biochem.*, **67**, 438–45

Gerber, L. D., Stein, S., Rubinstein, M., Wideman, J. and Udenfriend, S. *Brain Res.* (in press)

Ginzler, A. R., Levy, A. and Spector, S. (1976). *Proc. natn. Acad. Sci. U.S.A.*, **73**, 2132–6

Goldstein, A., Lowney, L. L. and Pal, B. K. (1971). *Proc. natn. Acad. Sci. U.S.A.*, **68**, 1742–7

Gruber, K. A., Stein, S., Brink, L., Radhakrishnan, A. and Udenfriend, S. (1976). *Proc. natn. Acad. Sci. U.S.A.*, **73**, 1314–8

Guillemin, R., Vargo, T., Rossier, J., Minick, S., Ling, N., Vale, W. and Bloom, F. (1977). *Science*, **197**, 1367–9

Hughes, J., Smith, T. W., Kosterlitz, H. W., Fothergill, L. A., Morgan, B. A. and Morris, H. R. (1975). *Nature*, **258**, 577–9

Klee, W. A. and Nirenberg, M. (1974). *Proc. natn. Acad. Sci. U.S.A.*, **71**, 3474–7

Krieger, D. T., Liotta, A. and Li, C. H. *Life Sci.*, (in press)

Li, C. H. and Chung, D. (1976). *Proc. natn. Acad. Sci. U.S.A.*, **73**, 1145–8

Mains, R. E., Eipper, B. A. and Ling, N. (1977). *Proc. natn. Acad. Sci. U.S.A.*, **74**, 3014–8

Roberts, J. L. and Herbert, E. (1977). *Proc. natn. Acad. Sci. U.S.A.*, **74**, 4826–30

Rossier, J., Vargo, T., Minick, S., Ling, N., Bloom, F. and Guillemin, R. (1977). *Proc. natn. Acad. Sci. U.S.A.*, **74**, 5162–5

Rubinstein, M., Stein, S., Gerber, L. D. and Udenfriend, S. (1977*a*). *Proc. natn. Acad. Sci. U.S.A.*, **74**, 3052–5

Rubinstein, M., Stein, S. and Udenfriend, S. (1977*b*). *Proc. natn. Acad. Sci. U.S.A.*, **74**, 4969–72

Rubinstein, M., Stein, S. and Udenfriend, S. (1978). *Proc. natn. Acad. Sci. U.S.A.*, **75**, 669–71

Stein, S., Böhlen, P., Stone, J., Dairman, W. and Udenfriend, S. (1973). *Archs Biochem. Biophys.*, **155**, 202–12

Udenfriend, S. (1977). *Fifth American Peptide Symposium*, La Jolla, California

Wahlström, A., Johansson, L. and Terenius, L. (1976). In *Opiates and Endogenous Opioid Peptides*, (ed. H. W. Kosterlitz). Elsevier/North Holland, Amsterdam

Wideman, J., Brink, L. and Stein, S. (1978). *Analyt. Biochem.* **86**, 670–8

Section One
Basic Studies

(B) Biosynthesis and degradation of endorphins

12
Metabolic regulation of β-endorphin levels in perspective

Neville Marks and Abel Lajtha (Institute of Neurochemistry, Rockland Research Institute, Ward's Island, New York, U.S.A.)

For a fuller understanding of the metabolism of specific peptides in perspective, it is important to review peptide metabolism in general in the brain—especially protein metabolism, since at any time almost all of the peptide bonds are present in proteins. The level of small peptides is very low in brain.

THE EXTENT OF PROTEIN TURNOVER

The fact that in adult as well as young brain radioactive amino acids are incorporated into proteins shows that proteins are synthesized even after growth ceases, and that this synthesis is balanced by an equivalent breakdown in the non-growing organ. The important question is whether such metabolic activity is characteristic of a major portion of the proteins. The present evidence indicates that most proteins are rapidly metabolized and only a very small fraction of the proteins of the brain are stable. We have labeled all brain proteins in mice by feeding the animals throughout their growth with a diet containing radioactive protein. When these animals reached adulthood the diet was replaced with a non-radioactive one, and approximately 98 per cent of the proteins lost their label (Lajtha and Toth, 1966), indicating that at least 98 per cent of the proteins are in a dynamic state, undergoing continuous and simultaneous synthesis and breakdown. Similar experiments have not been done with young brain, but the finding that the rate of protein breakdown in brain during growth is approximately twice that in the adult (Dunlop *et al.*, 1978) would indicate that also during growth most proteins undergo continuous turnover.

RATES OF CEREBRAL PROTEIN METABOLISM

Protein synthesis *in vivo* can be measured from rates of incorporation of amino acids if the experimental circumstances are such that the specific activity of the free amino acid precursor is known, and it can be kept constant over the experimental period. Protein metabolism is often studied by a single injection of a tracer dose of an amino acid. Such pulse-labeling results in a very rapidly changing specific activity in the precursor, making it impossible to calculate the rates of protein turnover. Several techniques have been used to keep specific activities of the precursors fairly constant; these include multiple injections (Austin *et al.*, 1972), constant or variable infusions (Garlick and Marshall, 1972; Seta *et al.*, 1973), injections of a large (flooding) dose (Dunlop *et al.*, 1975), injection of suspensions (Lajtha and Toth, 1978), and implanting of an amino acid pellet (Lajtha *et al.*, 1976). Precise knowledge of the specific activity under the above conditions is possible, but it does require the isolation of the amino acid. Whether the amino acids utilized for protein synthesis are compartmented in the brain, as has been indicated in the liver (Fern and Garlick, 1976), is not well established yet. Evidence indicates that under conditions where the specific activity in plasma and brain are close, and are kept constant for several hours, compartmentation is not significant (Dunlop *et al.*, 1975; Ames and Parks, 1976). This is important, since if the amino acid exists in several metabolic pools with differing specific activities, only one of which is used for protein synthesis, then the average does not indicate the specific activity of the true precursor, and so metabolic rate measurement can not be made from the measured average specific activity. An amino acid pool that is not directly used for protein synthesis is the lysosomal pool; the amino acids there are derived from protein breakdown and thus are not labeled like the amino acid taken up from the administered labeled pool in the plasma. This lysosomal pool may be smaller in the brain than it is in the liver, and in more rapid equilibrium with the rest of the intracellular free amino acid pool, owing at least in part to the lower metabolic rates of brain proteins. Under the conditions of our studies, incorporation was not influenced by the elevated amino acid levels (Dunlop *et al.*, 1975); therefore infusion or large-dose experiments can also be used. It seems that brain protein metabolism is not very sensitive to changes in amino acid levels (Roberts, 1974). The formation of activated amino acid is above saturation levels at physiological conditions and therefore is not influenced by fluctuations in amino acid concentrations. Specific proteins may be sensitive to changes in amino acid levels (Menkes, 1968). Therefore in many cases of aminoacidurias a general effect on brain protein metabolism is less likely than specific changes in a few compartments (Gaull *et al.*, 1975).

Table 12.1 Changes in amino acid incorporation with experimental time

Time	Protein metabolism, per cent per hour	
(h)	Newborn	Adult
0 - 0.5	2.03	0.67
0.5- 3	1.45	0.56
3 - 6	1.31	0.49
9 -12	1.24	0.40
24 -30	1.13	0.31

The incorporation of [^{14}C] tyrosine into brain proteins was measured under such conditions that the specific activity of the free amino acid was kept constant.

Incorporation was found to be time dependent in that the calculated rates of protein metabolism decreased with increasing experimental time (table 12.1). This is due to the heterogeneity of metabolism, since some proteins are metabolized rapidly, others more slowly. We estimated that in general the rapidly metabolized proteins comprise only a small fraction of the brain proteins—less than 5 per cent (Lajtha *et al.*, 1976). This small rapidly metabolized pool influences primarily the short-time results (giving then falsely high average values); longer-term experiments measure the metabolism of the main bulk of proteins. Many experiments measured the rates from short-time experiments, and the results are in good agreement (table 12.2); but it has to be emphasized that these rates are the averages of a small, active pool and a large, less active pool of proteins.

Table 12.2 Rates of brain protein synthesis

Method	Rate %/hour	Reference
Adult		
Pulse	0.61	Oja, 1967
Infusion	0.55	Seta *et al.*, 1973
Infusion	0.68	Garlick and Marshall, 1972
Glucose injections	0.80	Austin *et al.*, 1972
Gross injection	0.62	Dunlop *et al.*, 1975
Immature		
Pulse	2.0	Oja, 1967
Pulse	2.2	Dunlop *et al.*, 1975
Gross injection	2.1	Dunlop *et al.*, 1975

Changes of protein metabolism during development

Protein metabolism is not stable under all conditions—the best illustration is changes in synthesis and breakdown during growth. It has been well established that the rate of protein synthesis is greater in the immature brain (Roberts, 1977); this has been shown *in vivo* and *in vitro*. The numerous studies *in vitro* attempted to establish the factors in the synthetic mechanism that governs growth (Johnson, 1977). To study the rates of metabolism of the living brain, isolated systems are not very suitable; we found that the rates of protein metabolism are lower in isolated systems, especially those from adult brain. For example, in cerebellar slices from adult brain the incorporation was only 6 per cent of the incorporation into cortex proteins *in vivo* (Dunlop *et al.*, 1977). In some specific areas in the adult such as the retina or the pineal gland or in much of the brain in the newborn (Parks *et al.*, 1976; Dunlop *et al.*, 1977) incorporation in slices and *in vivo* are close, and such systems are therefore very suitable for studying protein metabolism under a wide range of experimental conditions not possible in the living animal.

The rate of synthesis of proteins in the immature brain is much greater than that needed for growth (for the net deposition of proteins) and therefore a considerable part of synthesis must be balanced by breakdown. Calculations show that the rate of breakdown is actually significantly higher in the immature brain than in the adult (table 12.3). This would indicate that in the immature brain the formed proteins undergo change—they are subsequently broken down and replaced by other newly formed proteins. This may also correspond to the disappearance of many cells at the time that growth in other cells occurs (Cowan, 1973).

Developmental changes in protein metabolism illustrate the heterogeneity of protein metabolism; it changes during development and is also different in various brain areas. This heterogeneity means that a wide spectrum of protein turnover rates exists (table 12.4). The calculations of half-life illustrated in table 12.4 are only approximations and are the averages of many different rates of metabolism. They show that the rapidly metabolized proteins constitute only a small fraction of the total; the turnover rates of the bulk (over 90 per cent) of the proteins are lower but still significant, and it is likely that most proteins 'turn over'— are broken down and resynthesized—many times during the lifetime of the organism. It seems that the increased rate of turnover in the immature brain is not confined to a small active pool, but that most proteins are metabolized faster compared with the adult. This then raises the possibility that the turnover rate of a protein species is not necessarily constant: it may change during development, possibly showing regional heterogeneity in metabolism, and its metabolism may be altered under other physiological or pathological conditions.

Table 12.3 Changes in brain protein metabolism during development

	Protein metabolism (%/hour)			
Age	Cerebral hemisphere		Cerebellum	
days	Synthesis	Breakdown	Synthesis	Breakdown
2	2.0	1.3	2.9	1.9
8	1.8	1.2	2.7	1.7
12	1.5	1.0	2.3	1.5
16	1.3	0.9	1.6	1.2
24	1.0	0.9	1.0	1.0
30	0.8	0.8	0.8	0.8

From Dunlop *et al.*, 1978.

Table 12.4 Calculated turnover rates of brain proteins

Animal	Pool	Pool size (% of total)	Turnover rates %/h	Turnover rates half-life, (h)
Rat newborn	fast	2	39	1.8
	slow	96	1.4	49
Mouse newborn	fast	0.3	400	0.2
	slow	97	1.6	44
Mouse adult	fast	5	7.4	10
	slow	93	0.25	280

From Lajtha *et al.*, 1978

The flux of amino acids and peptides in the brain

The size of the various metabolic pools of cerebral proteins and their turnover rates can be only crudely estimated. In spite of this, the estimates give us some idea of the rate of utilization of amino acids by incorporation into proteins and the rate of liberation of amino acids by protein breakdown. The turnover rates of most proteins are high enough, as mentioned already, to replace most proteins many times during the lifetime of the organism. The level of free amino acids is much lower than that of protein-bound amino acids; the ratio of free to protein-bound essential amino acid is 1:2–300 in most cases. Because of this the turnover rate of the free amino acids is several-hundredfold higher than the rate of protein turnover. This is illustrated in table 12.5 with arginine. It can be seen that the amount of arginine equivalent to that present in the cerebral free pool is incorporated into proteins in 40 min. If the total arginine pool is used for protein synthesis, this would indicate an approximate half-life of 20 min for the free arginine pool in protein metabolism. The half-life of leucine (table 12.6) is even less, again indicating the very high flux of amino acids from free to protein-bound form and back. Formation of proteins is not the only fate of amino acids, some of which participate in many other metabolic pathways and some of which, like leucine, are rapidly metabolized to other compounds. The pool of amino acids attached to tRNA is estimated to be much smaller (probably 1/10,000th or less) than that of the free amino acids; since this would indicate a half-life of aminoacyl-tRNA of a few seconds, or only a fraction of a second, the flux through tRNA is extremely rapid.

Table 12.5 Utilization of free arginine in protein turnover

	Protein fractions	
	Slow	Fast
Per cent of total protein in fractions	94	5
Turnover: half-life (hours)	240	10
Arginine content of proteins (μmol/g tissue)	28	1.5
Arginine incorporated into protein (μmol/g h)	0.08	0.07
Free arginine in brain (μmol/g tissue)	0.1	

0.1 μmol of free arginine incorporated into proteins in 40 min.

Table 12.6 Utilization of the cerebral free leucine pool

	Half-life (50% utilized (min))
Protein turnover, adult	11
Growth (net protein deposition), newborn	25
Protein synthesis, newborn	8.4
Metabolism, adult	5
Uptake from plasma, adult	3

Ratio of protein-bound to free leucine in brain: adult, 640, newborn, 170.
Ratio of plasma-free to brain-free leucine: adult, 1.3, newborn, 0.6.

Breakdown of opioid peptides

The potent action of β-endorphin (LPH_{61-91}) compared with other lipotropic fragments makes it of interest to determine whether its formation or inactivation play a part in altering behavior (Jacquet *et al.*, 1976; Jacquet and Marks, 1976; Gainer, 1977; Marks, 1978; Klee, 1977). Neurosecretory areas appear to contain intracellular enzymes capable of producing β-endorphin from β-LPH (see Graf, this volume), although these enzymes have not been well characterized. The existence of a precursor of β-LPH of larger molecular weight, along with evidence for a number of β-LPH fragments in pituitary (β-MSH; α and γ-endorphins) indicates that a number of enzymes are involved, some in sequential breakdown, many of which may participate in the metabolism of β-endorphin (Marks, 1978; Klee, 1977; Mains *et al.*, 1977). The questions concerning the action of such enzymes and the various factors that can enter into the processing and packaging of peptides are described in more detail elsewhere (Marks, 1978). Questions of interest in relation to endorphins are: (1) the sites for conversion and/or inactivation, (2) the role of transport processes, and (3) whether some of the intermediate peptides described are artifacts of extraction, or are intermediates in degradation. Evidence that enkephalin, and γ-endorphin in particular, are true breakdown products of β-endorphin has been reported (Austen *et al.*, 1977). There are some anomalies, since enkephalin, on the basis of radioimmunoassay is reported to be present in brain areas in concentrations that do not suggest a product–precursor relationship, unless exceptional transport factors are invoked (Rossier *et al.*, 1977). Lipotropic peptides undergo considerable change unless precautions are taken to prevent breakdown during storage and extraction of the tissues (Rubenstein *et al.*, 1977). This account briefly summarizes studies performed in this laboratory to measure breakdown of enkephalin and β-endorphin by brain extracts and the preparation of more stable derivatives.

Breakdown of enkephalin

Methods for studying breakdown of opioid peptides were identical to those used in comparable studies on luteinizing hormone releasing hormone (LHRH), Substance P, kinin-9, and somatostatin (Marks, 1978). They are based on measurements of the release of amino acids or peptides with time of incubation *in vitro*, since this has been shown to provide information on the primary and often rate-limiting points of cleavage. A number of the hypothalamic releasing factors have novel N and C-terminal end groups that limit the action of exopeptidases; therefore the primary points of cleavage are mediated by neutral endopeptidases releasing internal residues. This is substantiated by analogues with internal D-amino acids or other residues blocking the primary points of cleavage. Several such analogues have lower rates of breakdown and an enhanced activity *in vivo*.

Enkephalin has free N-(Tyr) and C-(Met) end groups, and is therefore a substrate for exopeptidases (Marks, 1978; Klee, 1977). Incubation with brain extracts causes release of Tyr and the remaining tetrapeptide fragment (Gly–Gly–Phe–Met) (table 12.7). Longer incubation periods lead to the release of Gly–Gly, Phe, and Met. The finding of Gly–Gly indicates the presence in brain of a slow-acting Gly–Gly dipeptidase dependent on the presence of Co^{2+} (Stern and Marks, 1978). Substitution of Gly in position 2 with D-Ala retarded breakdown, based on the release of the

Table 12.7 Breakdown of opioid peptides or analogues by mouse brain extracts

Substrate	Analogue	
Enkephalin	–	Tyr (85), Gly–Gly (45), Phe (45), Met (45), tetrapeptide
	D-Ala^2	Tyr (trace)
	D-Ala^3	Try (90), Gly (21), tetrapeptide
	D-Phe^4	Tyr (65), Gly (10), tetrapeptide
	D-Met^4	Tyr (82), Gly (4), tetrapeptide
	$-NH_2{}^5$	Tyr (50)
	D-Ala^2-$NH_2{}^5$	Tyr (trace)
Endorphin		Tyr (6), Phe (4), Ser (5), Glu (7), Lys (3), His (3), Ile (6), Leu (6)
	D Ala^2	Tyr (trace), Lys (6)

Peptides and their analogues were incubated, and the products analyzed as described previously (Marks *et al.*, 1977; Grynbaum *et al.*, 1977). The composition of the tetrapeptide was Gly–Gly–Phe–Met; analogues had the appropriate D-substituent. Products were those detected within 5 min of incubation at 37 °C.

Table 12.8 Stabilization of enkephalins to degradation: correlation with biological activity

(1) Substitutions that lead to loss of biological activity *in vitro* (guinea pig ileum, mouse vas deferens, or receptor binding assays)

Position 1: D-Tyr (or des-Tyr), O-methyl Tyr, Phe, sarcosine, L–DOPA, Trp, His

Position 2: Pro, sarcosine, D-Val, D-Phe

Position 3: D-Ala

Position 4: Gly, D-Phe

Position 5: D-Met

(2) Substitutions that lead to an enhancement of activity:

D-Ala^2.Met.NH_2 *†	D-Ala^2, D-Leu^5 *
D-Met^2.Pro NH_2 (or NHEt)†,‡	D-Ala^2, Met^5-carbinol*, †, ‡
D-Ala^2.Pro NH_2 (or NHEt)†	D-Ala^2, methyl Phe^4, Met (O)-carbinol*,†,‡
N-(methyl) Tyr^1 †	

*Activity measured † i.c., or ‡ when given systemically.
Summarized from Bradbury *et al.*, 1976; Coy *et al.*, 1976; Pert *et al.*, 1976; Baxter *et al.*, 1977; Grynbaum *et al.*, 1977; Roemer *et al.*, 1977 and Bajusz *et al.*, 1976.

N-terminal Tyr, but failed to prevent the action of carboxypeptidases, especially at longer incubation periods (table 12.7). The presence of Ala in position 2 and an amide grouping in position 5 gave a peptide that was not metabolized. The 'stabilized' pentapeptide not only retained activity *in vitro* but was active when administered directly into brain (Grynbaum *et al.*, 1977). Since pentapeptides are more easily synthesized than endorphins, stability is an important consideration for preparation of clinically useful agents. Table 12.8 lists some of these and demonstrates that substitution in position 2 and 3 by residues known to block the action of proteolytic enzymes in most cases enhances activity and in some cases equals the analgesic action of β-endorphin. Position 2 has been substituted with D-Ala, D-Met, and position 5 with amide (Met or Pro), D-Leu, and methionine sulfoxide. Alterations of position 1 with substituents such as D-Tyr, Phe, sarcosine, Trp, His, and DOPA generally lead to loss of activity, indicating the essentiality of the N-terminal Tyr grouping. We compared the biodegradation of analogues of enkephalin (table 12.7). Placement of a D-amino acid (Ala, Phe, or Met) in positions 3–5 failed to protect the N-terminal Tyr grouping, and would not therefore be expected to engender enhanced activity. Among the end products of these analogues was formation of a tetrapeptide resistant to brain carboxypeptidases.

Breakdown of β-endorphin

Our early studies were among the first to demonstrate a lower rate of breakdown of β-endorphin compared with enkephalin, when incubated under the same conditions with brain extracts (Marks *et al.*, 1977). This has been attributed to a conformation of β-endorphin resistant to brain exopeptidases, since the release of N-terminal Tyr is substantially smaller than in the case of the pentapeptide (table 12.7). The release, however, of trace levels of Tyr in the absence of residues adjacent to positions 65 and 66 suggests a direct action on β-endorphin rather than on some intermediate peptide such as LPH_{61-65} itself. The preferential release of amino acids from positions 76–80 indicates action by an endopeptidase with concomitant release of fragments such as γ and α-endorphins. The production of α-endorphin could result in secondary action by a carboxypeptidase on the released γ-fragment. Replacement of Gly in position 2 by D-Ala greatly reduced the release of N-terminal and internal amino acids, indicating a marked reduction in susceptibility to degradation. Mechanisms for breakdown or conversion of β-endorphin have not been fully delineated, and more than one pathway may exist, depending on the source of enzyme and the conditions used for study *in vitro* (pH, subcellular fraction). Smyth and co-workers reported production of trace amounts of enkephalin along with γ-endorphin upon incubation of β-endorphin with a washed synaptosomal membrane fraction in the presence of bacitracin at pH 7.4 (Austen *et al.*, 1977). The low rate of enkephalin production at physiological pH requires comment, since this may reflect on some aspects of processing *in vivo*. The possibility exists that enkephalin is not formed by cleavage of the 65–66 bond, but is the result of secondary cleavage of some intermediate fragment by carboxypeptidases.

CONCLUSION

In conclusion, we would like to emphasize the following points

(1) Protein metabolism in the brain is rapid. It is heterogeneous, but the majority of proteins have a half-life of 10 days or less and are therefore replaced several times during the lifetime of most species.

(2) Most proteins are metabolized at significant rates; very small amounts, if any, are stable. Turnover is extensive.

(3) The metabolic rates of peptides derived from protein are not known. The rapid and extensive metabolism of proteins produces continuously large amounts of peptides. Since the concentration of the peptide intermediates is very low, the further breakdown of peptides once formed from proteins must be much faster than that of the proteins—with a half-life in hours rather than days.

(4) The flux of amino acids from the free pool to proteins and back is very high, with half-lives in minutes. The half-lives of tRNA-bound amino acids are probably less than a second.

(5) The available evidence shows that proteinases are present in the brain in excess of that needed for protein turnover. Levels of peptidases are higher than those of proteinases. It seems likely that at least part of the enzymes or their substrates are occluded in some manner; bringing together or separating enzymes and substrates may be an important control step.

(6) The penetration and uptake of peptides into brain is small. This does, however, not exclude exogenous origin of some of the peptides in brain.

(7) A number of enzymes with varying properties, distribution, and substrate specificities participate in peptide and protein turnover. As proteins and peptides break down, their substrate specificity to these enzymes changes. The participation of enzymes in the sequential breakdown is complex.

We are just in the early stages in identifying the various peptides present in the brain, most of which are at very low levels. We are even less advanced in the search for the enzymes responsible for their formation and breakdown. Unlike with amino acid neurotransmitters, transport is unlikely to be a major factor in the control of the biological activity of neuropeptides. We must look for the enzymes, and the factors controlling enzyme activity, for the regulation of peptide composition of the brain.

ACKNOWLEDGEMENT

Work in the authors' laboratory was in part supported by P. H. S. grants NS03226 and NS12578. The authors want to thank Dr N. Kline for helpful discussions and support.

REFERENCES

Ames, A. III and Parks, J. M. (1976). *J. Neurochem.*, **27**, 1017–25

Austin, L., Lowry, O. H., Brown, J. G. and Carter, J. G. (1972). *Biochem. J.*, **126**, 351–9

Austen, B. M., Smyth, D. G. and Snell, C. R. (1977). *Nature*, **269**, 610–21

Bajusz, S., Ronai, A. Z., Szekely, J. I., Graf, L., Dumas-Koracs, Z. and Berzetei, I. (1976). *FEBS Lett.*, **76**, 91–2

Baxter, M. G., Goff, D., Miller, A. A. and Saunders, I. A. (1977). *Brit. J. Pharmac.*, **59**, 455P

Bradbury, A. F., Smyth, D. G. and Snell, G. R. (1976). *CIBA Found. Symp.*, **41**, 61–75

Cowan, W. M. (1973). In *Development and Aging in the Nervous System*, (ed. M. Rockstein). Academic Press, New York, pp. 19–34

Coy, D. H., Kastin, A. J., Schally, A. V., Morrin, G., Caron, N. G., Labrie, F., Walter, J. M., Fertel, R., Berntson, G. G. and Sandman, C. A. (1976). *Biochem. biophys. Res. Commun.*, **73**, 632–8

Dunlop, D. S., van Elden, W. and Lajtha, A. (1975). *J. Neurochem.*, **24**, 337–44

Dunlop, D. S., van Elden, W. and Lajtha, A. (1977). *J. Neurochem.*, **29**, 939–45

Dunlop, D. S., van Elden, W. and Lajtha, A (1978). *Biochem. J.*, **170**, 637–42

Fern, E. B. and Garlick, P. J. (1976). *Biochem. J.*, **156**, 189–92

Gainer, H. (ed.). (1977). *Peptides in Neurobiology,* Plenum Press, New York

Garlick, P. J. and Marshall, I. (1972). *J. Neurochem.,* **19**, 577–83

Gaull, G. E., Tallan, H. H., Lajtha, A. and Rassin, D. K. (1975). In *Biology of Brain Dysfunction* (ed. G. E. Gaull), Plenum Press, New York, pp. 47-143

Grynbaum, A., Kastin, A. J., Coy, D. H. and Marks, N. (1977). *Brain Res. Bull.,* **2,** 479–84

Jacquet, Y. and Marks, N. (1976). *Science,* **194**, 632–5

Jacquet, Y., Marks, N. and Li, C.–H. (1976). In *Opiates and Endogenous Opioid Peptides,* (ed. H. W. Kosterlitz), Elsevier, Amsterdam, pp. 411–4

Johnson, T. C. (1977). *J. Neurochem.,* **27**, 17–23

Klee, W. A. (1977). In *Peptides in Neurobiology,* (ed. H. Gainer), Plenum Press, New York, pp. 375–96

Lajtha, A., Latzkovits, L. and Toth, J. (1976). *Biochim. biophys. Acta,* **425**, 511–20

Lajtha, A. and Toth, J. (1966). *Biochem. biophys. Res. Commun.,* **23,** 294–8

Lajtha, A. and Toth, J. (1978). *Biochim. biophys. Acta* (in press)

Mains, R. E., Eipper, B. A. and Ling, N. (1977). *Proc. natn. Acad. Sci. U.S.A,* **74**, 3014–8

Marks, N. (1978). In *Frontiers in Neuroendocrinology,* Vol. 5, (eds. W. F. Ganong and L. Martini), Raven Press, New York, pp. 329–77

Marks, N., Grynbaum, A. and Neidle, A. (1977). *Biochem. biophys. Res. commun.,* **74,** 1552–9

Menkes, J. H. (1968). *Neurology,* **18**, 1003–8

Oja, S. S. (1967). *Annl Acad. Sci. Fenn.* **A5 131,** 1–18

Parks, J. M., Ames, A. III and Nesbett, F. B. (1976). *J. Neurochem.,* **27**, 987–97

Pert, C. B., Bowie, D. L., Fong, B. T. W. and Chang, J. -K. (1976). In *Opiates and Endogenous Opioid Peptides,* (ed. H. W. Kosterlitz). Elsevier, Amsterdam, pp. 79–102

Roemer, D., Buescher, H. H., Hill, R. C., Pless, J., Bauer, W., Cardinaux, F., Closse, A., Hauser, D. and Huguenin, R. (1977). *Nature,* **268**, 547–9

Roberts, S. (1974). In *Aromatic Amino Acids in the Brain. CIBA Found. Symp.,* **22**, American Elsevier, New York, pp. 299–324

Roberts, S. (1977). In *Mechanisms, Regulation and Special Functions of Protein Synthesis in the Brain,* (eds S. Roberts, A. Lajtha and W. H. Gispen). Elsevier, Amsterdam, (in press)

Rossier, J., Vargo, T. M., Minick, S., Ling, N., Bloom, F. E. and Guillemin, R. (1977). *Proc. natn. Acad. Sci. U.S.A.,* **74**, 5162–5

Rubenstein, M., Stein, S., Gerber, L. and Udenfriend, S. (1977). *Proc. natn. Acad. Sci. U.S.A.,* **74**, 3052–5

Seta, K., Sansur, M. and Lajtha, A. (1973). *Biochim. biophys. Acta,* **294**, 472–80

Stern, F. and Marks, N. (1978). *Trans. Am. Soc. Neurochem.*, **9**, 186

13
Coordinate synthesis and release of corticotropin and endorphin

Richard E. Mains and Betty A. Eipper (Department of Physiology, C240, University of Colorado Medical Center, Denver, Colorado, U.S.A.)

In the course of studies on the biosynthesis of adrenocorticotropin (ACTH) it was discovered that β-lipotropin (β-LPH) and β-endorphin [β-LPH_{61-91}] share a common biosynthetic precursor with ACTH. These initial findings are summarized and more recent work on the coordinate synthesis and release of ACTH and endorphin is presented.

ACTH is a peptide hormone which occurs in several forms with apparent molecular weights differing by more than a factor of six (Eipper and Mains, 1975; Mains and Eipper, 1976). In order to determine whether these various forms of ACTH are members of a biosynthetic pathway, it is necessary to introduce radioactive amino acids into ACTH-synthesizing tissue for a short period of time (pulse); the labeled amino acid is then replaced by unlabeled amino acid, and during the chase period (when no labeled proteins are synthesized) the fate of labeled proteins synthesized during the initial pulse incubation is determined. Labeled ACTH-containing molecules must then be isolated in good yield from each timed sample. The ACTH-secreting mouse pituitary tumor cell line (AtT-20/D-16v) developed by Furth (1955), Buonassisi *et al.* (1962) and Yasamura (1968) was used because it provides a homogeneous population of ACTH-synthesizing cells; immunochemical procedures were used to purify all ACTH-containing molecules from the tissue extracts in good yield in a single step.

The results of a pulse-chase experiment are summarized in figure 13.1 (Mains and Eipper, 1976). Identical microwells of AtT-20 cells were incubated in complete tissue culture growth medium containing [^{3}H] tyrosine for 20 min; one sample was harvested and the remaining microwells were rinsed and incubated for increasing periods of time in the same complete culture medium containing excess unlabeled tyrosine. Cell extracts were then immunoprecipitated with an affinity-purified ACTH antiserum and [^{3}H]-labeled ACTH-containing molecules were separated by SDS polyacrylamide gel electrophoresis. At short times only one form of ACTH is labeled; its apparent molecular weight in this particular gel system is 31 000 (hence the name 31K ACTH). At later times radioactivity appears in 23K ACTH (a biosynthetic intermediate) and then in 13K ACTH and 4.5K ACTH; the amount of label in each form of ACTH was determined for each time point and these data are plotted in figure 13.1. Experiments such as these clearly demonstrate that the various forms of ACTH represent different stages in a biosynthetic pathway. Several possible models for the conversion of 31K ACTH into the smaller corticotropins can be imagined; a scheme that is in agreement with all of the present data is shown in figure 13.2. The fact that 31K, 23K and 13K ACTH are all glycoproteins (4.5K ACTH is not) must be taken into account in thinking about the biosynthetic pathway (Eipper *et al.*, 1976).

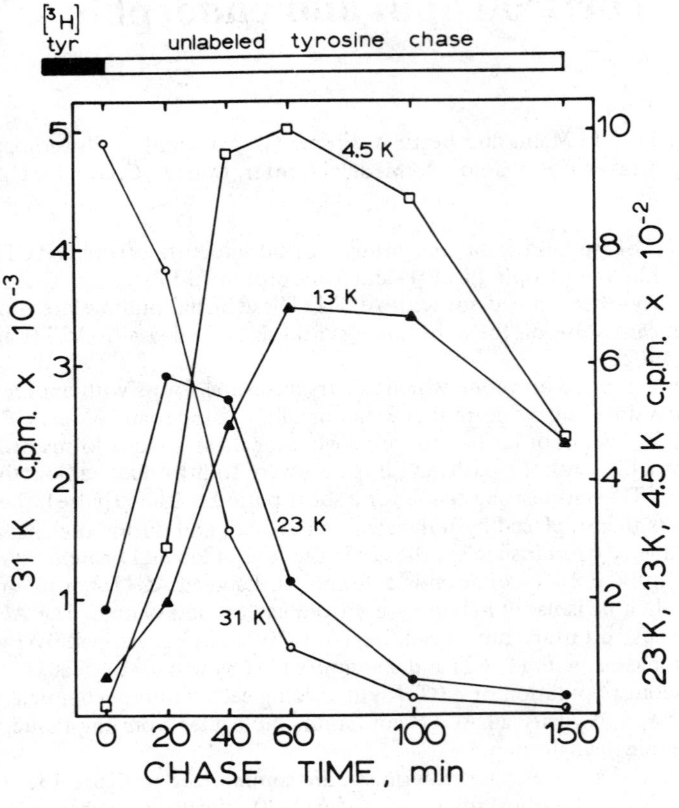

Figure 13.1 Corticotropin pulse-chase with [^{3}H] tyrosine. Six identical microwells of AtT-20/D-16v cells were incubated in a complete tissue culture medium in which [^{3}H] tyrosine (150 μM) replaced the usual unlabeled tyrosine for 20 min (Mains and Eipper, 1976). One microwell was harvested at the end of the pulse (at chase time = 0) and the remaining microwells were incubated in complete medium containing unlabeled tyrosine for varying periods of time. Cell extracts were immunoprecipitated with affinity-purified ACTH antiserum Bertha and analyzed by SDS polyacrylamide gel electrophoresis. The radioactivity in each form of ACTH for each timed extract was then summed from the gel data and is plotted here as a function of chase time.

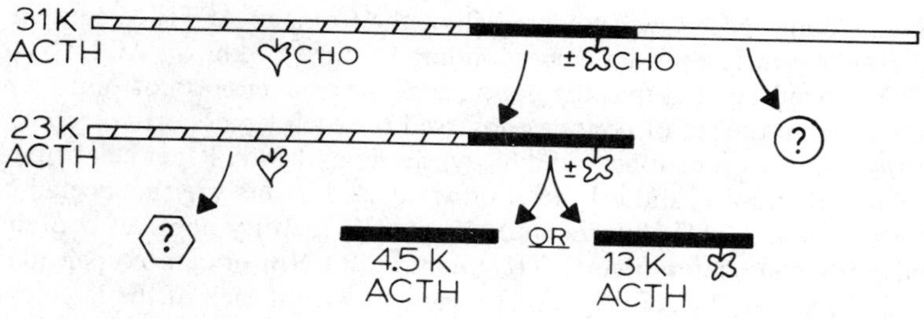

Figure 13.2 Biosynthetic processing of the ACTH precursor.

It is important to know whether the 31K ACTH molecule observed in intact cells is closely related to the initial gene product and whether ACTH synthesis in normal pituitary tissue is similar to that in AtT-20 cells. Since 31K ACTH labels linearly from approximately time zero for at least 30 min, any molecule preceding 31K ACTH in the biosynthetic sequence must be very short-lived (for example, a molecule with a 'pre' sequence). Roberts and Herbert (1977*a* and *b*) and Herbert *et al.* (this volume) have used several cell-free protein synthesizing systems to show that mRNA from AtT-20 cells directs the synthesis of a 28.5K ACTH molecule that is very similar to the 31K ACTH molecule observed in cells; oligosaccharide chains are not added in the cell-free systems. Similar studies using mRNA from bovine and rat pituitary tissue indicate that in normal pituitary tissue, ACTH is initially synthesized as a 30 000–35 000 dalton molecule (Nakanishi *et al.*, 1976; 1977).

We decided to study the structure of the various ACTH-containing molecules in order to address the following problems

(1) The 31K ACTH precursor is five or six times larger than the 39-amino acid polypeptide form of ACTH that has been purified from pituitary tissue. Do the non-corticotropin parts of the ACTH precursor have a biological function?

(2) Radioimmunoassays for the C-peptide of insulin (Tager *et al.*, 1975) and the COOH-terminal of parathyroid hormone (Segré *et al.*, 1974) have proved helpful in evaluating function of the endocrine pancreas and parathyroid gland. If a stable fragment of the ACTH precursor were secreted along with ACTH, it might provide a way to assess function of pituitary corticotropes.

(3) What enzymatic reactions occur at each step in the pathway?

(4) ACTH is synthesized in both the anterior and intermediate lobes of the pituitary; the steady-state pattern of ACTH-containing molecules in the two lobes is very different (Mains and Eipper, 1975). What enzymatic differences between ACTH-synthesizing cells in the two lobes could cause the observed differences?

As a first step in delineating the structure of the various forms of ACTH, we incubated AtT-20 cells with the desired [^{3}H]-labeled precursor (eleven different amino acids and four sugars have been used) and then isolated labeled ACTH-containing molecules by immunoprecipitation and gel filtration (Eipper and Mains, 1977; Mains *et al.*, 1977; Eipper and Mains, 1978). The purity of the pools obtained can be checked by SDS polyacrylamide gel electrophoresis (figure 13.3) and, if necessary, preparative polyacrylamide gel electrophoresis can be used to obtain pools containing a single form of ACTH (Roberts and Herbert, 1977*a*).

Since the sequence of the 39-amino acid form of ACTH appears to be highly conserved among species, we expected all of the forms of ACTH to contain tryptic and chymotryptic peptides corresponding to those of known $ACTH_{1-39}$ molecules. We also anticipated that the peptides of the smaller corticotropins would be contained within the set of peptides observed for each larger corticotropin, since the corticotropins are members of a biosynthetic pathway. Paper electrophoresis, paper chromatography, and gel-filtration were used to analyze the labeled peptides; in addition, ACTH antisera could be used to identify peptides containing particular antigenic determinants. Treatment with CNBr or carboxypeptidase A was used to localize the $ACTH_{1-39}$-like segment within each of the large corticotropins (Eipper and Mains, 1978).

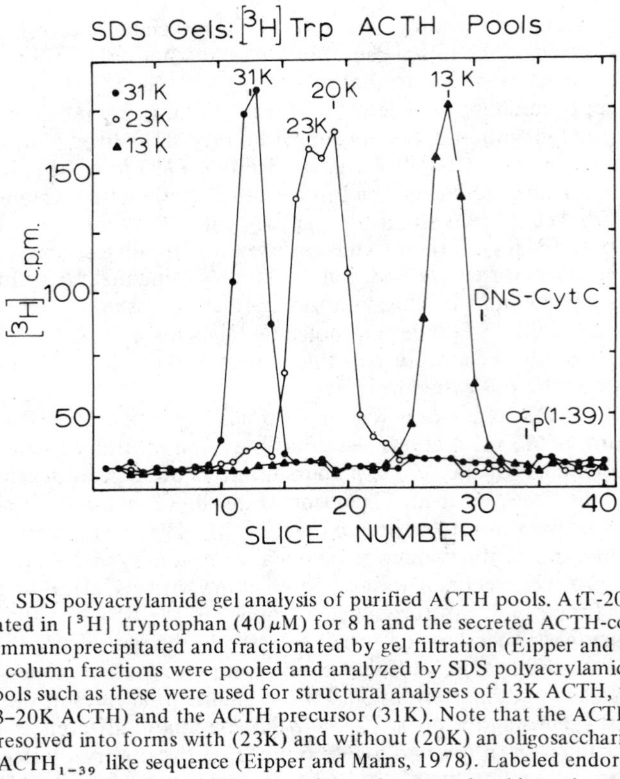

Figure 13.3 SDS polyacrylamide gel analysis of purified ACTH pools. AtT-20/D-16v cells were incubated in [^{3}H] tryptophan (40 μM) for 8 h and the secreted ACTH-containing molecules were immunoprecipitated and fractionated by gel filtration (Eipper and Mains, 1977). Aliquots of column fractions were pooled and analyzed by SDS polyacrylamide gel electrophoresis. Pools such as these were used for structural analyses of 13K ACTH, the ACTH intermediate (23–20K ACTH) and the ACTH precursor (31K). Note that the ACTH intermediate is partially resolved into forms with (23K) and without (20K) an oligosaccharide chain attached within the $ACTH_{1-39}$ like sequence (Eipper and Mains, 1978). Labeled endorphin-containing molecules can be prepared by a similar procedure using an endorphin antiserum. The method presently used to purify [^{3}H] labeled ACTH and endorphin-containing molecules begins with an endorphin immunoprecipitation step (which removes the ACTH/endorphin precursor) and thereby produces cleaner preparations of the ACTH intermediate (23–20K ACTH) (Eipper and Mains, 1978).

Using these techniques, the 4.5K ACTH synthesized by the tumor cells appears to be very similar to known $ACTH_{1-39}$ molecules. Studies on 13K ACTH (Eipper and Mains, 1977) indicate that it is simply a glycosylated $ACTH_{1-39}$-like peptide (figure 13.4); there are no peptide extensions at either end of the $ACTH_{1-39}$-like sequence in 13K ACTH. The mass of this glycosylated $ACTH_{1-39}$-like peptide appears to be 6700 ± 600 daltons (a 4600 dalton peptide plus a single 2400 ± 400 dalton oligosaccharide chain); SDS polyacrylamide gel electrophoresis often gives erroneously high apparent molecular weight estimates for glycoproteins (Segrest and Jackson, 1972; Weber *et al.*, 1972). In our experience, gel-filtration in 6 M guanidine HCl provides reasonably accurate molecular weight estimates for glycoproteins. It is not yet clear whether the peptide backbone of 13K ACTH is identical to that of 4.5K ACTH or whether there are slight differences in primary structure which may govern the addition or lack of addition of the sugar chain. There are precedents for both models: bovine and ovine ribonucleases occur in multiple forms consisting of a single primary sequence to which an oligosaccharide chain is sometimes added (Plummer and Hirs, 1963; Becker *et al.*, 1973); rat pancreatic islets contain two forms of rat proinsulin differing slightly in primary structure (Tager *et al.*, 1975). The structure of 13K ACTH (figure 13.4) means that conventional proteolytic processing cannot produce 4.5K ACTH from 13K ACTH and pulse-chase studies (figure 13.1) indicate that 13K ACTH does not have the properties expected of a precursor to 4.5K ACTH.

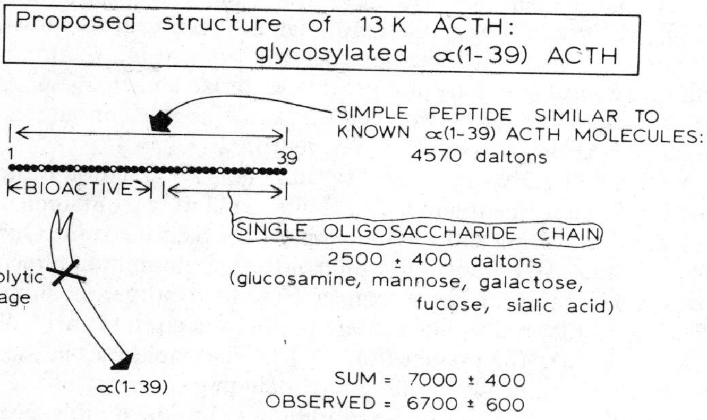

Figure 13.4 Structure of 13K ACTH. Analysis of [^{3}H] amino acid and [^{3}H] sugar labeled 13K ACTH indicates that 13K ACTH is simply a glycosylated $ACTH_{1-39}$-like molecule (Eipper and Mains, 1977). The mass of the $ACTH_{1-39}$-like peptide backbone (4600 daltons) plus the single oligosaccharide chain (2400 ± 400 daltons) fully accounts for the mass of 13K ACTH as determined by gel filtration in 6 M guanidine HCl (6700 ± 600 daltons). The sizes of small glycoproteins are often overestimated by SDS polyacrylamide gel electrophoresis (Segrest and Jackson, 1972; Weber *et al.*, 1972); gel-filtration in 6 M guanidine HCl has provided more accurate molecular weight estimates for glycoproteins.

The peptides of 31K ACTH and 23K ACTH labeled with particular amino acids were also analyzed (Eipper and Mains, 1978). The data indicate that the $ACTH_{1-39}$-like sequence is located at the COOH-terminal end of the 23K ACTH molecule (recall figure 13.2) and that most of the additional peptide present in 31K ACTH but absent from 23K ACTH is added to the COOH-terminal end of 23K ACTH (figure 13.2). Thus 31K ACTH could be converted into 13K ACTH (or 4.5K ACTH) plus two other peptide fragments with molecular weights of approximately 10 000. Two lines of evidence indicated that cells that synthesize ACTH often also synthesize β-LPH (or β-melanotropin (β-MSH), which is β-LPH_{41-58}): first, ACTH and β-LPH (or β-MSH) are released together in roughly equimolar amounts by normal pituitary tissue and by ectopic ACTH-secreting tumors (Gilkes *et al.*, 1975; Lowry *et al.*, 1976; Abe *et al.*, 1969; Hirata *et al.*, 1976); second, ACTH and β-LPH (β-MSH) can be localized in the same pituitary cells and in the same secretory granules by immunohistochemical techniques (Moriarty, 1973; Dubois *et al.*, 1973; Phifer *et al.*, 1974). We thus considered the possibility that part of the non-corticotropin region of 31K ACTH might consist of a peptide similar to known β-LPH molecules. It should be noted, before jumping to the conclusion that a common precursor for ACTH and β-LPH is inevitable, that although the many digestive enzymes of the exocrine pancreas fulfil the corelease and cellular localization criteria (Kraehenbuhl *et al.*, 1977), each enzyme is synthesized independently with its own 'pre' sequence and not as part of some giant common precursor molecule (Devillers-Thierry *et al.*, 1975).

Comparison of the peptide patterns of 31K ACTH and 23K ACTH labeled with methionine, lysine, arginine, threonine, tyrosine, phenylalanine, and tryptophan all indicated that the peptide segment cleaved from 31K ACTH during its conversion to 23K ACTH could be similar, although not identical, to known β-LPH molecules (Li and Chung, 1976*a*). The large peptide segment in question contained only one methionine residue in a tryptic peptide with size and charge properties similar to those of the β-LPH_{61-69} tryptic peptide; a methionine-containing tryptic peptide similar to β-LPH_{47-51} could not be identified.

To investigate directly the possibility that one 31 000 dalton protein contained both an ACTH-like segment and a β-LPH-like segment, we obtained endorphin antisera from Drs N. Ling and R. Guillemin of the Salk Institute. Our initial experiments showed that ACTH and endorphin antisera both immunoprecipitated equal amounts of a 31K molecule from samples of AtT-20 culture medium; in addition to the 31K molecule, endorphin antisera immunoprecipitate an 11.7K molecule and a 3.5K molecule. The presence of [^{3}H]-labeled molecules in each immunoprecipitate could be specifically abolished by including an excess of the appropriate synthetic peptide ($ACTH_{1-24}$ or β-$endorphin_{1-31}$) in the double antibody immunoprecipitation incubation (Mains *et al.*, 1977). Sequential immunoprecipitations with one antibody and then the other showed that no [^{3}H]-labeled 31K molecule remained for the second antibody to immunoprecipitate; this result implied that the two antisera were precipitating the same 31K molecule. A direct demonstration that 31K ACTH (the 31K molecule precipitated with an ACTH antiserum) and 31K endorphin (the 31K molecule precipitated with an endorphin antiserum) are the same molecule was obtained by comparing the tryptic and chymotryptic peptides of the two molecules labeled with several different [^{3}H] amino acids. An example of this type of analysis is shown in figure 13.5. The [^{3}H] phenylalanine-labeled chymotryptic peptides of 31K ACTH and 31K endorphin appear to be identical. Since a single molecule appears to contain antigenic determinants and peptides of both ACTH and β-endorphin, this molecule is referred to as 31K ACTH/endorphin.

The stars marked on the peptide patterns shown in figure 13.5 and 13.6 indicate the places where phenylalanine-labeled peptides are missing when the peptide patterns for 31K ACTH/endorphin and 23K ACTH are compared; these phenylalanine-containing chymotryptic peptides appear in 11.7K endorphin (a β-LPH-like molecule). Similar experiments have been carried out using tryptophan, methionine, leucine and arginine-labeled material (figure 13.7). In every case, comparison of the tryptic (or chymotryptic) peptide patterns of 31K ACTH/endorphin and 23K ACTH accurately predicts the peptides observed in 11.7K endorphin; in addition, the peptides of 11.7K endorphin have the size and charge properties expected of peptides obtained from a β-LPH-like molecule.

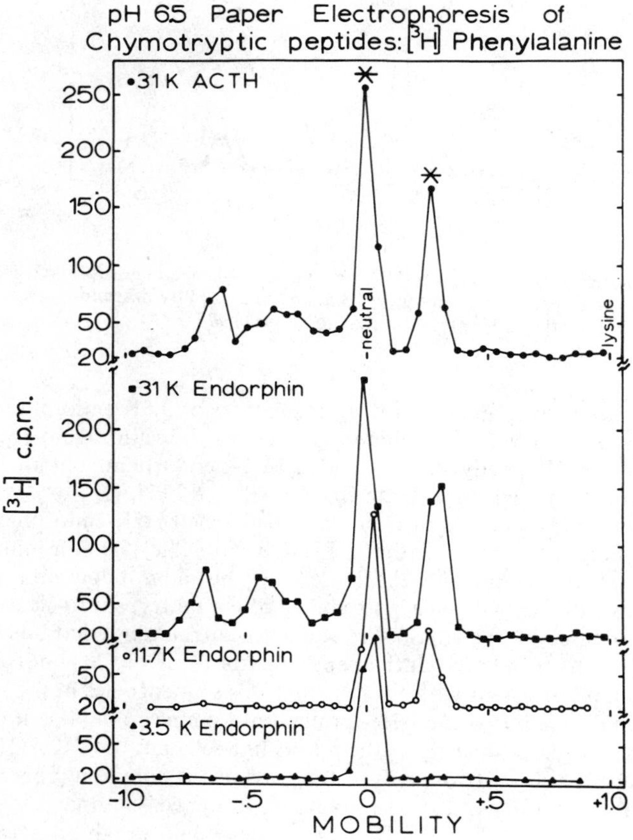

Figure 13.5 Paper electrophoresis of [^{3}H] phenylalanine-labeled chymotryptic peptides. AtT-20/D-16v cells were incubated in complete culture medium in which the usual phenylalinine was replaced with [^{3}H] phenylalanine (150 μM); secreted corticotropin and endorphin-containing molecules were purified by immunoprecipitation and gel-filtration (Mains *et al.*, 1977). Pools were digested with chymotrypsin (Eipper and Mains, 1977) and analyzed by paper electrophoresis. Comparison of the peptide patterns of 23K ACTH (not shown) and 31K ACTH indicated that peptides in the two starred positions were absent from 23K ACTH.

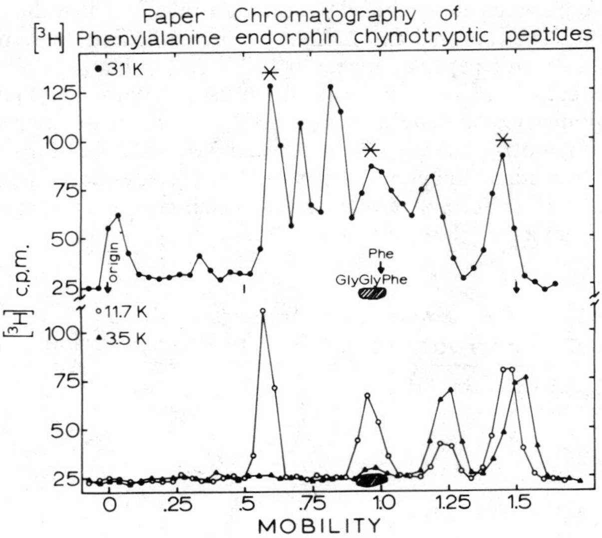

Figure 13.6 Paper chromatography of [^{3}H] phenylalanine-labeled endorphin chymotryptic peptides. Samples were prepared as in figure 13.5, and analyzed by descending paper chromatography in butanol/acetic acid/water (Eipper and Mains, 1977).

Analysis of the tryptic and chymotryptic peptides of 3.5K endorphin indicates that it is similar to known β-endorphin molecules. As shown in figure 13.6, chymotryptic digests of [^{3}H] phenylalanine-labeled 11.7K endorphin contain a labeled peptide that comigrates with synthetic Gly–Gly–Phe (β-LPH$_{62-64}$ or β-endorphin$_{2-4}$). Chymotryptic digests of phenylalanine-labeled 3.5K endorphin contain a peptide that comigrates with synthetic Tyr–Gly–Gly–Phe [β-endorphin$_{1-4}$; mobility relative to phenylalanine of 1.25, figure 13.6] but do not contain a peptide that comigrates with Gly–Gly–Phe. The ability of chymotrypsin to cleave a particular bond is affected by the amino acid sequence surrounding that bond (Smyth, 1967) and this difference between the peptide patterns of 11.7K endorphin and 3.5K endorphin is consistent with the fact that this sequence lies in the middle of a β-LPH-like molecule but at the NH_2-terminal of a β-endorphin-like molecule.

The ACTH$_{1-39}$-like segment plus the β-LPH-like segment of 31K ACTH/endorphin account for about two-thirds of the mass of the common precursor. As shown in figure 13.2, the peptide corresponding to the NH_2-terminal segment of the ACTH intermediate (23K ACTH) could be created during the conversion of this intermediate to the smaller forms of ACTH (13K ACTH or 4.5K ACTH depending upon the presence or absence of an oligosaccharide chain in the ACTH$_{22-37}$ region of the molecule). At present the only technique that can be used to identify such a peptide fragment is based on the 'difference of peptides' approach used to study the β-LPH-like molecule: most of the non-ACTH peptides observed in tryptic digests of labeled 23K ACTH should be present in such a fragment. Using this approach and an antiserum to general AtT-20 secretory proteins, we have been

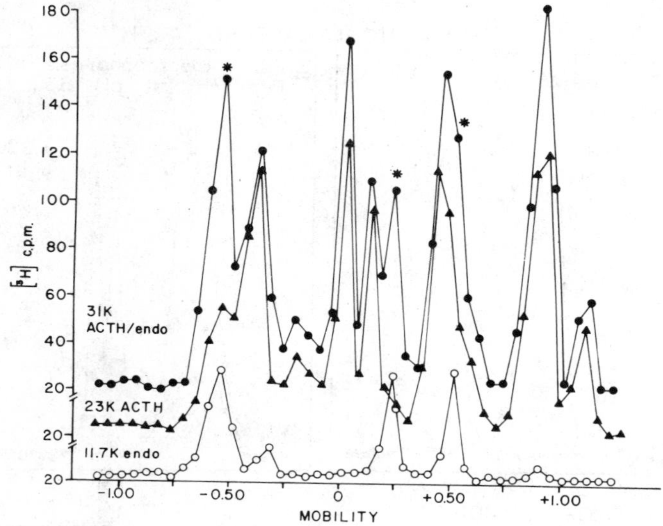

Figure 13.7 Paper electrophoresis of [^{3}H] arginine-labeled tryptic peptides. AtT-20/D-16v cells were incubated in [^{3}H] arginine-containing culture medium (150 μM arginine) for 8 h, and secreted corticotropin and endorphin-containing molecules were immunoprecipitated (see figure 13.5). The purified pools were digested with trypsin and analyzed by paper electrophoresis (pH 6.35). The ratio of radioactivity in the three major regions of the 11.7K endorphin analysis (negative: R_L = +0.25: R_L = +0.50) is 2.02:1.01:0.97, which suggests that there are four arginine residues in the mouse tumor cell β-LPH-like molecule.

able to identify a molecule (16K fragment) that appears to correspond to the NH_2-terminal region of 23K ACTH (or 31K ACTH/endorphin). Using a number of different labeled amino acids, the tryptic and chymotryptic peptides of 16K fragment plus those of 13K ACTH can be shown to account for all of the peptides of 23K ACTH (Mains and Eipper, 1978; Eipper and Mains, 1978). This 16K fragment can be recovered from culture medium in amounts roughly equimolar to the amount of 4.5K ACTH plus 13K ACTH recovered; apparently very little of this material is degraded. By comparing the tryptic peptides of [^{3}H] mannose-labeled 23K ACTH and 13K ACTH it can be predicted that 16K fragment is a glycopeptide (figure 13.8). On the basis of gel-filtration in 6 M guanidine HCl, the mass of the 16K fragment is 11 200 ± 500 daltons; as was the case for 13K ACTH (also a glycoprotein), SDS polyacrylamide gel electrophoresis does not provide an accurate estimate of molecular weight. The tryptic glycopeptides of sugar-labeled 31K ACTH/endorphin and 23K ACTH are very similar; this implies that 11.7K endorphin is not glycosylated and subsequent direct experiments indicate that this is true. Thus oligosaccharide chains can be attached to the ACTH/endorphin precursor at a site (or sites) in the 16K fragment and at a site in the COOH-terminal half of the ACTH-like segment. If the plasma half-life of the 16K fragment is sufficiently long, radioimmunoassays for plasma levels of the 16K fragment may prove to be clinically useful.

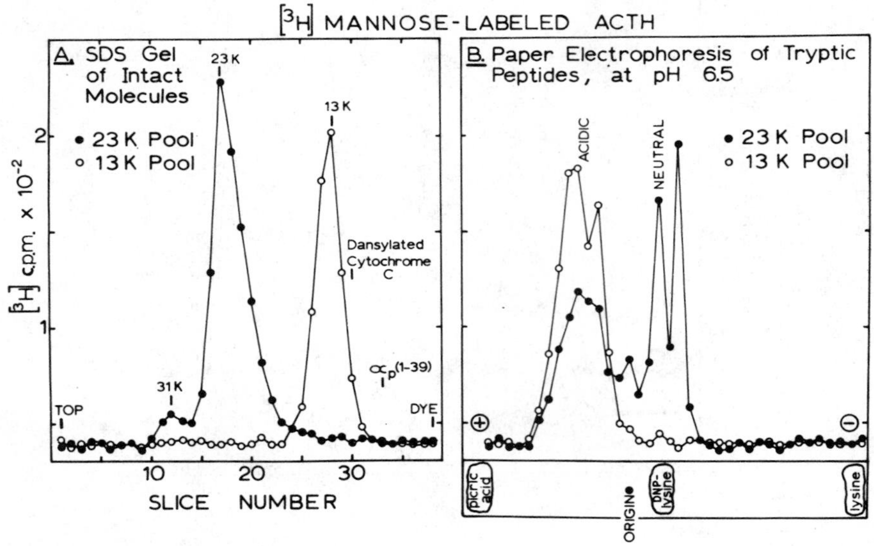

Figure 13.8 Analysis of [^{3}H] mannose-labeled corticotropins. A, AtT-20/D-16v cells were incubated in complete culture medium containing 5.5 mM glucose and 340 μM[^{3}H] mannose (Eipper *et al.*, 1976) for 8 h, and secreted [^{3}H] labeled ACTH-containing molecules were purified. SDS polyacrylamide gel electrophoresis was used to assess the purity of the pools of 23K and 13K ACTH. B, Pools of [^{3}H] mannose-labeled 23K ACTH and 13K ACTH were digested with trypsin and the peptides were analyzed by paper electrophoresis.

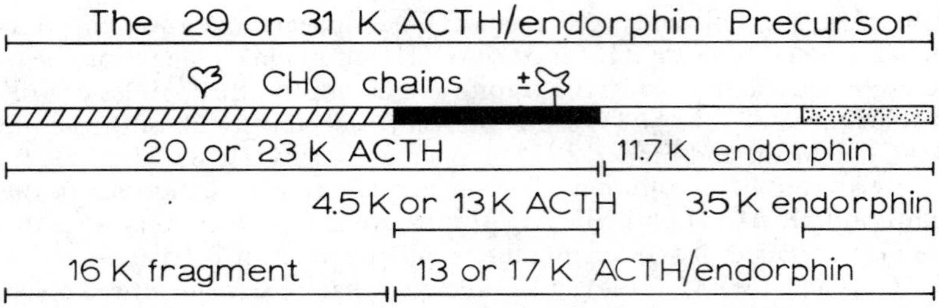

Figure 13.9 Model for the structure of the ACTH/endorphin precursor. The various cleavage products of the common precursor that have been observed are indicated; all cleavage products are identified by their apparent molecular weight on borate-acetate buffered SDS polyacrylamide gels and by the antigenic determinants they contain.

Studies such as those outlined above have made it possible to construct a model for the structure of the ACTH/endorphin precursor (figure 13.9) (Eipper and Mains, 1978). The existence of glycosylated (13K ACTH) and non-glycosylated (4.5K ACTH) $ACTH_{1-39}$-like molecules coupled with the fact that oligosaccharide chains can be attached to nascent peptide chains implies that the ACTH/endorphin precursor and the ACTH intermediate should consist of molecules with and without an oligosaccharide chain attached within their $ACTH_{1-39}$-like sequence. Prolonged SDS polyacrylamide gel electrophoresis can be used to resolve the ACTH/endorphin precursor and the ACTH intermediate into several different components (Roberts and Herbert, 1977; Eipper and Mains, 1978). Thus 31K ACTH/endorphin contains a glycosylated $ACTH_{1-39}$-like sequence and can be converted to 13K ACTH (through a 23K ACTH intermediate) plus 11.7K endorphin plus 16K fragment. The 29K ACTH/endorphin molecule does not contain a glycosylated $ACTH_{1-39}$-like sequence and is converted to 4.5K ACTH (through a 20K ACTH intermediate) plus 11.7K endorphin plus 16K fragment. The factors controlling addition or lack of addition of the oligosaccharide chains are not known.

The model shown in figure 13.9 predicts that smaller ACTH/endorphin peptides could be generated if the cleavages that normally occur to produce 13K ACTH (or 4.5K ACTH) take place in the opposite order. By searching for peptides that contain antigenic determinants for both ACTH and endorphin it is possible to detect a 17K ACTH/endorphin molecule (containing an oligosaccharide in its $ACTH_{1-39}$-like sequence) and a 13K ACTH/endorphin molecule. These smaller ACTH/endorphins account for only about 1 per cent of the total ACTH or endorphin present in AtT-20 culture medium (Eipper and Mains, 1978).

Another interesting consequence of the model in figure 13.9 is that 3.5K endorphin (the β-endorphin-like molecule) could be produced in a single step from the ACTH/endorphin precursor without the generation of a β-LPH-like intermediate (11.7K endorphin). Since the original reports on the structure of enkephalins and endorphins (Hughes *et al.*, 1975; Guillemin *et al.*, 1976; Li and Chung, 1976*b*; Bradbury *et al.*, 1976) it has been assumed that β-LPH served as the biosynthetic precursor to endorphins. The pulse-chase protocol described earlier was used to study endorphin biosynthesis. AtT-20 cells were incubated with [^{3}H] phenylalanine and samples were immunoprecipitated with an endorphin antiserum and analyzed by SDS polyacrylamide gel electrophoresis; both cell extracts and culture media were examined (Mains and Eipper, 1977). As expected, the ACTH/endorphin precursor is the only labeled endorphin-containing molecule present in the cells after a 15 min pulse label; after a 15 to 30 min chase period, the β-LPH-like 11.7K endorphin molecule appears in the cells. Labeled β-endorphin-like molecules (3.5K endorphin) appear after about half of the ACTH/endorphin precursor molecules have been converted to 11.7K endorphin; thus 11.7K endorphin appears to be an obligatory biosynthetic intermediate in the production of most of the β-endorphin-like 3.5K endorphin synthesized by the pituitary tumor cells. This result clearly does not imply that a β-LPH-like molecule will serve as an intermediate in the synthesis of β-endorphin in other tissues (such as the intermediate lobe of the pituitary or CNS tissue).

The pulse-chase data can also be used to quantitate the number of ACTH and endorphin-containing molecules produced from each molecule of ACTH/endorphin (Mains and Eipper, 1978). The number of phenylalanine residues in each form of ACTH and endorphin was determined by analysis of [^{3}H] phenylalanine-labeled peptides. This number was used to convert the amount of radioactivity in each hormonal form into a measure of the number of moles of each hormonal form. The data indicate that, for the AtT-20 pituitary tumor cells, essentially every ACTH/endorphin precursor molecule synthesized gives rise to an ACTH-containing molecule (23K ACTH, 13K ACTH, or 4.5K ACTH) and an endorphin-containing molecule (11.7K endorphin or 3.5K endorphin); no substantial degradation of either hormonal product is seen.

In the AtT-20 pituitary tumor cells, the time course of the processing of ACTH-related peptides and endorphin-related peptides differs (Mains and Eipper, 1978). After synthesis, the ACTH/endorphin precursor is stable inside the cells for approximately 30 min; it is then converted into 20K or 23K ACTH plus 11.7K endorphin with a half-time of about 10 to 15 min. The ACTH intermediate is rapidly converted into 4.5K ACTH or 13K ACTH (half-time of about 10 to 15 min); the endorphin biosynthetic intermediate (11.7K endorphin) is converted into 3.5K endorphin at a much slower rate (half-time of about 1 hour).

If other ACTH and/or endorphin synthesizing tissues in addition to pituitary utilize a similar biosynthetic pathway, variations in the processing mechanisms could account for preferential accumulation of specific cleavage products. Processing of the various hormone molecules after their release from their tissue of origin could also alter their molecular form and their biological effects.

The AtT-20 mouse pituitary tumor cells were used in these studies because they provide a simplified system in which to study ACTH and endorphin biosynthesis. As a first step in comparing the tumor cells with normal pituitary tissue, we fractionated tumor cell extracts and normal mouse anterior pituitary tissue extracts by SDS polyacrylamide gel electrophoresis and compared the distribution of immunoactive ACTH-containing and endorphin-containing molecules (figure 13.10). Normal pituitary tissue and the tumor cells contain the same major forms of ACTH (31K, 23K, 13K and 4.5K ACTH) and endorphin (31K, 11.7K and 3.5K endorphin). It seems likely, therefore, that the biosynthetic pathways observed in the tumor cells are also operating in normal anterior pituitary tissue. The major difference in the two tissues is that, in comparison to the amount of ACTH/endorphin precursor, the tumor cells are relatively depleted of the smaller products (13K and 4.5K ACTH; 11.7K and 3.5K endorphin). The fact that the tumor cells secrete their hormonal contents every 6 to 8 hours while normal anterior pituitary tissue secretes only a fraction of its ACTH content each day (Vale and Rivier, 1977) may explain the altered distribution. It is important to note that different ACTH and endorphin antisera show varying degrees of reactivity with the different high molecular weight forms of ACTH and endorphin; thus the profile of immunoactive material observed will depend on the antiserum used. The β-endorphin antiserum used in these studies (RB–100) can immunoprecipitate as much labeled ACTH/ endorphin precursor as the $ACTH_{11-24}$ antiserum used; however, when these antisera are used at a low concentration to carry out radioimmunoassays, the two antisera give different estimates for the concentration of ACTH/endorphin precursor. Differential sensitivity of insulin and parathyroid hormone antisera to their respective prohormones and cleavage products has been known for some time (Kitabchi, 1970; Habener *et al.*, 1976; Segre *et al.*, 1974; Tager *et al.*, 1975). The differential reactivity of various antisera to the different molecular forms of a hormone makes it very difficult to interpret estimates of immunoactive hormone levels in crude tissue extracts. For example, an antiserum to the COOH-terminal

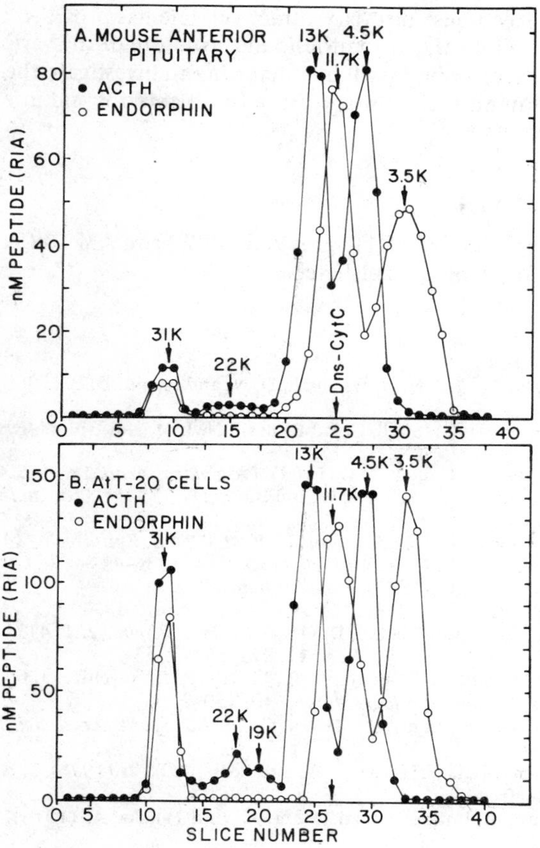

Figure 13.10 Tissue extract radioimmunoassays. Extracts of AtT-20 cells (1.1 mg of cell protein) and mouse anterior pituitary (2.4 lobes) were analyzed by SDS polyacrylamide gel electrophoresis; 2mm slices were eluted and then immunoassayed for ACTH (●; pmol porcine $ACTH_{1-39}$ equivalents/ml) and β-endorphin (○; pmol porcine β-endorphin equivalents/ml). In extracts of mouse anterior pituitary, 13K ACTH and 4.5K ACTH each account for 45 ± 3 per cent of the corticotropin immunoactivity; 11.7K endorphin and 3.5K endorphin each account for 47 ± 3 per cent of the endorphin immunoactivity. In tumor cell extracts, 13K ACTH and 4.5K ACTH each account for 37 ± 3 per cent of the corticotropin activity; 11.7K and 3.5K endorphin each account for 41 ± 3 per cent of the endorphin activity.

region of $ACTH_{1-39}$ is completely unreactive with the ACTH/endorphin precursor in both radioimmunoassay and immunoprecipitations; this antiserum does detect the ACTH intermediate and 13K ACTH. The lack of reactivity with the ACTH/endorphin precursor is presumably due to the presence of a peptide extension to the COOH-terminal side of the $ACTH_{1-39}$-like sequence in the common precursor (figure 13.9).

The AtT-20/D-16v mouse pitutiary tumor cell line has provided a great deal of useful information about the biosynthesis and structure of the various forms of endorphin and corticotropin. It will be interesting to investigate the biosynthesis of these molecules in normal pituitary tissue (both anterior and intermediate lobe tissue) and in brain tissue.

ACKNOWLEDGMENTS

This work was supported by NIH Grants AM 18929 and AM 19859. We thank Diane Honnecke for technical assistance.

REFERENCES

Abe, K., Nicholson, W. E., Liddle, G. W., Orth, D. N. and Island, D. P. (1969). *J. clin. Invest.*, **48**, 1580–5

Bradbury, A. F., Smyth, D. G., Snell, C. R., Birdsall, N. J. M. and Hulme, E. C. (1976). *Nature*, **260**, 793–5

Buonassisi, V., Sato, G. and Cohen, A. I. (1962). *Proc. natn. Acad. Sci. U.S.A.*, **48**, 1184–90

Devillers-Thierry, A., Kindt, T., Scheele, G. and Blobel, G. (1975). *Proc. natn. Acad. Sci. U.S.A.*, **72**, 5016–20

Dubois, P., Vargues-Regairaz, H. and Dubois, M. P. (1973). *Z. Zellforsch.*, **145**, 131–43

Eipper, B. A. and Mains, R. E. (1975). *Biochemistry*, **14**, 3836–44

Eipper, B. A. and Mains, R. E. (1977). *J. biol. Chem.*, **252**, in press

Eipper, B. A. and Mains, R. E. (1978). *J. biol. Chem.*, submitted

Eipper, B. A., Mains, R. E. and Guenzi, D. (1976). *J. biol. Chem.*, **251**, 4121–6

Furth, J. (1955). *Recent Prog. Horm. Res.*, **11**, 221–55.

Gilkes, J. J. H., Bloomfield, G. A., Scott, A. P., Lowry, P. J., Ratcliffe, J. G., Landon, J. and Rees, L. H. (1975). *J. clin. Endocr. Metab.*, **40**, 450–7

Guillemin, R., Ling, N. and Burgus, R. (1976). *C. r. hebd. Séanc. Acad. Sci. Paris Sér. D.* **282**, 783–5

Habener, J. F., Stevens, T. D., Tregear, G. W. and Potts, J. T., Jr (1976). *J. clin. Endocr. Metab.*, **42**, 520–30

Hirata, Y., Matsukura, S., Imura, H., Nakamura, M., and Tanaka, A. (1976). *J. clin. Endocr. Metab.*, **42**, 33–40

Hughes, J., Smith, T. W., Kosterlitz, H. W., Fothergill, L. A., Morgan, B. A. and Morris, H. R. (1975). *Nature*, **258**, 577–9

Kitabchi, A. E. (1970). *J. clin. Invest.*, **49**, 979–87

Kraehenbuhl, J. P., Racine, L. and Jamieson, J. D. (1977). *J. Cell Biol.*, **72**, 406–23

Li, C. H. and Chung, D. (1976*a*). *Proc. natn. Acad. Sci. U.S.A.*, **73**, 1145–8

Li, C. H. and Chung, D. (1976*b*). *Nature*, **260**, 622–4

Lowry, P. J., Rees, L. H., Tomlin, S., Gillies, G. and Landon, J. (1976). *J. clin. Endocr. Metab.*, **43**, 831–5

Mains, R. E. and Eipper, B. A. (1975). *Proc. natn. Acad. Sci. U.S.A.*, **72**, 3565–9

Mains, R. E. and Eipper, B. A. (1976). *J. biol. Chem.*, **251**, 4115–20

Mains, R. E. and Eipper, B. A. (1978). *J. biol. Chem.*, **252**, in press

Mains, R. E., Eipper, B. A. and Ling, N. (1977). *Proc. natn. Acad. Sci. U.S.A.*, **74**, 3014–8

Moriarty, G. C. (1973). *J. Histochem. Cytochem.*, **21**, 855–94

Nakanishi, S., Kita, T., Taii, S., Imura, H. and Numa, S. (1977). *Proc. natn. Acad. Sci. U.S.A.*, **74**, 3283–6

Nakanishi, S., Taii, S., Hirata, Y., Matsukura, S., Imura, H. and Numa, S. (1976). *Proc. natn. Acad. Sci. U.S.A.*, **73**, 4319–23

Phifer, R. F., Orth, D. N. and Spicer, S. S. (1974). *J. clin. Endocr. Metab.*, **39**, 684–92

Roberts, J. L. and Herbert, E. (1977*a*). *Proc. natn. Acad. Sci. U.S.A.*, **74**, 4826–30

Roberts, J. L. and Herbert, E. (1977*b*). *Proc. natn. Acad. Sci. U.S.A.*, **74**, 5300–4

Segre, G. V., Niall, H. D., Habener, J. F. and Potts, J. T., Jr (1974). *Am. J. Med.*, **56**, 774–84

Segrest, J. P., and Jackson, R. L. (1972). *Meth. Enzymol.*, **28B**, 54–63
Smyth, D. G. (1967). *Meth. Enzymol.*, **11**, 214–31
Tager, H. S., Rubenstein, A. H. and Steiner, D. F. (1975). *Meth Enzymol.*, **37**, 326–45
Vale, W. and Rivier, C. (1977). *Fedn. Proc.*, **36**, 2094–9
Weber, K., Pringle, J. R. and Osborn, M. (1972). *Meth. Enzymol.*, **26C**, 3–27
Yasamura, Y. (1968). *Am Zool.*, **8**, 285–305

14

Biosynthesis and processing of a common precursor to adrenocorticotropin and β-LPH in mouse pituitary cells

Edward Herbert, James L. Roberts*, Marjorie Phillips, Patricia A. Rosa, Marcia Budarf, Richard G. Allen, Paul F. Policastro, Thomas L. Paquette† and Michael Hinman
(Department of Chemistry, University of Oregon, Eugene, Oregon 97403, U.S.A.)

High molecular weight forms of ACTH have been detected in extracts of pituitary glands and pituitary tumor cells by Yalow and Berson (1971), Orth *et al.* (1973), Scott and Lowry (1974) and Eipper and Mains (1975). Fractionation of extracts of mouse pituitary cells (AtT-20/D-16v cell line) by SDS polyacrylamide gel electrophoresis has revealed the presence of four size classes of ACTH with apparent molecular weights of 31 000 (31K), 20–26 000 (20–26K), 12–15 000 (12–15K) and 4500 (4.5K) (Mains and Eipper, 1976). The 31K, 20-26K and 13–14K classes of ACTH are all glycosylated (Eipper *et al.*, 1976; Roberts *et al.*, 1978).

When mRNA from cultures of AtT-20/D-16v cells is translated in a reticulocyte cell-free protein synthesizing system, a species of ACTH is synthesized with an apparent molecular weight of 28 500 (Roberts and Herbert, 1977*a*). The same size ACTH molecule is made when polysomes from these cells are allowed to complete their nascent chains in the cell-free system (Roberts and Herbert, 1977*a*). The cell-free 28.5K ACTH is not glycosylated but contains all of the tryptic peptides present in the 31K ACTH glycoproteins observed in the tumor cells. Studies of the kinetics of labeling of ACTH glycoproteins with radioactive amino acids shows that the 31K ACTH proteins are the precursors of the lower molecular weight forms of ACTH found in the tumor cells (Mains and Eipper, 1976). Hence the 28.5K cell-free ACTH appears to be the primary translation product from which all the forms of ACTH in the AtT-20/D-16v cell line are derived.

Present Addresses: *Metabolic Research Unit, University of California Medical Center, San Francisco, California 94143, U.S.A.
†Department of Surgery, University of Washington School of Medicine, St Louis, Missouri 63110, U.S.A.

Tryptic peptide analysis of the cell-free product has revealed that it contains only one copy of α-$ACTH_{1-39}$ (Roberts and Herbert, 1977*a*) leaving a sequence of over 200 amino acids unaccounted for. Several kinds of studies suggested that β-LPH might be present in the same precursor molecule as ACTH. First, it had been shown by immunofluorescence techniques that ACTH and β-LPH are present in the same cells in the pituitary (Phifer *et al.*, 1974). Second, blood levels of β-melanocyte stimulating hormones (β-LPH_{41-58} and ACTH had been shown to rise and fall together under some circumstances (Abe *et al.*, 1967; 1969; Gilkes *et al.*, 1975). Finally the demonstration that β-endorphin is part of the structure of β-LPH (β-LPH_{61-91}) (Li and Chung, 1976) raised the possibility that coupled release of these hormones from a common precursor might account for the analgesic response that accompanies the rise in blood levels of ACTH during a stress response.

Hence, studies were undertaken to determine whether β-LPH is part of the sequence of the high molecular weight precursor to ACTH.

RELATIONSHIP OF ACTH AND β-LPH TO THE 28.5K POLYPEPTIDE

RNA was extracted from AtT-20/D-16v cells and translated in an mRNA-dependent reticulocyte cell-free system (prepared as described by Pelham and Jackson (1976)) in the presence of radioactive amino acids. The radioactive proteins were purified by double antibody immunoprecipitation with antisera specific for either ACTH (Herbert *et al.*, 1978) or β-endorphin (Guillemin *et al.*, 1977*a*). When the immunoprecipitates were analyzed by SDS polyacrylamide gel electrophoresis, only one labeled peak was observed as shown in figure 14.1 with an apparent molecular weight of 28 500.

Two approaches were used to show that the ACTH and β-endorphin antisera were binding to the same protein. First, the supernatant from an immunoprecipitation carried out with either the ACTH or β-endorphin antiserum was subsequently immunoprecipitated with the other antiserum. Analysis of the immunoprecipitates by SDS gel electrophoresis showed that all of the 28.5K cell-free product had been removed from the lysate by the first immunoprecipitation (table 2 in Roberts and Herbert, 1977*b*).

Further support for the identity of the proteins immunoprecipitated with the two antisera was provided by tryptic peptide mapping. After immunoprecipitation, the labeled ACTH and β-endorphin proteins were purified by SDS gel electrophoresis, eluted from the gels and digested with trypsin. The digests were fractionated by paper electrophoresis at pH 6.5 and by paper chromatography. Electrophoretic profiles of the tryptic peptides of [^{3}H] tryptophan and [^{35}S] methionine-labeled cell-free ACTH or β-endorphin show that the two proteins have very similar peptide content (figure 14.2). Hence, the peptide mapping studies and the immunological studies strongly suggest that the cell-free ACTH and β-endorphin molecules are the same. Paper chromatography of labeled peptides in a second dimension confirms the identity of the methionine (figure 14.2A) and tryptophan-labeled peptides (Roberts and Herbert, 1977*b*). Mains and Eipper (1977) have shown, by a similar approach, that 31K ACTH contains the sequence of β-endorphin

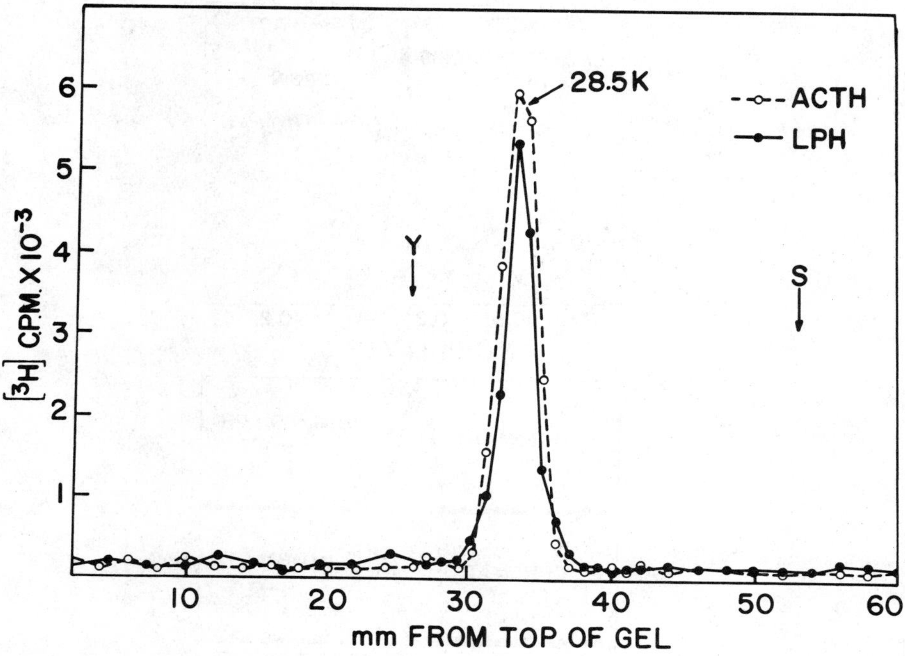

Figure 14.1 Size analysis of ACTH and β-LPH synthesized in the reticulocyte cell-free system. AtT-20/D-16v cells were grown to confluency in plastic roller bottles (Corning) in Dulbecco–Vogt Minimal Essential Medium (DMEM) with 5 per cent horse serum (Roberts and Herbert, 1977*a*), washed twice with serum-free DMEM, scraped from the bottles, and centrifuged. RNA was isolated from the cells as described by Roberts *et al.* (1977*a*) and incubated in the reticulocyte lysate system with [^{3}H] lysine (20 μM, 60 Ci/mmol, Amersham/Searle) as described by Roberts and Herbert (1977*a*). The product (~10 ng) was purified by immunoprecipitation using either ACTH antibody purified by affinity chromatography or β-endorphin antiserum (RB-100 of Guillemin *et al.* (1977*a*)). The entire immunoprecipitate (~80 μg protein) was subjected to SDS polyacrylamide gel electrophoresis on a 12 per cent Biophore gel. One millimeter slices were cut, eluted, and analyzed for [^{3}H] radioactivity in a triton-xylene fluor by liquid scintillation counting (efficiency ~40 per cent). Dansyl-yeast alcohol dehydrogenase and dansyl-soybean trypsin inhibitor (Y and S, arrows) were included as internal markers. Molecular weight was determined as previously described (Roberts and Herbert, 1977*a*).

Identification of ACTH and β-LPH peptides in cell-free product

The α_{1-24} sequence of ACTH and the β-MSH and β-endorphin sequences of β-LPH are highly conserved. Hence tryptic digests of porcine ACTH and β-endorphin and bovine β-MSH were used as sources of reference peptides for the identification of specific β-LPH and ACTH tryptic peptides in the labelled cell-free product.

The cell-free product synthesized under the direction of mRNA was labeled with 16 different radioactive amino acids in the reticulocyte cell-free system

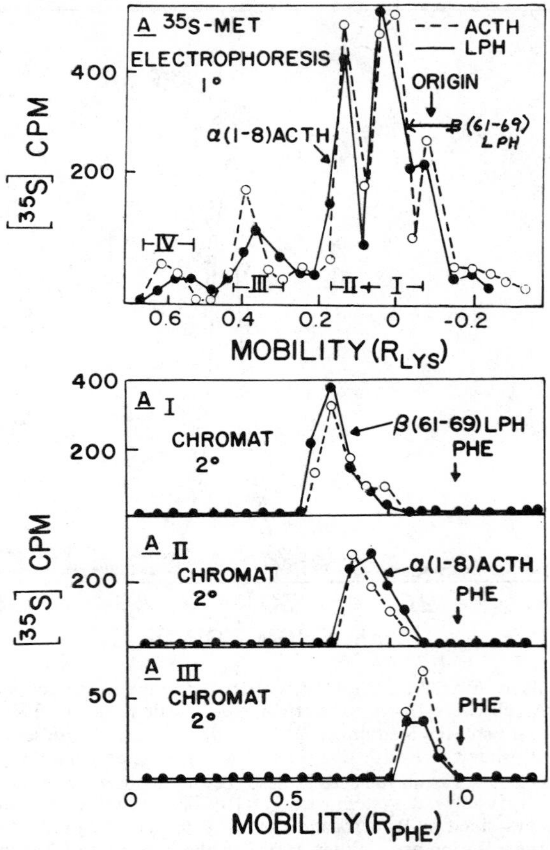

Figure 14.2 Similarity of tryptic peptides in cell-free ACTH and β-endorphin. A, Two dimensional separation of [^{35}S] methionine tryptic peptides of cell-free ACTH and β-endorphin; B, electrophoretic separation of [^{3}H] tryptophan tryptic peptides. Cell-free product was isolated with antiserum to ACTH or β-endorphin as in figure 14.1. The protein was eluted from the gel, precipitated with trichloroacetic acid, and the precipitate was dissolved in 100 μl of 0.1 M NH_4HCO_3, pH 8.5. The sample was treated with trypsin, lyophilized, and dissolved in 1 per cent acetic acid. For one dimensional analyses by electrophoresis (B) the peptides were spotted on 3-cm strips of Whatman 3MM paper. For two-dimensional analyses (A) duplicate samples were spotted in parallel, 2 cm and 5cm in from the edge of a 25 cm wide sheet of Whatman 3 MM paper. ε-DNP lysine, lysine, and picric acid were included as internal standards. Electrophoresis was done in pyridine: acetic acid: water, 10:35:90, pH 6.5, at 2000 V per 50 cm for ~1.5 h. A 3 cm strip, containing only one sample, was cut from the edge of the 25 cm sheet and sprayed with ninhydrin to locate lysine and ε-DNP lysine. The strip was cut into 8-mm slices, soaked in scintillation vials with 500 μl of 0.1 per cent SDS, 0.5 M urea for 6 h, 6 ml of fluor were added and the vials were counted. After determining the location of the labeled peptides, strips were cut from appropriate regions of the sheet as indicated in the upper panel in A and chromatographed in butanol: acetic acid: water, 4:1:5, upper phase with phenylalanine as an internal standard. Radioactivity was analyzed as above. Electrophoretic mobility was defined relative to lysine (ε-DNP lysine = 0 and lysine = 1). Chromatographic mobility was defined relative to phenylalanine (R_{Phe} = 1). Recovery of label off the paper was greater than 85 per cent in all cases.

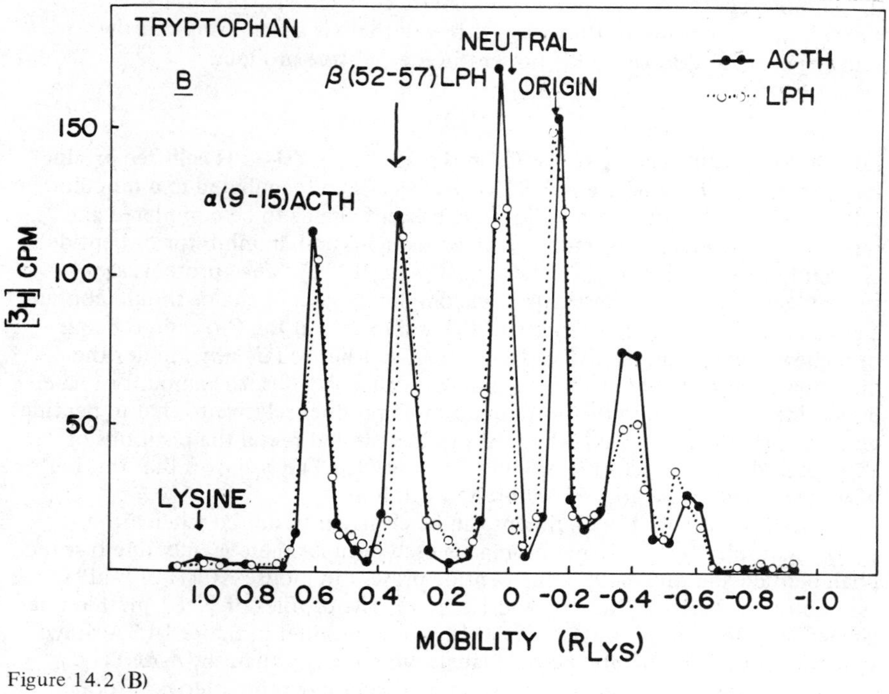

Figure 14.2 (B)

and the product was isolated as described in figure 14.1. Tryptic digests of the labeled proteins were analyzed by paper electrophoresis and by paper chromatography as in figure 14.2. The mobilities of these peptides during electrophoresis and chromatography were compared with the mobilities of the reference tryptic peptides derived from ACTH, β-MSH and β-endorphin (Roberts and Herbert, 1977*b*). With this approach it was possible to show that at least five of the reference tryptic peptides of β-MSH and β-endorphin were present in the 28.5K cell-free product. The identification of these peptides was confirmed by studies of the amino acid composition of the labeled peptides (Roberts and Herbert, 1977*a* and *b*). Four of the labeled peptides that have been identified by this approach are shown in figure 14.2A (α-$ACTH_{1-8}$ and β-LPH_{61-69}) and figure 14.2B (α-$ACTH_{9-15}$ and β-LPH_{52-57}).

Another point can be made from the peptide analyses shown in figure 14.2B. There are six radioactive peaks in the tryptophan-labeled peptide profile. Four of these peaks are of equal size and the other two sum to the equal of each of the other four (see Roberts and Herbert, 1977*a*). Since chromatography in a second dimension shows that the tryptophan-labeled peptides are homogeneous, the simplest interpretation is that there are five tryptophan peptides present, each having only one tryptophan residue. This suggests that all of the peptides, including those derived from ACTH and β-LPH, are present in the same number of copies in the cell-free product. The same analysis can be done for the methionine-labeled tryptic peptides (Roberts and Herbert, 1977*a, b*). The simplest interpretation of these results is that there is a single copy of the sequences of ACTH and β-LPH present in the cell-free product.

Location of β-LPH relative to ACTH in the 28.5K ACTH–LPH cell-free product
Polysomes were isolated from AtT-20/D-16v cells and incubated in a reticulocyte cell-free system to allow non-radioactive nascent chains to be completed and released in the presence of radioactive amino acids and an inhibitor of peptide chain initiation, aurintricarboxylic acid (Pestka, 1971). Since proteins are synthesized from N to C-terminus, the completed nascent chains should contain a gradient of labeled amino acid with the amino acid at the C-terminus being of highest specific radioactivity. The protein synthesized *de novo* under the direction of mRNA will not have a gradient of label. Thus, the amount of label in peptides derived from the polysome runoff product relative to that in peptides derived from the *de novo* synthesized product should reveal the positions of these peptides in the cell-free product. Dintzes (1961) has shown that this method of locating peptides works for rabbit hemoglobin.

The polysome runoff experiment can be clearly interpreted when either $[^3H]$ tryptophan or $[^{35}S]$ methionine is used because there is only one tryptophan peptide and one methionine peptide present in mouse ACTH or β-LPH (unpublished results of Roberts and Herbert). The profiles of $[^{35}S]$ methionine-labeled tryptic peptides of the polysome runoff product in figure 14.3A shows that the β-LPH_{61-91} tryptic peptide labels more heavily than the α-$ACTH_{1-8}$ tryptic peptide relative to the corresponding tryptic peptides derived from the *de novo* synthesized product. The ratio of c.p.m. in polysome runoff peptides relative to c.p.m. in *de novo* synthesized peptides is 0.5 and 2.0 for α-$ACTH_{1-8}$ and β-LPH_{61-91}, respectively. The conclusion is the same for the $[^3H]$ tryptophan-labeled tryptic peptides of the cell-free ACTH–LPH (figure 14.3B).

The same kind of studies have been done with isoleucine, leucine, valine, and phenylalanine-labeled cell-free product with similar results. These studies show that β-LPH is located carboxyterminal to ACTH and that ACTH is located carboxyterminal to the unidentified tryptic peptides in the profiles in figure 14.3.

STRUCTURE OF CELL-FREE ACTH–LPH

Since the precursor contains approximately 240 amino acids and ACTH and β-LPH together account for only half of the sequence, there are a number of possible arrangements of these two polypeptides in the precursor. Evidence from polysome runoff experiments suggest that ACTH is located near the middle of the precursor molecule and that β-LPH is next to ACTH and very near the carboxy terminal of the precursor. First, all of the non-α (1–39) and non-β (LPH) peptides appear from the pattern of label generated in the polysome runoff peptides (figure 14.3) to be located N-terminal to ACTH. The same kind of data also suggests that only a portion of one tryptic peptide (five or six amino acids long) is located C-terminal to β-LPH (unpublished results of Roberts and Herbert).

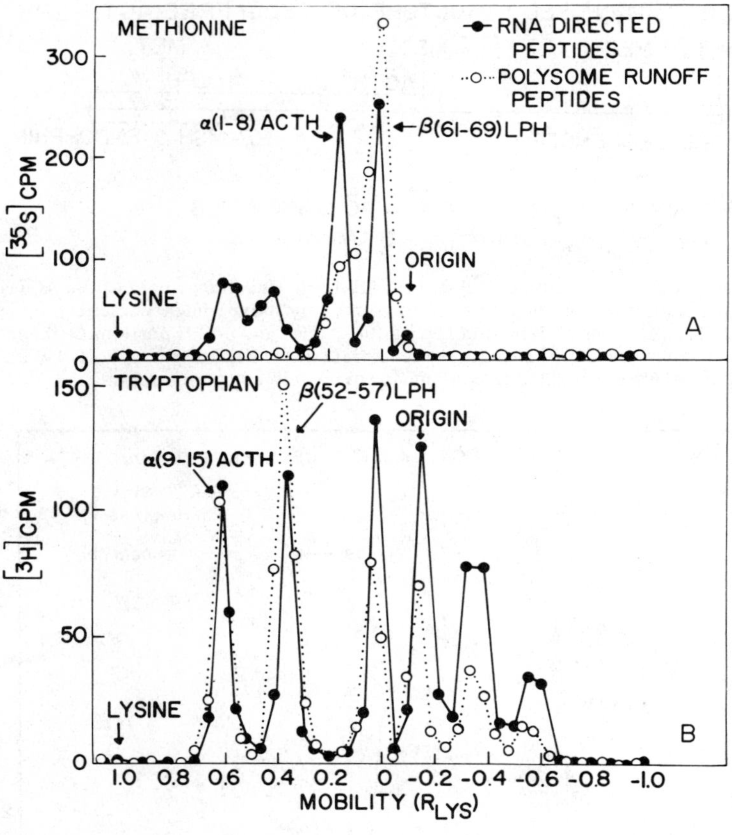

Figure 14.3 Profiles of methionine and tryptophan labelled peptides from the cell-free product made *de novo* and in polysome chain completion experiments. Cell-free ACTH was prepared as described in the methods section and in figure 14.1. The RNA-directed methionine-labelled peptides, α-$ACTH_{1-8}$ and β-LPH_{61-91} (A) contain 310 and 290 c.p.m., respectively. The corresponding runoff peptides contain 150 and 580 c.p.m. for ratios of 0.5 (150/310) and 2.0 (580/290). Tryptophan-labelled RNA-directed peptides, α-$ACTH_{9-15}$ and β-LPH_{52-57} (B) contain 190 and 170 c.p.m., respectively, and the corresponding runoff peptides contain 170 and 390 c.p.m. for ratios of approximately 0.9 (170/190) and 2.3 (390/170). [^{35}S] methionine (A) and [^{3}H] tryptophan (B) tryptic peptides of cell-free product synthesized *de novo* or in a polysome chain completion experiment.

These observations are summarized in the model of structure of the precursor in figure 14.4.

Cyanogen bromide (CNBr) can be used to cleave polypeptide chains specifically at methionine residues (Needleman, 1970). The above results show that there are three methionine residues in the cell-free precursor of ACTH and LPH (not counting the N-terminal initiator methionine). One methionine is in position 4 of ACTH and another in position 65 of β-LPH (Dayhoff, 1972). The methionine

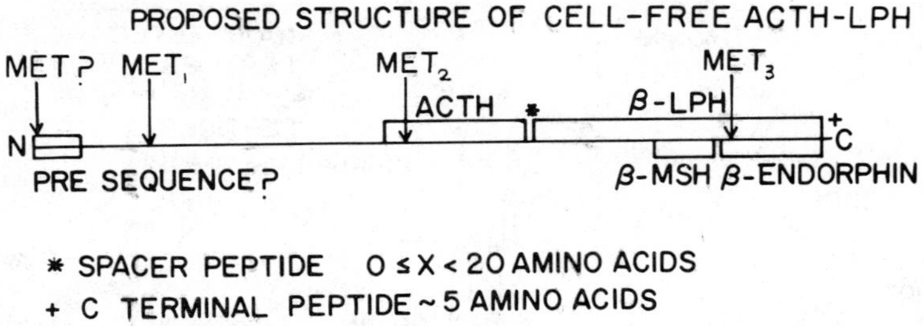

Figure 14.4 Model of structure of cell-free ACTH–LPH. The arrangement of the ACTH and β-LPH sequences is based on the results of polysome runoff experiments described in figure 14.3. The positions of Met² and Met³ in the ACTH and β-LPH portions of the molecule, respectively, were taken from the sequence data in the literature (Dayhoff, 1972). The 28.5K molecule is estimated to contain approximately 240 amino acids.

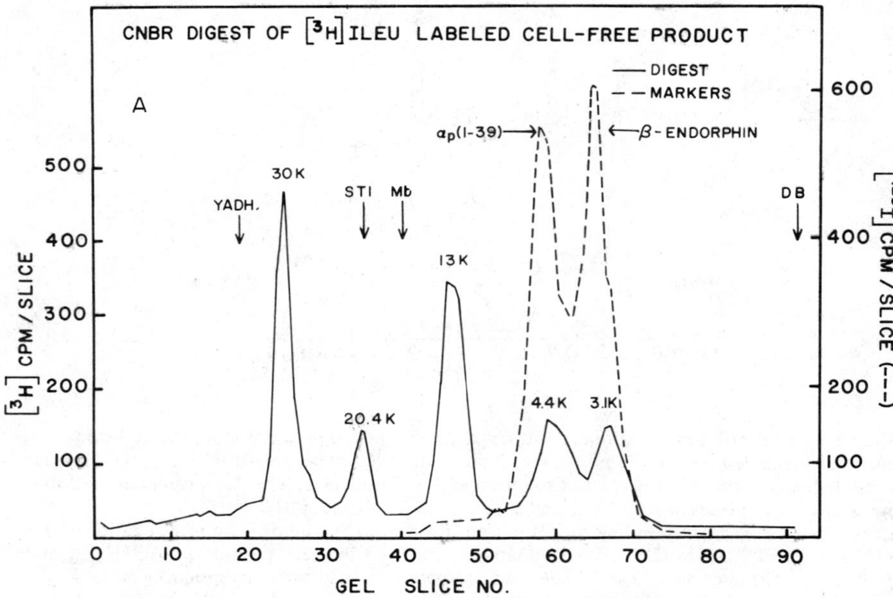

Figure 14.5 SDS gel electrophoresis profiles of [³H] isoleucine-labeled cyanogen bromide fragments from cell-free ACTH–LPH. Cell-free ACTH–LPH was prepared by incubating AtT-20/D-16v RNA in a modified reticulocyte cell-free system with either [³H] isoleucine (30 Ci/mmol, 200 μCi/incubation) (A) or [³H] lysine (30 Ci/mmol, 200 μCi/incubation) (B) as described. Cell-free ACTH–LPH was isolated from the lysate by immunoprecipitation with ACTH antiserum. Immunoprecipitates were dissolved in 70 per cent formic acid and reacted for 24 h at 20 °C with CNBr (10 mg/ml in acetonitrile) in 100-fold molar excess to methionine present in the immunoprecipitate. The reaction mixture was diluted to 10 per cent formic acid with water, lyophilized and analyzed in a SDS gel-electrophoresis system of 15 per cent polyacrylamide with 3.3 per cent *bis*-acrylamide to total acrylamide. Gels were sliced into 1-mm sections, eluted and counted (Roberts and Herbert, 1977*a*). YADH, yeast alcohol dehydrogenase; STI, soybean trypsin inhibitors, Mb, myoglobin; DB, dye band.

normally present at position 47 in β-LPH (the β-MSH methionine) is not present in the AtT-20 mouse ACTH-LPH precursor (Roberts and Herbert, unpublished observations). The third methionine is known to be located amino terminal to the ACTH methionine (figure 14.3A), and a more precise location can be assigned on the basis of analysis of CNBr cleavage products.

The cell-free product was labeled with a variety of radioactive amino acids, purified by immunoprecipitation, and reacted with CNBr. The cleavage products were separated by SDS gel electrophoresis as shown in figure 14.5 with isoleucine-labeled ACTH–LPH precursor. The CNBr fragments were further characterized by tryptic peptide analysis. These studies showed that a 4.5K CNBr fragment contains the tryptic peptide present at the amino terminal of the 28.5K precursor molecule, suggesting that the unidentified methionine is located approximately 40 amino acids from the amino terminal (figure 14.4). Thus, with the positions of the three methionines as shown in figure 14.4, one can predict the sizes of the fragments that should result from partial and complete CNBr digestion. The results in figure 14.5 are in good agreement with the predictions based on the positions of the methionines shown in figure 14.4. For example, the 3K fragment in figure 14.5 represents the Met^3 to carboxy terminal fragment whereas the 12–13K peak contains the fragment that results from the partial cleavage at Met^3 (the Met^2 to carboxy terminal fragment). Another method of confirming the identification of the CNBr fragments has been to label the precursor with amino acids known to be present in high proportions in different regions of ACTH and β-LPH and then determine the relative amounts of these amino acids present in different size CNBr fragments (by analyzing the amount of radioactivity under each peak).

RELATIONSHIP OF CELL-FREE PRODUCT TO ACTH–LPH PRECURSOR PROTEINS IN AtT-20/D-16v CELLS

Pulse chase experiments have shown that ACTH and β-LPH are synthesized as a 31K class of glycoproteins in AtT-20/D-16v cells. Using a 12 per cent Biophore SDS gel electrophoresis system, it has been possible to resolve 31K ACTH–LPH into three glycoprotein components of apparent molecular weight 29 000, 32 000 and 34 000, all of which contain ACTH and β-LPH (Roberts and Herbert, 1977*a*; Roberts *et al.*, 1978). Cell-free ACTH–LPH has been shown to contain all of the tryptic peptides present in the 29K ACTH–LPH precursor found in the tumor cells. In the experiment shown in figure 14.6, tumor cells were labeled with both $[^{35}S]$ methionine and $[^{3}H]$ glucosamine, (for a long enough time to achieve steady labeling of all of the forms of ACTH). The forms of ACTH were immunoprecipitated with ACTH antiserum and fractionated by SDS gel electrophoresis to determine the amounts of ^{35}S and ^{3}H they contain. The results show that all the forms of ACTH are glycosylated except for 4.5K ACTH and that the 29, 32 and 34K forms of ACTH–LPH can be resolved by this method. The ratio of $[^{3}H]$ glucosamine radioactivity to $[^{35}S]$ methionine radioactivity in the 29–34K region of the gel (figure 14.6) indicates that there is more carbohydrate (glucosamine) in the 32K and 34K forms than in the 29K form. (All of these forms have the same number of methionine residues). This was confirmed by doing a similar experiment with $[^{35}S]$ methionine and $[^{3}H]$ mannose

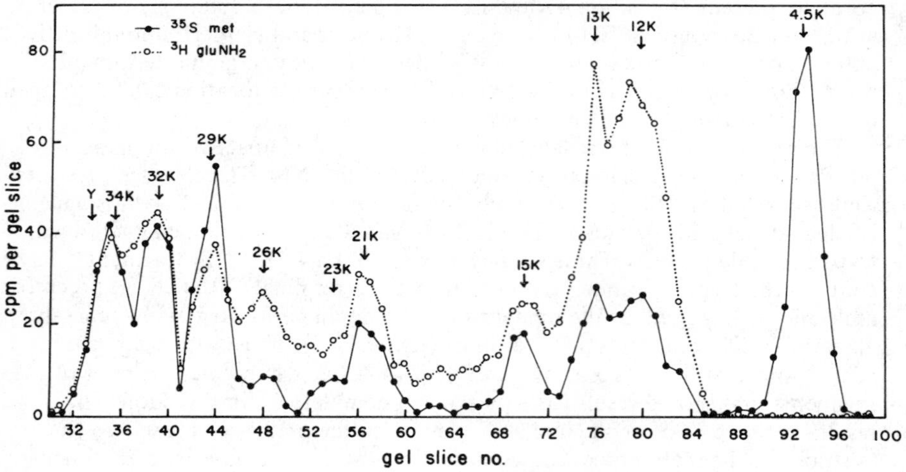

Figure 14.6 Distribution of glycosylated forms of ACTH in AtT-20/D-16v cells. AtT-20/D-16v cells were incubated in Falcon microtest wells for 90 min with 100 μCi [^{35}S] methionine and 300 μCi [^{3}H] glucosamine in 50 μl of low glucose Dulbecco-Vogt MEM with 10 per cent horse serum. Cells were extracted with 100 μl of 5 N acetic acid containing 5 mg per ml of bovine serum albumin and 1 mM each of freshly prepared phenyl methyl sulfonyl fluoride and iodoacetamide (Roberts *et al.*, 1978). The extracts were lyophilized and immunoprecipitated with an ACTH antiserum. The forms of ACTH were separated by SDS gel electrophoresis (12 per cent Biophore gels), sliced, eluted and counted (Roberts *et al.*, 1978) using a program for quenched [^{3}H]/[^{35}S]. [^{3}H] c.p.m. are adjusted for [^{35}S] cross-over and background has been subtracted. The [^{3}H] c.p.m. eluted from the gel were shown to be present as glucosamine by the following experiment. After hydrolysis at 100 °C for 4 h in an evacuated tube, the reduced [^{3}H] labeled material was shown to comigrate with authentic glucosamine during paper electrophoresis and paper chromatography (Roberts *et al.*, 1978). Y, yeast alcohol dehydrogenase marker.

(Roberts *et al.*, 1978). The same kind of analysis has been done with the immunoprecipitated forms of β-endorphin and it has been found that the 29, 32 and 34K forms are glycosylated but the 11.7K (β-LPH) and 3.5K (β-endorphin) forms are not.

These findings raise the possibility that the inital steps in processing of the primary translation product might be addition of sugars to this product to form the 29, 32 and 34K forms of the ACTH–LPH precursor seen in the cells.

EARLY EVENTS IN PROCESSING OF ACTH–LPH PRECURSORS IN AtT-20/D-16v CELLS

Pulse labeling studies with radioactive amino acids were performed with tumor cells to study early events in processing of the ACTH–LPH precursors. After 5 min of labeling with radioactive amino acids, ACTH proteins were purified by immunoprecipitation with the ACTH antiserum and SDS gel electrophoresis. Over 90 per cent of the radioactivity recovered from the gel is in 29K ACTH (figure 14.7).

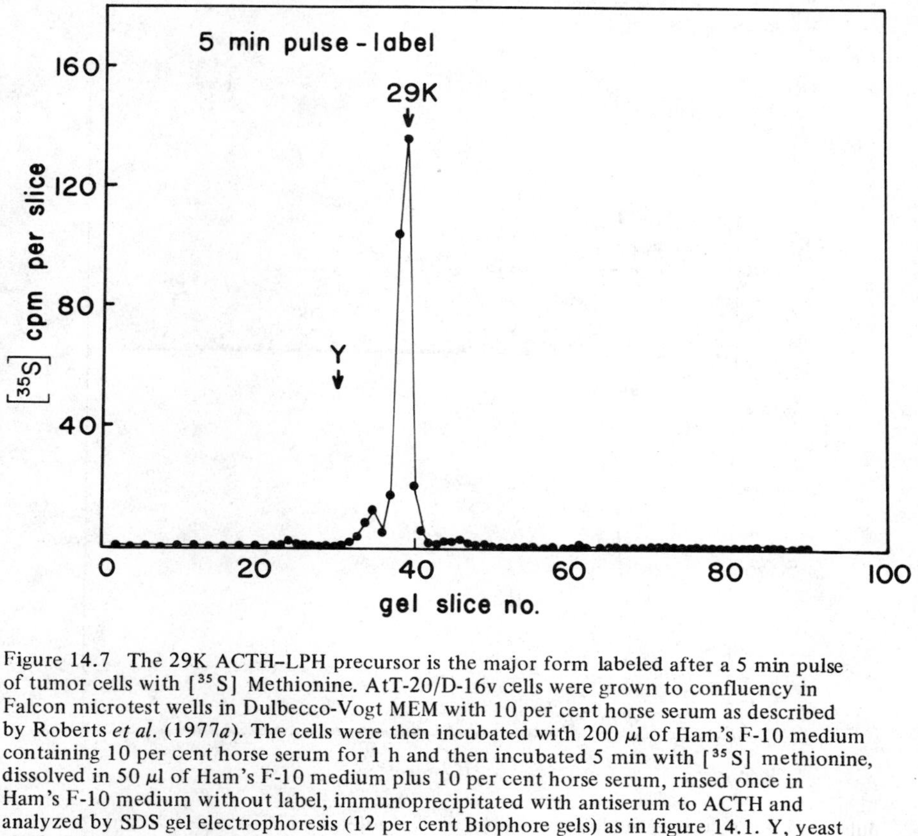

Figure 14.7 The 29K ACTH–LPH precursor is the major form labeled after a 5 min pulse of tumor cells with [^{35}S] Methionine. AtT-20/D-16v cells were grown to confluency in Falcon microtest wells in Dulbecco-Vogt MEM with 10 per cent horse serum as described by Roberts *et al.* (1977*a*). The cells were then incubated with 200 μl of Ham's F-10 medium containing 10 per cent horse serum for 1 h and then incubated 5 min with [^{35}S] methionine, dissolved in 50 μl of Ham's F-10 medium plus 10 per cent horse serum, rinsed once in Ham's F-10 medium without label, immunoprecipitated with antiserum to ACTH and analyzed by SDS gel electrophoresis (12 per cent Biophore gels) as in figure 14.1. Y, yeast alcohol dehydrogenase marker.

Cultures were then pulsed for 10 min with radioactive amino acids, and chased for varying periods of time with non-radioactive amino acids. The forms of ACTH and β-endorphin were purified by immunoprecipitation followed by SDS gel electrophoresis as described in figure 14.8. The results show that radioactivity in 29K ACTH–LPH chases more quickly than radioactivity in 32K ACTH–LPH and that radioactivity in 34K ACTH–LPH increases during the entire 30 minute chase period (figure 14.9). After 10 to 20 min, radioactivity appears in β-LPH and in two lower molecular weight forms of ACTH, 13K ACTH and 4.5K ACTH. No radioactivity appears in β-endorphin size material during the 30 min chase period. (Radioactivity does appear in β-endorphin size material later (Roberts *et al.*, 1978).)

The finding that the 32 and 34K forms of the precursor have more mannose and glucosamine than the 29K forms of the precursor (previous section and Roberts *et al.* (1978)) and the results of the pulse chase experiments suggest that

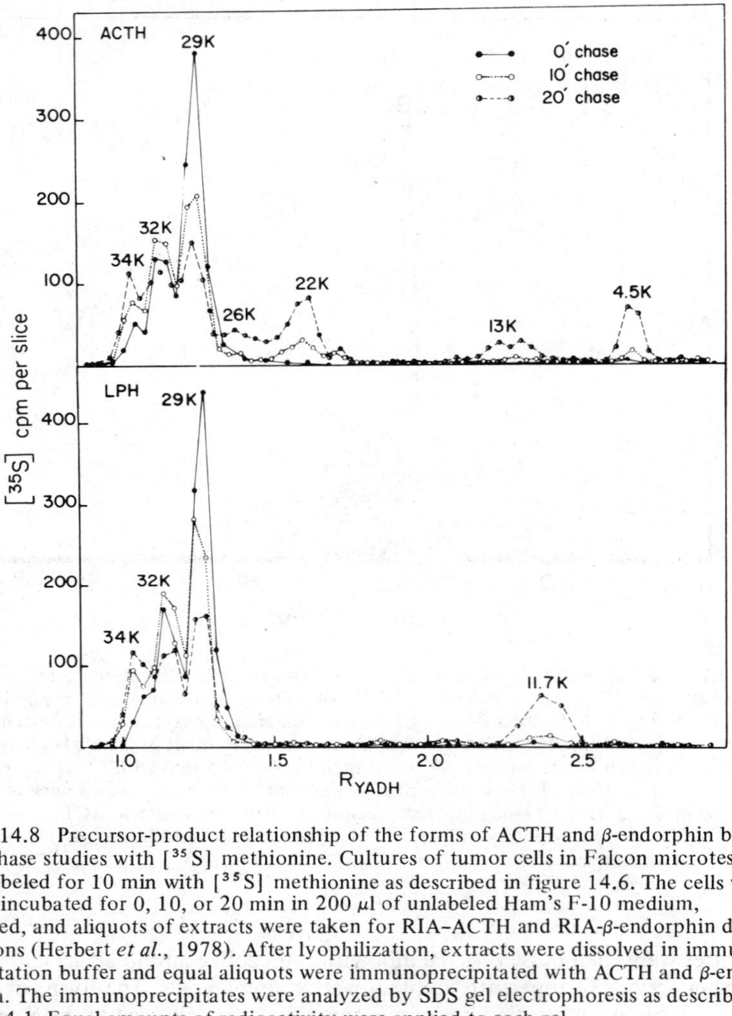

Figure 14.8 Precursor-product relationship of the forms of ACTH and β-endorphin by pulse chase studies with [^{35}S] methionine. Cultures of tumor cells in Falcon microtest wells were labeled for 10 min with [^{35}S] methionine as described in figure 14.6. The cells were rinsed, incubated for 0, 10, or 20 min in 200 μl of unlabeled Ham's F-10 medium, extracted, and aliquots of extracts were taken for RIA–ACTH and RIA-β-endorphin determinations (Herbert *et al.*, 1978). After lyophilization, extracts were dissolved in immunoprecipitation buffer and equal aliquots were immunoprecipitated with ACTH and β-endorphin antisera. The immunoprecipitates were analyzed by SDS gel electrophoresis as described in figure 14.1. Equal amounts of radioactivity were applied to each gel.

Gels were cut into 1-mm slices, eluted and radioactivity was determined (Roberts *et al.*, 1977*a*). For analysis of the material with an R_{YADH} of 1.4, every two slices were pooled, eluted and radioactivity determined as above. YADH, yeast alcohol dehydrogenase.

the 32 and 34K forms may be derived from the 29K form in the tumor cells by the further addition of sugars.

GLYCOPEPTIDE ANALYSIS OF THE ACTH–LPH PRECURSORS IN THE AtT-20/D-16v TUMOR CELLS

To understand better the relationship of the 29, 32 and 34K forms of the precursor to lower molecular weight forms of ACTH and β-LPH, a glycopeptide

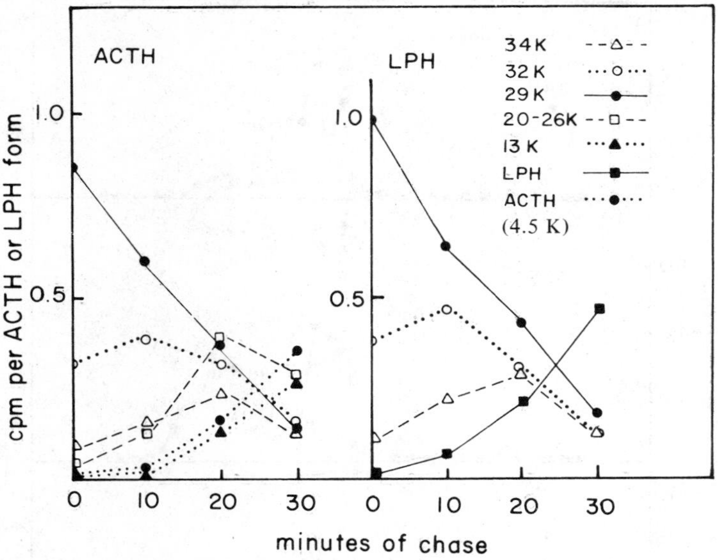

Figure 14.9 Time course of labeling of the forms of ACTH and β-endorphin. The total c.p.m. in the radioactive peaks in figure 14.8 were tabulated and replotted in this figure.

analysis of these forms was carried out. Tryptic peptides of cell-free ACTH–LPH were used as a reference point in these studies because the cell-free product is known not to contain any sugars (Roberts and Herbert, 1977*a*). Availability of unglycosylated peptides makes it possible to demonstrate shifts in mobilities of peptides due to the presence of carbohydrate. Cells were labeled with [^{3}H] glucosamine and the 29, 32 and 34K forms of ACTH–LPH precursor were isolated, digested with trypsin, and the peptides in the digests were separated by paper electrophoresis. The results in figure 14.10 show that all three forms of the precursor have in common the glycopeptides with mobilities of 0 and 0.1. However, only the 32K form has an acidic glycopeptide (mobility –0.25). The cell-free product (28.5K) does not label with [^{3}H] glucosamine.

In order to identify the acidic glycopeptide, tryptic digests of [^{3}H] phenylalanine and [^{3}H] tyrosine-labeled 29, 32 and 34K ACTH–LPH and the 28.5K cell-free ACTH–LPH forms were analyzed by paper electrophoresis. The results for the phenylalanine labeled tryptic peptides are shown in figure 14.11. The tryptic peptides of 29 and 28.5K ACTH–LPH have identical mobilities. The tryptic peptides of 32K ACTH are the same as those of 29 and 28.5K ACTH except for one acidic peptide which appears to have shifted mobility from –0.35 (R_{Lys}) in the 28.5K form to mobility –0.25 (R_{Lys}) in the 32K form. This peptide has been identified as the tryptic peptide containing the α_{22-39} sequence of ACTH (Roberts *et al.*, unpublished observations). A similar shift has been observed with tyrosine-labeled tryptic peptides from 29, 32 and 34K forms of the precursor (Roberts *et al.*, 1978). Because the acidic [^{3}H] glucosamine-labeled tryptic peptide derived from the 32K form has a mobility of –0.25 (R_{Lys}), the

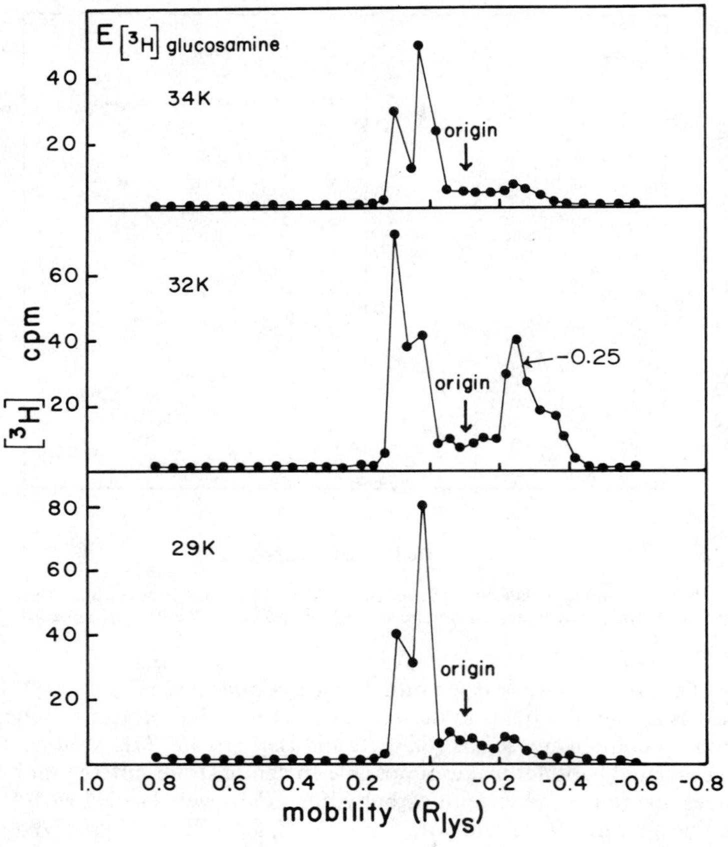

Figure 14.10 [^{3}H] glucosamine-labeled tryptic peptides in 29, 32 and 34K forms of ACTH–LPH. AtT-20/D-16v cells were labeled with [^{3}H] glucosamine, extracted, and the precursor forms of ACTH–LPH in the extracts were purified as described in figure 14.6. After elution from the SDS gels, the 29, 32 and 34K forms of ACTH–LPH were digested with trypsin and separated by paper electrophoresis and radioactivity in paper strips was determined as described in figure 14.2. Mobility was determined relative to lysine (R_{Lys} = 1.0) and the dinitrophenyl (DNP) derivative of lysine ($R_{DNP-Lys}$ = 0)

simplest explanation is that glycosylation alters the mobility of this peptide. It has recently been shown (Mains and Eipper, 1978) that 13K ACTH is the glycosylated form of 4.5K ACTH (α-ACTH$_{1-39}$ and that the glycopeptide derived from 13K ACTH by tryptic digestion is the α_{22-39} tryptic peptide.

The tryptic peptide profiles also show that the tryptic peptides of the 34K precursor form are similar to those of the 29 and 28.5K forms.

Additional peptide mapping studies (Roberts *et al.*, 1978) with tyrosine, tryptophan and methionine-labeled 29, 32 and 34K ACTH–LPH suggest that these forms have the same polypeptide backbone.

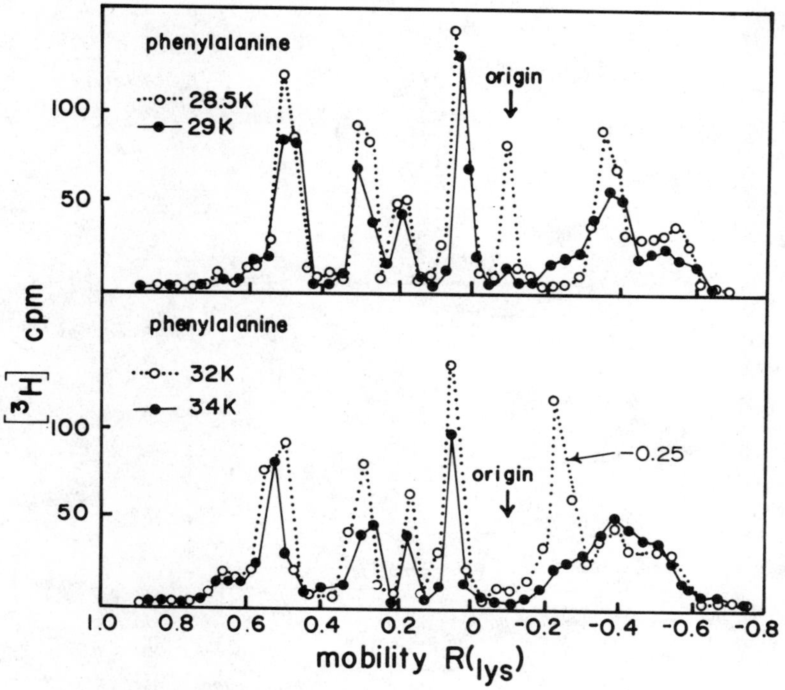

Figure 14.11 [^{3}H] phenylalanine-labeled tryptic peptides of 29, 32, 34 and 28.5K (cell-free) forms of ACTH–LPH. The [^{3}H] phenylalanine-labeled forms of ACTH–LPH were isolated as described in figures 14.1 and 14.6 (and in more detail in Roberts *et al.* (1978)). Tryptic peptide analysis was done as described in figure 14.2 and in figure 14.10. Mobilities were determined as described in figure 14.10.

COMPARISON OF ACTH AND β-ENDORPHIN FROM MOUSE PITUITARY AND AtT-20/D-16v CELLS

Mouse pituitaries were separated into anterior and intermediate-posterior lobes. Acetic acid extracts of the lobes and of tumor cells were fractionated by SDS gel electrophoresis. The gels were sliced, eluted, and the eluates were assayed for ACTH and β-endorphin by RIA (Guillemin *et al.*, 1977*a*; Allen *et al.*, 1978). The profiles of ACTH and β-endorphin immunoactivity coincide in the regions of the gels where the 29, 32 and 34K proteins are located (figure 14.12). Hence, the lobes of the pituitary appear to have the same precursor forms of ACTH and β-endorphin as the tumor cells. The proteins eluted in the lower molecular weight region of the gels contain either β-endorphin or ACTH, but not both. The lower molecular weight forms of ACTH and β-endorphin in the pituitary also correspond to lower molecular weight forms of these hormones seen in the tumor cell extracts.

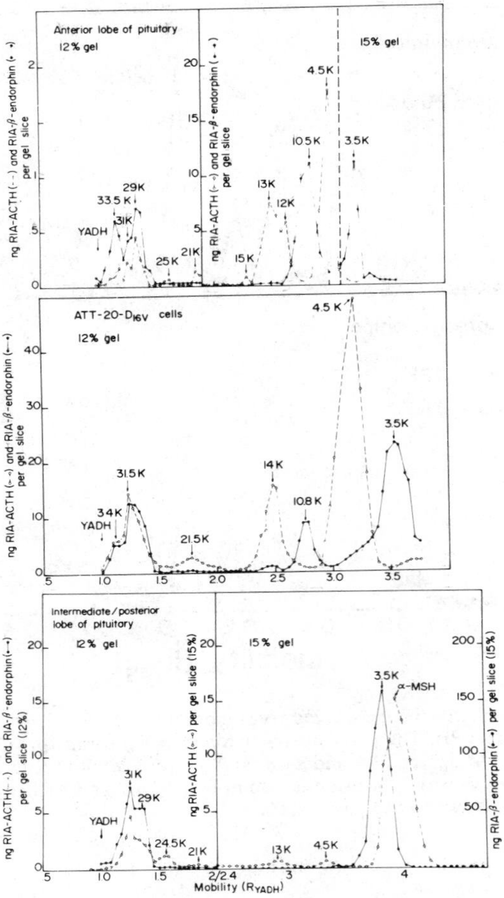

Figure 14.12 Forms of ACTH and β-endorphin in AtT-20/D-16v cells and anterior and intermediate-posterior lobes of mouse pituitary. AtT-20/D-16v cells were extracted in 5 N acetic acid (Herbert *et al.*, 1978). Pituitaries were removed from male adult mice by the procedure of Vale *et al.* (1972). The lobes were separated and anterior lobes were extracted individually as above. Intermediate-posterior lobes were pooled (20 in all) and extracted as above. Extracts were homogenized, heated 2 min at 100 °C, and centrifuged (Roberts *et al.*, 1978). Supernatants were lyophilized and redissolved in 50 μl of SDS-gel-buffer (Roberts *et al.*, 1977*a*) and applied to 12 per cent Biophore tube gels (10 cm). Aliquots of anterior lobe extract and intermediate-posterior lobe extract were also run on 15 per cent polyacrylamide gels. Samples were subjected to electrophoresis as described by Roberts *et al.* (in preparation). Gels were sliced in 1-mm sections and eluted (Roberts and Herbert, 1977*a*). Aliquots of the eluates were used for RIA with antisera to ACTH and β-endorphin as described by Herbert *et al.* (1978). In the upper panel the extract was run on 12 per cent gel. The lower panels are a composite of the two gel runs of lobe extracts; one done on a 12 per cent Biophore gel and the other on a 15 per cent gel. (Low molecular weight forms of ACTH and β-endorphin separate better on 15 per cent gels than on 12 per cent gels). RIA–ACTH and RIA–β–endorphin refer to the RIA results with the ACTH antiserum and the β-endorphin antiserum, respectively. YADH, Yeast alcohol dehydrogenase.

Almost all of the ACTH immunoactivity in the intermediate-posterior pituitary (excluding the activity in the α-MSH region which is believed to be due to cross-reactivity of α-MSH with the ACTH antiserum) is in the 29–34K forms of ACTH, whereas in the anterior pituitary the ACTH immunoactivity is mainly in the 13 and 4.5K forms of ACTH. Figure 14.12 also shows that β-endorphin immunoactivity is mainly in the form of β-LPH size material (11.7K) and β-endorphin (3.5K) in the anterior lobe, but predominantly in β-endorphin size material in the intermediate-posterior lobe. These results suggest that processing of the ACTH-LPH precursors is quite different in the two lobes of the pituitary.

It should also be noted that the distribution of immunoactive forms of ACTH and β-endorphin in the tumor cells is much closer to that seen in the anterior pituitary than in the intermediate-posterior pituitary.

COUPLED RELEASE OF ACTH AND β-LPH

If ACTH and β-LPH are derived from the same precursor molecule then the release of these hormones (and derivatives, β-endorphin and β-MSH) might be coupled. It has previously been shown (Herbert *et al.*, 1977) that dexamethasone inhibits ACTH release and that crude corticotropin-releasing factor (CRF) preparations (hypothalamic extracts) stimulates ACTH release in AtT-20/D-16v cultures. Hence, we have used D-16v cultures to determine whether release of the two

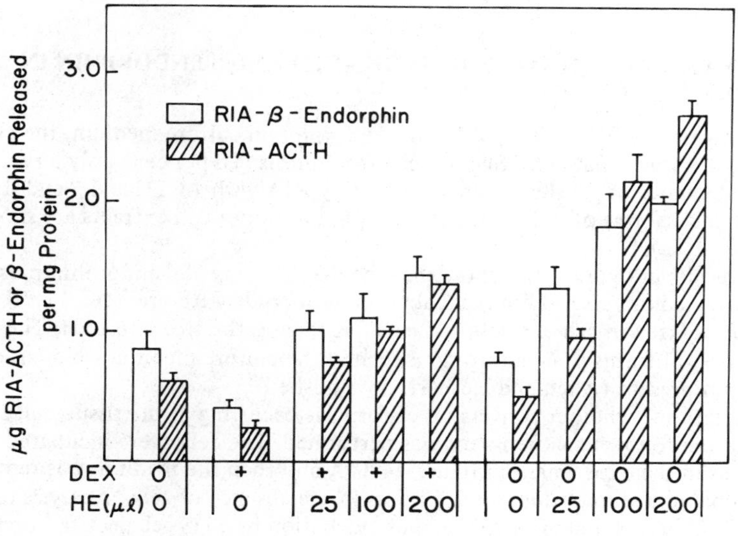

Figure 14.13 Effects of dexamethasone and hypothalamic extract on release of ACTH and β-endorphin activities in AtT-20/D-16v cultures. Cells were grown to half confluency in Dulbecco-Vogt MEM with 10 per cent horse serum (Herbert *et al.*, 1978) in 3.5 cm culture dishes containing 2.0 ml of medium. The medium was changed and cultures were incubated for 48 h with or without 1×10^{-6} M dexamethasone (DEX) with one change of medium at 24 h. The medium was replaced with 2.0 ml of serum-free test medium containing the amounts of rabbit hypothalamic extract (HE) shown below the histogram and the incubation was continued for 3.0 h. Medium was harvested and either frozen or assayed directly by RIA with ACTH and β-endorphin antisera (Herbert *et al.*, 1978).

hormones is coupled.

Cultures of D-16v cells were grown in the presence or absence of 1×10^{-6} M dexamethasone for 24–48 hours. These cultures were then incubated in the presence or absence of various amounts of crude hypothalamic extract from rabbit or mouse hypothalamus. The release of ACTH was measured by RIA with an ACTH antiserum that does not react with β-LPH or β-endorphin. Release of β-endorphin and β-LPH was measured with β-endorphin antiserum that does not react with ACTH. The β-endorphin antiserum reacts equally well with β-LPH and β-endorphin and almost as well with precursor forms of ACTH–LPH but does not react with ACTH or enkephalins (Guillemin *et al.*, 1977*a*).

The results in figure 14.13 show that D-16v cultures release ACTH activity and β-endorphin activity. The two activities rise and fall together in the culture medium in response to dexamethasone and hypothalamic extract suggesting that release of the two activities is coupled. Coupled release of ACTH and β-endorphin has also been observed in primary pituitary cell cultures from mouse pituitary (Allen *et al.*, 1978). However, this does not necessarily mean that the same number of moles of the two activities are released under all of the conditions studied. Further experiments are necessary to test this possibility.

(The crude CRF preparation used in this experiment contributed less than 2 per cent of the total RIA–ACTH and β-endorphin immunoactivity present in the culture medium.)

MOLECULAR WEIGHTS OF FORMS OF ACTH AND β-ENDORPHIN IN CULTURE MEDIUM

To investigate the forms of ACTH and β-endorphin in culture medium, the culture medium was fractionated by SDS gel electrophoresis (10 per cent polyacrylamide gels), and eluates of gel slices were analyzed by RIA with ACTH and β-endorphin antisera. (The forms of ACTH and β-endorphin in tumor cell extracts are shown in figure 14.12).

The results in figure 14.14 show that the major forms of β-endorphin present in culture medium after 3 hours incubation with crude CRF are 31K, 11.7K and 3.5K forms (seen in cell extracts). The 11.7K form is the size of β-LPH. The same distribution of forms of β-endorphin is seen in the culture medium when crude CRF is not present (Allen and Herbert, unpublished).

To determine whether conversion of forms is occurring in the tissue culture medium, the following experiment was performed. The cells were incubated for 3 hours as in the experiment in figure 14.14A and then the medium was removed and incubated a second time for 1.5 hours in the absence of cells. Analysis of the medium before and after the second incubation by SDS gel electrophoresis shows that there is no change in the distribution of the forms of β-endorphin (figure 14.14B).

The major forms of ACTH present in culture medium after 2 hours incubation with crude CRF are 13 and 4.5K ACTH (figure 14.14C). The distribution of ACTH forms in the culture medium is the same when crude CRF is not present (Allen *et al.*, 1978). Also, the 13 and 4.5K forms of ACTH are released when primary cell cultures from mouse anterior pituitary are incubated with or without vasopressin (Paquette and Herbert, 1978).

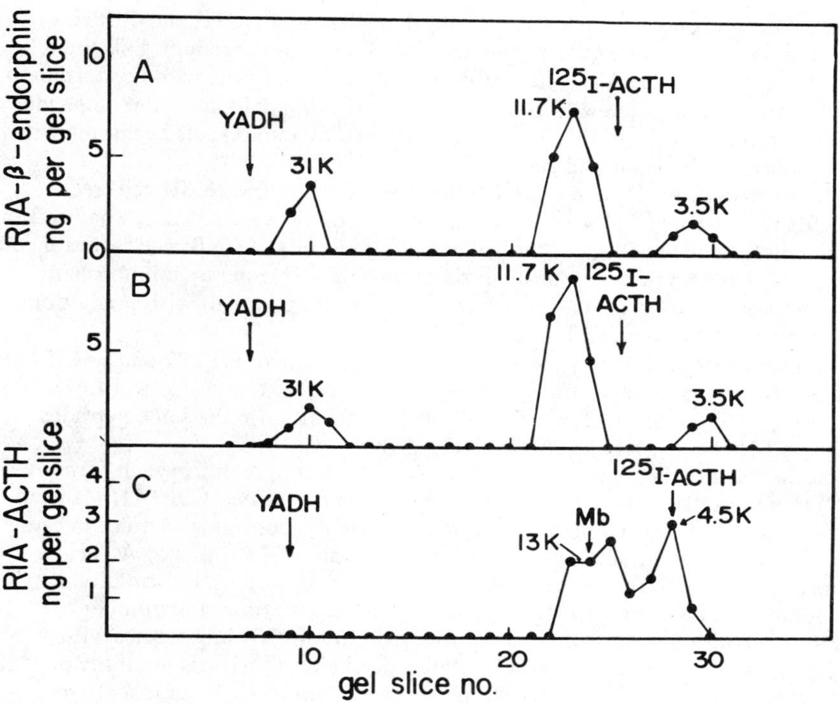

Figure 14.14 Forms of ACTH and β-endorphin present in tumor cell culture medium. Cultures were grown to half confluency and then incubated for 48 h with or without 1 × 10^{-6} M dexamethasone as described in figure 14.13. The medium was replaced with 2.0 ml of serum-free test medium containing 200 μl of rabbit hypothalamic extract where indicated and the incubation was continued for 3 h. Samples of medium were removed at 3 h (A). Half of the 3 h sample was incubated for another 1.5 h in the absence of cells (B). All of the samples of medium were fractionated by SDS gel electrophoresis on 10 per cent polyacrylamide tube gels (Allen *et al.*, 1978). The gels were sliced into 2 mm segments, the segments were eluted and the eluates were assayed with β-endorphin antiserum as described by Allen *et al.* (1978). Medium was harvested from another culture containing hypothalamic extract after a, 2 h incubation (C) and fractionated by gel electrophoresis as above. Eluates of gel slices were assayed for ACTH immunoactivity (C). The recoveries of immunoactivity from the gels ranged from 70–90 per cent of the total activity placed on the gel. The results in the graphs are for equal volumes of medium placed on the gels. The tissue culture dishes all had about the same amount of cell protein in them at the time of harvesting the medium (average variation of cell protein was less than ± 10 per cent). YADH, yeast alcohol dehydrogenase.

DISCUSSION

Two biologically active polypeptides, ACTH and β-endorphin, have been shown to be synthesized as part of a much larger precursor molecule in mouse pituitary tumor cells. The precursor appears to contain all of the conserved peptides of β-LPH and ACTH. The cell-free ACTH–LPH translation product is approximately

240 amino acids long (Roberts and Herbert, 1977*a*) and ACTH and β-LPH account for about half of the amino acid sequence of this product. Polysome runoff experiments indicate that β-LPH is located close to the carboxy terminal of the molecule and that ACTH is next to β-LPH in the middle of the molecule. As shown in figure 14.4, this leaves a long stretch of amino acids beginning with the N-terminal unaccounted for.

If one assigns ACTH and β-LPH definite positions in the 28.5K cell-free precursor molecule (figure 14.4) one can use CNBr cleavage to check the positions of the methionine residues in the molecule. The results of CNBr cleavage shown in figure 14.5 and tryptic peptide analysis of the CNBr fragments (unpublished observations of Roberts and Policastro) are in good agreement with predictions from the model in figure 14.4.

Three glycosylated forms of the ACTH–LPH precursor (29, 32 and 34K forms) are resolved by SDS gel electrophoresis of tumor cell extracts (figure 14.6). Tryptic peptide analysis shows that all of these forms have the same peptides (figures 14.10 and 14.11; Roberts *et al.*, 1978).

To determine the relative amounts of carbohydrate present in each form of ACTH and β-LPH, double label experiments were performed with [^{3}H] labeled sugars and [^{35}S] labeled methionine. Methionine is a convenient choice because the number of methionine residues is known for all of the forms of ACTH. Hence, one can determine the relative amounts of sugar in each form directly by comparing the ratio of [^{3}H] c.p.m. to [^{35}S] c.p.m. times the number of methionine residues present in each form. Continuous labeling studies with [^{3}H] labeled core sugars of carbohydrate side chains, ([^{3}H] glucosamine or [^{3}H] mannose) and [^{35}S] methionine show that the 32 and 34K precursors have more of these sugars than the 29K precursor (figure 14.6). When the same kind of studies are done with more peripheral sugars, fucose and galactose, only 13–15K ACTH becomes labeled, demonstrating that peripheral sugars are added after the precursors are processed to smaller molecular weight forms as shown in figure 14.15 (Roberts *et al.*, 1978). Finally, pulse chase studies with labeled amino acids show that 29K ACTH–LPH labels first and chases first (figures 14.7, 14.8 and 14.9). Taken together, these results suggest that glycosylation of the primary translation product to form 29K ACTH is a very early step in processing in the tumor cells and that the 32 and 34K forms arise by further glycosylation of the 29K form (figure 14.15). Proteolytic processing of the precursors to intermediate size ACTH fragments (20–23K ACTH) and β-LPH occurs as label chases into the 32 and 34K forms of the precursor (figures 14.8 and 14.9). Hence, 29K ACTH–LPH appears to be at a branch point in the pathway. It can be further glycosylated or processed proteolytically to smaller forms.

The 4.5 and 13K forms of ACTH are both end products of processing in the tumor cells. These forms are also major secretory products of the tumor cell (as shown in figure 14.14) and in primary pituitary cell cultures (Paquette and Herbert, 1978).

Formulation of separate processing pathways for 13 and 4.5K ACTH (figure 14.15) is based on glycopeptide analysis of all of the forms of ACTH. This analysis shows that the α-ACTH$_{22-39}$ peptide is glycosylated in 32K ACTH-LPH, 23K ACTH (an intermediate) and 13K ACTH (Mains and Eipper, 1978). The α-ACTH$_{22-39}$ peptide is not glycosylated in 29K ACTH–LPH, 20–21K ACTH

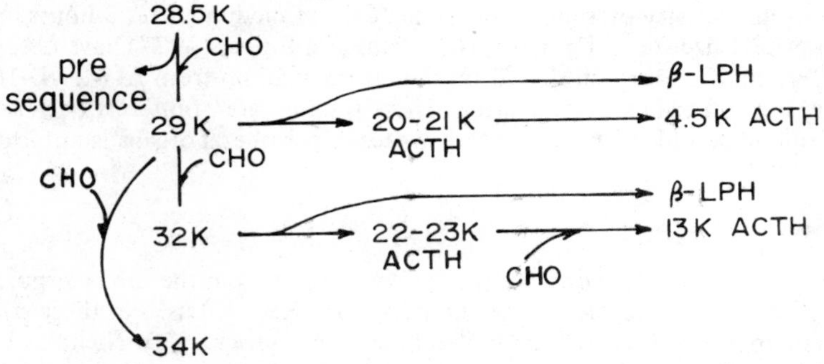

Figure 14.15 Processing pathways for ACTH–LPH precursors in AtT-20/D-16v cells.

and 4.5K ACTH. According to this model of processing the presence or absence of a carbohydrate side chain in the precursor determines whether the 13 or the 4.5K ACTH form is made. It is not known whether the two forms have different functions in the animal, but, if they do, then addition of carbohydrate side chains to 29K ACTH–LPH could play an important part in regulating the processes that 13 and 4.5K ACTH mediate.

The pulse chase studies with tumor cells (figure 14.8) show that a β-LPH-like molecule is the first form of β-endorphin cleaved out of the precursor. β-LPH is not glycosylated (Roberts *et al.*, 1978). β-LPH is also a major secretory product of the tumor cells. Cleavage of β-LPH from the carboxy terminal region of the precursor would also give rise to intermediate size forms of ACTH (20–23K ACTH). Hence, the pattern of processing in figure 14.15 is completely consistent with the assigned locations of ACTH and β-LPH in the precursor molecules in figure 14.4.

The presence of all of the forms of ACTH and β-endorphin in mouse pituitary provides some assurance that the processing pathways being studied are not tumor cell artifacts. It is interesting to note that the anterior and intermediate lobes of mouse pituitary appear to have the same forms of the ACTH–LPH precursor (29, 32 and 34K ACTH-LPH forms) but a very different distribution of lower molecular weight forms of ACTH and β-endorphin. This suggest that the processing of the precursors in the two lobes is quite different. It is known that the regulation of release of ACTH from the two lobes is also different. Release in the intermediate-posterior pituitary does not appear to be regulated by glucocorticoids as it is in the anterior pituitary. (Fischer and Moriarity, 1977).

Guillemin *et al.* (1977*b*) have shown that blood levels of β-endorphin and ACTH (immunoactivity) rise and fall together very rapidly after a rat is stressed by breaking its leg. The results in figure 14.13 show that levels of these two activities rise and fall together in tumor cell culture medium in response to addition of crude CRF and dexamethasone. A similar effect has been observed in primary cell cultures from mouse anterior pituitary with vasopressin and dexamethasone (Allen *et al.*, 1978). Coupled regulation of this kind would explain the results of Guillemin *et al.* (1977*b*). A surprising finding is that a major form of β-endorphin activity present in tumor cell culture medium after 3 hours incubation is β-LPH size form (figure 14.14). Mains and Eipper (1977) have observed both β-LPH and β-endorphin size forms in culture medium from AtT-20/D-16v cells after longer periods of incubation. These findings are of interest because the form of opiate peptide that acts on target sites in peripheral organs is not known.

ACKNOWLEDGEMENTS

β-melanocyte stimulating hormone (β-MSH) was a gift from the Ciba Corporation. Porcine β-endorphin and the endorphin antiserum (RB-100) used in these studies were a generous gift of Dr Roger Guillemin and his colleagues, Dr Nicholas Ling and Ms Vargo of the Salk Institute, La Jolla, California. This work was supported by National Institute of Health Grant AM 16879.

REFERENCES

Abe, K., Nicholson, W. E., Liddle, G. W. and Orth, D. N. (1967). *J. clin. Invest.*, **46**, 1609–20
Abe, K., Nicholson, W. E., Liddle, G. W., Orth, D. N. and Island, D. P. (1969). *J. clin. Invest.*, **48**, 1580–9
Allen, R. G., Hinman, M., Herbert, E., Shibuya, H. and Pert, C. (1978). *Proc. natn. Acad. Sci. U.S.A.*, (to be submitted)
Dayhoff, M. O. (1972). In *Atlas of Protein Sequence and Structure*, 5, D-194–7. National Biochemical Research Foundation, Washington, DC
Dintzes, H. M. (1961). *Proc. natn. Acad. Sci. U.S.A.*, 47, 247–61
Eipper, B. A. and Mains, R. E. (1975). *Biochemistry*, **14**, 3836–44
Eipper, B. A. and Mains, R. E. (1978). *J. biol. Chem.* (in press)
Eipper, B. A., Mains, R. E. and Guenzi, D. (1976). *J. biol. Chem.*, **251**, 4121–6
Fischer, J. L. and Moriarity, M. (1977). *Endocrinology*, **100**, 1047–53
Gilkes, J. J. H., Bloomfield, G. A., Scott, A. P., Lowry, P. J., Ratcliffe, J. G., Landon, J. and Rees, L. H. (1975). *J. clin. Endocr. Metab.*, **40**, 450–7
Guillemin, R., Ling, N., and Vargo, T. (1977*a*). *Biochem. biophys. Res. Commun.*, 77, 361–6
Guillemin, R., Vargo, T., Rossier, J., Scott, M., Ling, N., Rivier, C., Vale, W. and Bloom, F. (1977*b*). *Science*, **197**, 1367–9
Herbert, E., Allen, R. G. and Paquette, T. L. (1978). *Endocrinology*, **102**, 218–26
Li, C. H. and Chung, D. (1976). *Proc. natn. Acad. Sci. U.S.A.*, **73**, 1145–8
Mains, R. E. and Eipper, B. A. (1976). *J. biol. Chem.*, **251**, 4115–20
Mains, R. E. and Eipper, B. A. (1977). *Proc. natn. Acad. Sci. U.S.A.*, **74**, 3014–8
Mains, R. E. and Eipper, B. A. (1978). *J. biol. Chem.* (in press)
Needleman, S. B. (1970). In *Protein Sequence Determination.* (ed. S. B. Needleman), Springer-Verlag, New York
Orth, D. N., Nicholson, W. E., Mitchell, W. M., Island, D. P., Shapiro, M. and Byyny, R. L. (1973). *Endocrinology*, **92**, 385–93
Paquette, T. L. and Herbert, E. (1978). *Endocrinology* (submitted)
Pestka, S. (1971). *A. Rev. Microbiol.*, **25**, 487–562
Pelham, H. R. B. and Jackson, R. J. (1976). *Eur. J. Biochem.*, **67**, 247–56
Phifer, R. F., Orth, D. N and Spicer, S. S. (1974). *J. clin. Endocr. Metab.*, **39**, 684–92
Roberts, J. L. and Herbert, E. (1977*a*). *Proc. natn. Acad. Sci. U.S.A.*, **74**, 5300–4
Roberts, J. L. and Herbert, E. (1977*b*). *Proc. natn. Acad. Sci. U.S.A.*, **74**, 4826
Roberts, J. L., Phillips, M., Rosa, P. A. and Herbert, E. (1978). *Biochemistry* (in press)
Scott, A. P. and Lowry, P. J. (1974). *Biochem. J.*, **139**, 593–602
Vale, W., Grant, G., Amoss, M., Blackwell, R. and Guillemin, R. (1972). *Endocrinology*, **91**, 562–72
Yalow, R. S. and Berson, S. A. (1971). *Biochem. biophys. Res. Commun.*, **44**, 439–45

15

Enkephalin levels in mouse brain: diurnal variation, post-mortem degradation, and effect of cycloheximide

Steven R. Childers and Solomon H. Snyder
(Departments of Pharmacology and Experimental Therapeutics,
and Psychiatry and Behavioral Sciences,
Johns Hopkins University School of Medicine, Baltimore, Maryland 21205 U.S.A.)

Enkephalin was first isolated as a mixture of the two pentapeptides methionine enkephalin (met-enkephalin) and leucine enkephalin (leu-enkephalin) by its ability to inhibit electrically induced contractions of the guinea pig ileum (Hughes, 1975; Hughes *et al.*, 1976) and to compete with [^{3}H] opiate binding to rat brain membranes (Terenius and Wahlström, 1974; Pasternak *et al.*, 1975; Simantov and Snyder, 1976*a*). Although these assays have been useful in elucidating several properties of opioid peptides such as their regional (Hughes, 1975; Pasternak *et al.*, 1975) and subcellular distributions (Simantov and Snyder, 1976*b*), their lack of specificity makes it very difficult to distinguish the various opioid peptides from each other. Specific radioimmunoassays (RIA) for met and leu-enkephalin (Simantov *et al.*, 1977; Yang *et al.*, 1977) not only distinguish met and leu-enkephalin but also discriminate between enkephalin and the larger endorphin fragments of β-lipotropin (β-LPH). In this way enkephalin RIAs can detect changes in enkephalin levels which result from specific enkephalinergic metabolic processes in the brain.

The release of various pituitary hormones (Dunn *et al.*, 1972; Nokin *et al.*, 1972) is regulated by a circadian rhythm. The finding by Lutsch and Morris (1972) that the analgesic activity of morphine followed a diurnal rhythm led to the suggestion that endogenous opioids may also be released in a similar manner. Fredrickson *et al.* (1977) recently reported a diurnal rhythm in the hyperalgesia induced by naloxone and found that endogenous opioid activity was higher in mouse brain at 1500 hours than at 0800 hours. To test directly these results for enkephalin, we report the diurnal variation of met and leu-enkephalin levels in both rat and mouse brain.

Radioimmunoassay of brain enkephalin levels can also be used to assess the metabolism of enkephalin *in vivo*. Preliminary reports (Clouet and Ratner, 1976; Yang *et al.*, 1977) have demonstrated that intracerebral (i.c.) injection of several [^{3}H] amino acids results in the production of labeled enkephalin, thus suggesting that enkephalin synthesis may take place from amino acid precursors. However, these experiments have not determined the mechanism of enkephalin synthesis (whether synthesis occurs enzymatically or via ribosomes) or the rate of enkephalin turnover in the brain. The latter question is especially important in determining whether enkephalin acts quickly like a neurotransmitter released often, or slowly as a compound rarely utilized. In this report we attempt to assess enkephalin turnover by inhibiting its synthesis with injections of cycloheximide. In addition we measured the metabolism of enkephalin after death by assay of met and leu-enkephalin at various times *post mortem*.

MATERIALS AND METHODS

Radioimmunoassay of met and leu-enkephalin

Antisera to met-enkephalin (coupled to hemocyanin with glutaraldehyde) and leu-enkephalin (coupled with carbodiimide) were produced in rabbits as previously described (Simantov *et al.*, 1977; Childers *et al.*, 1977). These antisera were relatively specific: over 200-fold molar excess of one enkephalin was required to cross-react in the RIA of the other enkephalin. β-Endorphin did not cross-react with either serum at a concentration of 20 μM.

Enkephalin was extracted by homogenizing whole mouse brain in 5 ml of 0.1 N HCl and whole rat brain in 20 ml of 0.1 N HCl using a Brinkmann Polytron. The homogenates were then centrifuged at 4 °C for 10 min at 49 000*g*, and supernatants were lyophilized, neutralized, and centrifuged at 4 °C for 10 min. The supernatants were lyophilized again and samples were suspended in 0.8 ml of 50 mM sodium veronal buffer, pH 8.6. RIAs were conducted as previously described (Childers *et al.*, 1977) using 60 000 c.p.m. of either [^{3}H] met-enkephalin (17.4 Ci/mmol) or [^{3}H] leu-enkephalin (21 Ci/mmol; from New England Nuclear Corporation) along with antiserum and enkephalin standards or samples in a total volume of 0.25 ml.

Cycloheximide studies

Male Swiss albino mice (20–25 g) were anesthetized with i.p. injections of Equi-Thesin (Jensen-Salisbury Labs). Cycloheximide (Sigma Chemical Co.) was dissolved in saline at a concentration of 10 mg/ml, and 10 μl were injected i.c. at a depth of 2 mm in each of four sites: bilateral temporal and ventricular locations (Flexner *et al.*, 1963). Control mice received injections of 10 μl of saline in identical locations. Further studies indicated that a single series of injections was not sufficient to lower brain enkephalin levels (see Results); therefore, a second series of injections was performed 3 hours later in the same locations. In this procedure, the average mortality rate was 25–35 per cent.

Cerebral protein synthesis was determined by a modification of the method of Barondes *et al.* (1967). Mice were injected s.c. with 5 μCi of [^{3}H] leucine (5 Ci/mmol; New England Nuclear Corporation) and were killed 40 min later.

Brains were homogenized in 5ml of 0.1 N NaOH with the Polytron; 0.5 ml aliquots of each homogenate were added to 1.5 ml of cold 12 per cent TCA. The samples were centrifuged at 4 °C for 10 min at 49 000*g*, supernatants were discarded and pellets were washed with 1 ml of cold 10 per cent TCA. TCA was extracted from the pellets by three 1-ml washes with ether, and the pellets were dissolved in 0.5 ml of 0.1 N NaOH and radioactivity was determined in 10 ml of aqueous scintillation fluor. Protein synthesis was calculated by determining the ratio of TCA-precipitable radioactivity to total amount of radioactivity in the homogenate.

RESULTS

Diurnal variation of met and leu-enkephalin

To determine accurately the diurnal rhythm of enkephalin in brain, both rats (male Sprague-Dawley, 150–180 g) and mice (male Swiss albino, 20–25 g) were maintained at constant 12-hour light–darkness intervals for at least 1 week before killing. Animals were killed at 0630, 1100, and 1530 hours. Results (table 15.1) showed that there was no significant variation in met-enkephalin levels in either mouse or rat brain. There were slight, but significant, decreases in leu-enkephalin at 1530 hours in both species. When values for met and leu-enkephalin were added to provide total enkephalin values, no significant variation was detected in either species.

Table 15.1 Diurnal variation of enkephalin levels in whole rat and mouse brains

Time of death	Met-enkephalin (pmol/g)	Leu-enkephalin (pmol/g)
Rat Brain		
0630	600 ± 46	60 ± 7
1100	574 ± 79	77 ± 14
1530	570 ± 46	42 ± 9
Mouse Brain		
0630	1170 ± 120	115 ± 5
1100	1290 ± 180	98 ± 16
1530	1090 ± 100	82 ± 9

Animals were killed at the times indicated, brains were homogenized in 0.1 N HCl and extracted as described in Methods, and met and leu-enkephalin levels were determined by RIA. Data represent mean values ± s.e.m.

Post-mortem degradation of enkephalin

Enkephalin is extremely susceptible to proteolytic degradation, with a half-life of 1 min in brain homogenates at 37 °C (Hambrook *et al.*, 1976). However, enkeph-

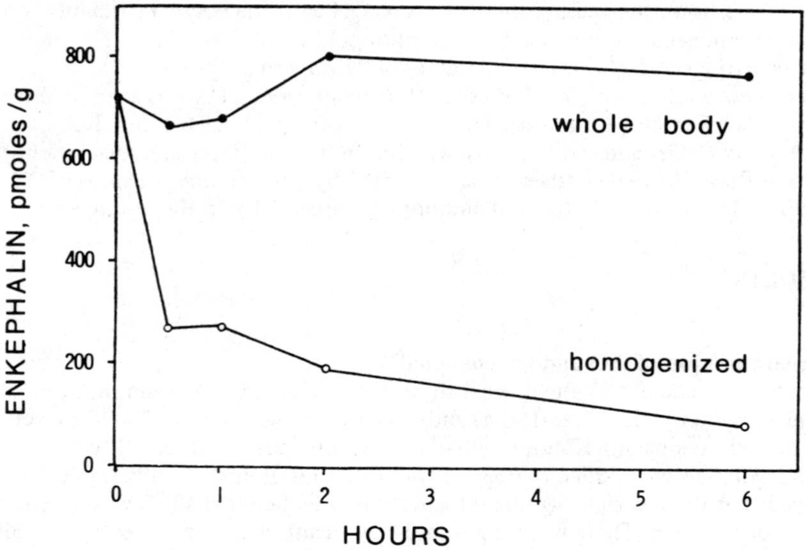

Figure 15.1 Post-mortem degradation of enkephalin in mice brains. One group of mice was killed, brains were homogenized in 4.5 ml water and incubated at 25 °C for the indicated times. Incubation was stopped by addition of 0.5 ml of 1.0 N HCl. The second group of mice was killed and remained undisturbed at room temperature. Brains were excised at the time indicated and homogenized in 5 ml of 0.1 N HCl. Met and leu-enkephalin levels were determined by RIA; data are expressed as the sum of met and leu-enkephalin levels.

alin may not normally be exposed to proteolytic enzymes in the cell and thus may be protected against degradation until released. To explore this possibility, enkephalin was assayed in mice brains subjected to two different post-mortem treatments. One group of mice was killed and brains were immediately homogenized in water and incubated at room temperature. Assay of met and leu-enkephalin (figure 15.1) revealed an immediate degradation of enkephalin, with approximately 70 per cent loss after 30 min. Enkephalin levels at 2 and 6 hours after death were close to the lower limits of sensitivity of the assay. In contrast, when the mice were killed and remained undisturbed, enkephalin levels remained fairly constant at least for 6 hours. Therefore, as long as cell structure remains intact, enkephalin is not appreciably degraded.

Inhibition of protein synthesis with cycloheximide

Cycloheximide, a potent inhibitor of protein synthesis, was injected i.c. in mice in an effort to halt production of met and leu-enkephalin and thereby measure their turnover in brain. Preliminary experiments revealed that enkephalin was remarkably resistant to such treatment. Assay of enkephlin levels 24 hours after one injection at four sites (100 μg cycloheximide per site) revealed no loss of met or leu-enkephalin (table 15.2), although this dose was sufficient to inhibit cerebral protein synthesis by 90 per cent for 2 hours (data not shown). The dose

Table 15.2 Enkephalin levels in mouse brain 24 hours after cycloheximide treatment

Injection	Met-enkephalin (pmol/g)	% control	Leu-enkephalin (pmol/g)	% control
A, 1 Injection series*				
Saline	1310 ± 150		136 ± 12	
Cycloheximide	1490 ± 320	113	122 ± 12	91
B. 2 Injection series†				
Saline	1440 ± 250		163 ± 10	
Cycloheximide	904 ± 61	63	113 ± 13	69

Mice were killed 24 hours after initial injections, and brains were extracted in 0.1 N HCl and met and leu-enkephalin were assayed by RIA as described in Methods.

*Group A mice were injected intracerebrally in two temporal sites and two ventricular sites with 10 μl (100 μg cycloheximide) per injection site.

†Group B mice were injected as above, followed by a second series of i.c. injections 3 hours later.

Data represent mean values ± s.e.m.

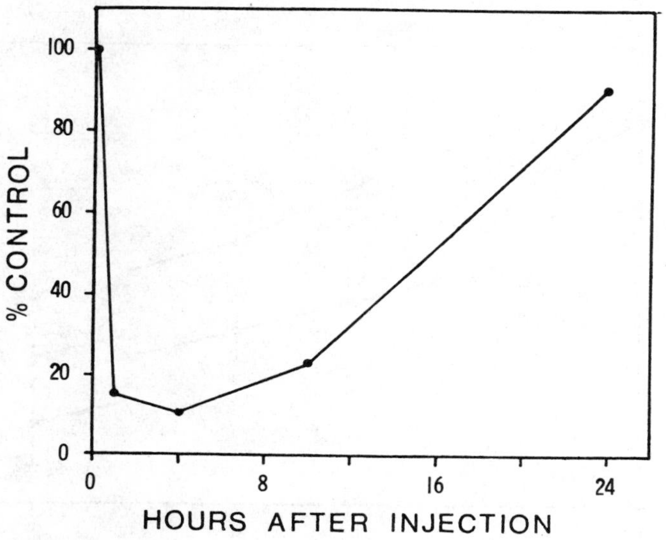

Figure 15.2 Inhibition of cerebral protein synthesis by cycloheximide. Mice were injected with two series of cycloheximide (100 μg/10 μl) at four cerebral sites. At various times mice were injected subcutaneously with 5 μCi of [^{3}H] leucine and protein synthesis was determined as described in Methods. Results are expressed as per cent of synthesis in brains of saline-injected mice.

of cycloheximide could not be increased because of toxicity, so a second injection of the same dose was given 3 hours later. This treatment resulted in a significant loss of enkephalin 24 hours after the first injection, with approximately 40 per cent loss of met-enkephalin and 30 per cent loss of leu-enkephalin (table 15.2). Analysis of cerebral protein synthesis following the two injections (figure 15.2) showed 90 per cent loss at 4 hours, 80 per cent loss at 10 hours and approximately normal synthesis at 24 hours.

Table 15.3 Effect of various doses of cycloheximide on enkephalin levels in mouse brain

μg Cycloheximide per injection site	Met-enkephalin (pmol/g)	% control	Leu-enkephalin (pmol/g)	% control
0	994 ± 65		112 ± 10	
25	937 ± 97	94	97 ± 9	87
50	771 ± 78	78	88 ± 13	79
100	828 ± 53	83	88 ± 6	79

Mice were injected i.c. with 10 μl of saline or cycloheximide at indicated doses in four sites as described in Materials and Methods. A second series of injections was performed 3 hours later, and mice were killed 24 hours after the first injection. Data represent mean values ± s.e.m.

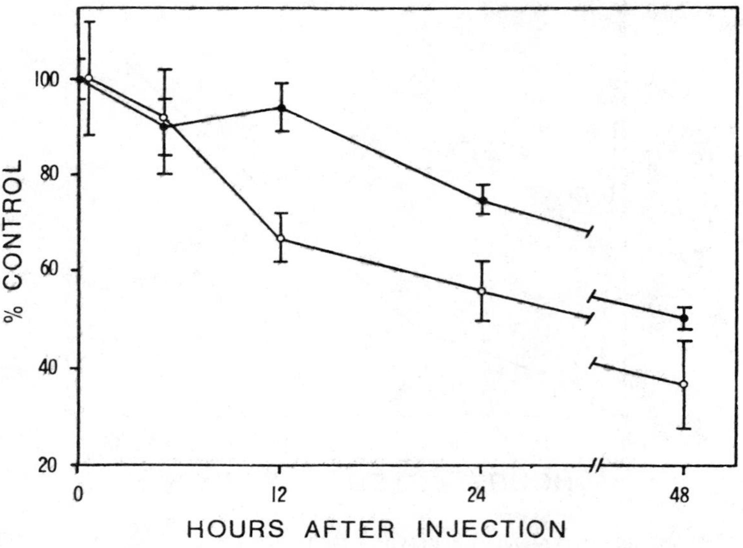

Figure 15.3 Time course of cycloheximide-induced decrease of met and leu-enkephalin. Mice were injected with two series of cycloheximide (100 μg/10 μl) at four cerebral sites. After killing at times indicated, brains were homogenized in 5 ml of 0.1 N HCl and met and leu-enkephalin levels were determined by RIA. Data represent percentage enkephalin levels in saline-injected mice.

The effect of cycloheximide on enkephalin levels was dose-dependent. Mice were given two series of injections as above, with each injection site receiving either 25, 50, or 100 μg cycloheximide per injection (table 15.3). Enkephalin levels 24 hours later were only slightly decreased with 25 μg cycloheximide; however, 50 μg provided a maximal response since no further decrease was seen with 100 μg cycloheximide.

The time course of enkephalin decrease after cycloheximide indicates a slow turnover (figure 15.3). No significant effect was seen on either met or leu-enkephalin levels at 5 hours, and leu-enkephalin remained unchanged at 12 hours while met-enkephalin decreased by approximately 30 per cent. Both peptides revealed significant decreases at 24 hours and further losses at 48 hours. Experiments are currently in progress to determine when enkephalin levels return to normal.

DISCUSSION

The finding that brain enkephalin levels are not appreciably affected by the time of killing indicates that, in these strains of mice and rats at least, there is no significant CNS diurnal rhythm of enkephalin. The suggestion (Fredrickson *et al.*, 1977) that brain opioid activity increases at 1500 hours is not supported by the present finding of a small decrease of leu-enkephalin at 1530 hours. The differences in the two studies may lie in the use of different opioid peptide assays as well as different strains of mice. It appears more likely that any diurnal rhythm of opioid peptides would involve β-endorphin, which is released from pituitary along with ACTH (Guillemin *et al.*, 1977).

The results of the post-mortem study support previous findings of the effect of microwave irradiation on brain enkephalin levels (Simantov *et al.*, 1977). Those experiments showed that microwave irradiation increased enkephalin levels in both live rats and in rats killed before irradiation. Such results are consistent with the idea that proteolytic degradation of enkephalin does not occur simply after death but begins rapidly as the brain is excised and homogenized without previous inactivation of enzymatic activity.

Injection of cycloheximide reduces brain enkephalin levels in a dose and time-dependent manner. These experiments suggest, but do not confirm, that enkephalin is synthesized ribosomally, although an alternative possibility—that cycloheximide halts production of an enkephalin-synthetic enzyme, cannot be eliminated. The slow onset of the cycloheximide effect suggests either that enkephalin is released at a slow rate or that much of the enkephalin in the cells is stored as a precursor which must be converted into enkephalin and released before any effect of protein synthesis inhibition can be seen. Perhaps these experiments can be most useful as a tool in measuring drug effects on enkephalin release which cannot be detected by assaying steady-state levels but which may become evident after enkephalin synthesis is stopped.

ACKNOWLEDGEMENTS

We thank Adele Snowman for technical assistance. The work was supported by USPHS grant DA01645 and USPHS postdoctoral grant MH07329 to S.R.C.

REFERENCES

Barondes, S. H. and Cohen, H. D. (1967). *Proc. natn. Acad. Sci. U.S.A.*, **58**, 157-64
Childers, S. R., Schwarcz, R., Coyle. J. T. and Snyder, S. H. (1978). *Advances in Biochemical Psychopharmacology*, vol. 18, *The Endorphins* (ed. E. Costa and M. Trabucchi), Raven Press, N.Y., pp. 161-74
Clouet, D. and Ratner, M. (1976). In *Opiates and Endogenous Opioid Peptides*, (ed. H. W. Kosterlitz) pp. 71-8, Elsevier, North-Holland, Amsterdam
Dunn, J. D., Arimura, A. and Schwing, L. E. (1972). *Endocrinology*, **90**, 29-36
Flexner, J. B., Flexner, L. B. and Stellar, E. (1963). *Science*, **141**, 57-9
Fredrickson, R. C. A., Burgis, V. and Edwards, J. D. (1977). *Science*, **198**, 756-8
Guillemin, R., Vargo, T., Rossier, J., Minick, S., Ling, N., Rivier, C., Vale, W. and Bloom, F. (1977). *Science*, **197**, 1367-9
Hambrook, J. M., Morgan, B. A., Rance, M. J. and Smith, C. F. C. (1976). *Nature*, **262**, 782-3
Hughes, J. T. (1975). *Brain Res.*, **88**, 295-308
Hughes, J., Smith, T., Kosterlitz, H. W., Fothergill, L. A., Morgan, B. and Morris, H. R. (1976). *Nature*, **258**, 577-9
Lutsch, E. F. and Morris, R. W. (1972). *Experientia*, **28**, 673-4
Nokin, M., Vekemano, M., L'Hermite, M. and Robyn, C. (1972). *Br. med. J.*, **3**, 561-6
Pasternak, G. W., Goodman, R. and Snyder, S. H. (1975). *Life Sci.*, **16**, 1765-9
Simantov, R. and Snyder, S. H. (1976*a*). *Proc. natn. Acad. Sci. U.S.A.*, **73**, 2515-9
Simantov, R. and Snyder, S. H. (1976*b*). *Molec. Pharmac.*, **12**, 987-98
Simantov, R., Childers, S. R. and Snyder, S. H. (1977). *Brain Res.*, **135**, 358-67
Terenius, L. and Wahlström, A. (1974). *Acta pharmac. scand.*, **35**, (suppl. 1), 55
Yang, H.-Y., Hong, J. S. and Costa, E. (1977). *Neuropharmacology*, **16**, 303-7
Yang, H.-Y. (1978). *Advances in Biochemical Psychopharmacology*, vol. 18, *The Endorphins* (ed. E. Costa and M. Trabucchi), Raven Press, N.Y., pp. 149-60

16
Proteolytic processing in the biosynthesis and metabolism of endorphins

László Gráf, Ágnes Kenessey, Sándor Bajusz, András Patthy,
András Z. Rónai and Ilona Berzétei
(Research Institute for Pharmaceutical Chemistry,
H-1325 Budapest, PO Box 82, Hungary)

All the brain and pituitary endorphins except leu-enkephalin identified to date appear to be β-lipotropin (β-LPH) fragments (Hughes *et al.*, 1975; Guillemin *et al.*, 1976; Li and Chung, 1976; Bradbury *et al.*, 1976; Gráf *et al.*, 1976*b*). Their structural relationships (figure 16.1) have stimulated our interest in the biosynthetic origin of these peptides. Theoretically, the release of β-endorphin from β-LPH requires a trypsin-like enzyme to split the molecule at Arg_{60}-Tyr_{61}. Among the naturally occurring endorphins, β-endorphin is the most potent, implying that it may be of special physiological significance in brain function. Met-enkephalin and pituitary endorphins of intermediate size might be formed from β-endorphin by further enzymatic cleavage. Their weak and transient effects *in vivo* give the impression that these opioid peptides may be intermediates in β-endorphin metabolism.

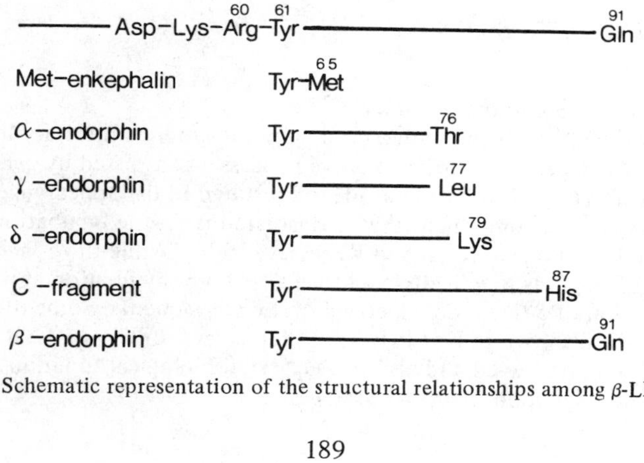

Figure 16.1 Schematic representation of the structural relationships among β-LPH and endorphins.

We describe here the results of our search for β-LPH-activating and β-endorphin-degrading proteinases of the pituitary and brain.

EXPERIMENTAL DETAILS

Porcine β-LPH and β-endorphin were prepared as described previously (Gráf and Cseh, 1968; Gráf *et al.*, 1976*a*). Bacitracin A was obtained from Dr A. Kótai (L. Eötvös University, Budapest). Pepstatin was a gift of Dr H. Umezawa (Institute of Microbial Chemistry, Tokyo). Soybean trypsin inhibitor and bovine pancreatic trypsin inhibitor (Kunitz) were the products of Calbiochem and G. Richter Factory, Budapest, respectively. Fragment LPH_{52-60} was prepared from a plasmin digest of β-LPH (Gráf, 1976). Tripeptide aldehyde inhibitors were synthesized by Bajusz *et al.* (1974, 1975).

For studies on the degradation of β-LPH, porcine anterior pituitary and rat brain homogenates were prepared as described previously (Gráf and Kenessey, 1976; Patthy *et al.*, 1977). Protein content was measured by Palladin's method (Palladin, 1961). For subcellular localization studies, porcine anterior pituitary and rat brain were homogenized in 0.32 M sucrose with a Potter–Elvehjem homogenizer and centrifuged according to Whittaker (1969). Protein content of the fractions was determined according to Lowry *et al.* (1951). Incubation of β-LPH with homogenates and subcellular fractions was performed in 0.05 M ammonium formate, pH 4.0, in 0.05 M ammonium acetate, pH 6.5 and in 0.05 M ammonium hydrogen carbonate, pH 8.0, at 37 °C with different β-LPH/homogenate ratios. Incubation was terminated by adding one volume of acetone to the aliquots taken. The pH of the samples (except those originated from the pH 4.0 incubation mixture) was adjusted to about 6 by the addition of acetic acid, and the supernatant fractions obtained were subjected to gel electrophoresis (Davis, 1964) and *in vitro* bioassays on longitudinal muscle strip of guinea pig ileum (GPI) and mouse vas deferens (MVD) (Rónai *et al.*, 1977).

To study the breakdown of β-endorphin in rat brain homogenate, Marks's method (Marks, 1977) was applied with some modifications (Patthy *et al.*, 1977). Amino acid analysis was carried out in a JEOL (JLC-5AH) automatic analyzer.

RESULTS AND DISCUSSION

Conversions of β-LPH in the pituitary

Porcine β-LPH was incubated with a crude porcine anterior pituitary homogenate at different pH values, and the breakdown process was assessed by gel electrophoresis (figure 16.2). Incubation at pH 6.5 resulted in the appearance of one main electrophoretic component that was isolated from the incubation mixture and identified as LPH_{1-77} (Gráf and Kenessey, 1976). While the conversion of β-LPH into LPH_{1-77} is practically exclusive at pH 6.5, incubation at pH 8.0 led to the formation of a few more electrophoretic components. Some of these were isolated and shown to be LPH_{1-46}, LPH_{1-60} and LPH_{1-79} (Gráf *et al.*, 1977*b*). The bonds cleaved and also the suggested biological function of these cleavages are indicated in figure 16.3.

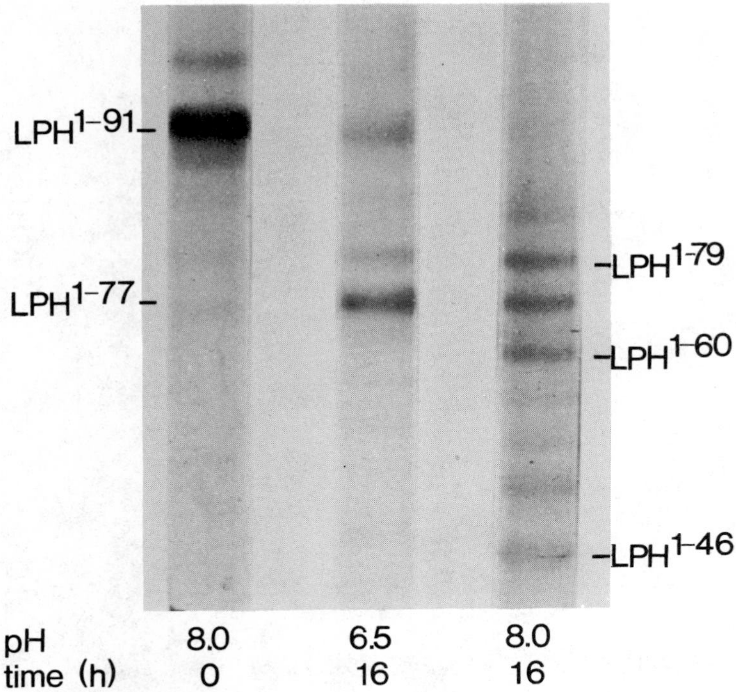

Figure 16.2 Effect of pH on the conversion of β-LPH by pituitary proteinases. The homogenate to β-LPH ratio was 1:1 (weight of the protein content per total weight, in all cases). Incubation time, pH and the gel electrophoretic components identified are indicated. Samples contained 100 μg of β-LPH.

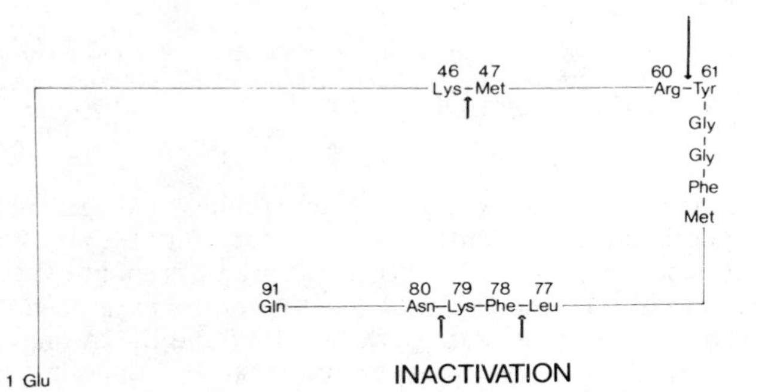

Figure 16.3 Schematic diagram of the β-LPH structure with the cleavage bonds indicated.

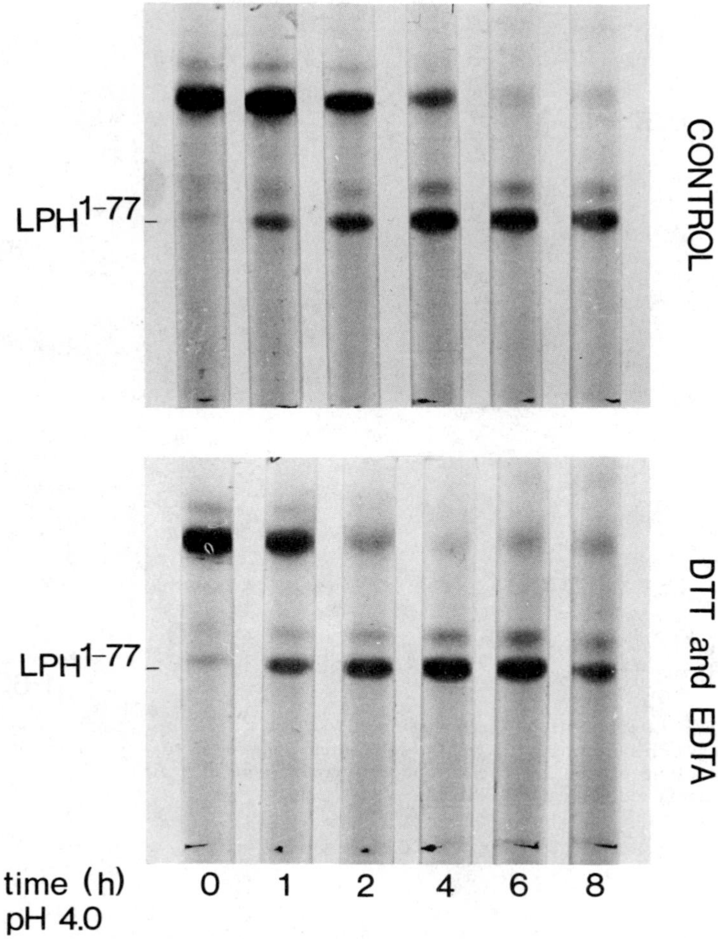

Figure 16.4 Time-course of the digestion of β-LPH with a pituitary homogenate to β-LPH ratio of 1:5 at pH 4.0 in the absence (control) and presence of 10 mM dithiothreitol (DTT) and 10 mM EDTA. Samples contained 100 μg of β-LPH

The pH dependence of β-LPH degradation by pituitary homogenate was studied and an optimum between pH 3.5–4.5 was found for the attack at Leu_{77}-Phe_{78}. The conversion of β-LPH into LPH_{1-77} at pH 4.0 is about twice as fast in the presence of DTT and EDTA than in the control experiment (figure 16.4). (On the basis of the potentiating effect of DTT and EDTA on this proteolytic process, we have suggested previously that the responsible endopeptidase is SH-dependent (Gráf and Kenessey, 1976; Gráf *et al.*, 1977*a*). Some characteristics of this pituitary proteinase revealed more recently are however, inconsistent with our original proposal.

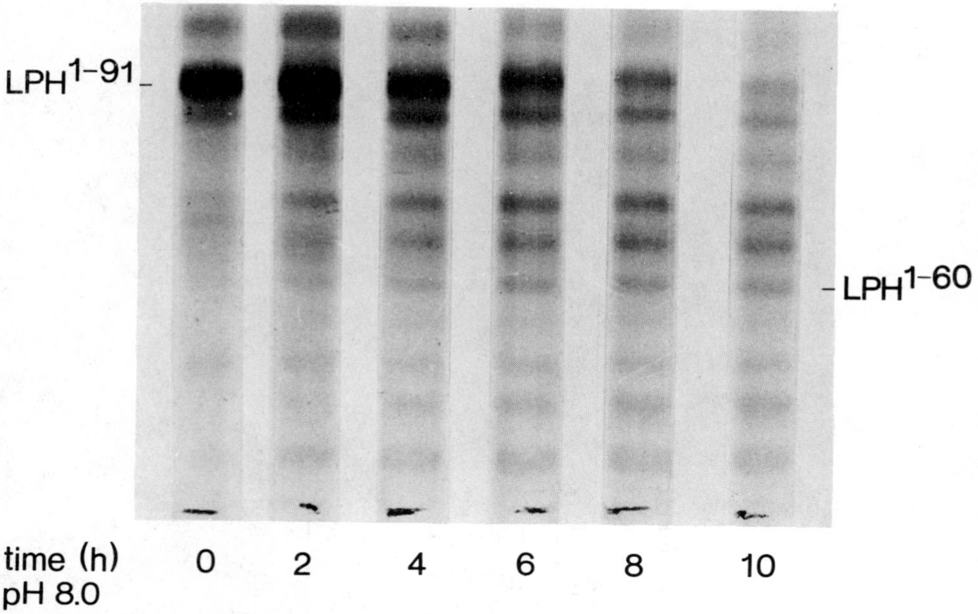

Figure 16.5 Time-course of the digestion of β-LPH with a pituitary homogenate to β-LPH ratio of 2:1 at pH 8.0 in the presence of 5×10^{-4} M bacitracin. Samples contained 200 μg of β-LPH.

The optimal pH for the cleavage of the critical Arg_{60}–Tyr_{61} bond in the β-LPH structure was estimated to be 8.0 under the usual incubation conditions. The time-course of the digestion at pH 8.0 revealed a gradual generation of LPH_{1-60} among other cleavage products (figure 16.5), and a concomitant release of opiate agonist activity as measured simultaneously on MVD and longitudinal muscle strip of GPI (figure 16.6). Incubations were carried out in the presence of 5×10^{-4} M bacitracin. The high MVD/GPI potency ratios of the incubation mixtures indicate the formation of opioid peptides shorter than β-endorphin (Rónai *et al.*, 1977). These biological data are in fair agreement with our finding that the Leu_{77}–Phe_{78} and Lys_{79}–Asn_{80} bonds of β-LPH are also split under these incubation conditions (figure 16.5).

To characterize further the pituitary endopeptidases, the effect of some potential enzyme inhibitors on the electrophoretically detectable conversions of β-LPH was examined at pH 8.0 and pH 4.0 (table 16.1). While bacitracin and soybean trypsin inhibitor affected none of the enzymatic cleavages tested, pancreatic trypsin inhibitor inhibited the attack of Arg_{60}–Tyr_{61} and Lys_{79}–Asn_{80} peptide bonds by the pituitary homogenate. LPH_{52-60}, originated from the N-terminal of the critical Arg_{60}–Tyr_{61} bond selectively inhibited this cleavage. Prompted by this observation a tripeptide aldehyde corresponding to residues 58–60 of the β-LPH sequence. Asp–Lys–Arg–H was synthesized and found to be a selective inhibitor of the activating enzyme at a minimum concentration of 3×10^{-5} M. When inhibitor concentration was increased by two orders of magni-

Table 16.1 Effect of some enzyme inhibitors on the breakdown of β-LPH in pituitary homogenate

Inhibitor	Cleavage sites			
	Lys_{46}–Met_{47}	Arg_{60}–Tyr_{61}	Leu_{77}–Phe_{78}	Lys_{79}–Asn_{80}
Bacitracin (10^{-3} M)	–	–	–	–
Soybean trypsin inhibitor (2×10^{-4} M)	–	–	–	–
Kunitz trypsin inhibitor (4×10^{-4} M)	–	+	–	+
LPH_{52-60} (3×10^{-4} M*)	–	+	–	–
Asp–Lys–Arg–H (3×10^{-5} M*)	–	+	–	–
Asp–Lys–Arg–H (3×10^{-3} M)	–	+	–	+
Pepstatin (10^{-6} M*)	–	–	+	–

*Minimum concentration at which complete inhibition could be achieved.

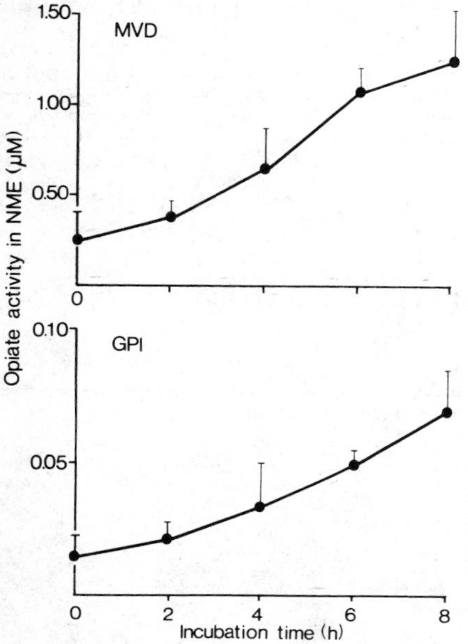

Figure 16.6 Release of opiate agonist activity (measured in the MVD and GPI tests) from β-LPH on incubation with pituitary homogenate under the conditions of figure 16.5. The opiate activity generated from 10^{-6} M β-LPH was characterized by equiactive doses of normorphine (NME) in μM.

tude, the cleavage of the Lys_{79}–Asn_{80} bond was also inhibited. Pepstatin proved to be a potent inhibitor of the Leu_{77}–Phe_{78} splitting endopeptidase at pH 4.0. This inhibition pattern (table 16.1) reveals some information regarding the biochemical nature of the β-LPH converting pituitary endopeptidases. The Arg_{60}–Tyr_{61} splitting enzyme appears to be a serine proteinase, but clearly different from trypsin and plasmin. The susceptibility of the Leu_{77}–Phe_{78} splitting endopeptidase to pepstatin implies its identity with a carboxyl proteinase, most probably cathepsin D.

These conclusions are supported by subcellular localization studies of these two enzymes (table 16.2). Porcine anterior pituitary subcellular fractions obtained by differential centrifugation were tested for β-LPH converting activity at pH 8.0 and pH 4.0. Both enzymes were found to be highly concentrated in the P_2 fraction, composed mainly of mitochondria, secretory granules and lysosomes. On hypo-osmotic shock of this fraction, the lipotropin-activating enzyme remained bound to some particles, whereas the Leu_{77}–Phe_{78} splitting acid proteinase was liberated into the soluble fraction. It must therefore be assumed that the lipotropin-activating enzyme is associated with secretory granule membranes, as the Leu_{77}–Phe_{78} splitting inactivating enzyme is of lysosomal origin.

Table 16.2 Subcellular localization of two β-LPH converting enzymes in porcine pituitary

	Endopeptidase splitting	
Fraction*	Arg_{60}–Tyr_{61}	Leu_{77}–Phe_{78}
P_1 (1×10^4 g min)	+	+
P_2 (3×10^5 g min)	+++	+++
P_3 (3×10^6 g min)	+	+
S_3	–	+
P_2 Lysis → P_2P (3×10^6 g min)	+++	+
P_2 Lysis → P_2S	–	+++

*Obtained by differential centrifugation.

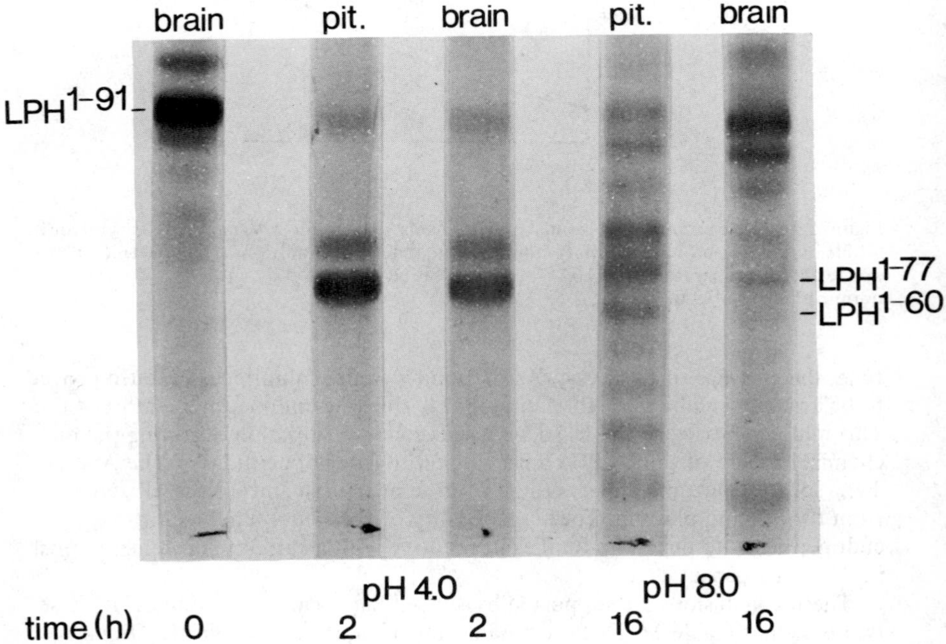

Figure 16.7 Conversions of β-LPH by porcine pituitary and rat brain homogenates at pH 4.0 (homogenate to β-LPH ratio was 1:2) and at pH 8.0 (homogenate to β-LPH ratio was 2:1), respectively. Samples contained 200 μg of β-LPH.

Breakdown of β-LPH and β-endorphin in the brain

In view of some recent data indicating the occurence of immunoreactive β-LPH and β-endorphin in different brain areas (LaBella *et al.*, 1977; Krieger *et al.*, 1977), we have assayed the brain for the presence of β-LPH converting endopeptidases. Incubation of porcine pituitary and rat brain homogenates with β-LPH at pH 4.0 led to the formation of the same fragment, LPH_{1-77}, indicating the presence of cathepsin D-like activity in both tissues (figure 16.7). At pH 8.0 however, β-LPH was degraded much more slowly in the brain homogenate than in that of pituitary. In addition, LPH_{1-60} did not show up in the incubation mixture containing brain homogenate. As a more sensitive assay for LPH activation, the release of opiate activity from β-LPH on incubation with P_2 fractions of pituitary and brain origin was measured in MVD (figure 16.8). As seen from the comparison, the crude synaptosomal brain preparation is a much less potent activator of β-LPH than is the crude secretory granule fraction of the pituitary. On the other hand, this relatively slight activating potency of the brain may have a functional significance in the biosynthesis of endorphins of non-hypophyseal origin.

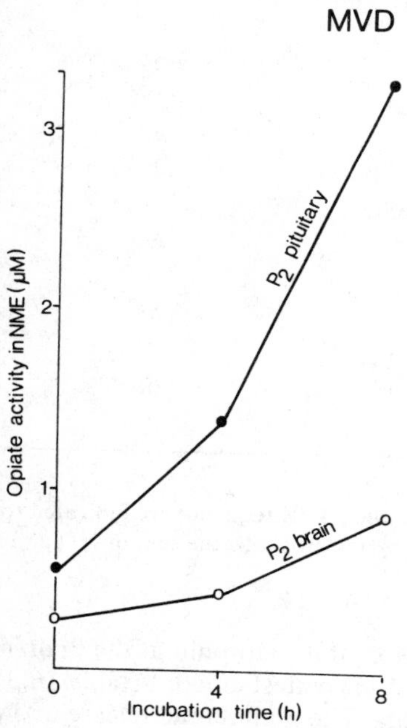

Figure 16.8 Release of opiate agonist activity (measured in the MVD test) from β-LPH on incubation with P_2 subcellular fractions (see table 16.2) of porcine pituitary and rat brain. The homogenate to β-LPH ratio was 2:1.

For further studies on the degradation of β-LPH and β-endorphin in rat brain homogenate at pH 7.5, Marks's strategy (Marks, 1977) was adopted; the release of amino acids from the polypeptides was determined with an amino acid analyzer. In accord with the results of our other approaches (figures 16.7, 16.8; Kenessey *et al.*, 1977), β-LPH appeared to be highly resistant to the degradative enzymes of the brain (table 16.3). This resistance also applies to the endorphin part of the molecule, and seems to be lost, at least partially, when β-endorphin is split from the β-LPH structure. The release of Thr and Ile, two residues present only in the β-endorphin portion of β-LPH, indicates the relative susceptibilities.

Table 16.3 Release of amino acids* from β-LPH and β-endorphin on incubation with rat brain homogenate

Amino acid†	β-LPH	β-endorphin
Lys	8	39
His	8	25
Arg	3	–
Asp	2	–
Thr (66, 72, 76)	5	27
Ser+Gln+Asn	4	26
Glu	6	27
Pro	0	25
Gly	2	24
Ala	4	29
Val	4	28
Met+MeSO	3	24
Ile (82)	6	27
Leu	5	48
Tyr	3	42
Phe	8	47
Trp	3	–

*Expressed in nmol per cent.

†Position numbers related to the β-LPH sequence are indicated for Thr and Ile; Ser, Gln and Asn were not separated by the analyzer; the sum of Met and its artifact, MeSO is given.

As to the biodegradation of β-endorphin in the brain homogenate, Tyr, Leu, Phe, and Lys are liberated in greatest amount (table 16.3). Marks *et al.* (1977) have published similar data. The preferential release of Tyr is clearly due to aminopeptidase action, whereas the high yields of Leu, Phe and Lys point to cleavages at internal sites in the molecule, presumably at the Leu_{77}–Phe_{78} and some lysyl bonds. Thus the simultaneous action of a cathepsin D-like proteinase, trypsin-like enzymes and exopeptidases seems to be reflected in the pattern of amino acid release. This view was checked by investigating the effect of exopeptidase, trypsin and cathepsin D inhibitors on the proteolysis of β-endorphin in rat brain homogenate (table 16.4). Both bacitracin and Boc-D-Phe-Pro-Arg-H, a selective serine proteinase inhibitor (Bajusz *et al.*, 1975), considerably inhibited the amino acid release, providing evidence that both exopeptidases and trypsin-like enzyme(s) are involved in the breakdown process (Patthy *et al.*, 1977). The reduced release of Tyr in the presence of Boc-D-Phe-Pro-Arg-H indicates that internal cleavages of the peptide chain may precede the removal of Tyr_{61} from the N-terminal by aminopeptidase action. Austen *et al.* (1977) have recently arrived at a similar conclusion. The addition of the inhibitory effects of

Table 16.4 Effect of various inhibitors* on brain β-endorphin-hydrolysing activity

Amino acid	Bacitracin	Boc–D-Phe–Pro–Arg–H	Boc–D-Phe–Pro–Arg–H + Bacitracin	Pepstatin
Lys	43	34	71	8
His	30	63	100	4
Thr	48	25	79	4
Ser + Gln + Asn	45	38	88	5
Glu	12	35	50	0
Pro	41	45	82	8
Gly	45	35	86	6
Ala	40	22	71	6
Val	31	35	65	6
Met	24	40	65	0
Ile	48	25	66	8
Leu	62	20	77	10
Tyr	33	18	63	2
Phe	38	23	61	12

*Values are percentage inhibition. The concentration of all the inhibitors was 5×10^{-4} M.

bacitracin and Boc–D-Pro–Arg–H, when a mixture of these two inhibitors is applied (table 16.4), clearly shows the different inhibitory mechanisms of these compounds, but by no means proves these two cleavage mechanisms to be exclusive in β-endorphin biodegradation.

Similarly, the lack of significant inhibitory effect of pepstatin on the breakdown (table 16.4) does not necessarily exclude the contribution of cathepsin D to the degradation process. In fact, we do have direct evidence for the cleavage of the Leu_{77}-Phe_{78} bond in β-LPH and β-endorphin at pH 7.5. In addition, we have recently developed a new synthetic inhibitor of the Leu_{77}-Phe_{78} splitting endopeptidase which is significantly active at pH 7.5, too (Bajusz *et al.*, to be published). As to the case of pepstatin, it may be speculated that the pH dependence of the catalytic activity and of the susceptibility of an enzyme to inhibitors may run divergently.

CONCLUSIONS

Mains *et al.* (1977) have recently reported a 31 000 dalton protein to be the common biological precursor to ACTH and the endorphins. The relatively high quantity of β-LPH and also the nearly equimolar amounts of β-LPH and β-endorphin in the pituitary gland (Gráf *et al.*, 1976*a*) suggest, however, that

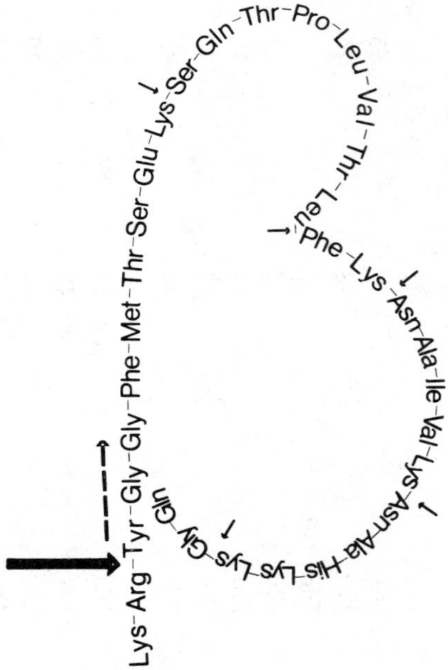

Figure 16.9 The amino acid sequence of porcine β-LPH between residues 59–91 (Gráf *et al.*, 1971). Arrows indicate proteolytic attacks on the polypeptide chain resulting in the activation of β-LPH (➔), biodegradation of β-endorphin (→) and complete inactivation of the shorter active fragments (--→).

endorphins are generated from β-LPH rather than directly from a larger precursor. Thus, the activating step appears to be the specific cleavage of the Arg_{60}–Tyr_{61} peptide bond in the β-LPH structure (figure 16.9). Crine *et al.* (1977) have recently shown that pituitary slices can synthesize β-endorphin *in vitro*. Now, we have provided evidence for the presence of an Arg_{60}–Tyr_{61} splitting endopeptidase in the crude secretory granule fraction of porcine and rat anterior pituitaries. Thus, the enzyme is easily accessible for β-LPH and other secreted hormones of the cell. It might be identical with the trypsin-like enzyme first reported by Adams and Smith (1951) in pituitary extracts, and shown by Tesar *et al.* (1969) to be associated with the small granule fraction of beef adenohypophysis. Physiological experiments to demonstrate the regulatory role of this enzyme in the activation of β-LPH are being carried out in our laboratory. Similarly, the physiological significance of the β-LPH activating potency detected in brain synaptosomes (figure 16.8) merits further investigation.

Our data cast light on the release mechanism of γ and α-endorphins first isolated and characterized by Guillemin *et al.* (1976). There is no doubt that these opioid peptides are cleavage products presumably formed by the action of lysosomal cathepsin D on β-endorphin, and by the subsequent removal of the newly formed C-terminal Leu_{77} by carboxypeptidase action (Gráf and Kenessey, 1976; Gráf *et al.*, 1977*a*; figure 16.4, table 16.1). Because of the high concentration of cathepsin D in the pituitary and the brain, and also the wide range of pH values at which it is active (Barrett, 1977, and references therein), the formation of these opioid peptides during any isolation procedure, in particular at acidic pH, can hardly be avoided. To explore the possible physiological significance of α and γ-endorphins, one must face a question of more general significance: does cathepsin D have a physiological role, a more specific one than the intracellular digestion of proteins? The strongest argument against its extracellular function is the failure of some authors to detect catalytic activity for cathepsin D at neutral pH (Day and Reid, 1976; Barrett, 1977). The pH range over which an enzyme may be active is, however, dependent on the substrate; β-LPH and β-endorphin were found to be susceptible to the cathepsin D-like proteinase at neutral pH also.

In our opinion, cleavages of the Leu_{77}-Phe_{78} and lysyl bonds by cathepsin D (or another carboxyl proteinase) and some trypsin-like degradative enzyme(s), respectively, represent an intermediate and rate-limiting phase in the β-endorphin metabolism (figure 16.9). By these cleavages, giving rise to the generation of α, γ, δ to perhaps ω-endorphins, the biologically essential Tyr_{61} appears to lose a great deal of its protection against aminopeptidase action (Gráf *et al.*, 1977*a*; Rónai *et al.*, 1977; Hollósi *et al.*, 1977). Thus, the removal of the N-terminal Tyr would seem to be the final inactivating step in the β-endorphin biodegradation (figure 16.9).

REFERENCES

Adams, E. and Smith, E. L. (1951). *J. biol. Chem.*, **191**, 651–61
Austen, B. M., Smyth, D. G. and Snell, C. R. (1977). *Nature*, **269**, 619–21
Bajusz, S., Barabás, É., Széll, E. and Bagdy, D. (1974). *Hungarian Patent*, No. 169, 870
Bajusz, S., Barabás, É., Széll, E. and Bagdy, D. (1975). In *Peptides: Chemistry, Structure*

and Biology, (eds R. Walter and J. Meinhofer), pp. 603–8. Ann Arbor Science Publishers, Ann Arbor

Barrett, A. J. (1977). In *Proteinases in Mammalian Cells and Tissues*, (ed. A. J. Barrett), pp. 209–48. North-Holland Publishing Company, Amsterdam/New York/Oxford

Bradbury, A. F., Smyth, D. G., Snell, C. R., Birdsall, N. J. M. and Hulme, E. C. (1976). *Nature,* **260**, 793–5

Crine, P., Benjannet, S., Seidah, N. G., Lis, M. and Chrétien, M. (1977). *Proc. natn. Acad. Sci. U.S.A.*, **74**, 1403–6

Davis, B. J. (1964). *Ann. N.Y. Acad. Sci.*, **121**, 404–27

Day, R. P. and Reid, I. A. (1976). *Endocrinology*, **99**, 93–100

Gráf, L. (1976). *Acta biochim. biophys. Acad. Sci. Hung.*, **11**, 267–77

Gráf, L., Barát, E., Cseh, G. and Sajgó, M. (1971). *Biochim. biophys. Acta,* **229**, 276–8

Gráf, L., Barát, E. and Patthy, A. (1976*a*). *Acta biochim. biophys. Acad. Sci. Hung.*, **11**, 121–2

Gráf, L. and Cseh, G. (1968). *Acta biochim. biophys. Acad. Sci. Hung.*, **3**, 175–7

Gráf, L., Cseh, G., Barát, E., Rónai, A. Z., Székely, J. I., Kenessey, Á. and Bajusz, S. (1977*a*). *Ann. N.Y. Acad. Sci.*, **297**, 63–85

Gráf, L. and Kenessey, Á. (1976). *FEBS Lett.*, **69**, 255–60

Gráf, L., Kenessey, Á., Berzétei, I. and Rónai, A. Z. (1977*b*). *Biochem. biophys. Res. Commun.*, **78**, 1114–25

Gráf, L., Székely, J. I., Rónai, A. Z., Dunai-Kovács, Zs. and Bajusz, S. (1976*b*). *Nature,* **263**, 240–2

Guillemin, R., Ling, N. and Burgus, R. (1976). *C. r. hebd. Séanc. Acad. Sci. Paris, Ser. D* **282**, 783–5

Hollósi, M., Kajtár, M. and Gráf, L. (1977). *FEBS Lett.*, **74**, 185–9

Hughes, J., Smith, T. W., Kosterlitz, H. W., Fothergill, L. A., Morgan, B. A. and Morris, H. R. (1975). *Nature,* **258**, 577–9

Kenessey, Á., Gráf, L. and Palkovits, M. (1977). *Brain Res. Bull.*, **2**, 247–50

Krieger, D. T., Liotta, A., Suda, T., Palkovits, M. and Brownstein, M. J. (1977). *Biochem. biophys. Res. Commun.*, **76**, 930–6

LaBella, F., Queen, G., Senyshyn, J., Lis, M. and Chrétien, M. (1977). *Biochem. biophys. Res. Commun.*, **75**, 350–7

Li, C. H. and Chung, D. (1976). *Proc. natn. Acad. Sci. U.S.A.*, **73**, 1145–8

Lowry, O. H., Rosebrough, N. J., Farr, A. L. and Randall, R. J. (1951). *J. biol. Chem.*, **193**, 265–75

Mains, R. E., Eipper, B. A. and Ling, N. (1977). *Proc. natn. Acad. Sci. U.S.A.*, **74**, 3014–8

Marks, N. (1977). In *Peptides in Neurobiology,* (ed. H. Gainer), pp. 221–58. Plenum Press, New York and London

Marks, N., Grynbaum, A. and Neidle, A. (1977). *Biochem. biophys. Res. Commun.*, **74**, 1552–9

Palladin, A. V. (1961). In *Regional Neurochemistry,* (eds. S. S. Kety and J. Elkes) pp. 8–11, Pergamon Press, Oxford

Patthy, A., Gráf, L., Kenessey, Á., Székely, J. I. and Bajusz, S. (1977). *Biochem. biophys. Res. Commun.* **79**, 254–9

Rónai, A. Z., Gráf, L., Székely, J. I., Dunai-Kovács, Zs. and Bajusz, S. (1977). *FEBS Lett.*, **74**, 182–4

Tesar, J. T., Koenig, H. and Hughes, C. (1969). *J. Cell Biol.* **40**, 225–35

Whittaker, V. P. (1969). In *Handbook of Neurochemistry,* (ed. A. Lajtha) pp. 327–64. Plenum Press, London.

17

Endogenous opioids: cold-induced release from pituitary tissue *in vitro*; extraction from pituitary and milk

Hansjörg Teschemacher, Katharina Csontos, Anton Westenthanner,
Viktor Brantl and Wolfgang Kromer* (Department of Neuropharmacology,
Max-Planck-Institut für Psychiatrie, Kraepelinstrasse 2,
8 Munich 40, F.G.R. and *Pharmacological Institute,
University of Munich, Nuβbaumstrasse 26, 8 Munich 2, F.G.R.)

All endogenous opioids identified so far are peptides–'endorphins'. Recently, however, endogenous opioids which might belong to another class of compounds have been detected in the blood. Both classes of endogenous opioids have been studied in this investigation. Pituitary opioid peptides were released from anterior lobe tissue on incubation between 0 and 15 °C, as reported for most of the pituitary hormones. β-endorphin and α and/or γ-endorphin were found in the incubation media. Using a hot glacial acetic acid extraction method, besides β-endorphin, an opioid with properties similar to those of the opioids detected in blood was extracted from bovine posterior pituitary lobes. To this class of endogenous opioids, apparently, also belongs a substance extracted from bovine and human milk.

Several pituitary hormones are released from pituitary tissue incubated at low temperatures. Vasopressin was found to be released on incubation below 15 °C of intact tissue (Hong and Poisner, 1974*a*), nerve endings (Baker and Hope, 1976), or neurosecretory granules (Hong and Poisner, 1974*b*) from the neurohypophysis. Adenohypophyseal hormones such as TSH, LH, FSH, ACTH and GH are released on incubation of anterior pituitary slices at 0°C; in contrast, very little release of prolactin was found (LaBella *et al.*, 1973). We also investigated whether one or several of the endorphins are released on incubation of pituitary tissue at low temperatures, in a similar manner to pituitary hormones such as ACTH.

Recently, endogenous opioids have been detected in blood (Pert *et al.*, 1976; Schulz *et al.*, 1977) and urine (Schulz and Wüster, 1977), which display properties quite different from those known for the endorphins identified so far. Our assumption that these endogenous opioids might pass from the blood into milk, which might explain the reported presence of opioid compounds in a casein hydrolysate (Wajda *et al.*, 1976) led us to search for endogenous opioids in the milk. We also tried to find such endogenous opioids in the pituitary.

METHODS

Cold-induced release of pituitary endorphins from anterior lobe tissue

Anterior lobes from porcine pituitaries transported from a local slaughterhouse to our laboratory at room temperature were pulled into pieces and incubated at various temperatures between 0 and 37 °C in Krebs–Ringer solution or other incubation media as indicated (one anterior lobe/ml medium). The samples were incubated for 10 min and subsequently centrifuged at 150 000*g* min at their incubation temperatures. The supernatants were frozen immediately on dry ice until their opioid activities were tested in the guinea pig ileum (GPI) 'strip' bioassay. The pellets were resuspended for the subsequent incubation period.

Extraction of endorphins from pituitary tissue

Endorphins were extracted from pituitary tissue using a hot glacial acetic acid method as described in detail by Teschemacher *et al.* (1975).

Extraction of compounds with opioid activity from milk

Milk was frozen on dry ice and lyophilized overnight. The residue was mixed with silicic acid (containing 13 per cent $CaSO_4$) and the mixture extracted with chloroform/methanol (2/1, v/v). The extract was centrifuged at 10 000*g* min. Supernatants were evaporated to dryness and the residues taken up into 1 ml of water for determination of opioid activities in the GPI bioassay.

Purification and characterization of endorphins extracted or released at 0 °C from pituitary tissue

Endorphins extracted from pituitary tissue using a hot glacial acetic acid extraction method or released from anterior pituitary lobes at 0 °C into Krebs–Ringer incubation medium were purified by gel filtration and ion exchange chromatography as described by Teschemacher *et al.* (1976) and Kromer *et al.* (1976). The materials thus purified on a DEAE Biogel A anion exchanger column were subjected to h.p.l.c. on a μ-Bondapak-C18 column, from which they were eluted using CH_3CN/HOAc mixtures in isocratic or gradient runs. Endorphins contained in the eluates of the μ-Bondapak-C18 column were identified by comparison with the elution times of reference compounds and by testing the sensitivity of the endorphins to aminopeptidase M. Purity was tested by peptide end group determination. (For a detailed description of the purification procedures see Westenthanner *et al.* (in preparation)).

Measurement of opioid activities
Endorphin activity in the incubation media and in crude or partially purified extracts was determined by bioassay using the GPI longitudinal muscle myenteric plexus 'strip' preparation. (For a description of the isolated preparation and stimulation parameters see Kosterlitz *et al.* 1970, and Schulz and Goldstein, 1972.) Opiate receptor binding was used as a further assay (Pert and Snyder, 1973).

RESULTS AND DISCUSSION

Cold-induced release of endorphins from anterior pituitary lobes
On incubation of pituitary tissue at 0 °C, most of the pituitary hormones are released into the incubation medium, as are also the endorphins (figure 17.1). This finding differs from that of Queen *et al.* (1976), who found only negligible amounts of endorphins to be liberated during density-gradient centrifugation at 4 °C.

The rate of endorphin release from anterior pituitary lobe tissue clearly depends on the composition of the incubation medium, as shown in figure 17.1 (see also Teschemacher *et al.*, 1977). When Tris-HCl buffer (25 mM) is added, the rate is not significantly changed compared with incubation in Krebs–Ringer solution alone but it is considerably enhanced when Krebs–Ringer solution is used from

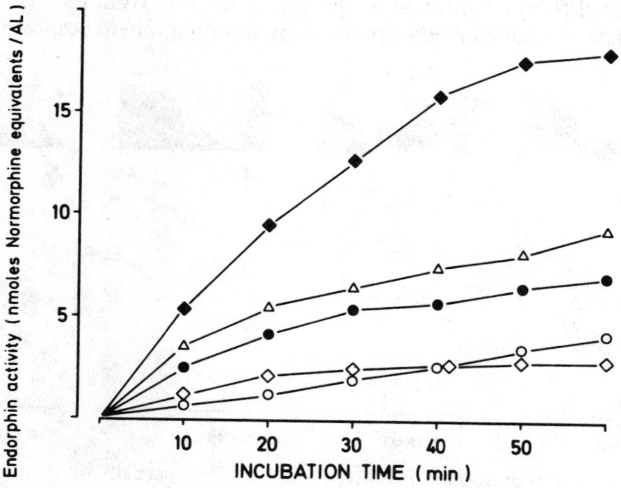

Figure 17.1 Endorphins released from anterior lobes of porcine pituitaries (pulled into pieces) on incubation at 0 °C. Incubation media: Krebs–Ringer solution (●) either without calcium chloride (◆) or with various additions: Tris-HCl, 25 mM (△), sucrose, 50 mM (○), calcium chloride, 5 mM (◇). Abscissa: Incubation time. Ordinate: Endorphin activity in the incubation media determined using the guinea pig ileum longitudinal muscle myenteric plexus preparation. Activities calculated by comparison with normorphine activities determined in the same assay system. Mean values of triplicates. Standard deviations (all below 20% of the mean values) omitted for sake of clarity.

which calcium has been omitted. In contrast, a significant decrease of the release rate is observed when sucrose (50 mM) or calcium (5 mM) are added to the Krebs–Ringer solution. These changes in the composition of the incubation medium have been reported to induce almost the same effects on the cold-induced release of vasopressin from neurohypophyseal tissue (Hong and Poisner, 1974*a*, 1974*b*; Baker and Hope, 1976).

The mechanism of this release process as well as the mechanisms by which it can be influenced, are unknown. Depletion of intracellular calcium stores and more or less nonspecific disturbance of membrane structures of the secretory granules have both been discussed. The latter interpretation has been considered in view of inhibition of the cold-induced release process by lauryl alcohol, which is thought to stabilize the granules by restoring the lipid composition of the membrane (Hong and Poisner, 1974*b*).

Purification and subsequent characterization of the endorphin activity found in the Krebs–Ringer solution after 0 °C incubation showed that β-endorphin was among the endorphins released. α and/or γ-endorphin are also released as well as another endorphin of unknown structure.

Extraction of endogenous opioids from pituitary and milk

Posterior lobes of bovine pituitaries were extracted using a hot glacial acetic acid method. The extract was subjected to gel filtration on a Biogel P4 column. Two materials with opioid activity were eluted from the column. Material I ($V_0 \times 1.3$), as can be judged from its chromatographic behavior and from its resistance to aminopeptidase contained β-endorphin as a major component responsible for the

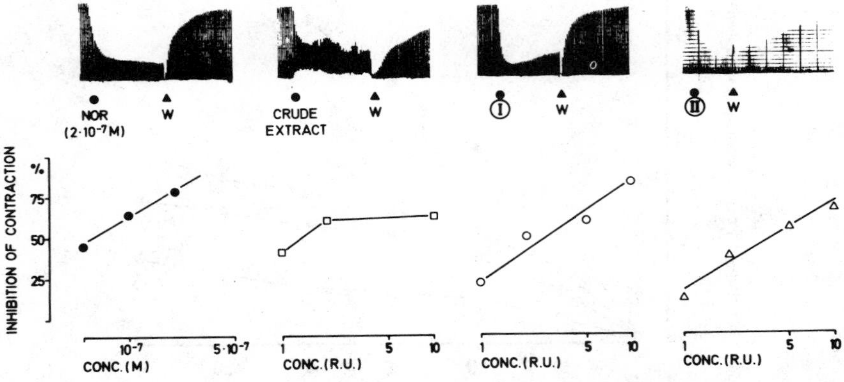

Figure 17.2 Activities of normorphine (NOR) and crude or partially purified extracts from bovine posterior pituitary lobes in the GPI longitudinal muscle myenteric plexus preparation ('strip'). The crude extract is a hot glacial acetic acid extract. I and II, Materials with opioid activity eluted from a Biogel P4 column (I: $V_0 \times 1.3$; II: $V_0 \times 3.1$) used for purification of the crude extract.

Upper panel: Effects of normorphine and crude or partially purified extracts on the guinea pig ileum 'strip'. W. Preparation washed.

Lower panel: Dose–response relationships. Ordinate, inhibition of contraction of the electrically stimulated guinea pig ileum 'strip'. Abscissae, concentration. Concentration of crude extract and materials I and II is expressed in relative units (R.U.).

opioid activity of material I. Material II was not purified further, since it was very unstable.

In figure 17.2, the opioid activity of the crude extract and materials I and II is compared with that of normorphine in the GPI bioassay. The onset of effect is very fast with normorphine and material I (β-endorphin) and the wash-out time is very short for both compounds. In contrast, material II takes effect more slowly and the wash-out time is very long. The influence of both I and II on the kinetics of the effect elicited by the crude extract can be seen in figure 17.2. The lines on the lower panel representing dose–response relationships run in parallel for normorphine and for material I and II. This is not the case with the crude extract as a result of a principle interfering with its opioid effects by stimulating the 'strip' preparation. The slower onset of effect and the very long wash-out time observed with material II, in contrast to material I (β-endorphin) or normorphine, indicate that this material might belong to that class of endogenous opioids which has been found in the blood (Pert *et al.*, 1976; Schulz *et al.*, 1977) and for which this behavior is characteristic (Schulz *et al.*, 1977).

Because those endogenous opioids found in the blood might pass into the milk, we looked for such material in human and bovine milk. We did in fact find such endogenous opioids which displayed opioid behavior in the GPI 'strip' preparation and in opiate receptor binding assays (Teschemacher *et al.*, 1978). These opioids possessed physicochemical properties quite similar to those of the opioids found in the blood and also proved resistant to Pronase (Schulz *et al.*, 1977). However, the variations between individuals and within individuals in the levels of these 'lactorphins' seem to be very high and, moreover, over periods of several months they could not be demonstrated in the milk. Since such opioids, might be taken up in food, such as milk or milk products, they might not originate in all cases from the organism in which they were detected. Therefore we proposed to call these natural but possibly, exogenous opioids 'exorphins' (Teschemacher *et al.*, 1977; Terenius, 1978).

REFERENCES

Baker, R. V. and Hope, D. B. (1976). *J. Neurochem.*, **27**, 197–202

Hong, J. S. and Poisner, A. (1974*a*). *Endocrinology*, **94**, 234–40

Hong, J. S. and Poisner, A. (1974*b*). *Neuroendocrinology*, **16**, 165–77

Kosterlitz, H. W., Lydon, R. J., Watt, A. J. (1970). *Br. J. Pharmac.*, **39**, 398–413

Kromer, W., Bläsig, J., Westenthanner, A., Haarmann, I. and Teschemacher, H. (1976). In *Opiates and Endogenous Opioid Peptides*, (ed. H. W. Kosterlitz), Elsevier/North-Holland Biomedical Press, Amsterdam, pp. 1–8

LaBella, F. S., Dular, R. and Vivian, S. (1973). *Endocrinology*, **92**, 1571–4

Pert, C. B. and Snyder, S. H. (1973). *Science*, **179**, 1011–4

Pert, C. B., Pert, A. and Tallman, J. F. (1976). *Proc. natn Acad. Sci. U.S.A.*, **73**, 2226–30

Queen, G., Pinsky, C. and LaBella, F. (1976). *Biochem. biophys. Res. Commun.*, **72**, 1021–7

Schulz, R. and Goldstein, A. (1972). *J. Pharmac. exp. Ther.*, **183**, 404–10

Schulz, R. and Wüster, M. (1977). *Eur. J. Pharmac.*, **43**, 383–4

Schulz, R., Wüster, M. and Herz, A. (1977). *Life Sci.*, **21**, 105–16

Terenius, L. (1978). In *The Bases of Addiction*. Dahlem Workshop, 1977, in press

Teschemacher, H., Opheim, K. E., Cox, B. M. and Goldstein, A. (1975). *Life Sci.*, **16**, 1771–6

Teschemacher, H., Bläsig, J. and Kromer, W. (1976). *Naunyn-Schmiedeberg's Arch. Pharmac.*, **294**, 293–5

Teschemacher, H., Brantl, V. and Haarman, V. (1978). *Naunyn-Schmiedeberg's Arch. Pharmac.,* **302,** Suppl. R60
Teschemacher, H., Westenthanner, A., Kromer, A., Csontos, K. and Haarmann, I. (1977). *Naunyn-Schmiedeberg's Arch. Pharmac.,* 297, Suppl. II, R53
Wajda, I. J., Neidle, A., Ehrenpreis, S. and Manigault, I. (1976). In *Opiates and Endogenous Opioid Peptides,* (ed. H. W. Kosterlitz), Elsevier/North-Holland Biomedical Press, Amsterdam, pp. 129–36

18

Exorphins: peptides with opioid activity isolated from wheat gluten, and their possible role in the etiology of schizophrenia

Werner A. Klee, Christine Zioudrou* and Richard A. Streaty (Laboratory of General and Comparative Biochemistry National Institute of Mental Health Bethesda, Maryland 20014, U.S.A.)

Endogenous opioid peptides, the endorphins (including enkephalin) are extremely potent substances which exert their effect at concentrations in the nanomolar range (Hughes *et al.*, 1975; Lord *et al.*, 1977; Klee, 1977). Furthermore, even though endorphin receptors are very specific, many structural variations are tolerated, albeit often with some loss of potency (Terenius *et al.*, 1976*a*; Ling and Guillemin, 1976; Chang *et al.*, 1976; Coy *et al.*, 1976; Schiller *et al.*; 1977, Agarwal *et al.*, 1977; Beddell *et al.*, 1977). Nevertheless, peptides with as little as 1 per cent of the activity of enkephalin will still be potent and could have profound pharmacological effects. Food proteins which happen to contain the appropriate peptide sequences, related to but not necessarily identical with those of the enkephalins could therefore be a natural source of opioid peptides. Such peptides might logically be called 'exorphins', since they are exogenously derived substances with morphine-like activity. We have found exorphin activity in pepsin digests of wheat gluten, a protein known to be a primary factor in the pathology of celiac disease, and postulated by Dohan (1966*a*) to be also involved in the etiology of schizophrenia.

Similarities between the behavioral anomalies of children with celiac disease (also known as gluten enteropathy) and those of schizophrenia led Dohan (1966*a*) to examine the role of cereal proteins, especially wheat gluten, in the pathology of schizophrenia. His findings can be summarized as follows:

(1) There is a greater than chance association between the occurence of celiac disease and schizophrenia in the same individual. Thus, there may be a genetic trait in common leading to each syndrome.

*Visiting Scientist from the Nuclear Research Center 'Demokritos,' Aghia Paraskevi, Attikis, Athens, Greece.

(2) Epidemiological studies of schizophrenia admissions to mental hospitals during the Second World War, when there were large variations in wheat and rye consumption, showed a direct correlation between wheat and rye consumption and schizophrenia, but not other forms of mental illness (Dohan, 1966*b*).

(3) Schizophrenic patients were shown in two separate clinical studies to improve more readily when kept on gluten-free diets and to relapse somewhat when gluten was reintroduced into the diet without the knowledge of the patient, or the observer (Dohan and Grassberger, 1973; Singh and Kay, 1976).

Evidence has been presented previously to suggest that endorphins may be involved in schizophrenia (Terenius *et al.*, 1976*b*; Jacquet and Marks, 1976; Bloom *et al.*, 1976). We now demonstrate the presence of endorphin-like activity (exorphins) in peptides derived from wheat gluten. Interaction of exorphins, derived from wheat, with brain opiate receptors could serve as a biochemical mechanism which accounts for Dohan's clinical findings.

A closer examination of receptor specificity

Receptors are characterized by the specificity with which they recognize the appropriate ligands. Often, very minor structural alterations can effect changes in receptor binding affinities of three or more orders of magnitude, or alternatively, transform an agonist into an antagonist. The opiate receptor, which is perhaps more appropriately thought of as the endorphin or enkephalin receptor is, of course, no exception. The data presented in the upper portion of table 18.1 show that the potency of a series of methionine enkephalin analogues may be varied by a factor of 100 by minimal structure changes. The addition of an arginine residue to the amino group of tyrosine, or removal of the phenolic hydroxyl group results in drastic reduction of potency in the adenylate cyclase assay performed with

Table 18.1 Potencies of some enkephalin analogues as inhibitors of adenylate cyclase in homogenates of neuroblastoma × glioma hybrid cells*.

	K_i (nM)
Tyr–Gly–Gly–Phe–Met	12
Tyr–Gly–Gly–Phe–Met–Thr	30
Arg–Tyr–Gly–Gly–Phe–Met	1 000
Phe–Gly–Gly–Phe–Met	1000
Tyr–Gly–Gly–Phe–Leu	25
Tyr–Ala–Gly–Phe–Leu	1500
Tyr–Gly–Ser–Phe–Leu	2400
Tyr–Gly–Phe–Leu	6500
Tyr–Ser–Gly–Phe–Leu	30 000
Tyr–D-Ala–Gly–Phe–Met–NH_2	12
Tyr–L-Ala–Gly–Phe–Met–NH_2	400
Tyr–D-Ala–Gly–N-Me-Phe–Met-ol	200

*Determined as described by Sharma *et al.* (1975).

homogenates of neuroblastoma × glioma NG108–15 hybrid cells. Thus, the endorphin receptors are exquisitely sensitive to some types of structural variation in enkephalin analogues. On the other hand, as demonstrated by data in the middle and lower portions of table 18.1 some structural alterations in enkephalin analogues are associated with only relatively small decreases in potency. Thus, D-amino acids can replace glycine in position 2 (as well as methionine in position 5) (Beddell *et al.*, 1977; Pert *et al.*, 1976) with little or no change in potency. Other types of substitution, L-alanine for glycine 2, for example, are more deleterious, but the resulting peptides still have easily measurable activity. In fact, because of the extraordinary potency of enkephalin, even a peptide with a 100-fold decrease in potency is still highly active. If such a peptide were to reach the brain in micromolar concentrations, it would be expected to have profound effects.

Adenylate cyclase and the mouse vas deferens assays

The neuroblastoma × glioma adenylate cyclase assay is a sensitive and convenient method of measuring opioid peptide action (Klee and Nirenberg, 1976). An important feature of the assay is that specificity can be demonstrated with naloxone reversal. The electrically stimulated mouse vas deferens (Hughes *et al.*, 1975) shares the sensitivity and naloxone reversibility of the adenylate cyclase assay and, in our work, we use the two test systems concurrently. We have found that all effects of the exorphins in the adenylate cyclase assay are also observed with the mouse vas deferens.

Table 18.2 Comparison of the potencies of endorphins and morphine as inhibitors of neuroblastoma × glioma adenylate cyclase and of the mouse vas deferens

	Adenylate cyclase K_i (nM)	Vas deferens ID_{50} (nM)
Met-enkephalin	12	12
α-Endorphin	250	30
β-Endorphin	150	80
Morphine	1500	500

Hughes *et al.* (1975) were able to isolate and characterize the enkephalins largely because of the favorable properties of the mouse vas deferens assay. As shown in table 18.2, potency data obtained with a series of endorphins using the vas deferens assay (Lord *et al.*, 1976) are remarkably similar to data obtained using the adenylate cyclase assay in our own laboratories. Particularly striking is the observation that enkephalin is more potent, by a factor of 5–10 than is β-endorphin (LPH_{61-91}) or any lipotropin fragment of intermediate length. In most other tests, enkephalins are weaker than β-endorphin, perhaps because of the more important role of proteolytic degradation in most other opiate assay systems.

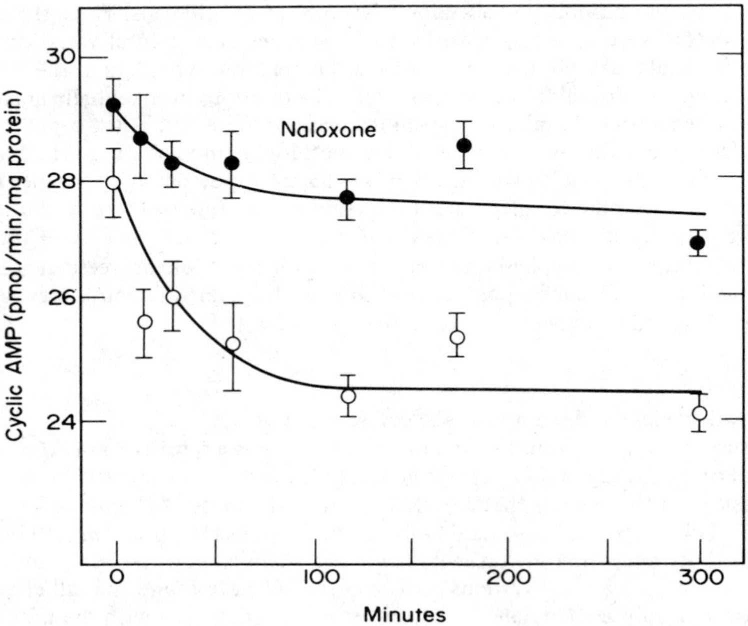

Figure 18.1 Exorphin activity in a pepsin digest of gluten as a function of time of treatment with pepsin. Activity was determined as the effect of the gluten digest upon the adenylate cyclase present in homogenates of neuroblastoma × glioma hybrid NG108–15 cells, assayed in the presence (solid symbols) or in the absence (open symbols) of 0.1 mM naloxone. Wheat gluten (ICN), 50 mg/ml in 0.1 N HCl was treated with pepsin (Worthington), 1.25 mg/ml at 37 °C for the times shown. The reaction was terminated by the addition of 1 M Tris (150 μl/ml) to bring the pH to 7.5. Aliquots of 20 μl of each time point were tested for their effects upon the activity of adenylate cyclase in a standard 100 μl reaction mixture as described by Sharma *et al.* (1975). The error bars represent standard errors for triplicate determinations.

Accordingly, peptic digests of proteins containing the appropriate amino acid sequences would be expected to contain peptides with an amino-terminal tyrosine residue and, perhaps, with opioid activity. We have found that pepsin digests of wheat gluten contain opioid activity. The time-dependent production of naloxone-reversible inhibitory activity of adenylate cyclase by the action of pepsin on gluten is shown in figure 18.1. The inhibitory activity generated, although relatively small, is highly significant and was observed in each of the five pepsin digests of wheat gluten we have prepared to date. One interesting feature of these digests is that a stimulatory activity is also observed, even in the zero time points. Thus, when pepsin digests of gluten were tested in the neuroblastoma × glioma adenylate cyclase it was found that they contain two kinds of activities. A crude peptide mixture is observed to stimulate the activity of the enzyme, and the addition of nalozone results in an even greater stimulation and thus uncovers a masked inhibitory action. The data shown in table 18.3 illustrate this point, and show further that the effect of naloxone has the appropriate stereospecificity. Only (–)-naloxone stimu-

Exorphins in pepsin digests of wheat gluten

Pepsin, the major proteolytic enzyme of the stomach is the only protease which can preferentially hydrolyze peptide bonds involving aromatic amino acids of the type

$$\ldots \text{—X— Tyr —Y} \ldots$$

to yield peptides with amino terminal aromatic amino acids of the type

$$NH_2 \text{ — Tyr — Y} \ldots \qquad \text{(Fruton, 1971).}$$

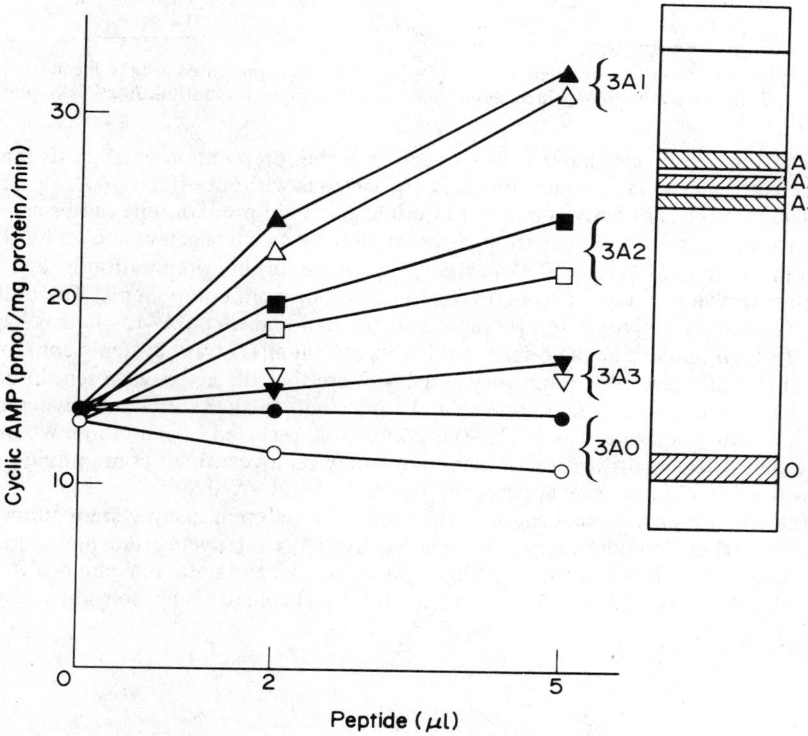

Figure 18.2 Activity of partially purified gluten peptides in the adenylate cyclase assay. The peptides were resolved by silica gel chromatography and the fractions eluted from preparative silica gel plates correspond to the four major components shown in the diagram. Assays were performed in quadruplicate, and standard errors were near 0.5 pmol cyclic AMP/min/mg protein.

Before application to the silica gel plates, the pepsin digest of gluten was purified by adsorption on to polystyrene beads (Bio-Rad SM-2) followed by elution with isopropanol. After removal of the solvent, the peptides from 100 g of gluten were dissolved in 25 ml H_2O. The equivalent of 5 ml of this solution was applied to the silica plate and chromatography was performed using *n*-butanol: methanol: 20 per cent NH_4OH (80:20:20) the bands were eluted with 90 per cent methanol, and after removal of the solvent, the eluted material was dissolved in 1 ml H_2O for assay.

Table 18.3 Stereospecificity of the reversal of exorphin activity by naloxone

Sample	Adenylate cyclase activity* pmol cyclic AMP/min/mg protein — Additions: None	(–)-Naloxone	(+)-Naloxone
Buffer	14.7	14.9	14.7
3A–0	13.0	15.6	12.0
3A–1	33.9	36.6	33.4
3A–2	21.7	22.5	21.5
3A–3	14.7	16.3	14.4

*Determined as described by Sharma *et al.* (1975). The values presented are the mean of quadruplicate determinations which show standard errors of ±0.6 pmol/min/mg. Naloxone was 0.1 mM.

lates in the presence of a partially purified exorphin preparation whereas its inactive enantiomer (+)-naloxone (Iijima *et al.*, 1978) is without effect.

The two types of activity present in crude exorphin preparations can be separated from one another by partition chromatography on silica gel, as shown by the data presented in figure 18.2. A partially purified exorphin preparation is separated by preparative thin layer chromatography into four main components. The bulk of the stimulatory activity migrates rapidly as the band labelled 3A–1, whereas band 3A–0 which remains at the origin in this (but not in all) solvent systems contains only naloxone-reversible inhibitory activity. Note that the activity present in band 3A–1 is not affected by naloxone except for a slight further stimulation whereas the inhibitory activity of band 3A–0 is completely reversed by naloxone. We believe that further purification of band 3A–1 may remove a small contamination with the exorphin activity apparently present in band 3A–2.

Exorphin preparations behave in the mouse vas deferens assay system almost exactly as they do in the adenylate cyclase assay. Thus, relatively crude preparations stimulate the contractions of the mouse vas deferens, and naloxone elicits a further stimulation (figure 18.3A). After purification by chromatography on silica, the

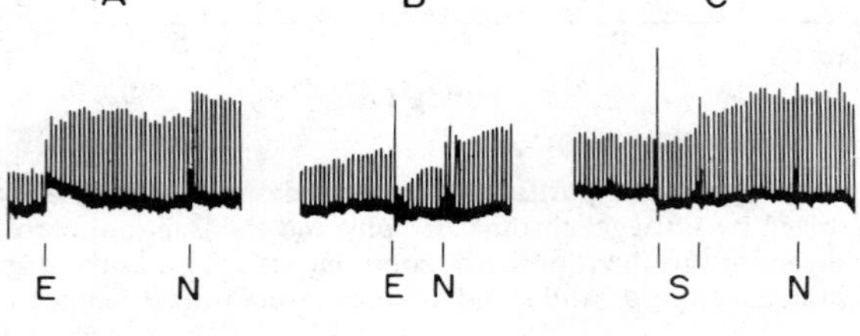

Figure 18.3 Assay of peptides from wheat gluten with the electrically stimulated mouse vas deferens. In part A, 50 μl of crude exorphin (the polystyrene column eluate, see legend to figure 18.2) was applied at E and 50 μl of 10^{-4} M naloxone at N. In part B, 50 μl of a purified exorphin (band 3A–0) was applied at E and 50 μl naloxone at N. In part C, 50 μl of band 3A–1 was applied (in 20 + 30 μl portions at the arrows marked S and 50 μl of naloxone at N. The assay was performed essentially as described by Henderson *et al.* (1972). The bath volume was 5 ml.

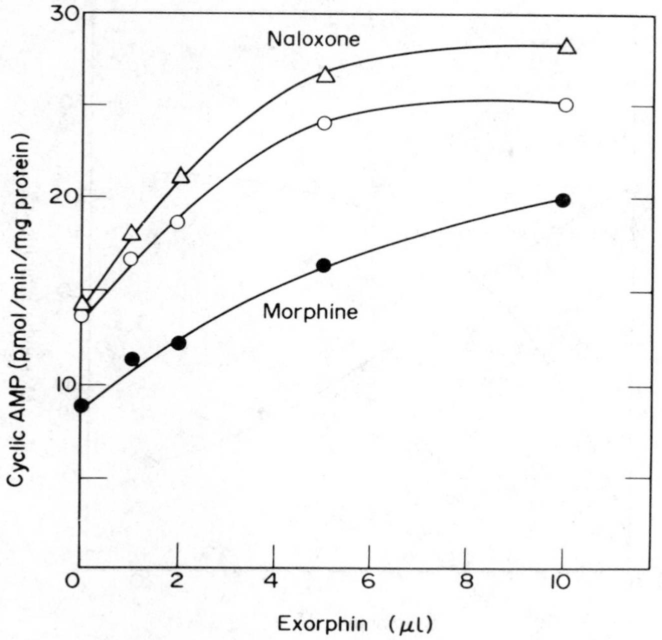

Figure 18.4 Activity of a partially purified pepsin digest of gliadin in the adenylate cyclase assay. Gliadin was treated with pepsin for 2 h as described for gluten in figure 18.1. The peptide mixture for 100 g of gliadin, after adsorption on and elution from polystyrene beads was dissolved in 5 ml water, brought to pH 7.5 with NaOH, and assayed in the presence and absence of 10^{-4} M naloxone.

partially purified exorphin (corresponding to 3A-0 of figure 2) inhibits contractions and the inhibition is reversed by naloxone (figure 18.3B) whereas the fast moving material (corresponding to 3A-1 of figure 18.2) shows stimulatory activity which is relatively insensitive to naloxone (figure 18.3C).

Exorphin can also be prepared from gliadin, the major, alcohol-soluble, protein component of wheat gluten. A partially purified exorphin prepared from a peptic digest of gliadin stimulates adenylate cyclase, as shown in figure 18.4, and the stimulation is enhanced by naloxone as seen before with gluten digests. Such partially purified exorphin preparations have properties reminiscent of those of mixed agonist opiates. As shown in figure 18.5, morphine inhibition of adenylate cyclase is decreased by the exorphin preparation at concentrations at which the exorphin itself has inhibitory effects upon opiate receptors.

DISCUSSION

We have shown that wheat gluten, as well as one of its major components, gliadin, on digestion with pepsin releases material which inhibits the neuroblastoma × glioma adenylate cyclase assay as well as the electrically stimulated contractions of the

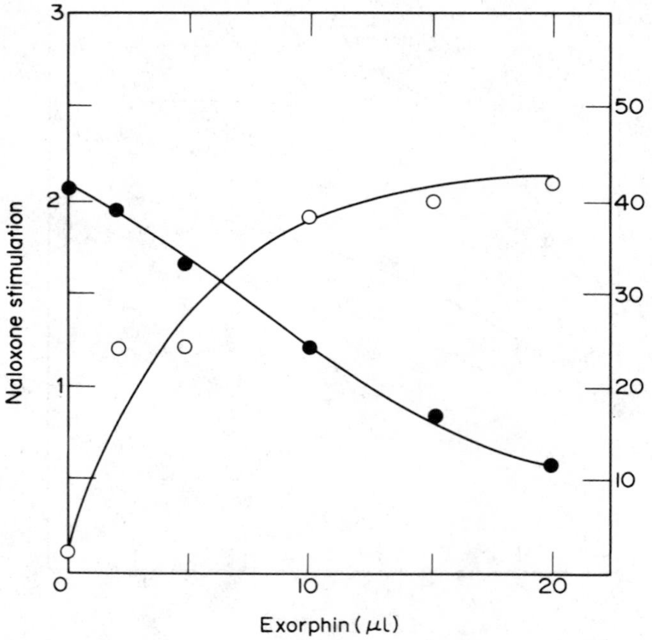

Figure 18.5 Exorphin isolated from a pepsin digest of gliadin (see figure 18.4) acts as a morphine antagonist in the adenylate cyclase assay. The ability of this partially purified exorphin to inhibit adenylate cyclase activity (as measured by naloxone stimulation (○) of the assay) appears to be accompanied by its ability to diminish the inhibitory effect of morphine (●) in the same assay. The concentrations of drugs used were: morphine, 10 μM and nalozone, 100 μM. Naloxone stimulation is expressed as pmol/min/mg protein of cyclic AMP produced over the control value.

mouse vas deferens. These inhibitory activities are reversed by (–)-naloxone (but not by (+)-naloxone) and are therefore morphine-like. We have chosen to call the material carrying this activity exorphin since it is derived from exogenous sources, is morphine-like and, apparently, peptide in nature.

In the partially purified state, exorphin preparations also contain a substance which has activities opposite to those of morphine. Such preparations although they have morphine-like effects, also behave as antagonists of morphine. This type of mixed agonist/antagonist behavior is similar in some respects to that of substances such as cyclazocine and nalorphine. Interestingly, such mixed agonists occasionally produce profound dysphoria, bordering upon psychosis, in patients, effects which are reversed by naloxone (Jaffe and Martin, 1975). The combination of stimulatory and inhibitory substances present in the peptide fragments of gluten may be responsible for the proposed relationship between wheat gluten and schizophrenia.

We have examined pepsin digests of a number of proteins other than gluten and gliadin. Most were found to be inert in our assay systems. These included ovalbumin, ribonuclease and pepsin itself. Exorphin activity has been observed in pepsin digests of bovine serum albumin and casein. Conceivably this activity may be due to endorphins, bound to the protein, which are released on pepsin treatment. Further studies will be needed to characterize this material. No evidence of the stimulatory activity present in crude exorphin preparations was found in pepsin digests of proteins other than gluten or gliadin. Wajda *et al.* (1976) have reported that a commercially prepared hydrolysate of casein contains material which inhibits the guinea pig ileum and that the inhibition is partially reversed by naloxone. We have found that the ileum is relatively insensitive to exorphin inhibition as well as to stimulation by wheat gluten peptides. Nevertheless, milk is often also withheld in gluten free diets used to treat celiac disease or in the study of schizophrenic patients (Dohan *et al.*, 1969). Some other cereal proteins, particularly rye gluten, might be expected to have exorphin activity if the proposed relationship between celiac disease and schizophrenia is valid.

Both exorphin and the stimulatory component of gluten peptide mixtures behave as very hydrophobic peptides. They are adsorbed on to polystyrene beads from aqueous solutions (as are the enkephalins and endorphins) and have chromatographic properties similar to those of the enkephalins on silica. Furthermore, amino acid analysis of partially purified peptides associated with exorphin or stimulatory activity shows a predominance of leucine and isoleucine, the presence of phenylalanine and tyrosine and the almost complete absence of charged amino acids. Thus, both types of peptide might be expected to traverse biological membranes. including the blood-brain barrier (Rapaport, 1976) with relative ease.

Our experiments have provided a plausible biochemical mechanism by which wheat gluten could be a factor in the pathology of schizophrenia. Pepsin digestion of gluten, in the stomach, will generate a class of hydrophobic peptides, the exorphins, which, when they reach the brain, will interact with endorphin receptors as agonists. Also present in gluten are stimulatory factors which antagonize morphine action. In view of the profound behavioral effects of β-endorphin (Bloom *et al.*, 1976; Jacquet and Marks, 1976) either the exorphins alone, or a combination of the two active principles of gluten digests could, as well, cause behavioral changes which, in the extreme, might be diagnosed as schizophrenia. We believe, therefore, that serious clinical evaluation of the thesis put forward by Dohan (1966*a*, *b*), relating wheat gluten and schizophrenia, is warranted.

REFERENCES

Agarwal, N. S., Hruby, V. J., Katz, R., Klee, W. and Nirenberg, M. (1977). *Biochem. biophys. Res. Commun.*, **76**, 129–35

Beddell, C. R., Clark, R. B., Hardy, G. W., Lowe, L. A., Ubatuba, F. B., Vane, J. R., Wilkinson, S., Chang, J-K., Cuatrecasas, P. and Miller, R. J. (1977). *Proc. R. Soc.*, **B 198**, 249–65

Bloom, F., Segal, N., Ling, H. and Guillemin, R. (1976). *Science*, **194**, 630–2

Chang, J. K., Fong, B. T. W., Pert, A. and Pert, C. B. (1976). *Life Sci.*, **18**, 1473–81

Coy, D. H., Kastin, A. J., Schally, A. V., Morin, O., Caron, N. G., Labrie, F., Walker, J. M., Fertel, R., Berutson, G. G. and Sandmer, C. A. (1976). *Biochem. biophys. Res. Commun.*, **73**, 632–8

Dohan, F. C. (1966*a*). *Acta psychiat. scand.*, **42**, 125–52

Dohan, F. C. (1966*b*). *Acta psychiat. scand.*, **42**, 1–23

Dohan, F. C. and Grasberger, J. C. (1973). *Am. J. Psychiat.*, **130**, 685–8

Fruton, J. S. (1971). In *The Enzymes* (ed. P. D. Boyer), Vol. III, Third Edition. Academic Press, New York, pp. 120–64

Henderson, G., Hughes, J. and Kosterlitz, H. W. (1972). *Br. J. Pharmac.*, **46**, 764–6

Hughes, J., Smith, T. W., Kosterlitz, H. W., Fothergill, L. A., Morgan, B. A. and Morris, H. R. (1975). *Nature,* **258**, 577–9
Iijima, I., Minamikawa, J., Jacobson, A. E., Brossi, A., Rice, K. C. and Klee, W. A. (1978). *J. med. Chem.,* (in press)
Jacquet, Y. and Marks, N. (1976). *Science,* **194**, 632–5
Jaffe, J. H. and Martin, W. R. (1975). In *The Pharmacological Basis of Therapeutics,* (eds. L. S. Goodman and A. Gilman) Fifth Edition, Macmillan, New Jersey, pp. 245–83
Klee, W. A. (1977). In *Peptides in Neurobiology,* (ed. H. Gainer). Plenum Press, New York, pp. 375–96
Klee, W. A. and Nirenberg, M. (1976). *Nature,* **263,** 609–12
Ling, N. and Guillemin, R. (1976). *Proc. natn. Acad. Sci. U.S.A.,* **73**, 2895–8
Lord, J. A. H., Waterfield, A. A., Hughes, J. and Kosterlitz, H. W. (1977). *Nature,* **267**, 495–9
Pert, C. B., Pert, A., Chang, J.-K. and Fong, B. T. W. (1976). *Science,* **194**, 330–2
Rapaport, S. I. (1976). *Blood-Brain Barrier in Physiology and Medicine.* Raven Press, New York, 316 pp
Schiller, P. W., Yam, C. F. and Lis, M. (1977). *Biochemistry,* **16**, 1831–8
Sharma, S. K., Nirenberg, M. and Klee, W. A. (1975). *Proc. natn. Acad. Sci. U.S.A.,* **72**, 590–4
Singh, M. M. and Kay, S. R. (1976). *Science,* **191**, 401–2; *ibid.,* **194**, 449–50
Terenius, L., Wahlström, A., Lindeberg, G., Karlsson, S. and Ragnarsson, Y. (1976*a*). *Biochem. biophys. Res. Commun.,* **71**, 175–87
Terenius, L., Wahlström, A., Lindström, L. and Widerlöv, E. (1976*b*). *Neurosci. Lett.,* **3**, 157–62
Wajda, I. J., Neidle, A., Ehrenpreis, S. and Manigault, I. (1976). In *Endogenous Opioid Peptides,* (ed. H. W. Kosterlitz), North Holland, Amsterdam, pp. 129–36

19
Release and inactivation of opioids in the guinea pig ileum

José M. Musacchio, Margarita M. Puig and Gale L. Craviso (Department of Pharmacology New York University School of Medicine
550 First Avenue New York, New York 10016, U.S.A.)

The electrically stimulated myenteric plexus-longitudinal muscle (MPLM) preparation is generally recognized as a reliable and sensitive bioassay for opiates and opiate-like peptides. We have recently demonstrated the release of endorphins from this preparation (Puig *et al.*, 1977*a*) by using the same MPLM strip as both the source of endorphins and the bioassay to detect their opiate-like effects. We have also established the existence of cross-tolerance between the electrically induced release of endorphins and morphine (Puig *et al.*, 1977*b*). Subsequently, we have studied the general characteristics of the endorphin release by investigating different parameters of electrical stimulation as well as the effects of other procedures.

Even though the MPLM preparation is known to contain enkephalins (Smith *et al.*, 1976), we had been unable to detect them in the perfusate fluid after electrical stimulation at 10 Hz. This prompted us to study the degradation of enkephalins in different preparations of the guinea pig ileum (GPI). Our paper will consist of two parts—the electrically induced release of endorphins and the inactivation of enkephalins.

ELECTRICALLY INDUCED RELEASE OF ENDORPHINS

We were puzzled by the lack of effect of naloxone on the contractions of the MPLM induced by electrical stimulation at 0.1 Hz, especially since the output of acetylcholine by the same preparation, stimulated at 0.017 Hz in the presence of physostigmine, is increased 35 per cent by the addition of 10^{-7} M naloxone (Waterfield and Kosterlitz, 1975). We thought that perhaps the effects of naloxone could not be demonstrated directly on the contractility of the ileum because the frequencies of stimulation used to demonstrate the effects of opiates might not be appropriate to release endorphins. Therefore, we combined periods of stimulation at different frequencies and durations with the basal stimulation at 0.1 Hz and we found that stimulating at 10 Hz for several minutes produced an inhibitory res-

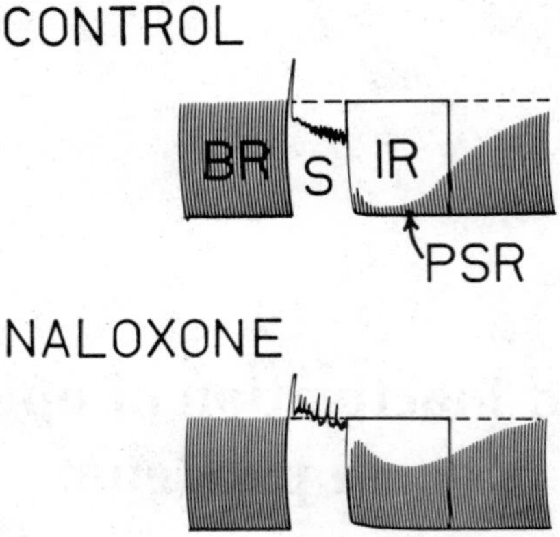

Figure 19.1 Inhibition of the twitch response of the MPLM strip preparation by stimulation at 10 Hz for a period of 3 min. The basal response (BR) and the post-stimulatory response (PSR) correspond to the area of contractions produced by stimulation at 0.1 Hz for 5 min before and after the period of stimulation (S). The inhibitory response (IR) is obtained by subtracting the PSR from the BR. The control MPLM strip was placed in Krebs-bicarbonate solution, and another strip from the same animal in Krebs with 5×10^{-7} M naloxone. The figure represents the first period of stimulation of a typical experiment, and the inhibitory responses shown are of the same magnitude as the average of several identical experiments. For additional details see Puig *et al.* (1977*a* and 1978).

ponse (IR) which was in great part reversed by naloxone (Puig *et al.*, 1977*a*). Figure 19.1 illustrates this phenomenon.

The specificity of the IR was further investigated by studying the reversal produced by other opiate antagonists such as naltrexone and two benzomorphan derivatives, GPA 1843 (*N*-allyl-β-9-methyl-5-phenyl-2′ hydroxy-6, 7-benzomorphan) and GPA 1847, the inactive (+)-isomer of GPA 1843. The EC_{50} for each antagonist was calculated from dose–response curves (Puig *et al.*, 1977*a*). Table 19.1 lists these values and shows the relative potencies of these antagonists in reversing the electrically induced inhibitory response compared with their potencies in reversing the effects of normorphine in the same tissue. From these experiments we concluded that: (1) opiate antagonists of different chemical structure such as naloxone and naltrexone (oximorphone derivatives) and GPA 1843 (a

Table 19.1 Relative potencies of narcotic antagonists to reverse the normorphine and the electrically evoked inhibition of the myenteric plexus–longitudinal muscle preparation

	Electrically evoked*		Normorphine produced†	
	EC_{50} (nM)	Nx/*x*	K_e (nM)	Nx/*x*
Naloxone (Nx)	25	1	1.20	1
Naltrexone	10	2.5	0.38	3.16
GPA 1843	150	0.16	19.8	0.06
GPA 1847	10 000	0.0025	1190.0	0.001

*Data from Puig *et al.* (1977*a*).
†Data from Kosterlitz *et al.* (1973).

benzomorphan) can reverse the electrically induced IR. (2) The reversal of the IR is stereospecific as demonstrated by the negligible activity of GPA 1847, the (+)-isomer when compared with GPA 1843, the (–)-isomer. (3) The order of potency of the different antagonists is identical to that needed to reverse the inhibitory effects of normorphine in the same preparation. (4) The IR is reversed by the different antagonists with an EC_{50} which is well within the concentration at which these drugs exert their specific antagonistic effects. However, it can be observed that the concentrations of the antagonists necessary to inhibit the electrically induced IR are consistently a few-fold higher than those necessary to antagonize normorphine. The reason for this difference is not apparent at present.

All the characteristics of the IR demonstrate that electrical stimulation of the MPLM preparation at 10 Hz produces a specific activation of opiate receptors. The inescapable conclusion from these experiments is that electrical stimulation releases an endogenous ligand for the opiate receptor. Endorphin release has also been demonstrated by other *in vitro* studies. Smith *et al.* (1976) have reported a small potassium-induced calcium-dependent release of enkephalins from rat brain synaptosomes and GPI, and Schulz *et al.* (1977*b*) have detected enkephalins after low frequency stimulation of the MPLM. There is also indirect evidence for the release of opiate-like substances in the CNS. Electrical stimuation of the periaqueductal grey matter of several animals has been shown to produce an analgesia that has some of the characteristics of opiate analgesia such as partial reversal by naloxone and development of tolerance (Akil *et al.*, 1972; 1976; Mayer and Hayes, 1975; Adams, 1976; Hosobuchi *et al.*, 1977). However, stimulation-produced analgesia is a very complex phenomenon and conflicting reports indicate that the naloxone reversal can only be obtained under certain conditions and to a certain degree (Pert and Walter, 1976). Moreover, Yaksh *et al.* (1976) have been unable to antagonize with naloxone the elevated nociceptive thresholds resulting from electrical stimulation of the mesencephalic central grey matter. Aside from these controversies, additional evidence strongly suggesting a release of endorphins has been provided by reports in which naloxone has been shown to exert effects of its own *in vivo*. Jacob *et al.* (1974) and Frederickson *et al.* (1976) have pretreated mice with naloxone and found that their pain threshold was lowered in the hotplate test.

General characteristics of the inhibitory response

Effects of naloxone

In the previous section we have indicated that naloxone produces a considerable blockade of the IR elicited by stimulation at 10 Hz. However, quantitation of this blockade is difficult because the magnitude of the IR is also a function of the number of times that the preparation is stimulated. To circumvent this problem, two MPLM strips obtained from the same animal were mounted in identical chambers under the same conditions. The control strip was in contact with normal Krebs and the other with 5×10^{-7} M naloxone in the Krebs solution. The results of these experiments, as illustrated in figure 19.2, clearly show that the magnitude of the IR under control conditions and in the presence of naloxone decreases as a

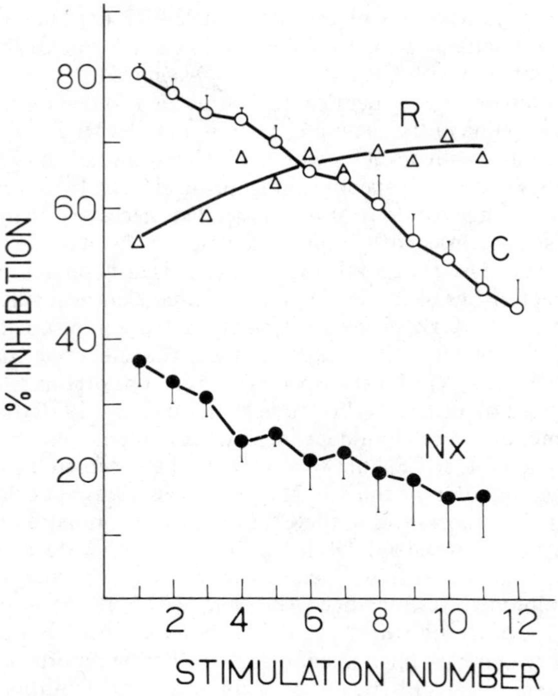

Figure 19.2 Effect of naloxone on the inhibitory response produced by electrical stimulation of the MPLM strip preparation at 10 Hz. Control (C) and naloxone (Nx) curves were obtained by stimulation of two strips from the same guinea pig. Naloxone was added to the Krebs-bicarbonate solution at a concentration of 5×10^{-7} M, and kept in contact with one strip throughout the experiment. Each strip was continuously stimulated at a frequency of 0.1 Hz and every 30 min was stimulated at 10 Hz for 3 min. Total number of stimulatory periods was 12. In the figure, each point represents the mean values of four experiments and the vertical bars indicate the s.e. All the points from the control curve were significantly different from the corresponding points of the naloxone curve with a $P < 0.001$. R, per cent reversal of the inhibitory response produced by naloxone and represents the percentage of the IR which is due to the release of endorphins (Puig *et al.*, 1977*a*). Ordinate: per cent inhibition of the basal response (also referred to as the IR). Abscissa: cycle of stimulation in which the response was obtained.

function of the number of times the preparation is stimulated. The IR under control conditions decreased from 81 to 51 per cent after 10 stimulations and in the presence of naloxone from 37 per cent to 16 per cent. Therefore, the reversal induced by naloxone has to be calculated in reference to the proper control. Additional experiments have indicated moreover, that the decrease in the IR is not only a function of the number of stimulatory periods but also of the amount of time elapsed since the preparation was mounted (Puig *et al.*, 1978). Figure 19.2 also illustrates the naloxone reversal calculated as the percentage of the IR that is reversed by the opiate antagonist. Thus, the naloxone reversal measures the percentage of the IR that is mediated by endorphins.

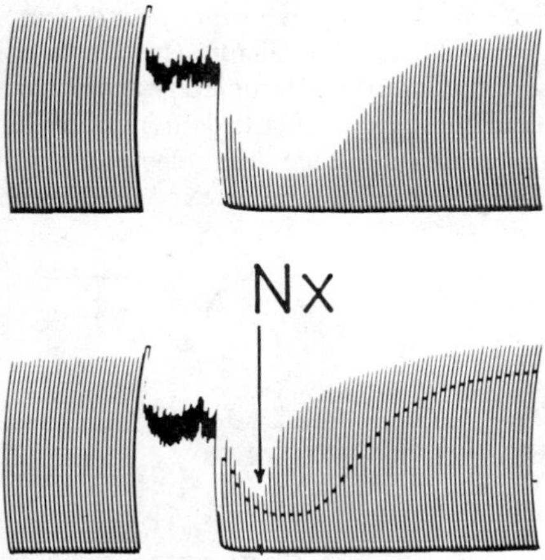

Figure 19.3 Effect of naloxone added after the stimulatory period. The upper graph illustrates the control inhibitory response obtained after stimulation at 10 Hz for a period of 3 min; this response is also represented in the lower graph by a dotted line. The lower graph demonstrates the reversal of the inhibitory response obtained when naloxone (5×10^{-7} M) was added to the organ bath 90 s after the stimulatory period.

Although the effects of naloxone in reversing the IR are more accurately quantitated in the way described, they can also be demonstrated by adding the naloxone after the IR is apparent (figure 19.3). This is an important point because it demonstrates that the opiate antagonist has access to the sites where endorphins are released by electrical stimulation.

Effects of different parameters of stimulation

The magnitude and duration of the IR are also functions of the frequency of the electrical pulses applied and of the total duration of the stimulation. The maximal IR is obtained when the MPLM is stimulated at 20 Hz. Stimulation at 25 and 30 Hz does not produce a significant increase in the IR, at least under the experimental conditions that we have used (Puig *et al.*, 1977*a* and 1978). It is noteworthy that the frequencies of stimulation used in our experiments are comparable to the firing rates of other autonomic nerves (Koizumi and Brooks, 1972; Kunze, 1972).

Increasing the duration of the stimulatory period also enhances the duration and magnitude of the IR. Near maximal inhibition is obtained by a stimulatory period of 5 min at 10 Hz. Longer stimulatory periods do not significantly prolong the IR. It seems that at this time a steady-state situation is achieved in which the rate of combination of the released endorphin with the opiate receptor is balanced by the rate of diffusion or destruction of the endogenous ligand. Since stimualtion for 5 min produces a complete inhibition of the basal contractions elicited at 0.1 Hz, reliable quantitation of the phenomenon can be achieved only by using shorter periods of stimulation. With the parameters used in our system, 3 min of stimulation at 10 Hz results in approximately 80 per cent inhibition of the basal contractions at 0.1 Hz during the five min immediately following the stimulatory period. (For details see figure 19.1).

Effects of calcium-free Krebs, washing and other procedures

Replacement of the normal Krebs with calcium-free Krebs containing 1 mM EGTA during the stimulatory period at 10 Hz completely abolishes the IR, as shown in figure 19.4. The results of these experiments demonstrate that the IR is calcium-dependent; this is consistent with the idea that electrical stimulation of the MPLM strip produces the release of endorphin by an exocytotic process.

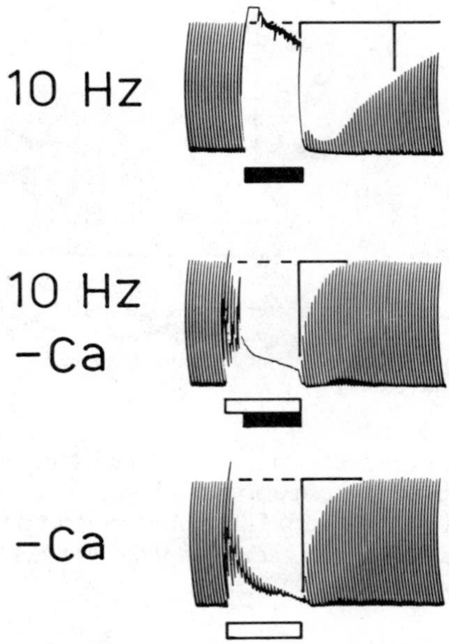

Figure 19.4 Effect of calcium-free Krebs on the inhibitory response. The graph at the top shows the control IR produced by stimulation at 10 Hz for a period of 3 min in Krebs-bicarbonate solution. In the center graph, the preparation was stimulated in a similar way, but in the presence of calcium-free Krebs which contained 1 mM EGTA (10 Hz, minus Ca). The bottom graph demonstrates the effect of calcium-free Krebs on the basal contractions (elicited by stimulation at 0.1 Hz) for a period of 4 min (minus Ca). Open bars indicate the time (4 min) during which the preparation was in contact with calcium-free 1 mM EGTA Krebs. Solid bars indicate the time (3 min) during which the preparation was stimulated at a frequency of 10 Hz. The experiment was replicated three times.

One of the most striking characteristics of the IR is its resistance to washing; washing at very high rates does not produce any effect whether started before, during or after the stimulatory period at 10 Hz. In contrast, the inhibition produced by met or leu-enkephalin is easily washable with the half-life of the met-enkephalin opiate receptor complex being only 10 s (Puig *et al.*, 1978). Similar results have been obtained previously by Schulz and Herz (1976). We have also found that the half-life of the β-endorphin opiate receptor complex determined by the same method is 85 s (Puig *et al.*, 1978). There are three possible explanations for the relatively long lasting duration of the electrically elicited opiate-like inhibition. One is that there is a diffusion barrier for the endorphins released by nerve stimulation. This possibility can be disregarded because the opiate receptors which bind the exogenous ligand are immediately accessible to naloxone added to the organ bath (see figure 19.3). In addition, it has been demonstrated that lanthanum ion and ruthenium red rapidly penetrate all the regions of the myenteric plexus including synaptic gaps (Bursztajn and Gershon, 1977). The second possibility is that the stimulatory period at 10 Hz has triggered a sustained period of neuronal activity that releases endorphins throughout the IR. To examine this possibility, we performed a series of experiments that should have disrupted this hypothetical process of long-lasting neuronal activation. These experiments consisted of perfusing either ice cold Krebs or calcium-free manganese-containing modified Krebs for 1 min immediately after the stimulatory period. Even though in control experiments these two buffers immediately stopped all evidence of neuronal activity in the preparation, they failed to alter the duration of the IR which was measured after replacement with normal Krebs (Puig *et al.*, 1978). The third possible explanation for the long lasting duration of the IR and its resistance to wash off is that the released endorphin dissociates very slowly from the myenteric plexus opiate receptor. This is a distinct possibility because our experiments demonstrate that the release of endorphins takes place during the stimulatory period and not afterwards. As already mentioned, enkephalins and β-endorphin have relatively fast offset rates from the receptor. Therefore, the endorphin released by field stimulation from the GPI myenteric plexus during our experiments may not be identical to the enkephalins described by Hughes *et al.* (1975) or to human β-endorphin. It is possible that the endorphin that mediates the electrically induced IR is similar to the long acting endogenous opioid recently found in the blood and in the fluid bathing MPLM strips of the guinea pig (Schulz *et al.*, 1977*a*).

Other components of the IR

Other inhibitory mechanisms mediated by adrenergic and purinergic neurotransmitters probably also play a part in the IR. Initial experiments designed to study the adrenergic component of the IR were performed with MPLM strips obtained from guinea pigs that were treated with i.p. injections of reserpine (2.5 mg/kg) 48 and 24 hours before the experiment. Because the changes obtained in the IR were inconsistent we decided to study the effects of 6-hydroxydopamine (6-OHDA), which destroys catecholamine-containing neurons (Thoenen and Tranzer, 1968; Furness *et al.*, 1970) without affecting serotonin-containing neurons. The decrease in the IR produced by 6-OHDA, even though consistent, was of very small magnitude (Puig *et al.*, 1978). This of course cannot be interpreted as an indication of the relative importance of catecholamines and endorphins in the regulation of intestinal motility. Attempts to identify a purinergic component in the IR were not made because there are not specific purinergic blocking agents available (Burnstock, 1975).

Cross tolerance to morphine

The IR of MPLM strips obtained from morphine-tolerant guinea pigs is markedly decreased when compared with that obtained from placebo-implated animals (figure 19.5). The IR was 80.5 ± 2.4 per cent (n = 9) in strips obtained from placebo-implanted animals and 54.9 ± 4.4 per cent (n = 11) in strips from mor-

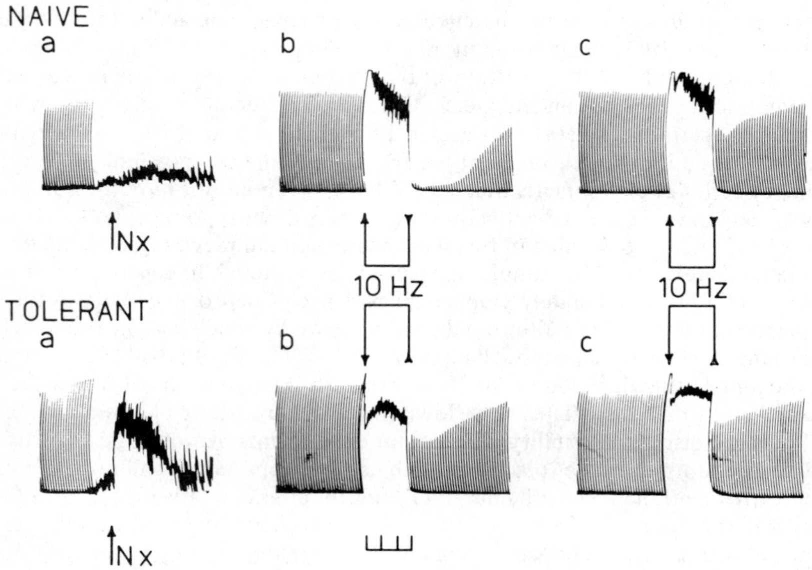

Figure 19.5 Response of the MPLM strip preparation from naive (top) and from tolerant (bottom) guinea pigs. Male guinea pigs were made tolerant to morphine by subcutaneous implantation of 75 mg morphine-base pellets. Control (naive) animals were implanted with placebo pellets. For details see Puig *et al.* (1977*b*) and Puig *et al.* (1978). Panel (a) represents a challenge with 10^{-7} M naloxone (Nx) added 1 min after the stimulation at 0.1 Hz was interrupted. Panel (b) shows the effect of changing the frequency of stimulation from 0.1 to 10 Hz for 3 min. Panel (c) shows the same effect as panel (b) in the presence of 5×10^{-7} M naloxone. The horizontal calibration is 1 min per division.

phine-implanted animals. These differences were statistically significant ($P < 0.001$) and they were seen throughout 10 successive stimulatory periods. In contrast, in the presence of naloxone, the IR was 42.6 ± 3.5 per cent and 31.4 ± 2.1 per cent, respectively. These differences were not statistically significant from each other but they were different from the IR obtained in the absence of naloxone (Puig *et al.*, 1978).

Our experiments demonstrate that there is cross-tolerance between morphine and the endorphin that mediates the IR. Waterfield *et al.* (1976) have found that the vas deferens of mice and the MPLM of guinea pigs which are made tolerant to morphine are cross-tolerant to met-enkephalin. This cross-tolerance has also been demonstrated at the neuronal level (Zieglgansberger *et al.*, 1976). Conversely animals which have been made tolerant to opiate-like peptides (Loh *et al.*, 1976; Wei and Loh, 1976) are cross-tolerant to morphine. Furthermore, enkephalins have been shown to produce in glioma × neuroblastoma cell cultures an increase in adenylate cyclase that is thought to be associated with opiate tolerance and dependence (Lampert *et al.*, 1976; Brand *et al.*, 1976).

INACTIVATION OF ENKEPHALINS

Since the myenteric plexus is known to contain enkephalin (Elde *et al.*, 1976; Smith *et al.*, 1976), we thought that the endorphins which were being released in our experiments could be the enkephalin pentapeptides. However, even though Schulz *et al.* (1977*b*) have reported the release of enkephalin from the MPLM, our attempts to identify enkephalin in the tissue bath after stimulation at 10 Hz had been unsuccessful. We felt, therefore, that if enkephalin was being released, it might have been almost completely destroyed by tissue peptidases before we could detect it (Craviso and Musacchio, 1977).

We, as well as other investigators, have previously demonstrated that GPI tissue preparations contain enzymes which degrade the enkephalin pentapeptides (Hughes, 1975; Terenius and Wahlström, 1975, Puig *et al.*, 1977*c*). We undertook the present study in order to characterize the nature of the enzymes responsible for enkephalin degradation in the ileum (Craviso and Musacchio, unpublished work).

Mode of inactivation of enkephalin

Labeled met or leu-enkephalin was incubated with MPLM strips or with intact ileum segments in Krebs bicarbonate buffer maintained at 37 °C and gassed with 95 per cent O_2–5 per cent CO_2. At the end of the incubation the tissue was removed; HCl was added which contained cold enkephalin and tyrosine as carriers. Aliquots from each incubation were spotted on silica gel plates and analyzed by thin-layer chromatography (t.l.c.). The radioactivity in the areas corresponding

Table 19.2 Degradation of [^{3}H] met-enkephalin and [^{3}H] leu-enkephalin by MPLM strip leaching enzymes

	Solvent 1			Solvent 2		
	0	20	60 min	0	20	60 min
Met-enkephalin spot	897	200	43	903	186	98
Tyrosine spot	56	990	1088	105	864	943
Totals	953	1190	1131	1008	1050	1041
Leu-enkephalin spot	2753	846	438	2434	581	139
Tyrosine spot	165	2101	2908	125	2091	2435
Totals	2918	2947	3346	2559	2672	2574

Peptidase activity was assayed in the Krebs medium surrounding MPLM strips by removing the tissue and incubating aliquots of the Krebs with 2×10^{-8} M ([^{3}H] tyrosyl-3, 5)-met-enkephalin or ([^{3}H] tyrosyl-3, 5)-leu-enkephalin at 37°C for 20 or 60 min; 0 min samples were incubated at 0 °C. At the end of the incubation, HCl was added which contained cold enkephalin and tyrosine as carriers. Aliquots from each incubation were spotted on silica gel plates. The plates were developed in *n*-butanol: acetic acid: ethyl acetate: water; 1:1:2:1 (solvent 1) or chloroform: methanol: ammonium hydroxide; 60:30:5 (solvent 2) and sprayed with ninhydrin. The radioactivity in the areas corresponding to enkephalin and tyrosine was determined by liquid scintillation spectrometry. The results are expressed as c.p.m. and represent the values obtained from one experiment. The experiment was repeated several times and similar results were obtained.

to enkephalin and tyrosine was determined. For both tissue preparations almost all of the radioactivity lost from the enkephalin spot could be accounted for as free tyrosine, indicating that the pentapeptides were cleaved at the tyrosyl–glycine bond. Degradation at the carboxyl end was not apparent.

By removing the tissue, incubating aliquots of the Krebs medium with labeled enkephalin and analyzing the products by t.l.c., we found that considerable peptidase activity leached out of both tissue preparations into the surrounding Krebs medium. The results depicted in table 19.2 for the MPLM strip leaching enzymes demonstrate that the major degradation product is free tyrosine. Similar results were obtained for the enzymes leaching out of intact ileum segments.

We investigated many compounds which might act as inhibitors of enkephalin degradation by the leaching enzymes from MPLM strips or intact ileum segments. Several of these are listed in table 19.3. As can be seen, only *o*-phenanthroline, 8-OH-quinoline and hexachlorophene completely inhibited both leaching peptidase activities. It is also apparent that there are differences in the degree of inhibition produced by the various compounds; that is, bacitracin, puromycin and EDTA inhibit very well the myenteric plexus strip leaching enzymes but have relatively little effect on the intact ileum leaching enzymes. On the basis of these results, we concluded that the enzymes were different.

Table 19.3 Inhibition (per cent) of [^{3}H] met-enkephalin destruction by ileum leaching enzymes

	MPLM strip leaching enzymes	Intact ileum leaching enzymes
Met-enkephalin 10^{-4}M	80	47
Bacitracin 100 μg ml^{-1}	85	34
Puromycin 5×10^{-5} M	93	21
Lima bean trypsin inhibitor 100 μg ml^{-1}	41	–
EDTA 10^{-3} M	85	29
o-Phenanthroline 10^{-3} M	100	98
8-OH-quinoline 10^{-3} M	100	100
Hexachlorophene 10^{-3} M	100	100

Aliquots of the Krebs medium surrounding MPLM strips and intact ileum segments were incubated in 25 mM HEPES buffer, pH 7 with 2×10^{-8} M [^{3}H] met-enkephalin for 30 min at 37 °C in the presence and absence of the various inhibitors. Enzyme activity was adjusted so that control samples degraded 30–40 per cent of the labeled enkephalin in this time period. The incubations were terminated by the addition of HCl which contained cold enkephalin and tyrosine as carriers. The amount of enkephalin degradation was quantitated by t.l.c. as described in table 2 using solvent 1. All values represent the average of duplicate determinations. The experiment was repeated several times and similar results were obtained.

Nature of the leaching enzymes

Since in all probability the leaching enzymes from both tissue preparations were either from broken cells and/or serum in vascular and extravascular spaces, we studied enkephalin degradation in guinea pig serum and in a 100 000*g* supernatant fraction from MPLM strips and compared them to the leaching enzymes; a 100 000 *g* supernatant fraction from guinea pig brain was also included in the comparison. We found that the enzymes from the serum and supernatant fractions were also able to degrade enkephalin at the N-terminal tyrosine. Based on their sensitivities to the various compounds which acted as inhibitors of enkephalin degradation, the 100 000 *g* supernatant fraction enzymes appeared to be different from the serum enzymes. As table 19.4 demonstrates, bacitracin, puromycin and EDTA are good inhibitors of the supernatant fraction enzymes but poor inhibitors of the serum enzymes; hexachlorophene, *o*-phenanthroline and 8-OH-quinoline completely inhibited all of the enzymes. In comparing these results to those obtained for the leaching enzymes it was apparent that the MPLM leaching enzymes were similar to the 100 000 *g* supernatant fraction enzymes whereas the intact ileum leaching enzymes were similar to those found in the serum.

The leaching enzymes of the MPLM strip and intact ileum and enzymes from the 100 000 *g* MPLM strip supernatant and the serum were subjected to Sephadex G-200 gel filtration to see if we could further demonstrate differences or similarities among the enzymes from these four sources. Figure 19.6 shows the Sephadex

Table 19.4 Inhibition (per cent) of [^{3}H] met-enkephalin destruction by serum and 100 000 *g* supernatant fraction enzymes

	100 000 *g* Supernatant brain	100 000 *g* Supernatant strip	Serum
Met-enkephalin			
10^{-4} M	85	81	36
Bacitracin			
100 μg ml^{-1}	86	88	12
Puromycin			
5×10^{-5} M	99	99	8
Lima bean trypsin inhibitor			
100 μg ml^{-1}	8	22	–
EDTA			
10^{-3} M	90	84	11
o-Phenanthroline			
10^{-3} M	100	100	100
8-OH-quinoline			
10^{-3} M	100	100	97
Hexachlorophene			
10^{-3}M	100	100	100

The experiment was carried out as described in table 19.3. The amount of enzyme activity from each source was adjusted so that control samples degraded 30–40 per cent of the labeled enkephalin in 30 min at 37 °C. All values represent the average of duplicate determinations. The experiment was repeated several times and similar results were obtained.

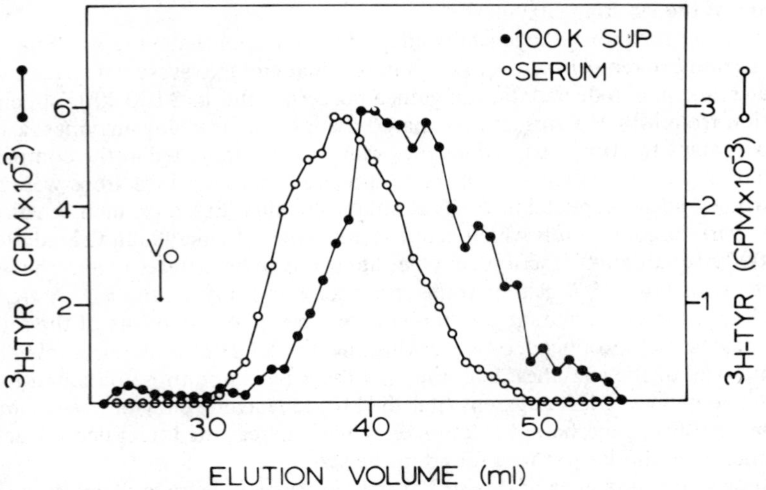

Figure 19.6 Sephadex G-200 elution patterns of the 100 000 *g* MPLM strip supernatant fraction enzymes (100 K Sup) and the serum enzymes. Each enzyme preparation in a volume of 0.4 ml was applied to a Sephadex G-200 column (0.9 × 31 cm) equilibrated with 50 mM Tris-HCl, pH 6.8, 100 mM sodium chloride. Fractions of 0.8 ml were collected by reverse flow and enkephalin degrading activity in each fraction was determined as described in table 19.3.

G-200 profile of the serum and MPLM strip supernatant enzymes. On the basis of their respective elution profiles, the enzymes appear to be different. To explore further this difference and to see if the two enzyme preparations were homogeneous, different peak fractions from each were assayed in the presence of EDTA, puromycin and bacitracin. We found that early and late peak fractions of the 100 000 *g* supernatant enzymes exhibited the same sensitivity to the inhibitors as the enzyme preparation before gel filtration. This same result was obtained for different peak fractions of the serum enzymes; that is, the serum enzymes off G-200 exhibited the same sensitivity to bacitracin, EDTA and puromycin as the serum preparation before gel filtration. Therefore, we concluded that the supernatant and the serum enzymes are different and that each enzyme preparation appears to be homogeneous at least with regard to its enkephalin degrading activity and sensitivity to inhibitors.

Figure 19.7 compares the 100 000 *g* strip supernatant Sephadex G-200 profile to that of the MPLM strip leaching enzymes. The peaks coincide indicating that the enzymes may have similar molecular weights. When assaying the early and late portions of the peak activity of the strip leaching enzymes in the presence of bacitracin, EDTA and puromycin, it was found that they differed in their sensitivities to the various inhibitors. This is demonstrated in table 19.5. The early enzyme activity, based on the amount of inhibition to the various compounds, is similar to that displayed by serum peptidases; the late eluting enzyme activity is similar to the strip 100 000 *g* supernatant activity. Therefore, as these results demonstrate, there are at least two different enzymes responsible for enkephalin degradation in

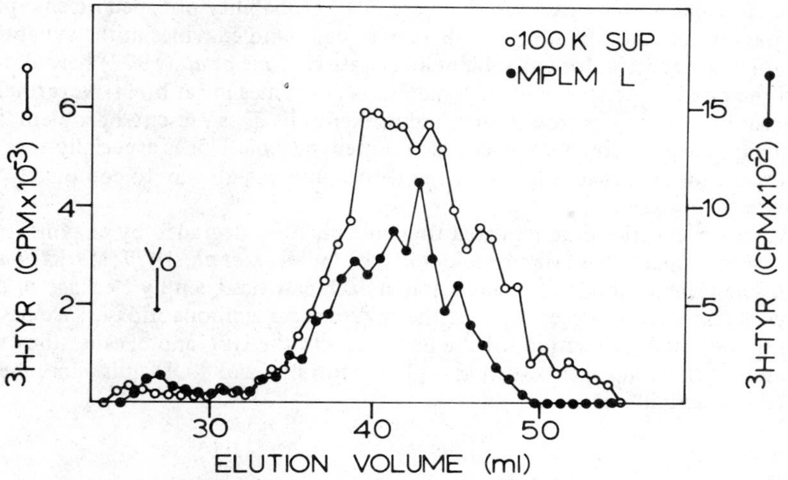

Figure 19.7 Sephadex G-200 elution patterns of the 100 000 *g* MPLM strip supernatant fraction enzymes (100 K Sup) and the MPLM leaching enzymes (MPLM L). Gel filtration and assay of enzyme activity was carried out as described in figure 19.6.

the organ bath surrounding the MPLM strip preparation—one from broken cells, the other from serum.

The Sephadex G-200 profile of the intact ileum leaching enzymes was compared with that of the serum enzymes. The peaks coincided and when testing different fractions of peak activity of the leaching enzymes in the presence of bacitracin, EDTA and puromycin, we found no differences in sensitivity to these inhibitors. The sensitivity of the various inhibitors throughout the peak was similar to that shown for the serum enzymes suggesting that the enzymes which leach out of this preparation into the organ bath are homogeneous and similar to serum enkephalin degrading enzymes.

Table 19.5 Inhibition (per cent) of MPLM strip leaching enzymes in different Sephadex G-200 fractions

	Early fraction (No. 48 = 38 ml)	Late fraction (No. 57 = 45 ml)
Met-enkephalin 10^{-4} M	52	100
Bacitracin 100 μg ml^{-1}	39	97
Puromycin 5×10^{-5} M	50	100
EDTA 10^{-3} M	55	100

Enkephalin degrading activity in early and late fractions from the experiment illustrated in figure 19.7 was measured in the presence and absence of the various inhibitors as described in table 19.3. Each value represents the average of duplicate samples.

The enzymes we have just described are in all probability not specific enkephalin degrading enzymes. In addition, there may be bound enzymes in the synaptic cleft which are specific for enkephalin inactivation. Lane *et al.* (1977) have described the possible existence of such membrane enzymes in rat brain. Nevertheless, the presence of enzymes from serum and broken cells does present a problem if enkephalin release is to be studied in ileum preparations. This is especially true since even after extensive washing of the tissues, there is no way to completely eliminate their presence.

Several laboratories have reported that enkephalin is degraded by enzymes in many tissue preparations (Hambrook *et al.*, 1976; Meek *et al.*, 1977; Marks *et al.*, 1977). The primary mode of inactivation in each case has been by cleavage of the tyrosyl-glycine bond, suggesting that the enzymes are aminopeptidases. We have found similar modes of action for the peptidases in the GPI, and because they are inhibited by chelating agents such as *o*-phenanthroline and 8-OH-quinoline, they may also be metalloenzymes.

Enkephalin analogues as peptidase inhibitors

Because of the presence of peptidases, enkephalin release in GPI preparations could best be studied if enzyme inhibitors were available. Although we have found several compounds, namely *o*-phenanthroline, hexachlorophene and 8-OH-quinoline, which completely inhibit the destruction of enkephalin by enzymes from serum and broken cells, these could not be used in the endorphin release experiments because when present in the organ bath, these compounds caused the MPLM strip to lose its contractility. Therefore, other less toxic inhibitors were sought.

We tested several enkephalin analogues as potentially specific inhibitors of enkephalin degradation. Table 19.6 lists some of the analogue tested and shows their

Table 19.6 Effect of several enkephalin analogues on the inhibition of serum enkephalin degrading enzymes

Peptide	Per cent inhibition
Tyr–Gly–Ser–Phe–Leu	55
Tyr–Ala–Gly–Phe–Leu	72
Tyr–Pro–Gly–Phe–Leu	48
Tyr–Gly–Gly–D-Phe–Leu	59
Tyr–Gly–D-Ala–Phe–Leu	69
Tyr–D-Ala–D-Ala–Phe–Leu	7
Tyr–D-Ala–D-Pro–Phe–Leu	32
Tyr–D-Ala–Gly–D-Phe–Leu	0
Try–D-Ala–Gly–Leu–Leu	0
Try–Ala–Ala–Phe–Leu	73
Tyr–Gly–Gly–Phe–Met*	47
Tyr–Gly–Gly–Phe–Leu*	63

The experiment was carried out as described in table 19.3. The amount of serum enzyme activity was adjusted so that control samples degraded 30–40 per cent of the labeled enkephalin in 30 min at 37 °C. All values represent the average of duplicate determinations. The concentration of each peptide in the incubation mixure was 10^{-4} M. *Natural enkephalin pentapeptides.

effects on serum enkephalin degrading enzymes. As is clearly seen, none of the analogues was an effective inhibitor. Since it has been demonstrated that many of these analogues can be degraded by enzymes during the opiate receptor binding assay (Beddell *et al.*, 1977), most probably they are acting as competitive enzyme substrates in our assay. Those analogues that are resistant to degradation, namely any analogues with D-alanine as the second residue (Pert *et al.*, 1976; Miller *et al.*, 1977), do not inhibit enzyme activity.

CONCLUSIONS

The electrical stimulation of the GPI MPLM strip elicits a complex IR. This response can be modified within certain limits by altering the frequency and duration of the stimuli.

The IR is calcium dependent; it cannot be attenuated by washing and is mediated by several components. The main component is opiate-like in nature and contributes to 55–70 per cent of the IR. There are at least two additional components, one of them adrenergic and a third one that has not been identified.

The opiate-like component is thought to be mediated by an endorphin which has slower offset rates than enkephalin or human β-endorphin.

There is cross-tolerance between morphine and the opiate-like component of the IR.

The guinea pig ileum contains peptidase activity that rapidly destroys enkephalin. Considerable peptidase activity leaches out of the preparation into the surrounding Krebs medium.

The leaching peptidase activity comes from the MPLM broken cells and from the serum. All the enzymes can be inhibited by *o*-phenanthroline, 8-OH-quinoline and hexachlorophene. The peptidases from broken cells are much more sensitive to EDTA, puromycin and bacitracin than the serum peptidases.

ACKNOWLEDGEMENTS

This work was supported in part by USPHS grants MH 29591. DA-00351, and by Hoffmann-LaRoche Inc. José M. Musacchio is a recipient of a PHS Research Scientist Award MH 17785. Margarita M. Puig received an award from the Fundación Universitaria Agustín Pedro y Pons, Barcelona, Spain. We thank Endo Laboratories for providing us with naloxone hydrochloride and naltrexone hydrochloride and Dr W. D. Cash and Dr F. H. Clarke of Ciba-Geigy Corp. for the GPA 1843 and GPA 1847 compounds. We also thank Dr Richard J. Miller and Dr Pedro Cuatrecasas from Wellcome Research Laboratories for several of the peptides used in this study.

REFERENCES

Adams, J. E. (1976). *Pain,* **2**, 161–6

Akil, H., Mayer, D. J. and Liebeskind, J. C. (1972). *C. r. hebd. Séanc. Acad. Sci. Paris,* **274**, 3603–5

Akil, H., Mayer, D. J. and Liebeskind, J. C. (1976). *Science,* **191**, 961–2

Beddell, C. R., Clark, R. B., Hardy, G. W., Lowe, L. A., Ubatuba, F. B., Vane, J. R., Wilkinson, S., Chang, J.-K., Cuatrecasas, P. and Miller, R. J. (1977). *Proc. R. Soc. Lond.,* **198**, 249–65

Brand, M., Fisher, K., Moroder, L., Wunsch, E. and Hamprecht, B. (1976). *FEBS Lett.*, **68**, 38–40
Burnstock, G. (1975). In *Handbook of Psychopharmacology,* (eds L. L. Iversen, S. D. Iversen and S. H. Snyder), 5, Plenum Press, New York, pp. 131–94
Bursztajn, S. and Gershon, M. D. (1977). *J. Physiol., Lond.*, **269**, 17–31
Craviso, G. L. and Musacchio, J. M. (1977). *Soc. Neurosci. Abstr.*, **3**, 289
Elde, R., Hökfelt, T., Johansson, O. and Terenius, L. (1976). *Neuroscience,* **1**, 349–51
Frederickson, R. C. A., Nickander, R., Smithwick, R. H. and Norris, F. H. (1976). In *Opiates and Endogenous Opioid Peptides,* (ed. H. W. Kosterlitz) Elsevier/North-Holland Biomedical Press, Amsterdam, pp. 239–46
Furness, J. B., Campbell, G. R., Gillard, S. M., Malmfors, T., Cobb, J. L. S. and Burnstock, G. (1970). *J. Pharmac. exp. Ther.*, **174**, 111–22
Hambrook, J. M., Morgan, B. A., Rance, M. J. and Smith, C. F. C. (1976). *Nature,* **262**, 782–3
Hosobuchi, Y., Adams, J. E. and Linchitz, R. (1977). *Science,* **197**, 183–6
Hughes, J. (1975). *Brain Res.*, **88**, 295–308
Hughes, J., Smith, T. W., Kosterlitz, H. W., Fothergill, L. A., Morgan, B. A. and Morris, H. R. (1975). *Nature,* **258**, 577–9
Jacob, J. J., Tremblay, E. C. and Colombel, M. C. (1974). *Psychopharmacology,* **37**, 217–23
Koizumi, K. and Brooks, C. McC. (1972). *Ergeb. Physiol.*, **67**, 1–68
Kosterlitz, H. W., Lord, J. A. H. and Watt, A. J. (1973). In *Agonist and Antagonist Actions of Narcotic Analgesic Drugs,* (eds H. W. Kosterlitz, H. O. J. Collier and J. E. Villareal) University Park Press, Baltimore, pp. 45–61
Kunze, D. L. (1972). *J. Physiol., Lond.*, **222**, 1–15
Lampert, A., Nirenberg, M. and Klee, W. A. (1976). *Proc. natn. Acad. Sci. U.S.A.*, **73**, 3165–7
Lane, A. C., Rance, M. J. and Walter, D. S. (1977). *Nature*, **269**, 75–6
Loh, H. H., Tseng, L. F., Wei, E. and Li, C. H. (1976). *Proc. natn. Acad. Sci. U.S.A.*, **73**, 2895–8
Marks, N., Grynbaum, A. and Neidle, A. (1977). *Biochem. biophys. Res. Commun.*, **74**, 1552–9
Mayer, D. J. and Hayes, R. L. (1975). *Science,* **188**, 941–3
Meek, J. L., Yang, H.–Y. T. and Costa, E. (1977). *Neuropharmacology,* **16**, 151–4
Miller, R. J., Chang, J.-K. and Cuatrecasas, P. (1977). *Biochem. biophys. Res. Commun.*, **74**, 1311–7
Pert, C. B., Pert, A., Chang, J.-K. and Fong, B. T. W. (1976). *Science,* **194**, 330–2
Pert, A. and Walter, M. (1976). *Life Sci.*, **19**, 1023–32
Puig, M. M., Gascon, P., Craviso, G. L. and Musacchio, J. M. (1977*a*). *Science,* **195**, 419–20
Puig, M. M., Gascon, P. and Musacchio, J. M. (1977*b*). *Eur. J. Pharmac.*, **46**, 205–6
Puig, M. M., Gascon, P., Craviso, G. L., Bjur, R. A., Matsueda, G., Stewart, J. M. and Musacchio, J. M. (1977*c*). *Archs int. Pharmacodyn. Ther.*, **226**, 69–80
Puig, M. M., Gascon, P., and Musacchio, J. M. (1978). *J. Pharmac. exp. Ther.*, (in press)
Schulz, R. and Herz, A. (1976). *Life Sci.*, **19**, 1117–28
Schulz, R., Wuster, M. and Herz, A. (1977*a*). *Life Sci.*, **21**, 105–16
Schulz, R., Wuster, M., Simantov, R., Snyder, S. and Herz, A. (1977*b*). *Eur. J. Pharmac.*, **41**, 347–8
Smith, T. W., Hughes, J., Kosterlitz, H. W. and Sosa, R. P. (1976). In *Opiates and Endogenous Opioid Peptides,* (ed. H. W. Kostertitz). Elsevier/North-Holland Biomedical Press, Amsterdam, pp. 57–62
Terenius, L. and Wahlström, A. (1975). *Acta physiol. scand.*, **94**, 74–81
Thoenen, H. and Tranzer, J. P. (1968). *Naunyn-Schmiedebergs Arch. Pharmakol. exp. Path.*, **261**, 271–88
Waterfield, A. A. and Kosterlitz, H. W. (1975). *Life Sci.*, **16**, 1787–92
Waterfield, A. A., Hughes, J. and Kosterlitz, H. W. (1976). *Nature,* **260**, 624–5
Wei, E. and Loh, H. (1976). *Science,* **193**, 1262–3
Yaksh, T. L., Yeung, J. C. and Rudy, T. A. (1976). *Life Sci.*, **18**, 1193–8
Zieglgansberger, W., Fry, J. P., Herz, A., Moroder, L. and Wunsch, E. (1976). *Brain Res.*, **115**, 160–4

20
Dynamics of [Met^5]– enkephalin storage in rat striatum

H.-Y. T. Yang, J. S. Hong, W. Fratta and E. Costa
(Laboratory of Preclinical Pharmacology, National Institute of Mental Health, Saint Elizabeth's Hospital, Washington, DC 20032, U.S.A.)

In 1975, Hughes *et al.* isolated and chemically characterized from brain tissue two pentapeptides–[Met^5] and [Leu^5]-enkephalin–which bind to opiate receptors with high affinity. Since then, these two endogenous ligands for opiate receptors have been intensively investigated histochemically (Hökfelt *et al.*, 1977), biochemically (Simantov *et al.*, 1976), physiologically (Nicoll *et al.*, 1977) and pharmacologically (Hong *et al.*, 1977*c*). Currently, it is believed that they may function as neurotransmitters or neuro-modulators; however, the exact physiological role of enkephalins still remains unclear. To assess the role of enkephalin in neurophysiological and behavioral functions as well as in the establishment of morphine tolerance and dependence, it would be helpful to measure whether and how the synthesis and catabolism of enkephalin changes in various conditions *in vivo*. To this end it is essential to know the structure of the biological precursor of [Met^5] and [Leu^5]-enkephalin. While we do not have any information with regard to [Leu^5]-enkephalin, we know that in pituitary and hypothalamus there are two possible precursors of [Met^5]-enkephalin. These are β-lipotropin (β-LPH) (Li *et al.*, 1965; LaBella *et al.*, 1977) and β-endorphin (Bradbury *et al.*, 1976; Li *et al.*, 1976; Ling *et al.*, 1976). Met-enkephalin occurs at positions 61–65 of β-lipotropin and 1–5 of β-endorphin. Whether these two larger peptides are precursors of [Met^5]-enkephalin has been discussed. To obtain more direct information and to better understand the compartmentalization and regulation of [Met^5]-enkephalin biosynthesis, we have studied the incorporation of radioactive glycine, tyrosine and methionine into [Met^5]-enkephalin *in vivo*.

METHODS

Labeling of [Met^5]-enkephalin with radioactive amino acids

[^{3}H] Tyrosine (51 mCi/mmol) or [^{3}H] glycine (15 mCi/mmol), 150 μCi in 30 μl saline, was infused at constant rates into brain lateral ventricle of conscious

Sprague-Dawley male rats (150–200 g) over 30 min. At various times after infusion was terminated, rats were killed by focused microwave irradiation (Guidotti *et al.*, 1974). Various brain regions were extracted with 0.1 N CH_3-COOH and the extracts were neutralized with 1 N NaOH and the radiolabeled [Met^5]-enkephalin was isolated and purified by antiserum-affinity column chromatography.

Affinity column chromatography with [Met^5]-enkephalin
The immobilized antiserum or control serum was prepared by conjugating the partially purified [Met^5]-enkephalin directed antiserum or control serum to Sepharose 2B with cyanogen bromide. The antiserum or control serum-Sepharose conjugate was then packed into polypropylene columns. The tissue extracts in 0.2 M Tris buffer at pH 7.4 containing 0.1 per cent albumin and 0.06 per cent dextran were applied to the affinity columns. The columns were washed with the same buffer until the eluants were free of radioactivity. The enkephalin immunoreactive material was subsequently eluted with 2 N CH_3COOH. In parallel, the same tissue extracts were applied to control serum-Sepharose affinity column chromatography and the radioactivity eluted by 2 N CH_3COOH was used as the blanks to calculate the labeled [Met^5]-enkephalin immunoreactive material.

Identification of radiolabeled [Met^5]-enkephalin
The 2 N CH_3COOH extracts were mixed with synthetic [Met^5]-enkephalin, lyophilized and extracted with absolute ethanol. The ethanol extracts were subjected to silica gel G thin-layer chromatography (t.l.c.) and compared with synthetic [Met^5]-enkephalin.

Radioimmunoassay of [Met^5]-enkephalin after thin-layer chromatography
Striatum from rats killed by focused microwave irradiation was extracted with absolute ethanol and the extract was fractionated by silica gel G thin-layer chromatography. [Met^5]-enkephalin immunoreactive material was eluted from silica gel by 0.1 N CH_3COOH, neutralized with 1 N NaOH and radioimmunoassayed for [Met^5]-enkephalin (Yang *et al.*, 1977).

RESULTS

As shown in figure 20.1, [Met^5]-enkephalin was quantitatively retained by antiserum–Sepharose column but not by control serum–Sepharose. The [Met^5]-enkephalin adsorbed by the affinity column was not washed out by repeated washings with a very large amount of the buffer but was readily eluted with 2 N CH_3COOH. The fraction obtained at this step is referred to as [Met^5]-enkephalin immunoreactive material.

As the first step in testing the possibility of incorporation of radioactive amino acid into [Met^5]-enkephalin *in vivo*, we have examined the incorporation of [^3H] tyrosine or [^3H] glycine into the [Met^5]-enkephalin immunoreactive fraction. The highest concentration of [Met^5]-enkephalin is in striatum (Hong *et al.*, 1977*b*);

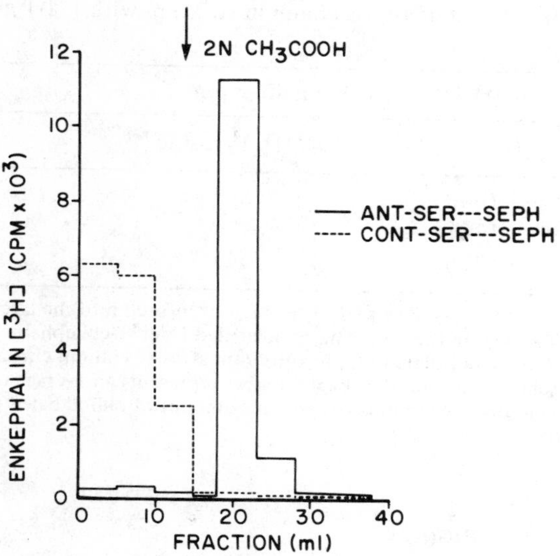

Figure 20.1 Isolation of [Met^5]-enkephalin by antiserum affinity column chromatography. The tissue extract from two pairs of striata mixed with [^3H] [Met^5]-enkephalin (about 12 000 c.p.m.) was applied to the antiserum Sepharose column or control serum Sepharose column and eluted with buffer solution and 2 N CH_3COOH as described in the text.

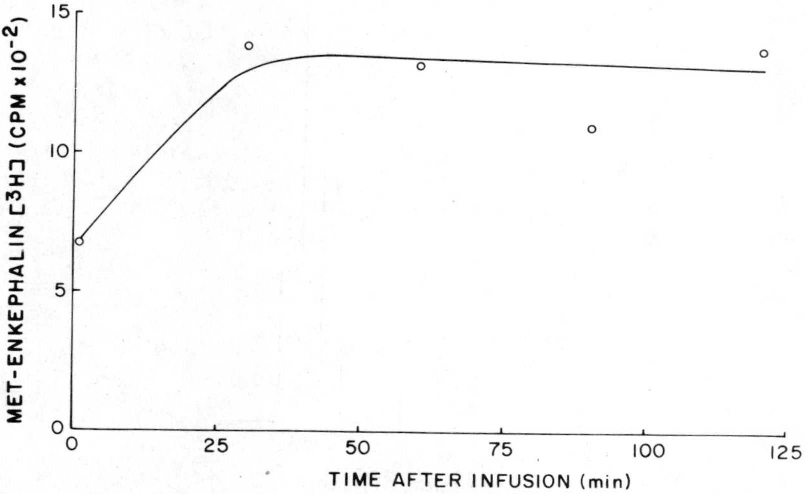

Figure 20.2 Incorporation of [^3H] tyrosine into [Met^5]-enkephalin immunoreactive peptide. A dose of 150 μCi [^3H] tyrosine was infused into the lateral ventricle of the rat brain as described in the text. The radiolabeled [Met^5]-enkephalin immunoreactive material was isolated by the affinity column chromatography. Each point represents radioactivity from two rats and is the average of two duplicate samples (average of four affinity columns). The tissue used in this study was whole brain minus striatum and cerebellum.

Table 20.1 Labeling of [Met^5]-enkephalin in striatum with [^{3}H] glycine or [^{3}H] tyrosine

	[^{3}H] [Met^5]-enkephalin c.p.m.	
Time (min)	[^{3}H] Glycine	[^{3}H] Tyrosine
0	1080	377
15	1301	
30	1278	511

A dose of 150 μCi of [^{3}H] glycine or [^{3}H] tyrosine was infused into the lateral ventricle of the rat brain as described in the text. The radiolabeled [Met^5]-enkephalin immunoreactive material was isolated by the antiserum affinity column chromatography and measured by a scintillation counter. Each number represents an average of results from four affinity columns. Each number represents amount of radiolabeled [Met^5]-enkephalin from two rats.

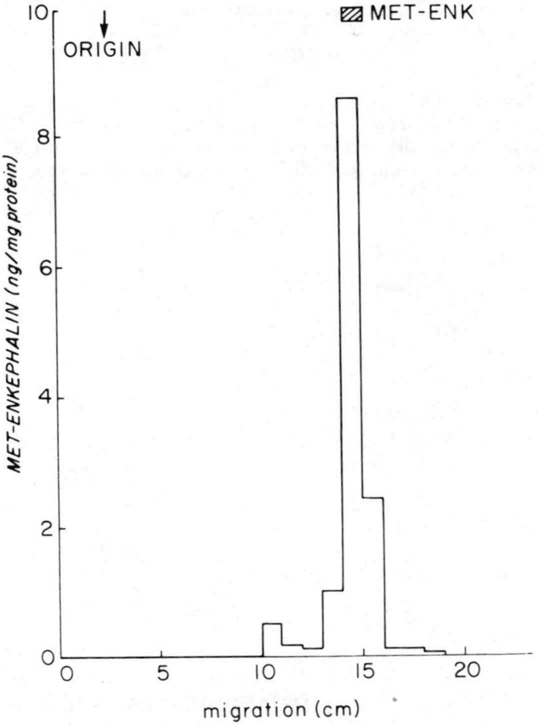

Figure 20.3 Identification of [Met^5]-enkephalin immunoreactive peptide by radioimmunoassay after silicia gel G thin-layer chromatography. Ethanol extract from one pair of striata as described in the text was applied to a silica gel thin-layer plate. The plate was developed with the solvent (*n*-butanol: acetic acid: H_2O, 60:15:25). The peptides were eluted and assayed as described in the text.

moreover, it was shown that striatum contains a considerable number of [Met^5]-enkephalin interneurons (Hong *et al.*, 1977*a*). Thus, striatum and the rest of the brain apart from the cerebellum were chosen for this study. As shown in table 20.1, incorporation of [^{3}H] glycine into [Met^5]-enkephalin was demonstrated in striatum. When [^{3}H] tyrosine was infused, radiolabeled [Met^5]-enkephalin immunoreactive material formed was very small. In the rest of the brain, the radiolabeling of [Met^5]-enkephalin immunoreactive material with [^{3}H] tyrosine was clearly observed (figure 20.2).

In order to examine the molecular nature of [Met^5]-enkephalin immunoreactive material, the brain extract was fractionated by silica gel G t.l.c. and various fractions eluted from silica gel were radioimmunoassayed for [Met^5]-enkephalin. As shown in figure 20.3, the main fraction measured by the radioimmunoassay was [Met^5]-enkephalin; however, an additional [Met^5]-enkephalin immunoreactive fraction which migrated slower than [Met^5]-enkephalin was observed. The size of the extra peak seems to vary from time to time, perhaps due

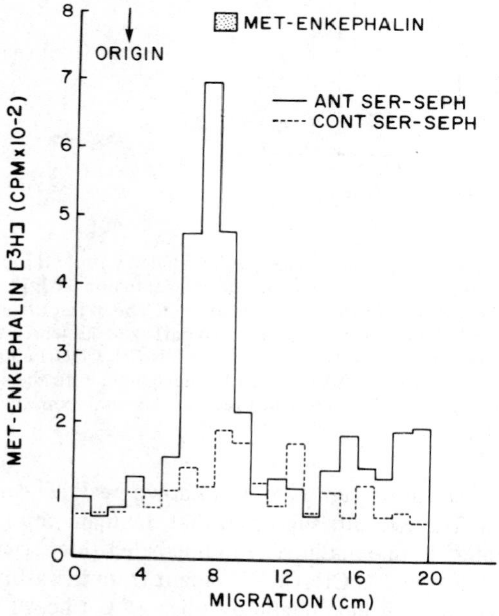

Figure 20.4 Identification of [^{3}H] [Met^5]-enkephalin by silica gel G thin-layer chromatography after intracerebroventricular infusion with [^{3}H] tyrosine. Four rats were infused with [^{3}H] tyrosine as described in the text. The animals were killed 30 min after the termination of the infusion by a focused microwave irradiation. The extract from striatum was divided into two. One portion was applied to the antiserum–Sepharose column and the other portion to the control serum–Sepharose column. The columns were eluted with buffer followed by 2 N CH_3COOH. The 2 N CH_3COOH eluants were lyophilized, extracted with ethanol and applied to silica gel G plates. The t.l.c. was developed with two different solvents (*n*-butanol: acetic acid: H_2O; 60:15:25) and (cyclohexane:benzene:methanol, 15:85:2) in the same direction. The silica gel was removed from the plates and measured for radioactivity with a scintillation counter.

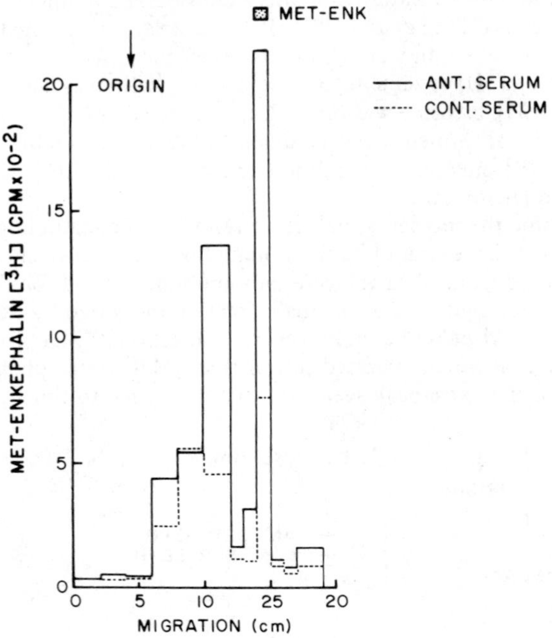

Figure 20.5 Identification of [^{3}H] [Met^5]-enkephalin labeled with [^{3}H] glycine by silica gel thin-layer chromatography after intracerebroventricular infusion with [^{3}H] glycine. Two rats were infused with [^{3}H] glycine as described in the text. The extract from whole brain devoid of striatum and cerebellum was divided into two parts and subjected to affinity column chromatography as described in figure 20.3. The 2 N CH_3COOH eluant was examined for radiolabeled [Met^5]-enkephalin by silica gel G t.l.c. developed with the solvent (*n*-butanol: acetic acid:H_2O, 60:15:25). The silica gel was removed from the plates and measured for radioactivity.

to the lower affinity of the antiserum to this unknown peak. The nature of this peak is not yet known. These results suggested that the main peptide adsorbed by the antiserum is [Met^5]-enkephalin. The radiolabeled [Met^5]-enkephalin immunoreactive fraction (the 2 N CH_3COOH eluant from the affinity column) was examined for [^{3}H] [Met^5]-enkephalin by silica gel G t.l.c. As shown in figure 20.4, [^{3}H] [Met^5]-enkephalin was detected in the radiolabeled immunoreactive fraction when rat was infused with [^{3}H] tyrosine. When glycine was used for radiolabeling, in addition to [Met^5]-enkephalin, another radioactive compound which migrated slower than [Met^5]-enkephalin in silica gel G t.l.c. was observed (figure 20.5).

DISCUSSION

The experimental results indicated that labeling of [Met^5]-enkephalin with radioactive tyrosine and glycine *in vivo* is possible if the radioactive amino acid is infused i.v.t. and at constant rate over a long period (30 min). By pulse i.v.t. injection of [^{3}H] phenylalanine, we have failed to observe the formation of radiolabeled [Met^5]-enkephalin immunoreactive material. In contrast, slow perfusion with [^{3}H] methionine yielded radioactive [Met^5]-enkephalin. Table 20.1 shows that labeling of [Met^5]-enkephalin immunoreactive fraction tends to increase after the termination of radioactive amino acid infusion. Recently, we have studied the incorporation of [^{3}H] glycine into [Met^5]-enkephalin specifically and the same tendency was observed. Radiolabeled [Met^5]-enkephalin was still detected 2 hours after the end of [^{3}H] glycine infusion (figure 20.5). Although the mechanism of enkephalin synthesis still remains unclear, this preliminary result seems to agree with the view that there are two precursors of [Met^5]-enkephalin: the radioactive amino acid is first incorporated into a small pool of precursor which turns over rapidly and which is then incorporated into a large pool of a second precursor. The latter is then converted into [Met^5]-enkephalin; this second process appears to be slower than the first in normal physiological conditions. β-LPH and β-endorphin are less likely to represent these hypothetical precursors because their quantities in rat striatum are negligible (Fratta *et al.*, unpublished observation). Although β-LPH and β-endorphin cannot be detected in rat striatum we cannot exclude the possibility that β-LPH or β-endorphin may be the [Met^5]-enkephalin precursor present in a small compartment which turns over at relatively fast rate.

In conclusion, it is possible *in vivo* to radiolabel the [Met^5]-enkephalin present in striatum. With further refinement of this technique, it may be possible to estimate and compare the relative rate of *in vivo* [Met^5]-enkephalin biosynthesis in various experimental conditions.

REFERENCES

Bradbury, A. F., Smyth, D. G. and Snell, C. R. (1976). *Biochem. biophys. Res. Commun.*, **69**, 950–6

Guidotti, A., Cheney, D. L., Trabucchi, M., Doteuchi, M. and Wang, C. (1974). *Neuropharmacology*, **13**, 1115–22

Hökfelt, T., Elde, R., Johansson, O., Terenius, L. and Stein, L. (1977). *Neurosci. Lett.*, **5**, 25–31

Hong, J. S., Yang, H.-Y. T. and Costa, E. (1977*a*). *Neuropharmacology*, **16**, 451–3

Hong, J. S., Yang, H.-Y. T., Fratta, W. and Costa, E. (1977*b*). *Brain Res.*, **134**, 383–6

Hong, J. S., Yang, H.-Y. T., Fratta, W. and Costa, E. (1977*c*). *J. Pharmac. exp. Ther.* (in press)

Hughes, J., Smith, T. W., Kosterlitz, H. W., Fothergill, L. A., Morgan, B. A. and Morris, H. R. (1975). *Nature*, **258**, 577–9

LaBella, F., Queen, G. and Senyshyn, I. (1977). *Biochem. biophys. Res. Commun.*, **75**, 350–7

Li, C. H., Barnafi, L., Chretien, M. and Chung, D. (1965). *Nature*, **208**, 1093–4

Li, C. H. and Chung, D. (1976). *Proc. natn. Acad. Sci. U.S.A.*, **73**, 1145–8

Ling, N., Burgus, R. and Guillemin, R. (1976). *Proc. natn. Acad. Sci. U.S.A.*, **73**, 3942–6

Nicoll, R. A., Siggins, G. R., Ling, N., Bloom, F. E. and Guillemin, R. (1977). *Proc. natn. Acad. Sci. U.S.A.*, **74**, 2584–8

Simantov, R. and Snyder, S. H. (1976). In *Opiates and Endogenous Opioid Peptides*, (ed. H. W. Kosterlitz), Elsevier/North-Holland Biomedical Press, Amsterdam

Yang, H.-Y. T., Hong, J. S. and Costa, E. (1977). *Neuropharmacology*, **16**, 303–7

Section One

Basic Studies

(C) Functions and Interactions of Endorphins

21
Structure–activity relationships of β-endorphin by synthesis – 1977

Choh Hao Li (Hormone Research Laboratory, University of California
San Francisco, California 94143, U.S.A.)

During isolation of melanotropins from camel pituitary glands (Li *et al.*, 1975), we were unable to find β-LPH, but obtained an untriakontapeptide (Li and Chung, 1976*a*) with an amino acid sequence identical to the COOH-terminal 31-residues of ovine lipotropin (β_s-LPH_{61-91}) (Li and Chung, 1976*b* and figure 21.1). The peptide possesses very low lipotropic activity but significant opiate activity (Li and Chung, 1976*a*), as displayed in a preparation of guinea pig ileum (GPI) and in the opiate receptor binding assay (Cox *et al.*, 1976). This untriakontapeptide was designated β-endorphin (Li and Chung, 1976*a*). A similar untriakontapeptide with opiate activity was obtained from porcine (Bradbury *et al.*, 1976; Gráf *et al.*, 1976), ovine (Chrétien *et al.*, 1976) and bovine (Li *et al.*, 1977) pituitary glands.

Isolation of human β-endorphin has also been reported (Chrétien *et al.*, 1976; Li *et al.*, 1976*a*). From 1000 frozen human glands, only 3 mg of the peptide were obtained (Li *et al.*, 1976*a*). Structural analysis (Li *et al.*, 1976*a*) established that the amino acid sequence of the human peptide is identical to the COOH-terminal 31-amino acid fragment of β_h-LPH (see figure 21.2). Figure 21.2 presents the amino acid sequence of β-endorphin from various species. The only variations occur in residues 23, 27, and 31.

Both camel (Li *et al.*, 1976*b*) and human (Li *et al.*, 1977*b*) β-endorphin have been synthesized by the improved procedures of the solid-phase method. The brominated styrene-1 per cent divinylbenzene polymer was used for the synthesis of β_h-endorphin. Figure 21.3 presents the synthetic scheme for the human β-endorphin. A yield of 32 per cent was achieved based on starting resin. The opiate activity of the synthetic product was comparable to that of the natural peptide by the GPI assay. It was found that the opiate activity of the synthetic camel and human β-endorphin is identical even though their amino acid sequences are slightly different (see figure 21.2).

Structure–Activity relationship by chemical or enzymic treatment

Opiate activities of β-endorphin after chemical or enzymic treatment as measured in the GPI and rat brain receptor assays have been investigated by Doneen *et al.*

	5 10
Human:	H-Glu-Leu-Thr-Gly-Gln-Arg-Leu-Arg-Gln-Gly-
Ovine:	H-Glu-Leu-Thr-Gly-Glu-Arg-Leu-Glu-Gln-Ala-
Porcine:	H-Glu-Leu-Ala-Gly-Ala-Pro-Pro-Glu-Pro-Ala-

15 20
Asp-Gly-Pro-Asn-Ala-Gly-Ala-Asn-Asp-Gly-
Arg-Gly-Pro-Glu-Ala-Gln-Ala-Glu-Ser-Ala-
Arg-Asp-Pro-Glu-Ala-Pro-Ala-Glu-Gly-Ala-

25 30
Glu-Gly-Pro-Asn-Ala-Leu-Glu-His-Ser-Leu-
Ala-Ala-Arg-Ala-Glu-Leu-Glu-Tyr-Gly-Leu-
Ala-Ala-Arg-Ala-Glu-Leu-Glu-His-Gly-Leu-

35 40
Leu-Ala-Asp-Leu-Val-Ala-Ala-Glu-Lys-Lys-
Val-Ala-Glu-Ala-Glu-Ala-Ala-Glu-Lys-Lys-
Val-Ala-Glu-Ala-Gln-Ala-Ala-Glu-Lys-Lys-

45 50
Asp-Glu-Gly-Pro-Tyr-Arg-Met-Glu-His-Phe-
Asp-Ser-Gly-Pro-Tyr-Lys-Met-Glu-His-Phe-
Asp-Glu-Gly-Pro-Tyr-Lys-Met-Glu-His-Phe-

55 60
Arg-Trp-Gly-Ser-Pro-Pro-Lys-Asp-Lys-Arg-
Arg-Trp-Gly-Ser-Pro-Pro-Lys-Asp-Lys-Arg-
Arg-Trp-Gly-Ser-Pro-Pro-Lys-Asp-Lys-Arg-

65 70
Tyr-Gly-Gly-Phe-Met-Thr-Ser-Glu-Lys-Ser-
Tyr-Gly-Gly-Phe-Met-Thr-Ser-Glu-Lys-Ser-
Tyr-Gly-Gly-Phe-Met-Thr-Ser-Glu-Lys-Ser-

75 80
Gln-Thr-Pro-Leu-Val-Thr-Leu-Phe-Lys-Asn-
Gln-Thr-Pro-Leu-Val-Thr-Leu-Phe-Lys-Asn-
Gln-Thr-Pro-Leu-Val-Thr-Leu-Phe-Lys-Asn-

85 91
Ala-Ile-Ile-Lys-Asn-Ala-Tyr-Lys-Lys-Gly-Glu-OH
Ala-Ile-Ile-Lys-Asn-Ala-His-Lys-Lys-Gly-Gln-OH
Ala-Ile-Val-Lys-Asn-Ala-His-Lys-Lys-Gly-Gln-OH

Figure 21.1 The primary structure of ovine, porcine and human β-lipotropin

(1977). As shown in table 21.2, acetone-treated β_h-endorphin, cyclized between Tyr^1-Gly^2 by a bridge which incorporates the amino group of Tyr^1, displayed only 1 per cent (GPI) and 2 per cent (opiate receptor assay) of β_h-endorphin activity. β_h-endorphin dansylated at its C-terminal glutamic acid residue, showed a modest decline in opiate activities. Whereas its amino terminal tyrosine may be essential, the carboxy terminal glutamic acid residue appears to contribute little directly to the interaction of β_h-endorphin with opiate receptors. In addition, conversion of Met^5 to 5-hormoserine abolished the opiate activities of β_h-endorphin.

Hydrolysis of β_h-endorphin with chymotrypsin diminished considerably its potency in both assays. Chymotrypsin can be expected to cleave β_h-endorphin at Phe^4 as well as at other aromatic residues. Trypsin digestion yielded lower activity in both assay systems, whereas carboxypeptidase did not change the activity at all.

```
                                    5                    10
HUMAN:            H-TYR-GLY-GLY-PHE-MET-THR-SER-GLU-LYS-SER-

                                   15                    20
                    GLN-THR-PRO-LEU-VAL-THR-LEU-PHE-LYS-ASN-

                                   25                        31
                    ALA-ILE-ILE-LYS-ASN-ALA-TYR-LYS-LYS-GLY-GLU-OH

PORCINE:                  VAL            HIS.              GLN-OH

CAMEL,OVINE,BOVINE:       ILE            HIS               GLN-OH
```

AMINO ACID SEQUENCE OF HUMAN, PORCINE, CAMEL, OVINE, AND

BOVINE β-ENDORPHINS

Figure 21.2 The amino acid sequence of β-endorphin from various species.

Table 21.1 Opiate activities of β_c-endorphin and derivatives

Preparation	Relative potency in	
	Guinea pig ileum	Brain opiate receptor binding
β_h-endorphin	1.00	1.00
Met-enkephalin	0.25	0.34
Normorphine	0.65	–
Acetone treated-β_h-endorphin	0.01	0.02
(Dansylated-Glu^{31})-β_h-endorphin	0.76	0.75
Formic acid-treated-β_h-endorphin	1.00	1.00
(5-homoserine)-β_h-endorphin	<0.01	0.01
β_h-endorphin: carboxypeptidase A digest	1.00	1.00
β_h-endorphin: chymotryptic digest	0.13	0.03
β_h-endorphin: tryptic digest	0.71	0.61
β_c-endorphin: leucine aminopeptidase digest	0.97	0.93
Met-enkephalin: leucine aminopeptidase digest	<0.01	0.01

N^{α}-Boc-(Bzl)-Glu-Resin

↓
1. TFA-CH_2Cl_2, 15 min
2. N-methylmorpholine
3. preformed symmetrical anhydride of Boc-Gly (CF_3CH_2OH to 20%)

Boc-Gly-(Bzl)-Glu-Resin

↓
1. TFA-CH_2Cl_2, 15 min
2. N-methylmorpholine
3. preformed symmetrical anhydride of Boc-AA (CF_3CH_2OH to 20%)

Fully protected β_h-endorphin

↓
1. TFA-CH_2Cl_2, 15 min
2. N-methylmorpholine

Protected β_h-endorphin with free α-NH_2 group

↓
1. HF, anisole, 0°, 75 min

Crude β_h-endorphin

↓
1. Sephadex G-10, 0.5 N HOAc
2. CMC chromatography
3. partition chromatography on G-50

β_h-Endorphin (32% yield)

Figure 21.3 The synthetic scheme of human β-endorphin. Resin, brominated styrene resin (1% divinylbenzene); side-chain protecting groups: Lys, Z(o-Br); His, Boc; Asp, Bzl; Thr, Bzl; Ser, Bzl; Glu, Bzl and Tyr(o-Br). Boc, *t*-butyloxycarbonyl; Bzl, benzyl; TFA, trifluoracetic acid; AA, amino acid.

β_c-endorphin was susceptible to very limited hydrolysis with leucine aminopeptidase as indicated by liberation of only trace amounts of tryrosine detected by amino acid analysis. As shown in table 21.1, this enzyme digest of β_c-endorphin showed only slight diminution of opiate activity; in contrast, met-enkephalin, which showed stoichiometric hydrolysis of the Tyr^1-Gly^2 bond, lost all activity after leucine aminopeptidase digestion. Therefore, the amino terminal residue of β_c-endorphin appears to differ from that of met-enkephalin by being protected from exopeptidase attack.

Synthetic analogues with various amino acid residues in positions 1, 2, 4 and 5
Tables 21.2 and 21.3 summarize the *in vivo* and *in vitro* opiate activities of synthetic analogues with various amino acid residues in positions 1, 2, 4 and 5 (Yamashiro *et al.*, 1977; Yamashiro *et al.*, 1978). It may be noted that substitutions of Tyr^1 with its D-isomer; the residue in position 2 with Ser, Ala, D-Leu or D-Lys; position 4 with D-Phe or position 5 with D-Met, Pro, Leu or D-Leu decreases the activity. Substitution of Gly^2 with D-Ala retains full analgesic activity. The synthetic analogue containing the leu-enkephalin segment has only 17 per cent of the analgesic activity of the parent molecule and replacement of Leu with its D-isomer lowers the activity to only 0.2 per cent. Apparently, residue 5 in the β-endorphin structure is very important for its analgesic activity.

Table 21.2 Opiate activity of synthetic β_c-endorphin with D-amino acids in positions 1, 2, 4 and 5

Synthetic peptides	Relative potency	
	Guinea pig ileum assay	i.v.t. in mice
β_c-endorphin	100	100
[D-Tyr^1]-β_c-endorphin	<1	0.5
[D-Ala^2]-β_c-endorphin	43	100
[D-Phe^4]-β_c-endorphin	4	<0.3
[D-Met^5]-β_c-endorphin	4	1

Table 21.3 Opiate activity of synthetic β-endorphin with substitutions in positions 2 and 5

Synthetic peptides	Relative potency	
	Guinea pig ileum assay	i.v.t. in mice
β_h-endorphin	100	100
[Ser^2]-β_c-endorphin	13	<0.3
[Ala^2]-β_c-endorphin	6	12
[D-Leu^2]-β_c-endorphin	12	48
[D-Lys^2]-β_c-endorphin	8	15
[Pro^5]-β_h-endorphin	<0.01	0.6
[Leu^5]-β_h-endorphin	18	17
[D-Leu^5]-β_h-endorphin	<0.01	0.2
[D-Ala^2, D-Leu^5]-β_h-endorphin	3	8

Synthetic analogues with shortened peptide chains

In order to explore the contribution of the 'non-enkephalin' segment of β-endorphin to its biological behavior, three analogues (Li *et al.*, 1977*c*) of β-endorphin have been synthesized by variations of the solid phase method: β_c-endorphin$_{(1-5)-(28-31)}$, β_c-endorphin$_{(6-31)}$ and β_h-endorphin$_{(1-5)-(16-31)}$.

It was found that only β_c-endorphin$_{(1-5)-(16-31)}$ exhibited significant analgesic activity with a relative potency compared to the parent peptide of 0.3 per cent (table 21.4); analgesia was partially but not completely blocked by naloxone (3 mg/kg); the duration of analgesia was shorter after naloxone injection. In addition to the inhibition of the tail-flick response, mice became extremely hyperactive to sound and touch, attempting to jump out of their cages and escape. The analgesic response and hyperactivity lasted 10 to 20 min. However, the hyperactive response was not antagonized by pretreatment with naloxone (3 mg/kg), indicating that the response is not mediated through opiate-like mechanisms.

β_c-endorphin$_{(1-5)-(28-31)}$ was not active at a dose of 42.5 μg. β_c-endorphin$_{(6-31)}$ at doses of 42.5 and 85 μg produced analgesia in one out of five and four out of eleven mice, respectively. Increasing the dose to 170 μg did not enhance the analgesic activity. It was reported (Li *et al.*, 1977*d*) previously that inhibition of transmurally stimulated contraction of GPI by this peptide was not blocked by naloxone. Inhibition of the tail-flick response by β_c-endorphin$_{(6-31)}$ in some mice did not appear to be an opioid action.

The opiate activity (Li *et al.*, 1977*d*) of the synthetic peptides as assayed *in vitro* by the GPI method is presented in figure 21.4. It may be seen that β_c-endorphin$_{(1-5)-(16-31)}$ is more active *in vitro* than the parent molecule,

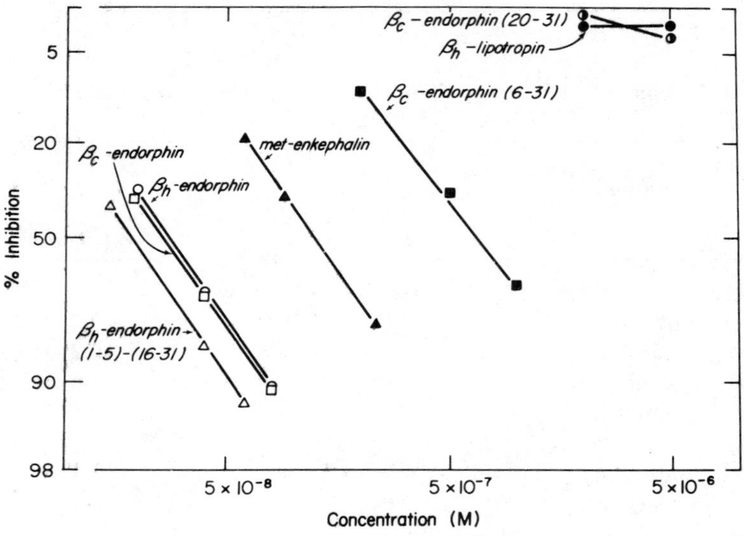

Figure 21.4 Guinea pig ileum assay of synthetic β-endorphin and its fragments.

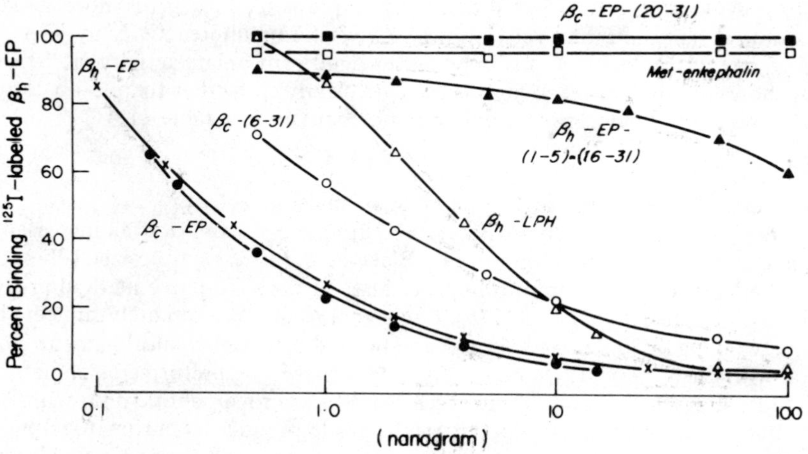

Figure 21.5 Radioimmunoassay of human β-endorphin. Final dilution of guinea pig antiserum was 1:3000. EP, endorphin.

but shows very weak analgesic activity in the *in vivo* assay. The lack of correlation between the *in vitro* and *in vivo* assay results has also been observed in earlier studies (Yamashiro *et al.*, 1977) with other synthetic analogues of β_c-endorphin.

By radioimmunoassay (RIA) of β_h-endorphin (Li *et al.*, 1977*d*), β_c-endorphin gave a completely parallel and almost identical inhibition curve. β_c-endorphin$_{(16-31)}$ also exhibited a parallel inhibition curve but had 40 per cent immunoreactivity as compared with β_c-endorphin (figure 21.5). On the other hand β_c-endorphin$_{(1-5)\ +\ (16-31)}$ showed very weak cross-reaction. It may be noted that β_h-LPH, which contains the complete amino acid sequence of β_h-endorphin, had only 10 per cent immunoreactivity. Figure 21.5 also shows that β_c-endorphin$_{(20-31)}$ and met-enkephalin (β_c-endorphin$_{(1-5)}$) did not show any cross-reactivity. Thus it is probable that β-endorphin$_{(6-15)}$ or β-endorphin$_{(6-31)}$ represents the antigenic determinant of β-endorphin.

Table 21.4 Biological activity of synthetic β-endorphin with shortened peptide chains

Synthetic peptides	Relative potency: Guinea pig ileum assay	i.v.t. in mice	Immunoreactivity by RIA
β_c-endorphin	100	100	100
β_c-endorphin$_{(6-31)}$	4	<0.1	40
β_h-endorphin$_{(1-5)\ -\ (16-31)}$	135	0.3	nil
β_c-endorphin$_{(1-5)\ -\ (28-31)}$	<0.001	<0.1	nil

It is evident from figure 21.4 that β_c-endorphin$_{(1-5)+(16-31)}$ is more active than the parent molecule, yet it shows very weak immunoreactivity by RIA (see figure 21.5). Met-enkephalin possesses significant opiate activity *in vitro* but shows no immunoreactivity. These data clearly show that there is no correlation between opiate activity and immunoreactivity (see table 21.4).

Synthesis of an analogue with an increase in analgesic activity

In an effort to delineate the structural requirements for full or even increased opiate activity of human β-endorphin, Blake *et al.* (1978) synthesized (Phe^{27}, Gly^{31})-β_h-endorphin by improved procedures of the solid-phase method previously described Li *et al.* (1977*b*). Boc-glycyl resin was alternately subjected to deblocking in 55 per cent trifluoroacetic acid-methylene chloride, neutralization with diisopropylethylamine, and coupling with the preformed symmetrical anhydride of the Boc amino acid. Treatment of the final peptide resin with liquid HF, followed by purification of the crude product by chromatography on carboxymethylcellulose and partition chromatography on Sephadex G-50 gave the highly purified peptide. The synthetic peptide was characterized by amino acid analysis of acid hydrolysates and enzyme digests, paper electrophoresis, and thin layer chromatography.

The opiate activity of (Phe^{27}, Gly^{31})-β_h-endorphin, as assayed *in vitro* and *in vivo*, is summarized in table 21.5. It may be noted that the synthetic analogue is more potent than the parent molecule by these assays. The duration of analgesic activity after i.v. injection appeared to be shorter than after i.v.t. injection. To our knowledge, the peptide is the first synthetic analogue of β_h-endorphin to possess a greater analgesic activity *in vivo* than the natural peptide. It should be noted that the positions (27 and 31) of substitution in the peptide correspond to the positions where amino acid sequences of human (Li *et al.*, 1976*a*) and camel (Li and Chung, 1976*a*) β-endorphin differ. The comparable analgesic potencies of β_c and β_h-endorphin (Li *et al.*, 1976*a*) led us to conclude that the Tyr and His residue at position 27 could be substituted by Phe, and the Glu or Gln residue at position 31 could be substituted by Gly without deleterious effect on biological potency. The results support this belief. In fact, the analgesic potency of the synthetic analogue I by i.v. administration is somewhat greater than that of the natural peptide (table 21.5).

Table 21.5 Opiate activity of synthetic [Phe^{27}, Gly^{31}]-β_h-endorphin

Synthetic peptide	Relative potency: Guinea pig ileum assay	i.v.t.	i.v.
β_h-endorphin	100	100	100
[Phe^{27}, Gly^{31}]-β_h-endorphin	128	119	148

CONCLUSION

Among various fragments of β-LPH having opiate activity, only β-endorphin exhibits potent analgesic activity by i.v. injections. In addition, it is the most active peptide when administered directly into the brain. (Kline *et al.*, 1977; Catlin *et al.*, 1977; Su *et al.*, 1978, Hosobuchi and Li, 1978). Recent clinical studies indicate that synthetic β_h-endorphin (Li *et al.*, 1977*b*) is active in patients with severe pain, narcotic abstinence, schizophrenic behavior and deep depression by i.v. injections. Future structure-activity investigations of β_h-endorphin may lead to the development of a peptide with long-acting and/or oral-active properties for extensive clinical studies.

ACKNOWLEDGEMENT

I thank Drs D. Yamashiro, J. Blake, S. Lemaire, D. Chung, B. A. Doneen, A. J. Rao, W. C. Chang, L-F. Tseng, and H. H. Loh for their contributions to these investigations. Experimental work was supported in part by NIHM Grant MH 30245 and the Hormone Research Foundation.

REFERENCES

Blake, J., Tseng, L-F., Chang, W. C. and Li, C. H. (1978). *Int. J. Pept. Prot. Res.* (in press)
Bradbury, A. F., Smyth, D. G. and Snell, C. R. (1976). *Biochem. biophys. Res. Commun.* **69**, 950–6
Catlin, D. H., Hui, K. K., Loh, H. H. and Li, C. H. (1977). *Commun. Psychopharmac.* (in press)
Chrétien, M., Benjannet, S., Dragon, N., Seidah, N. G. and Lis, M. (1976). *Biochem. biophys. Res. Commun.*, **72**, 472–8
Cox, B. M., Goldstein, A. and Li, C. H. (1976). *Proc. natn. Acad. Sci. U.S.A.*, **73**, 1821–3
Doneen, B. A., Chung, D., Yamashiro, D., Law, P. Y., Loh, H. H. and Li, C. H. (1977). *Biochem. biophys. Res. Commun.*, **74**, 656–62
Gráf, L., Barat, E. and Patthy, A. (1976). *Acta biochim. biophys. Acad. Sci. Hung.*, **11** (2–3), 121–2
Hosobuchi, Y. and Li, C. H. (1978). *Commun. Psychopharmac.* (in press).
Kline, N. S., Li, C. H., Lehmann, H. E., Lajtha, A., Laski, E. and Cooper, T. (1977). *Archs gen. Psychiat.*, **34**, 1111–3
Li, C. H. and Chung, D. (1976*a*). *Proc. natn. Acad. Sci. U.S.A.*, **73**, 1145–8
Li, C. H. and Chung, D. (1976*b*). *Nature*, **260**, 622–4
Li, C. H., Chung, D. and Doneen, B. A. (1976*a*). *Biochem. biophys. Res. Commun.*, **72**, 1542–7
Li, C. H., Danho, W. O., Chung, D. and Rao, A. J. (1975). *Biochemistry*, **14**, 947–52
Li, C. H., Lemaire, S., Yamashiro, D., and Doneen, B. A. (1976*b*). *Biochem. biophys. Res. Commun.*, **71**, 19–25
Li, C. H., Rao, A. J., Doneen, B. A. and Yamashiro, D. (1977*d*). *Biochem. biophys. Res. Commun.*, **75**, 576–80
Li, C. H., Tan, L. and Chung, D. (1977*a*). *Biochem. biophys. Res. Commun.*, **77**, 1088–93
Li, C. H., Yamashiro, D., Tseng, L-F. and Loh, H. H. (1977*b*). *J. med. Chem.*, **20**, 325–8
Li, C. H., Yamashiro, D., Tseng, L-F. and Loh, H. H. (1977*c*). *Int. J. Pept. Prot. Res.* (in press)
Su, C. Y., Lin, S. H., Wang, Y. T., Li, C. H., Loh, H. H., Chen, C. S., Hung, L. H., Lin, C. S. and Lin. B. C. (1978). *J. Formosan med. Assoc.* (in press).
Yamashiro, D., Li, C. H., Tseng, L-F. and Loh, H. H. (1978). *Int. J. Pept. Prot. Res.* (in press)
Yamashiro, D., Tseng, L-F., Doneen, B. A., Loh, H. H. and Li, C. H. (1977). *Int. J. Pept. Prot. Res.*, **10**, 159–66

22

β-endorphin: stimulation of DNA-dependent RNA formation

Horace H. Loh, Nancy M. Lee and Choh Hao Li*
(Departments of Pharmacology and Psychiatry and Hormone Research Laboratory*, University of California, San Francisco, California 94143, U.S.A.)

Many hormones have been shown to alter gene expression with resultant stimulation of protein and/or RNA synthesis in target cells and, in some instances, inhibition of protein synthesis (Hamilton, 1968; Tata, 1970). We report here that β-endorphin (Li and Chung, 1976*a*), a fragment of pituitary hormone β-lipotropin (β-LPH) (Li and Chung, 1976*b*) with an amino acid sequence corresponding to residues 61–91, directly stimulates brain chromatin-dependent UTP incorporation into RNA.

Table 22.1 shows that synthetic β-endorphin (Li *et al.*, 1976) causes an increase in template activity of deproteinized DNA. The reaction is sensitive to rifampicin and actinomycin D when bacterial RNA polymerase is used. [^{3}H] UTP incorporation (with or without β-endorphin) was temperature dependent; at 0 °C, only a small percentage of incorporation occured. Stimulation of template activity by the peptide required the presence of both the template and RNA polymerase.

Figure 22.1 shows that with brain chromatin as template and *Escherichia coli* RNA polymerase as enzyme, UTP incorporation is linear with respect to the amount of chromatin added up to 16 μg of DNA with or without β-endorphin. The reaction is also sensitive to actinomycin D and rifampicin.

Table 22.2 shows that β-LPH (Li and Chung 1976*b*) is also active in promoting RNA formation on deproteinized DNA. Synthetic β-melanotropin (β-MSH) (Li *et al.*, 1975), with a sequence corresponding to residues 41–58 of β-LPH (Li and Chung, 1976*b*), is only weakly active. Met-enkephalin (Hughes *et al.*, 1975), with a sequence corresponding to residues 61–65 of β-lipotropin, is inactive in this system. In a previous study, chromatin from oligodendroglial nuclei taken from mice given chronic morphine treatment showed an increase in template activity (Lee *et al.*, 1975). β-endorphin and its related peptides have been shown to possess morphine-like activities in various systems (Terenius and Wahlström, 1975; Hughes, 1975; Loh *et al.*, 1976; Pasternak *et al.*, 1975; Simantov and Snyder, 1976). In all studies reported, β-endorphin fulfilled the criteria for an endogenous opiate. How-

Table 22.1 Effect of β-endorphin and other compounds on template activity of deproteinized DNA

Temperature (°C)	Addition	Concentration	% of [^{3}H] UTP incorporation
	None		100
	β-Endorphin	5.8 x 10^{-5} M	202
37	β-Endorphin + rifampicin	5.8 x 10^{-5} M + 0.4 μg/ml	0
	β-Endorphin actinomycin D	5.8 x 10^{-5} M + 40 μg/ml	0
	None	—	0
0	β-Endorphin	5.8 x 10^{-5} M	16

Experimental procedures were as described in figure 22.1.

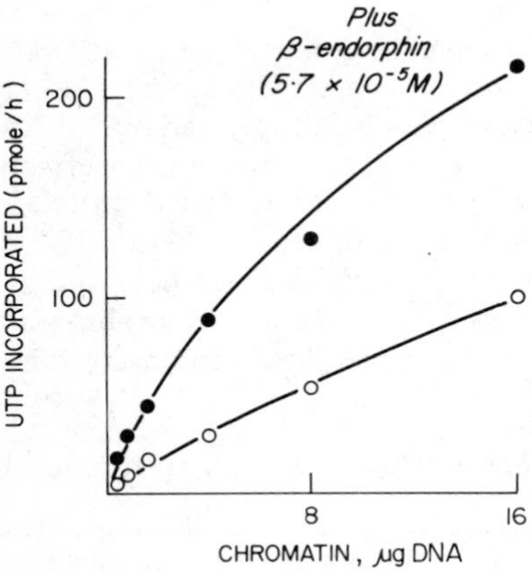

Figure 22.1 Effect of β-endorphin on [^{3}H] UTP incorporation with different amounts of mouse brain chromatin. Brain chromatin was isolated according to Lee *et al.* (1975). Three units of *E. coli* K–12 RNA polymerase were incubated in 0.25 ml, at 37 °C for 60 min. The reaction mixture contains Tris-HCl, 80 mM (pH 8.3, 23° C), 100 mM NaCl, 4 mM $MgCl_2$, 2 mM $MnCl_2$, 6 mM DTT, 20 μg bentonite, 0.1 mM each of GTP, ATP, CTP and UTP with 0.4 μCi [^{3}H] UTP, and with or without 5.8 × 10^{-5} M β-endorphin. The reaction was stopped by the addition of 1 ml of 10 per cent trichloroacetic acid containing 5 per cent sodium pyrophosphate and 150 μg bovine serum albumin. After 15 min at 0 °C, the precipitates were filtered on glass fiber filters (Whatman GF/C) and washed five times with 9 ml 5 per cent TCA + 3 per cent PPi and once with 2 ml of cold ethanol. The filters were dried and counted in 9 ml Scintiverse. Background incorporation without added DNA was always less than 20 per cent of the total counts and was, therefore, subtracted from the total incorporation. Experiments were carried out in triplicate and the data presented are the mean of three assays.

Table 22.2 Effect of β-endorphin and related peptides on template activity of calf thymus DNA

Peptides	Concentration (10^{-5} M)	Specific activity ([^{3}H] UTP incorporated, nmol/mg DNA)	% Stimulation
No addition	0	1.02	0
β-LPH	6	2.30	125
β-Endorphin	0.011	1.0	0
	0.11	1.31	29
	3.0	1.89	85
	6.0	2.30	125
β-MSH	3	1.71	15
	6	1.33	30
Met-enkephalin	6	1.07	5
	20	1.12	10

Experimental procedures were as described in figure 22.1.

ever, the present study revealed that morphine sulfate, (at concentrations up to 10^{-4} M) had no effect on template activity *in vitro*. Moreover, stimulation of template activity by β-endorphin is not reversed by 10^{-4} M naloxone.

Table 22.3 shows that β-endorphin is much more effective in stimulating brain chromatin template activity than in stimulating deproteinized DNA or liver chromatin. At concentrations as low as 10^{-9} M or 10^{-8} M, β-endorphin increased brain chromatin-dependent RNA formation, whereas, if liver chromatin or deproteinized DNA was used as template, β-endorphin was only effective at 10^{-6} M or higher. This phenomenon has been observed in both mouse and rat.

Table 22.3 Effect of β-endorphin on RNA formation using DNA liver chromatin or brain chromatin as template

β-Endorphin concentration (M)	% Stimulation		
	DNA	Liver chromatin	Brain chromatin
0			
10^{-9}	0	0	24
10^{-8}	0	0	34
10^{-7}	0	0	40
10^{-6}	29	15	45
10^{-5}	76	—	78

Experimental procedures were as described in figure 22.1 except that the incubation time was 20 min.

To ascertain that the stimulation of template activity of β-endorphin is not due to the use of bacterial enzymes, one of the RNA polymerases isolated from mouse brain oligodendroglial nuclei (Stokes *et al.*, 1977) was used. Figure 22.2 shows that when peak I RNA polymerase is used in lieu of bacterial enzymes, DNA-dependent RNA formation is also stimulated by β-endorphin. This and the fact that low concentrations of β-endorphin (10^{-7} M or lower) can stimulate only brain chromatin, and not liver chromatin or deproteinized DNA, indicates that β-endorphin is indeed affecting the brain chromatin and not the enzyme. Since chromatin contains proteins which are thought to regulate gene transcription, it is possible that β-endorphin may interact with such brain chromatin proteins in some specific way to increase template activity.

The rate of RNA formation from DNA template depends on many factors, one of which is the number of available initiation sites. To check the effect of β-endorphin on initiation, [^{3}H] UTP incorporation in the presence of three nucleotides–GTP, ATP and UTP–and low salt was measured. Under these conditions, RNA polymerase can bind to the template and initiate the reaction but

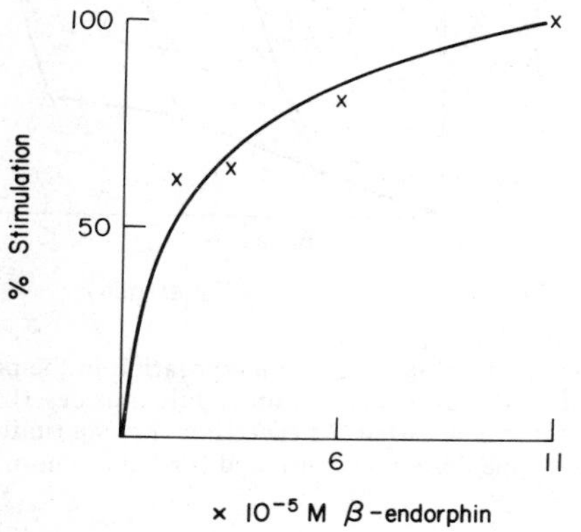

Figure 22.2 Effect of β-endorphin on RNA formation with brain RNA polymerase. The experimental procedure is as described in figure 22.1.

without the fourth nucleotide, transcription does not continue (Cedar, 1976), thus allowing one to measure the number of initiation sites available for enzyme binding. The addition of high salt [0.3 M $(NH_4)_2SO_4$] after the initiation reaction is started prevents further chain initiation by enzyme molecules (Hyman and Davidson, 1970). Figure 22.3 reveals that in the presence of β-endorphin, the number of initiation sites is actually decreased. However, as the reaction is allowed to continue (for 5 min more each time) it proceeds much more rapidly in the presence of β-endorphin than in the control. So, although β-endorphin can actually decrease the number of initiation sites on DNA, it may stimulate template activity by affecting the rate of propagation and/or termination.

This study is the first to demonstrate that β-endorphin affects DNA-dependent RNA synthesis. Although the stimulation of transcription by β-endorphin

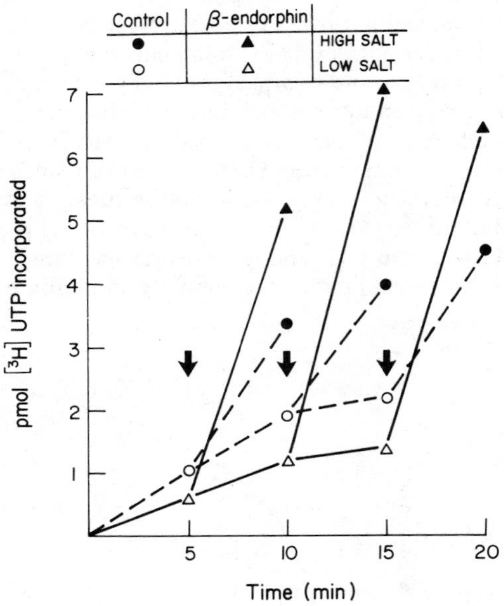

Figure 22.3 Effect of β-endorphin on UTP incorporation in the presence of three nucleotide triphosphates. The experimental procedure is as described in figure 22.1 except that ATP, GTP and UTP only are used. At each time interval (indicated by arrows), 0.3 M $(NH_4)_2SO_4$ is added and incubation is continued for 5 more min.

is organ specific, the true function of β-endorphin in the body is still unknown. The molecular mechanism and the consequences of stimulation of template-dependent RNA formation by β-endorphin have not been fully elucidated. Whether or not the effect of β-endorphin on template activity *in vitro* is of physiological significance remains to be determined.

Acknowledgements

This study was supported in part by NIDA Grant DA-00564. H. H. Loh and N. M. Lee are recipients of NIMH and NIDA Research Scientist Career Development Awards, K2-DA-70554 and 5-KO2-DA-00020, respectively. We thank Barbara Halperin for editorial assistance.

References

Bobel, G. and van Potter, R. (1966). *Science,* **154,** 1662–3

Cedar, H. (1976). *Nucleic Acids Res.,* **3**, 1659–70

Hamilton, T. H. (1968). *Science,* **161**, 649–61

Hughes, J. (1975). *Brain Res.,* **88**, 295–308

Hughes, J., Smith, T. W., Kosterlitz, H. W., Fothergill, L. A., Morgan, B. A. and Morris, H. R. (1975). *Nature,* **258**, 577–9

Hyman, R. W. and Davidson, N. (1970). *J. molec. Biol.,* **50**, 421–38

Li, C. H. and Chung, D. (1976*a*). *Proc. natn. Acad. Sci. U.S.A.,* **73**, 1145–8

Li, C. H. and Chung, D. (1976*b*). *Nature,* **260**, 623–4

Li, C. H., Lemaire, S., Yamashiro, D. and Donee, B. A. (1976). *Biochem. biophys. Res. Commun.,* **71**, 19–25

Li, C. H., Yamashiro, D. and Lemaire, S. (1975). *Biochemistry,* **14**, 953–6

Lee, N. M., Ho, I. K. and Loh, H. H. (1975). *Biochem. Pharmac.* **24**, 1983–7

Loh, H. H., Tseng, L. F., Wei, E. and Li, C. H. (1976). *Proc. natn. Acad. Sci. U.S.A.,* **73**, 2895–6

Pasternak, G. W., Goodman, R. and Snyder, S. H. (1975). *Life Sci.,* **16**, 1765–9

Simantov, R. and Snyder, S. H. (1976). *Life Sci.,* **18**, 781–8

Stokes, K. B., Lee, N. M. and Loh, H. H. Biochem. Pharmacol. (Submitted)

Tata, J. R. (1970). In *Biochemical Action of Hormones,* (ed. G. Litwach), Vol. **1**, Academic Press, New York

Terenius, L. and Wahlström, A. (1974). *Acta pharmac. tox.* (Suppl. 1), **35,** 55

Terenius, L. and Wahlström, A. (1975). *Acta physiol. scand.,* **94**, 74–81

23
Studies on endorphin function in animals and man

Avram Goldstein and B. M. Cox (Stanford University and Addiction Research Foundation, Palo Alto, California 94304, U.S.A.)

Endorphin activity in tissue extracts can be estimated by bioassay or by radioimmunoassay (RIA). The high sensitivity of radioimmunoassay is essential to measure the very low concentrations of endorphin in body fluids such as plasma. However, for peptides containing more than five to ten amino acids, there is no *a priori* reason why the features of the peptide conferring biological reactivity should necessarily also confer immunological reactivity. In the case of β-endorphin, it has already been shown that antisera raised to this peptide also cross-react with peptides with related structure, but without opioid activity (Li *et al.* , 1977). The receptor-binding assay (where displacement of radioactive opiate ligands from opiate receptor binding sites in brain membranes is measured) is far less sensitive than RIA, but is relatively specific for opioid substances. In the following studies on pituitary endorphin, we have routinely used the receptor-binding assay. It is likely that most of the activity measured in the gland extracts results from β-endorphin, but we have clear evidence that in bovine and porcine pituitaries at least one other active opioid peptide is also present. If this material is also present in rat pituitary, it presumably contributes to the measured activity.

CONDITIONS AFFECTING PITUITARY ENDORPHIN CONTENT

In making measurements of gland endorphin content, it is important that the amounts of recovered activity are not artifactually elevated by the post-mortem cleavage of precursor peptides such as β-lipotropin (β-LPH), or reduced by post-mortem enzymatic degradation of endorphin to less active or inactive peptides. There are indications that opioid activity in pituitary may be generated by incubation of the gland in cold aqueous media (Teschemacher, 1977; Baizman and Cox, 1978). To minimize post-mortem changes in activity, the gland must be dispersed in a denaturing solvent such as acetone, or glacial acetic acid–acetone mixtures, as soon as possible after killing.

Endorphins are present in the pituitary gland in high concentrations (Teschemacher *et al.,* 1975; Ross *et al.,* 1977). In both bovine and rat pituitaries most of the material with opioid activity has an apparent molecular weight in the range 3000 to 3500 daltons (Ross *et al.*, 1977). It is likely that the peptide β-endorphin is responsible for a significant part of this activity. In bovine pituitary, the highest concentration of opioid activity, as measured by assay on the isolated guinea pig ileum preparation, was found in the pars intermedia, although an almost equal total quantity of endorphin activity was recovered from the pars distalis (Ross *et al.*, 1977). A similar distribution has been observed in the rat when activity was assayed by receptor-binding assay (Baizman and Cox, 1978). Thus in both rat and cattle the distribution of endorphin activity within the pituitary is qualitatively similar to the distribution of two other pituitary peptides, β-LPH and β-melanotropin (β-MSH).

The posterior lobe (containing the pars intermedia and pars nervosa) of the pituitary of a mature male albino rat was found to contain opioid activity equivalent to about 260 pmol (0.9 μg) of β-endorphin, while the anterior lobe (pars distalis) contained activity equivalent to about 220 pmol (0.75 μg) of β-endorphin. In mature female rats the anterior lobe of the pituitary is substantially larger than in male rats of equivalent age or weight. Here, the endorphin content of the anterior lobe is equivalent to as much as 330 pmol (1.1 μg) of β-endorphin (Baizman and Cox, 1978).

In pituitary cell lines in culture, there is evidence that β-LPH and adrenocorticotropin (ACTH) are derived from a common precursor peptide (Mains *et al.*, 1977). In view of the presumed common origin of at least one endorphin (β-endorphin), ACTH, and α-MSH and β-MSH, it was of interest to determine whether the function of pituitary endorphin was regulated in a manner similar to that of MSH or ACTH. We first considered the ontological development of pituitary endorphin.

The amount of endorphin activity in the pituitaries of both male and female neonatal rats was substantially lower than that observed in mature animals. A four to sixfold increase to adult levels in both anterior and posterior lobe endorphin content occured rather sharply between the fifth and tenth week after birth (Baizman and Cox, 1978). The MSH content of male rat neurointermediate lobe also shows a substantial rise at about the same time after birth (table 23.1). Thus there appears to be a close temporal relationship in the development of synthetic and/or storage processes for pituitary endorphin and MSH.

These results led us to examine systems that might function in the neural control of pituitary endorphin. Some stimuli appear to have similar effects on both MSH and endorphin storage and release processes. Thus administration of hypertonic solutions of sodium chloride has been shown to induce release of MSH from the pituitary gland (Cyrkowicz and Traczyck, 1975) and to modify gland content of MSH (Kastin, 1967; Howe and Thody, 1970). In our studies, administration of 2 per cent sodium chloride in the drinking water resulted in a decline of pituitary endorphin content in most of the rats studied (Baizman, Osman and Cox, in preparation). Thus this stimulus probably provokes a release of both MSH and endorphin into the circulation.

However, other procedures appear to indicate that there is a differential neural control over these substances. The pars intermedia, where both MSH and endorphin activity is concentrated, receives innervation from the paraventricular nucleus of the hypothalamus (Howe, 1973). Lesions of the paraventricular nucleus have been reported to affect pituitary levels of MSH (Taleisnik *et al.*, 1967; Howe

Table 23.1 Changes in endorphin and MSH content of neurointermediate lobe of male rats with age

	Endorphin content*		MSH content†	
Time after birth	ID_{50} units/gland	ID_{50} units/mg	Units/gland	Units/mg
3–4 weeks	—	—	503 ± 132	912 ± 153
5 weeks	1.21 ± 0.31	2.06 ± 0.30	1929 ± 311	2848 ± 221
10–12 weeks	7.77 ± 0.99	7.45 ± 1.02	6526 ± 436	4228 ± 253
24–30 weeks	9.97 ± 2.79	4.55 ± 1.04	10,472 ± 3122	5430 ± 1412

*One ID_{50} unit represents the amount of endorphin activity producing 50 per cent inhibition of [^{3}H] etorphine stereospecific binding under defined assay conditions, and is approximately equivalent to 25 pmol of β-endorphin. (Baizman and Cox, unpublished data).

†Taken from Howe and Thody (1969).

Reported values are means ± s.e.m.

and Thody, 1969) and elevate circulating levels of the hormone (Carrillo *et al.*, 1973; Thody, 1974). However, 7 days after complete bilateral lesions of the paraventricular nuclei, pituitary endorphin content was not significantly different from control values (Baizman, Osman and Cox, in preparation). Suckling in lactating rats also failed to affect pituitary endorphin content, although this stimulus has been reported to reduce pituitary MSH content by 50 per cent (Taleisnik and Orias, 1966).

There is evidence that some stimuli will release both endorphin and ACTH from pituitary (Guillemin *et al.*, 1977). ACTH release can be provoked by both noxious and non-noxious stimuli. In our laboratory we have found that both the application of repeated inescapable electric footshock over a period of 30 min, and the complete physical immobilisation of rats over a period of 3 h (a non-painful stress) reduced the endorphin content of the pituitary gland. Although it has not so far been possible to demonstrate by bioassay the presence in circulating blood of any material that can be unambiguously identified as an endorphin of pituitary origin, β-endorphin-like immunoreactive material has been identified in rat plasma (Guillemin *et al.*, 1977). The concentration of this material was shown to increase in parallel with the rise in plasma ACTH following the application of a severe stress. We have recently confirmed that application of footshock results in about a two-fold elevation of the circulating level of β-endorphin-like immunoreactive material.

Both footshock and physical restraint reduced the anterior lobe endorphin content by 40-50 per cent. The high variance of neurointermediate lobe values would preclude the demonstration of a statistically significant decline of this magnitude. However, inspection of mean values does not suggest that a decline in content occured. In contrast, after sodium chloride loading, more than 75 per cent of treated rats had neurointermediate lobe levels more than two standard deviations below the control mean value. Significant depletion was also observed in the anterior lobe. It seems probable that endorphin stores in the neurointermediate and anterior lobes are regulated by separate control mechanisms. In view of the different vascular and nervous connections of these two parts of the pituitary, it is difficult to envisage a common regulatory system. Since man, unlike lower vertebrates including some primates, does not possess a separate pars intermedia with unique neural and vascular supply, it is possible that stimuli that specifically induce endorphin release from the pars intermedia of lower animals may be ineffective as endorphin releasers in man.

We have examined the effects of acute and chronic administration of morphine on the pituitary content of endorphins in rats. Neither morphine, administered s.c. at 10 mg/kg 1 hour before killing, nor naloxone (1 mg/kg, given 30 min before killing) had any effect. Gland levels of endorphin were also unaffected by s.c. implantation of morphine pellets 3 days before killing. Administration of naloxone to rats implanted with morphine pellets resulted in the appearance of typical opiate withdrawal symptoms, including jumping, head twitching, wet shakes, and diarrhea, but did not significantly lower the gland endorphin level (table 23.2). Effects of opiate treatment or opiate withdrawal upon pituitary endorphin may be measured more appropriately by determining the circulating levels of endorphin. Such experiments are in progress.

Table 23.2 Effects of opiate drug administration on pituitary gland endorphin content

Treatment	Endorphin content, ID_{50} units per gland Anterior lobe	Neurointermediate lobe
Controls	12.8 ± 2.3 (5)	5.3 ± 1.5 (5)
Morphine, 10 mg/kg, 1 h	10.9 ± 1.6 (6)	6.8 ± 2.1 (6)
Naloxone, 1 mg/kg, 30 min	10.3 ± 2.5 (6)	4.3 ± 0.6 (6)
Chronic morphine, 3 days*	12.2 ± 1.5 (6)	4.3 ± 0.8 (6)
Chronic morphine, 3 days, followed by naloxone, 1 mg/kg, 30 min	9.7 ± 1.2 (6)	3.6 ± 0.5 (5)
Placebo pellets, 3 days†	13.0 ± 1.6 (5)	7.4 ± 2.0 (4)

*The rats were implanted s.c. with five morphine pellets, each containing 75 mg of morphine base, 3 days before the experiment.
†Placebo pellets contained no morphine. In other respects, the rats were treated in the same way as the rats chronically treated with morphine.

EXPERIMENTS WITH NALOXONE

Depletion of endorphin from the pituitary and its appearance in the circulating blood in response to certain stimuli, as reported in the preceding section, cannot reveal a physiological function as long as the target organ for circulating endorphin remains unknown. Administration of β-endorphin or of metabolically stable enkephalins is unable, in principle, to prove a physiological function, since many neurohumoral and hormonal substances produce pathological effects when injected systemically or into the CNS. On the other hand, blocking the specific receptors of a given system should yield valid information, from the resulting abnormalities, concerning the system's physiological function. Provided the dosage of the blocking agent is high enough to saturate the receptors, observed changes may be interpreted as due to abolition of the system's function. Negative results strongly suggest that the system is not functional under the conditions studied.

We began experiments with naloxone in animals even before the endogenous ligands of the opiate receptors were identified. In view of the known hyperthermic effects of opiates at low doses in the rat, we tested the hypothesis that an endogenous opioid might exert a tonic influence on the maintenance of body temperature. Thus, we expected naloxone to cause a fall in body temperature. A small but significant hypothermic effect was found at naloxone doses known to be effective in antagonizing exogenous opiates (Goldstein and Lowery, 1975).

Since analgesia is a prominent effect of opiates, we supposed that an endogenous opioid might tonically modulate the sensitivity to noxious inputs, and therefore we expected naloxone to lower the nociceptive threshold. Experiments were carried out with trained rats in a shock avoidance procedure (Goldstein *et al.*, 1976). Random shock intensities were delivered to a grid floor, and the frequency of pole-jumps was measured automatically. At low shock intensity, the animals did not jump, presumably because the stimulus was not perceived as noxious. At high intensity, the animals jumped at every shock. The shock intensity producing escape behavior half the time was a precise measure of the nociceptive threshold. This was unaffected by naloxone at all doses up to 25 mg/kg s.c., a dose above which generalized behavioral deficits ensued. In this same paradigm, morphine (2.5 and 10 mg/kg) dramatically raised the threshold, and this effect was completely abolished by naloxone. Similar negative effects of naloxone (up to 10 mg/kg) have been reported recently by Dykstra and McMillan (1977) in shock titration experiments with squirrel monkeys.

Negative results have also been obtained in humans subjected to experimental pain. El-Sobky *et al.* (1976) showed that the response of normal volunteers to a painful electric shock was unaltered by 0.4 mg of naloxone i.v. Grevert and Goldstein (1977*a*) demonstrated, in 12 subjects, using a double-blind design with saline and naloxone up to 10 mg i.v., that there was no alteration of the subjective rating of pain intensity, with ischemic exercise pain as the stimulus. Moreover, there were also virtually no changes in mood, as measured on a standardized mood scale. The single significant change observed at $P < 0.05$—an increase in anxiety—could not be replicated subsequently; it was presumably a chance phenomenon (Grevert and Goldstein, 1978). In the replication, with 12 additional subjects, virtually identical negative results were again found for the ischemic pain ratings, the mood scales, and the Addiction Research Center MBG (morphine, benzedrine group) scale, which is sensitive to euphoria induced by opiates. In a third experiment, with 18 more subjects, cold-water immersion pain was studied. The dosage of naloxone was again as high as 10 mg i.v., the order of administration was strictly counterbalanced, vials were coded, and all the procedures were double-blind. Once more there were no effects on perception of pain intensity, mood scales, or MBG scale.

Sometimes an informative experiment can be conducted with a single subject, provided the design is rigorous. We have reported such an experiment, designed to see if naloxone had any effect on sexual arousal, penile erection, ejaculation, or orgasm (Goldstein and Hansteen, 1977). The logic was dictated by the reported subjective experiences, said to be like sexual orgasm, when addicts use opiates intravenously. If enkephalinergic neurons have an essential role in some part of the process leading to sexual satisfaction, this process should be disrupted by naloxone. As in experiments with pain, it was absolutely essential that neither the subject nor the experimenter know the sequence of injections. Vials coded only with random serial numbers were prepared by a third person having no contact with the experiment. On the same night of the week for twelve successive weeks, an injection was given i.v., and the subject then masturbated to orgasm in privacy. Saline, 3 mg naloxone, and 10 mg naloxone were given, each on four separate occasions. There were no significant effects. We concluded, pending confirmation in more subjects, that the opioid peptides do not play an essential part in the physiological processes under examination here.

It has been suggested that it may require a great deal more naloxone to compete with an endogenous ligand than to compete with an exogenous one (Hughes and Kosterlitz, 1977). Recent experimental data have shown, however, that low doses of naloxone are quite able to antagonize certain effects likely to be due to endorphins. In humans, for example, analgesia produced by brain stimulation was blocked by single doses of 0.2 mg (Adams, 1976). Likewise, a dose of 0.8 mg reduced thresholds for tooth stimulation pain in subjects experiencing acupuncture analgesia (Mayer *et al.,* 1977). In a patient with congenital insensitivity to pain, a dose of 0.8 mg caused a large and rapid reduction of the nociceptive reflex threshold (Dehen *et al.,* 1977; J. C. Willer, personal communication).

In animals naloxone at 4 mg/kg strikingly increased the frequency of acetic acid-induced writhing in rats (Kokka and Fairhurst, 1977). In the experiments of Jacob *et al.* (1974), and in our replication of those experiments (Grevert and Goldstein, 1977*b*) naloxone doses as low as 0.1 mg/kg reduced the latency for mice to jump off a hot plate (a response to a relatively prolonged and severe noxious stimulus), while doses up to 10 mg/kg had no effect on the paw-lick latency (an early response to the noxious stimulus). Similar findings were reported recently by Frederickson *et al.* (1977).

Finally, in the studies of Shaar *et al.* (1977) and of Bruni *et al.* (1977), wherein enkephalin analogues stimulated the release of growth hormone and prolactin from rat pituitary (as do the opiates), naloxone alone, at 0.2 mg/kg, had the opposite effect, reducing the basal output of these hormones. Thus, an apparent tonic stimulation by an endorphin system was readily blocked by a very low naloxone dose.

At present, therefore, it appears that certain functions likely to be mediated by endorphins are indeed altered by naloxone, at low doses, whereas others are not. For those functions unaltered by naloxone, it may be concluded tentatively that no endorphin, large or small, has a significant role. We are currently investigating the possibility that some effects of naloxone may have a slow onset of action, and therefore might have escaped detection in experiments of short duration.

As matters now stand, it would appear that only intense and prolonged noxious stimulation may activate an antinociceptive endorphin system, as in our 30-min continuous footshock in rats, or our leaving mice on a hot plate until they jump. One can even argue from the evolutionary standpoint that instantaneous suppression of pain would be disadvantageous. Only after acute pain has triggered appropriate responses would there be survival value in suppressing the noxious character of the stimulus and the associated anxiety and fear responses.

HUMAN RESEARCH ON ENDORPHIN FUNCTION AND MALFUNCTION

There is an established state of the art in clinical pharmacology, the end product of many years of experience on the part of a great many investigators (Goldstein *et al.,* 1974). Experimental designs and biostatistical standards and procedures are routine. We are no longer in the Middle Ages, when simple observations and anecdotal results sufficed. Fspecially in behavioral, psychological, and psychiatric research, where subjective phenomena are under investigation, experiments that lack adequate safeguards against subjective bias are, *a priori*, invalid. Double-blind placebo-controlled trials are the *sine qua non* of sound experimentation in these fields.

It is reasonable to conduct a few preliminary trials with a new agent in an open fashion for the purpose of gaining experience and confidence, and to see what happens in order better to plan the details of a definitive experiment. If the outcome is manifestly negative, one may wish to abandon the whole approach. If the outcome seems indicative of positive effects, the conclusive double-blind trials can then be initiated. The results of uncontrolled preliminary trials should not under any circumstances be published; if the agent in question really has effects, the data for convincing publication will be obtained soon enough.

The first report of ameliorative effects of naloxone in schizophrenia was very promising (Gunne *et al.*, 1977). Subsequent double-blind studies, however, failed to substantiate the earlier dramatic improvements, although some patients did improve slightly, especially several hours after the naloxone injection (Janowsky *et al.*, 1977; Volavka *et al.*, 1977; Emrich *et al.*, 1977; Davis *et al.*, 1977).

More recently, an anecdotal report has appeared concerning effects of β-endorphin, given in remarkably small doses i.v. on schizophrenics and depressed psychotics (Kline *et al.*, 1977). The extraordinary thing about this is that a considerable supply of the rare and expensive synthetic β-endorphin was committed to an experiment that could not, in principle yield decisive results.

Whether or not β-endorphin turns out to have some effect in psychoses is beside the point here. To raise public hopes without sound scientific evidence will serve science poorly in the long run. Rigorous double -blind clinical trials require very little additional effort. We hope that future clinical investigations of endorphin function and malfunction will adhere to the same rigorous standards that have come to characterize the best clinical trials in other fields of medicine.

ACKNOWLEDGEMENTS

Some of the investigations reported here were supported by grant DA-1199 from the National Institute on Drug Abuse. We are grateful to Drs Priscilla Grevert, E. R. Baizman, and O. H. Osman, and to Maureen Ross for permission to cite some of their findings, and to Rekha Padhya for technical assistance.

REFERENCES

Adams, J. E. (1976). *Pain,* **2**, 161–6

Baizman, E. R. and Cox, B. M. (1978). *Life Sci.* (in press)

Bruni, J. F., Van Vugt, D., Marshall, S. and Meites, J. (1977). *Life Sci.*, **21**, 461–6

Carrillo, A. J., Kastin, A. J., Dunn, J. D. and Schally, A. V. (1973). *Neuroendocrinology,* **12** 120–8

Cyrkowicz, A. and Traczyck, W. Z. (1975). *J. Endocr.*, **66**, 85–91

Davis, G. C., Bunney, W. E. Jr., de Fraites, E. G., Kleinman, J. E., van Kammen, D. P., Post, R. M. and Wyatt, R. J. (1977). *Science,* **197**, 74–7

Dehen, H., Willer, J. C., Boureau, F. and Cambier, J. (1977). *Lancet,* **ii**, 293–4

Dykstra, L. A. and McMillan, D. E. (1977). *J. Pharmac. exp. Ther.*, **202**, 660–9

El-Sobky, A., Dostrovsky, J. O. and Wall, P. D. (1976). *Nature,* **263**, 783–4

Emrich, H. M., Cording, C., Pirée, S., Kölling, A., v. Zerssen, D. and Herz, A. (1977). *Pharmakopsychiat.*, **10**, 265–70

Frederickson, R. C. A., Burgis, V. and Edwards, J. D. (1977). *Science,* **198**, 756–8

Goldstein, A., Aronow, L. and Kalman, S. M. (1974). In *Principles of Drug Action: The Basis of Pharmacology,* Chap. 14. John Wiley and Sons, New York

Goldstein, A. and Hansteen, R. W. (1977). *Archs gen. Psychiatr.*, **34**, 1179–80

Goldstein, A. and Lowery, P. J. (1975). *Life Sci.*, **17**, 927–32.

Goldstein, A., Pryor, G. T., Otis. L. S. and Larsen, F. (1976). *Life Sci.*, **18**, 599–604

Grevert, P. and Goldstein, A. (1977*a*). *Proc. natn. Acad. Sci. U.S.A.*, **74**, 1291–4

Grevert, P. and Goldstein, A. (1977*b*). *Psychopharmacology*, **53**, 111–3

Grevert, P. and Goldstein, A. (1978). *Science,* **199**, 1093–5
Guillemin, R., Vargo, T., Rossier, J., Minick, S., Ling, N., Rivier, C., Vale, W. and Bloom, F. (1977). *Science,* **197**, 1367–9
Gunne, L. M., Lindström, L. and Terenius, L. (1977). *J. Neural Transmission,* **40**, 13–9
Howe, A. (1973). *J. Endocr.,* **59**, 385–409
Howe, A. and Thody, A. J. (1969). *J. Physiol.,* **203**, 159–71
Howe, A. and Thody, A. J. (1970). *J. Endocr.,* **46**, 201–8
Hughes, J. and Kosterlitz, H. W. (1977). *Br. med. Bull.,* **33**, 157–61
Jacob, J. J., Tremblay, E. C. and Colombel, M. C. (1974). *Psychopharmacologia,* **37**, 217–23
Janowsky, D. S., Segal, D. S., Abrams, A., Bloom, F. and Guillemin, R. (1977). *Psychopharmacology,* **53**, 295–7
Kastin, A. J. (1967). *Fedn Proc.,* **26**, 255
Kline, N. S., Li, C. H., Lehmann, H. E., Lajtha, A., Laski, E. and Cooper, T. (1977). *Archs gen. Psychiatr.,* **34**, 1111–3
Kokka, N. and Fairhurst, A. S. (1977). *Life Sci.,* **21**, 975–80
Li, C. H., Rao, A. O., Doneen, B. A. and Yamashiro, D. (1977). *Biochem. biophys. Res. Commun.,* **75**, 576–80
Mains, R. E., Eipper, B. A. and Ling, N. (1977). *Proc. natn. Acad. Sci. U.S.A.,* **74**, 3014–8
Mayer, D. J., Price, D. D. and Rafii, A. (1977). *Brain Res.,* **121**, 368–72
Ross, M., Dingledine, R., Cox, B. M. and Goldstein, A. (1977). *Brain Res.,* **124**, 523–32
Shaar, C. J., Frederickson, R. C. A., Dininger, N. B. and Jackson, L. (1977). *Life Sci.,* **21**, 853–60
Taleisnik, S. and Orias, R. (1966). *J. Endocr.,* **78**, 522–6
Taleisnik, S., De Olmos, J., Orias, R. and Tomatis, M. E. (1967). *J. Endocr.,* **39**, 485–92
Teschemacher, H. (1977). *Naunyn-Schmiederberg's Arch. Pharmak.,* **297**, 851–2
Teschemacher, H., Opheim, K. E., Cox, B. M. and Goldstein, A. (1975). *Life Sci.,* **16**, 1771–6
Thody, A. J. (1974). *Neuroendocrinology,* **16**, 323–31
Volavka, J., Mallya, A., Baig, S. and Perez-Cruet, J. (1977). *Science,* **196**, 1227–8

24

Analgesia, catatonia and changes in core temperature induced by opiates and endorphins: a comparison

Albert Herz and Julia Bläsig (Department of Neuropharmacology, Max-Planck-Institut für Psychiatrie, Kraepelinstrasse 2, 8 Munich 40, G. F. R.)

Since the detection of met and leu-enkephalins as endogenous opiate receptor ligands (Hughes *et al.*, 1975) several other endogenous opioids, or endorphins, have been discovered and many synthetic derivatives of such compounds have become available. There are many parallels between the pharmacological actions of the endorphins and the opiate alkaloids. Some studies, however, have indicated that differences not attributable to variations in pharmacokinetic properties appear to exist not only between these two groups of compounds but also between individual opioid peptides (Bloom *et al.*, 1976; Jacquet and Marks, 1976). Such differences might be expected, at least in part, to arise from actions at different types of opiate receptors (Martin *et al.*, 1976; Lord *et al.*, 1977). The purpose of the present study was, therefore, to compare the effects of a representative series of opioid peptides and opiate alkaloids on nociception, general motor behavior and body temperature. Results obtained during the measurement of body temperature prompted some preliminary investigations into the possible role of endorphins in stress-induced hyperthermia.

METHODS

Male Sprague-Dawley rats, weighing about 200 g, were used throughout. They were housed six to a cage, allowed free access to food pellets and tap water and kept at an environmental temperature of 22 ± 1 °C, with a 12-h light cycle. Analgesia was measured by using the 'vocalization test', in which vocalization is induced by electrical stimulation of the root of the tail, by means of a bipolar clamp electrode. The different degrees of catatonia (also described as 'rigidity', 'immobility' or 'catalepsy' by others) were distinguished according to the following criteria: a score of 1 was given if the catatonic posture, held by gripping a 15-cm high horizontal bar with the forepaws for 30 s, could be interrupted by a tactile or acoustic stimulus; a score of 2 was given if this abnormal posture remained uninterrupted; a score of 3 was given when the rats displayed loss of the righting reflex, coupled with extreme muscle rigidity and stupor. The presence of muscle rigidity was checked by flexion of the hindlimbs.

For the temperature studies the rats were carried in their home cages through the open air into the experimental room, 24 h before the start of the experiment. During this pre-experimental period the thermistor probe was inserted several times into the rectum, so that the animals became used to the measurement procedure. The conditions of this room were identical to those in the animal house (22 ± 1 °C).

At the start of the experiment the rats were put individually into open plastic boxes. Core temperature was measured with a digital thermometer (Technoterm 2500, Sekundenthermometer) by means of a thermistor probe inserted 5 cm into the rectum. Rats were allowed to adapt to the new surroundings for 2 hours during which at least three measurements were performed to obtain baseline temperature. All experiments started at 0800 h. For the stress experiments naive rats were used that had not been handled before. The first temperature was recorded in the animal house. Directly after this measurement rats received an i.p. injection of either saline or naloxone, were put back into their home cages, transported through open air (~ 100 m, ~ 5 °C), and put into the plastic boxes in the experimental room. The temperature was then recorded at 30 min intervals.

For intraventricular (i.v.t.) injections, cannulae were implanted into the right lateral ventricle, under pentobarbitone anesthesia, at least 1 week before the experiment. The injection volume, applied by microsyringe, was 5 μl. Only one experiment was performed in each animal.

Substances used

β-Endorphin (a gift of Dr C. H. Li, San Francisco, or purchased from Peninsula Laboratories, San Carlos, California),
[D-Ala^2-Met^5]-enkephalinamide (Peninsula Laboratories, San Carlos, California),
[D-Ala^2-D-Leu^5]-enkephalin (Dr S. Wilkinson, Welcome Laboratories, Beckenham, England),
FK33-824 (D-Ala^2, MePhe^4, Met-(O)^5-ol) (Dr Roemer, Sandoz AG, Basel, Switzerland)
Sufentanyl (Janssen, Beerse, Belgium)
Etorphine (Reckitt and Sons, Kingston upon Hull, U.K.)
Morphine hydrochloride (Merck, Darmstadt, Germany)
Methadone hydrochloride (Hoechst, Frankfurt/M., Germany)
Naloxone hydrochloride (Endo Laboratories, Garden City, New York, U.S.A.).
In case of salts, the doses refer to the base.

RESULTS AND DISCUSSION

Analgesia and catatonia

Figure 24.1 shows the dose–response curves for analgesia (above) and catatonia (below) as obtained after i.v.t. administration of the opioid peptides and opiate alkaloids. On a molar basis the met-enkephalin derivative FK33–824 proved to be most effective in both tests, the potency of this drug exceeding those of even the extremely effective opiates, etorphine and sufentanyl. As can be seen the steepness of the individual curves and the order of potencies of the substances to induce analgesia and catatonia are rather similar. Only in the case of morphine is the curve for catatonia rather flat, since high scores for catatonia, associated with loss of the righting reflex, were rarely induced by this drug.

almost equipotent to M

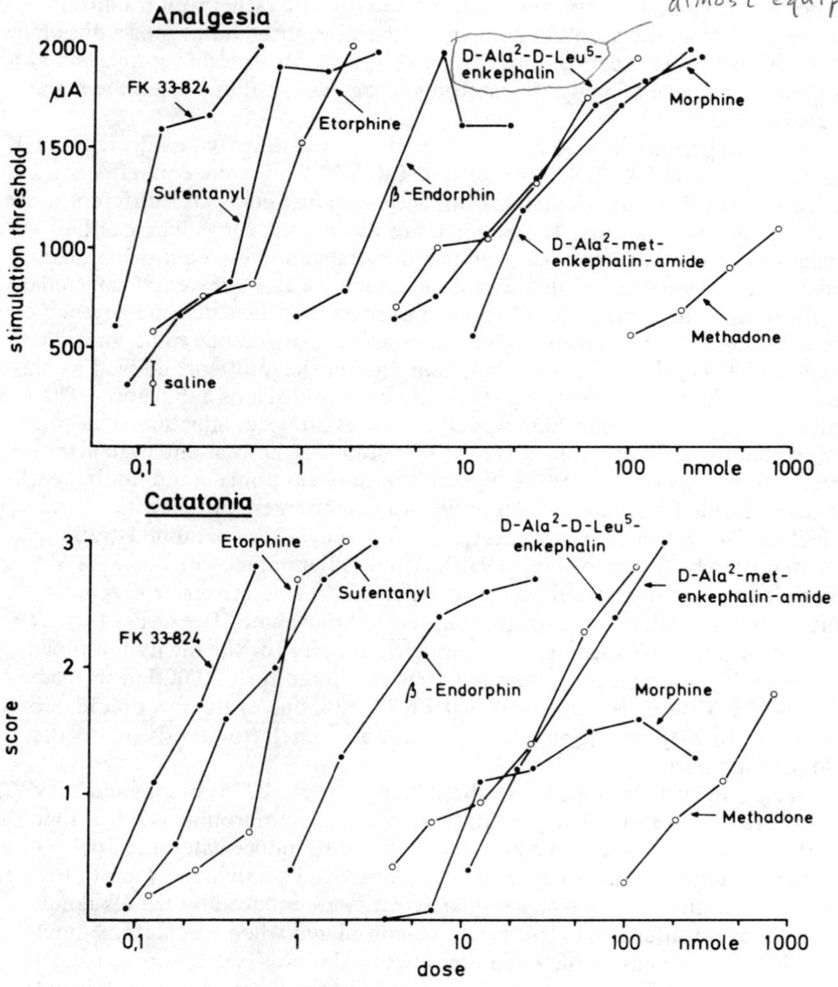

Seems to be a nice rank-order corr. bet. analgesia + catatonia scores.

Figure 24.1 Analgesia (above) and catatonia (below) induced by i.v.t. injection of opioids in rats. Saline controls normally vocalize at a stimulation threshold of 300 μA and do not fulfil any of the criteria for catalepsy. The points represent the mean maximum value obtained, with at least eight rats per dose. The time at which the maximum effects were observed was similar for both analgesia and catatonia and occurred 30–60 min after injection, depending on the substance used.

In table 24.1 the potencies of these substances for induction of analgesia and catatonia are compared directly. For each substance two different degrees of analgesia and catatonia are correlated with each other. The first quotient represents the correlation between the doses necessary to increase pain threshold up to 1 mA (threefold baseline threshold) and to elicit catatonia score 1, and the second quotient the correlation between the doses necessary to increase pain threshold up to 1.5 mA and to elicit catatonia score 2. The effective doses for induction of both degrees of analgesia and catatonia correspond rather well for all substances, although the absolute potency of the substances varies over a dose range of more than three orders of magnitude. Morphine fits into this correlation as long as the lower degree of analgesia/catatonia is regarded, but not when the higher degree is considered.

Similar experiments were performed in which the drugs were injected s.c. Of the peptides, only FK33–824 was tested. Table 24.2 gives the equi-effective dosages of the drugs as calculated from dose–response curves for different degrees of analgesia and catatonia. The potencies of these drugs for inducing either analgesia or catatonia have been compared by calculating the quotient: dose inducing a given degree of analgesia/dose inducing a given degree of catatonia.

From these dose–response relations it appears that the catatonic potency of the substances in comparison to their analgesic potency tends to be somewhat smaller after s.c. than after i.v.t. injection, in that the quotients derived by this latter procedure are closer to one than those derived after s.c. injection. The low catatonic potency of morphine was also obvious after s.c. injection. Thus the corresponding dose response curve for this drug is rather flat and even after injection of massive dosages the highest degree of catatonia could not be reached.

The peptide FK33–824 which proved to be extremely potent after i.v.t. injection showed an enormous decrease in potency after s.c. administration, as also reported by Roemer *et al.* (1977). Whereas the potency of FK33–824 exceeded that of sufentanyl after i.v.t. injection, its effectiveness after s.c. injection was similar to that of methadone and morphine. The ratio of i.v.t. to s.c. injected equi-effective dosages approached unity for the highly lipophilic compounds etorphine and sufentanyl, but amounted to 1:20 000 in the case of FK33–824. Thus it would appear that FK33–824, one of the few opioid peptides that are effective upon systemic injection, penetrates poorly across the blood–brain barrier.

In agreement with previous studies (Barnett *et al.*, 1975; Bloom *et al.*, 1976), the above results show that the catatonic potency of morphine is lower than that of the opioid peptides. Nevertheless, the ability to induce catatonia does not, as previously implied (Bloom *et al.*, 1976), appear to be a unique property of the endorphins, since qualitatively similar effects were induced by the alkaloids etorphine and sufentanyl. This has to be considered when speculating about a possible involvement of such peptides in mental illness (see Bloom *et al.*, 1976; Jacquet *et al.*, 1977). One probable explanation for the comparably low catatonic effectiveness of morphine is the fact that this drug possesses (non-specific?) excitatory effects not shared by other opiates (Jacquet *et al.*, 1976; Jacquet *et al.*, 1977). These excitatory effects could prevent the development of a high degree of catatonia.

Table 24.1 Equi-effective doses (nmol) of opioids for induction of analgesia and catatonia after i.v.t. injection

	Increase in pain threshold		Catatonia (C)		Quotients: analgesia/catatonia	
	1 mA	1.5 mA	1	2	1 mA/C1	1.5 mA/C2
Sufentanyl	0.4	0.55	0.23	0.7	1.74	0.78
Etorphine	0.57	0.95	0.55	0.77	1.04	1.23
Morphine	11.2	33.0	12.3	–	0.91	<0.12
Methadone	560.0	–	320.0	–	1.75	–
FK33–824	0.09	0.125	0.12	0.3	0.75	0.42
β-Endorphin	2.3	4.1	1.4	4.3	1.64	0.95
[D-Ala^2-D-Leu^5]-enkephalin	10.0	33.0	14.0	41.0	0.72	0.80
[D-Ala^2-Met^5]-enkephalinamide	14.0	48.0	13.0	55.0	1.08	0.87

Normal pain threshold in rats, ~ 0.3 mA.

Table 24.2 Equi-effective doses (μmol/kg) of opioids for induction of analgesia and catatonia after s.c. injection

	Increase in pain threshold		Degrees of catatonia (C)			Quotients: analgesia/catatonia	
	1 mA	1.5 mA	1	2	3	1 mA/C1	1.5 mA/C2
Sufentanyl	0.00065	0.002	0.0016	0.0046	0.007	0.41	0.44
Etorphine	0.004	0.007	0.006	0.016	0.04	0.67	0.44
Methadone	9.5	16.0	19.0	60.0	100.0	0.5	0.27
Morphine	12.0	27.0	42.0	155.0	>500.0	0.29	0.17
FK33–824	9.0	15.5	12.0	22.0	34.0	0.75	0.70

Normal pain threshold in rats, ~ 0.3 mA.

Effects of opioids on core temperature

Effect of opiates on core temperature have been the subject of a great variety of studies. Though there are many discrepancies in detail, there seems to be a general agreement that, in rats, low doses of opiates cause an increase and higher doses a decrease in core temperature (see Lotti, 1973; Cox *et al.*, 1976). The few data so far available for opioid peptides point to both hypo- (Bloom *et al.*, 1976; Tseng *et al.*, 1977) and hyperthermic effects (Lal *et al.*, 1976; Huidobro-Toro *et al.*, 1977; Arrigo Reina *et al.*, 1977) but fail to establish dose–response relations and do not compare these effects on core temperature with the incidence of other pharmacological actions.

The present experiments, by comparing the effects of opioid peptides and opiate alkaloids on body temperature, clearly showed that both groups of substances have biphasic effects on temperature; producing hyperthermia at low dosages and hypothermia at high dosages. The hyperthermia induced by both groups of opioids was independent of ambient temperature and inducable by all substances tested, whereas the hypothermia was consistently induced only in a cold environment and only by doses, which caused marked behavioral and respiratory depression. Of particular interest was the finding that hyperthermia was

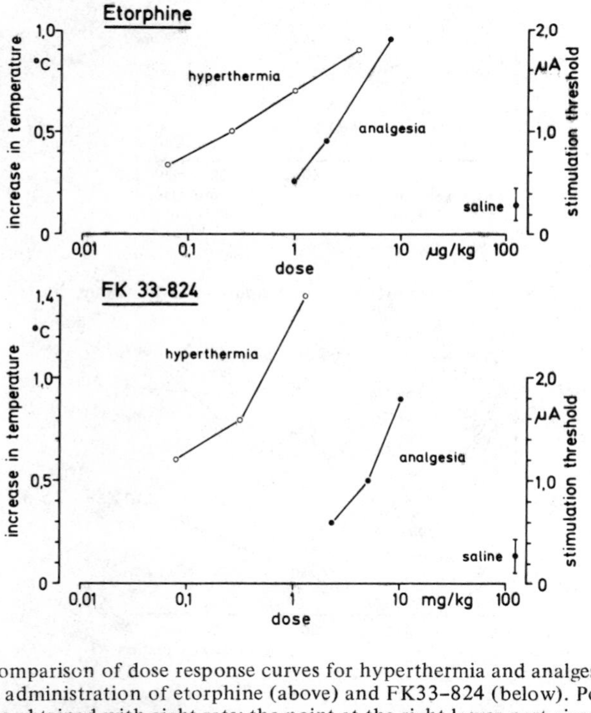

Figure 24.2 Comparison of dose response curves for hyperthermia and analgesia as induced by s.c. administration of etorphine (above) and FK33–824 (below). Points represent means obtained with eight rats; the point at the right lower part gives the pain threshold of saline controls ± s.d.; left ordinate gives the increase in temperature, obtained after subtraction of the slight increase induced by saline injection alone; right ordinate gives the stimulation threshold, at which animals vocalized in response to electrical stimulation of their tails.

induced by doses considerably lower than those necessary for eliciting analgesia, as shown for s.c. administered etorphine and FK33-824 (figure 24.2). Similar results, in principle, were obtained when the opioid peptides were injected i.v.t. In these experiments, however, the control injection of pyrogen-free saline or water alone often had a considerable hyperthermic effect, which caused difficulties in obtaining dose-response curves for this effect of the opioids.

Effects of opiate antagonists on emotional hyperthermia

The fact that hyperthermia can be induced by extremely low doses of opioids, which do not have any overt effects on behavior, suggests that this effect could be a primary one of significance for a possible physiological role of endorphins.

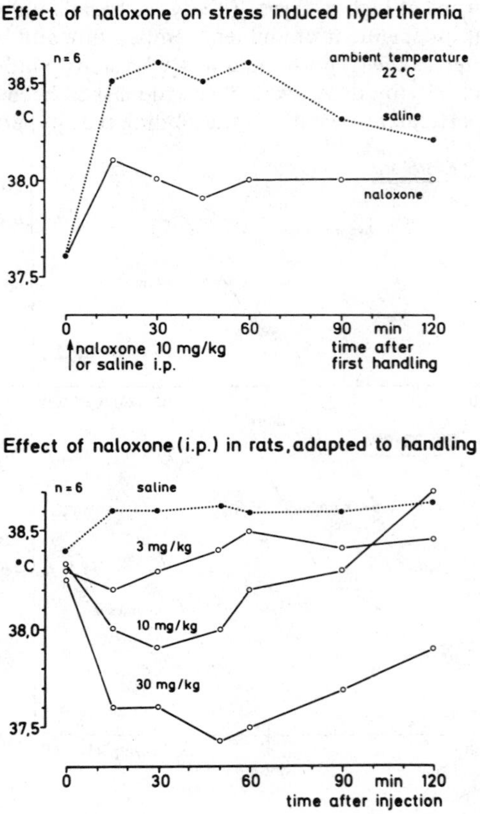

Figure 24.3 The figure demonstrates the effects of naloxone in preventing stress-induced hyperthermia (above) and in reducing the increased baseline temperature in rats accustomed to stress (below). Points represent means of six experiments. For details of the experiments see the Methods section.

The hypothesis that endorphins may be involved in adaptation to cold has been recently tested and rejected by Goldstein and Lowery (1976). In their experiments naloxone had the same slight hypothermic effect under conditions of chronic cold stress as in a normal ambient temperature, suggesting that endorphins were not responsible for preventing heat dissipation in a cold environment. This finding raised the possibility that stimuli other than cold might trigger endorphin-induced hyperthermia.

Current interest in the relation between endorphins and stress (Madden *et al.*, 1977; Frederickson, 1977; Guillemin *et al.*, 1977; Akil *et al.*, 1977) has prompted us to study whether or not endorphins are responsible for emotional hyperthermia (Briese and Quijada, 1970) in rodents. This rise in temperature is usually an undesirable effect which makes temperature studies very difficult for unexperienced experimenters.

During our studies, it was observed that the temperature of previously unhandled naive rats rose by more than a degree within minutes of moving them to a new environment for measurement of core temperature. After this initial measurement, a single dose of naloxone could partially antagonize the subsequent increase in core temperature (see figure 24.3). Furthermore, in rats that had adapted for at least 24 hours to the new environment and to the handling procedure, naloxone caused a dose-dependent decrease in the newly established core temperature.

Although the non-availability of the (+)-stereoisomer of naloxone did not allow tests of the specificity of this naloxone effect, these findings strongly suggest a participation of endorphins in emotional hyperthermia. Interestingly, naloxone has also been reported to be only partially capable of antagonizing stress-induced analgesia (Madden *et al.*, 1977), which points to the complexity of such phenomena and to the possible involvement of additional mechanisms other than those mediated by endorphins.

SUMMARY

A comparison of the abilities of some representative opioid peptides and opiate alkaloids to induce analgesia, catatonia and changes in body temperature revealed no significant differences between these two groups of drugs. With the exception of morphine, effects on pain and motor behavior ran closely parallel. Hyperthermia, however, was induced at considerably lower doses. The hypothermic effects of opioids were induced consistently only in a cold environment and were associated with marked behavioral depression. These findings suggest that hyperthermia may be a primary action of opioids, of significance for the possible physiological role of endorphins. In support of this suggestion it was shown that opiate antagonists prevent emotional hyperthermia.

ACKNOWLEDGEMENT

Supported by Bundesministerium für Jugend, Familie and Gesundheit, Bonn. The authors wish to thank Ms U. Bäuerle for technical assistance.

REFERENCES

Akil, H., Watson, S. J., Berger, P. A. and Barchas, J. D. (1978). In *'Endorphins', Advances in Biochemical Psychopharmacology,* **18**, (eds E. Costa and M. Trabucchi). Raven Press, New York, 125–90

Arrigo Reina, R., Scoto, G., Spadaro, C., and Ferri, S. (1977). Joint meeting of *German and Italian Pharmacologists, Venezia, Oct. 4–6, 1977,* Programme Abstracts

Barnett, A., Goldstein, J., Fiedler, E. and Taber, R. (1975). *Eur. J. Pharmac.,* **30**, 23–8

Bloom, F., Segal, D., Ling, N. and Guillemin, R. (1976). *Science,* **194**, 630–2

Briese, E. and de Quijada, M. G. (1970). *Acta physiol. Lat-Am.,* **20**, 97–102

Cox, B., Ary, M., Chesarek, W. and Lomax, P. (1976). *Eur. J. Pharmac.,* **36**, 33–9

Goldstein, A. and Lowery, P. J. (1975). *Life Sci.,* **17**, 927–31

Frederickson, R. C. A. (1977). *Life Sci.,* **21**, 23–42

Guillemin, R., Vargo, T., Rossier, J., Minick, S., Ling, N., Rivier, C., Vale, W. and Bloom, F. (1977). *Science,* **197**, 1367–9

Hughes, J., Smith, T., Kosterlitz, H. W., Fothergill, L. A., Morgan, B. A. and Morris, H. R. (1975). *Nature,* **258**, 577–9

Huidobro-Toro, J. P., Meglio, M. and Way, E. L. (1977). *Pharmacologist,* **19**, 189

Jacquet, Y. F., Carol, M. and Russel, I. S. (1976). *Science,* **192**, 261–3

Jacquet, Y. F. and Marks, W. (1976). *Science,* **194**, 632–5

Jacquet, Y. F., Klee, W. A., Rice, K. C., Jijima, J. and Minamikawa, J. (1977). *Science,* (in press)

Lal, H., Miksic, S. and Smith, N. (1976). *Life Sci.,* **18**, 971–6

Lord, J. A. H., Waterfield, A. A., Hughes, J. and Kosterlitz, H. W. (1977). *Nature,* **267**, 495–9

Lotti, V. J. (1973). In *The Pharmacology of Thermoregulation*, Karger, Basel, pp. 382–94

Madden, J., Akil, H., Patrick, R. L. and Barchas, J. D. (1977). *Nature,* **265**, 358–60

Martin, W. R., Eades, C. G., Thompson, J. A., Huppler, R. E. and Gilbert, P. E. (1976). *J. Pharmac. exp. Ther.,* **197**, 517–32

Roemer, D., Buescher, H. H., Hill, R. C., Pless, J., Bauer, W., Cardinaux, F., Closse, A., Hauser, D. and Huguenin, R. (1977). *Nature,* **268**, 547–9

Tseng, L., Loh, H. H. and Li, C. H. (1977). *Biochem. biophys. Res. Commun.,* **74**, 390–6

25

Behavioral and biochemical effects of FK 33-824, a parenterally and orally active enkephalin analogue

Irl Extein, Frederick K. Goodwin, Alfred J. Lewy, Ronald I. Schoenfeld
Layla R. Fakhuri, Mark S. Gold and D. Eugene Redmond Jr*
(Clinical Psychobiology Branch, National Institute of Mental Health, Bethesda, Maryland 20014, and *Department of Psychiatry, Yale University School of Medicine, New Haven, Connecticut 06510, U.S.A.)

The pentapeptide FK33–824 is a synthetic analogue of the naturally occurring met-enkephalin (Roemer *et al.*, 1977). This compound was synthesized in a successful effort to enhance the potency and systemic absorption of met-enkephalin (figure 25.1). As reviewed throughout this book, there is a growing body of laboratory and clinical evidence that the endorphins have a role in many important CNS functions. It follows that the clinical effects of a drug such as FK33–824, which exhibits the spectrum of action of the endorphins and can be synthesized and administered with relative ease, should be carefully investigated.

In this chapter we will review the basic pharmacology of FK33–824. We will discuss the effects of administration of this synthetic pentapeptide by Sandoz, Ltd to normal volunteers in Europe. We will also report some behavioral and biochemical studies undertaken in our laboratory, preparatory to planned double-blind controlled clinical investigation of the effect of FK33–824 on psychiatric patients in the United States.

FK33–824 was prepared by fragment condensation methods as an analogue of met-enkephalin (Roemer *et al.*, 1977) (figure 25.1). At position two, D-alanine replaced glycine. An N-methyl group was added to the phenylalanine at position four. The sulfur of methionine at position five was oxidized to a sulfoxide, and the carboxyl group was changed to a carbinol. These modifications were designed to make the compound more resistant to degradation by peptidases.

FK33–824 has been investigated in a wide range of pharmacological tests (Roemer *et al.*, 1977; R. C. Hill, unpublished. It binds *in vitro* to opiate receptors and has many opiate-like properties. It is a respiratory depressant and inhibitor of gut motility. It possesses potent analgesic properties lasting up to 5 hours after parenteral administration and exhibits analgesic activity when given orally

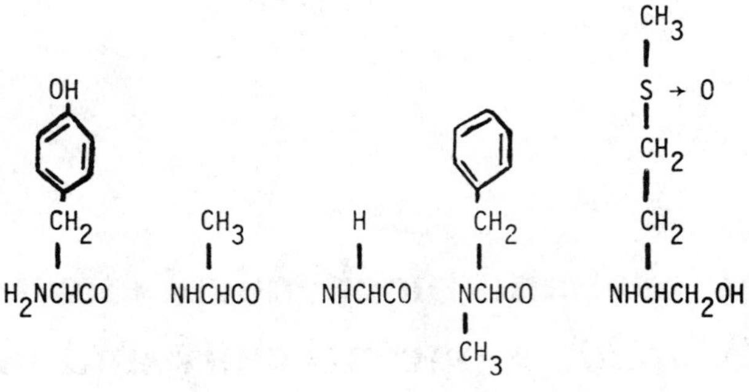

Tyr-D-Ala-Gly-MePhe-Met (O)-ol

FK 33-824

Tyr-Gly-Gly-Phe-Met-OH

Methionine Enkephalin

Figure 25.1 Structure of FK33–824 and methionine-enkephalin (Roemer *et al.*, 1977).

Table 25.1 Relative analgesic doses of FK33–824 and related compounds (Roemer *et al.*, 1977; Tseng *et al.*, 1976).

	Displacing [^{3}H]-naloxone binding *in vitro* in rats	Mouse				Monkey	
		i.c.v.	i.v.	s.c.	p.o.	i.v.	s.c.
Morphine	1	1	1	1	1	1	1
Met-enkephalin	1.67	30.3	∞	∞	∞	∞	∞
β-endorphin	0.42	0.023	0.27	–	∞	–	–
FK33–824	0.17	0.001	0.11	0.23	0.25	1	2.5

(table 25.1). When injected intracerebroventricularly (i.c.v.) into the mouse, FK33–824 (on a molar basis) is 30 000 and 1 000 times more potent an analgesic than met-enkephalin and morphine respectively and 23 times more active than β-endorphin. It is also about four times more active as an analgesic than morphine after subcutaneous (s.c.) administration to mice and rats. Orally, in the mouse, it is two to three times less potent an analgesic than morphine. When administered parenterally to Rhesus monkeys, FK33-824 has about half the analgesic potency of morphine. Naloxone antagonizes FK33-824 analgesia in a reversible competitive manner. FK33-824 exhibits tolerance to its own analgesic effect and cross tolerance with the analgesic effect of morphine. It possesses no morphine antagonistic properties. Repeated administration of FK33-824 produces a mild degree of physical dependence. FK33-824 is self-administered by drug-naive Rhesus monkeys at doses of 0.1 mg/kg intravenously (i.v.) and above. At doses below this, there was evidence that the monkeys had a mild aversion to the drug.

So far, we have described FK33-824 as a morphine-like drug. There are probably other effects of morphine that will be discovered or rediscovered as a result of the renewed interest in opiates following the discovery of the endorphins. However, it is also possible that endorphin and related synthetic analogues such as FK33-824 will have pharmacological properties different from morphine. Recent work suggesting the existence of more than one type of opiate receptor (Lord *et al.*, 1976) provides a framework for exploring a spectrum of opiate-like drugs with different actions.

FK33-824 causes CNS effects that are similar to, but not identical to those exhibited by morphine (R. C. Hill, unpublished). In behavioral tests in the mouse, FK33-824 shows predominantly inhibitory effects though a stimulatory component is also detectable. Morphine has a similar activity spectrum with the difference that the stimulatory component is much more marked than after FK33-824.

When administered parenterally to the rat in doses of approximately 30 mg/kg and above, FK33-824 produces a catatonia-like state of rigid immobility (Roemer *et al.*, 1977; R. C. Hill, unpublished). This state is very similar to that described in rats after intracerebral (i.c.) (Jacquet and Marks, 1976) and i.c.v. (Bloom *et al.*, 1976) administration of endorphin. In contrast to the well-documented morphine catalepsy in rats which is abolished by low doses of apomorphine, FK33-824-induced catatonia is reversed only by larger doses. Also, the muscle akinesia produced by morphine may differ qualitatively from that produced by endorphins and endorphin analogues (Bloom *et al.*, 1976; Browne and Segal, 1977; R. C. Hill, unpublished).

The akinetic state in rats caused by high doses of opiates and endorphins has been compared to catatonic schizophrenia, as well as to neuroleptic-induced catalepsy (Jacquet and Marks, 1976; Bloom *et al.*, 1976). There is a report of efficacy of acute administration of β-endorphin to patients with schizophrenic psychosis and depression (Kline *et al.*, 1977). In addition, there is a report (Gunne *et al.*, 1977) that others have failed to replicate (Davis *et al.*, 1977) that the narcotic antagonist naloxone has antipsychotic activity in humans, which is hypothesized to be mediated through the inhibition of endorphin activity. In view of this evidence suggesting a possible role for endorphins in the etiology or treatment of schizophrenia, there has been considerable interest in the interaction of FK33-824 with brain dopamine (DA), a monoamine neurotransmitter thought to be involved in the etiology and pharmacotherapy of schizophrenia. There is evidence (Lal, 1975) that the acute administration of opiate drugs results in an inhibition of DA effects, as measured by increased DA turnover, stimulation of prolactin (PRL) release, inhibition of conditioned avoidance, and antagonism of apomorphine and amphetamine effects. Enkephalin receptors have been identified on dopaminergic neurons in rat striatum (Pollard *et al.*, 1977) and β-endorphin has been shown *in vitro* to inhibit the release of striatal DA (Loh *et al.*, 1976). Opiates interact with norepinephrine, serotonin, and acetylcholine as well (Eidelberg, 1976). FK33-824 increases the metabolism of DA, norepinephrine, and serotonin, as measured by levels of 3, 4-dihydroxyphenylacetic acid (DOPAC), 3-methoxy-4-hydroxy-phenylglycol (MHPG), and 5-hydroxyindoleacetic acid (5-HIAA) in rat brain (R. C. Hill, unpublished). The drug stimulates PRL secretion in the rat brain (R. C. Hill, unpublished) and man (Graffenried *et al.*, 1978). These results suggest that FK33-824 may have neuroleptic-like actions.

After animal toxicity studies showed FK33-824 to be relatively safe, a preliminary single-blind placebo controlled study of its effects in normal male volunteers was conducted in Europe by Sandoz, Ltd (Graffenried *et al.*, 1978). After administration of FK33-824 in doses from 0.1 to 1.0 mg s.c. or intramuscularly (i.m.), no significant changes in pulse, blood pressure, respiratory rate, temperature, electrocardiogram or routine laboratory values were noted. Reported side effects included flushing, feelings of heaviness in the limbs and pressure on the neck and chest, as well as increased bowel sound and diarrhea. The feeling of heaviness seemed to be predominant. It was experienced as uncomfortable, reaching peak intensity after 5 min and lasting up to an hour. FK33-824 caused an elevation of serum PRL and growth hormone (GH) in human volunteers.

Because of our interest in the potential usefulness of FK33-824 in psychiatric illness, we are studying FK33-824 in several animal paradigms thought to be predictive of psychotropic actions. These include conditioned avoidance and apomorphine-induced stereotypy in rats, and behavioral, neuroendocrine, and CSF monoamine metabolite changes in monkeys. Each of these paradigms can be used to determine the effect of the drug on monoamine systems, especially on dopamine. Classic neuroleptic drugs, such as chlorpromazine or haloperidol, inhibit conditioned avoidance, inhibit apomorphine stereotypy, raise PRL levels and raise 3-methoxy-4-hydroxyphenylacetic acid (HVA) in the brain and CSF.

PRELIMINARY RESULTS

Behavioral Observations in the Rat

There is some confusion in the literature in the terms used to describe the akinetic state induced by high doses of opiates and endorphins. This state has been compared to neuroleptic-induced catalepsy (Jacquet and Marks, 1976), and has been contrasted to neuroleptic catalepsy by emphasising the rigidity (Browne and Segal, 1977; Bloom *et al.*, 1976). We have compared the akinetic state induced by neuroleptics with that induced by low doses of morphine and FK33-824.

Male Sprague-Dawley rats weighing 220-250 g were allowed food and water *ad libitum.* A 12 hour light-12 hour dark cycle was maintained. Rats were injected during the light hours, and behavioral observations were made using a modified rating system (Jacquet and Marks, 1976; Bloom *et al.*, 1976). Single doses of FK33–824 and morphine (1–30 mg/kg s.c.), and haloperidol (3 mg/kg s.c.) were administered to drug-naive rats. In another experiment, daily injections of FK33–824 (30 mg/kg s.c.) were administered to individually housed rats at the same time for five consecutive days.

The optimal dose of FK33–824 (30 mg/kg s.c.), morphine (30 mg/kg s.c.), and haloperidol (3 mg/kg s.c.) was selected as the dose which would reliably produce maximum catatonia/catalepsy. The acute behavioral effects of these high doses are presented in table 25.2. The antinociceptive effect, reflected in decreased corneal reflex and tailpinch response, was very pronounced after FK33–824 and morphine, much less so after haloperidol. All three drugs decreased the startle response and almost eliminated spontaneous motility. The most interesting differences among the three drugs were in their production of rigidity.

Table 25.2 Behavioral effects of FK33–824 (30 mg/kg s.c.), morphine, (30 mg/kg s.c.), and haloperidol (3 mg/kg s.c.) in the rat. Dosages were selected as the optimal dose to reliably produce maximum catatonia/catalepsy.

	FK33–824	Morphine	Haloperidol
Righting and corneal reflexes	↓↓↓	↓↓↓	↓↓
Tailpinch response	↓↓↓	↓↓↓	↓↓
Motility: induced (startle)	↓↓	↓↓	↓↓
Motility: spontaneous	↓↓↓	↓↓↓	↓↓↓
Rigidity	↑↑↑↑	↑↑	↑
Molding	↑↑	↑↑	↑↑

FK33–824 caused a rigid state similar to that described in rats administered β-endorphin i.c. Morphine caused less rigidity, and haloperidol much less, despite the fact that they had a similar profound effect on spontaneous movement. These observations are consistent with the report that neuroleptic-induced akinesia is less characterized by rigidity than is β-endorphin-induced akinesia (Browne and Segal, 1977). Figure 25.2 contrasts the rigidity produced by FK33–824 with that produced by haloperidol. With all three drugs the limbs of the rats could be molded. This has been thought of as analogous to the waxy flexibility of human catatonia, but was difficult to rate. In summary, the akinetic state induced by FK33–824 cannot be explained simply as that characteristic of a dopamine antagonist like haloperidol. Both the high and low dose effects of FK33–824 may be somewhat different from those of morphine as well.

After repeated daily injections of a catatonia-producing dose of FK33–824 (30 mg/kg s.c.) an interesting sequence of behavior was observed (figure 25.3). Tolerance developed over several days to most of the effects, including antinociceptive and sedative effects and rigidity. However, stereotypic gnawing, reminiscent of DA stereotypy, became more intense and appeared sooner after the injection over the five days. Behavioral activation best described as 'play', reminiscent of morphine activation, appeared on day 3 and then decreased in intensity. The changes in stereotypy and activation suggest changes in sensitivity of the receptors with which FK33–824 is interacting.

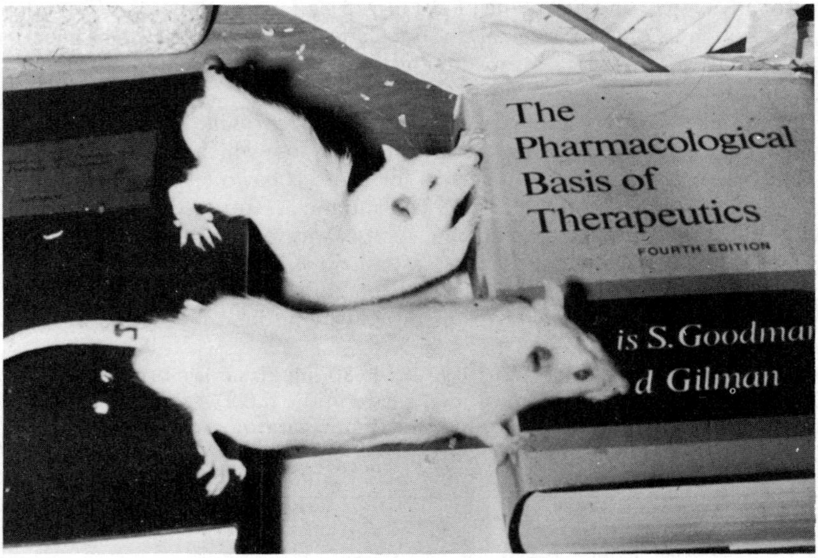

Figure 25.2 Photograph showing the difference between the rigidity induced by FK33–824 (30 mg/kg s.c.) (*bottom*) and haloperidol (3 mg/kg s.c.) (*top*) in the rat.

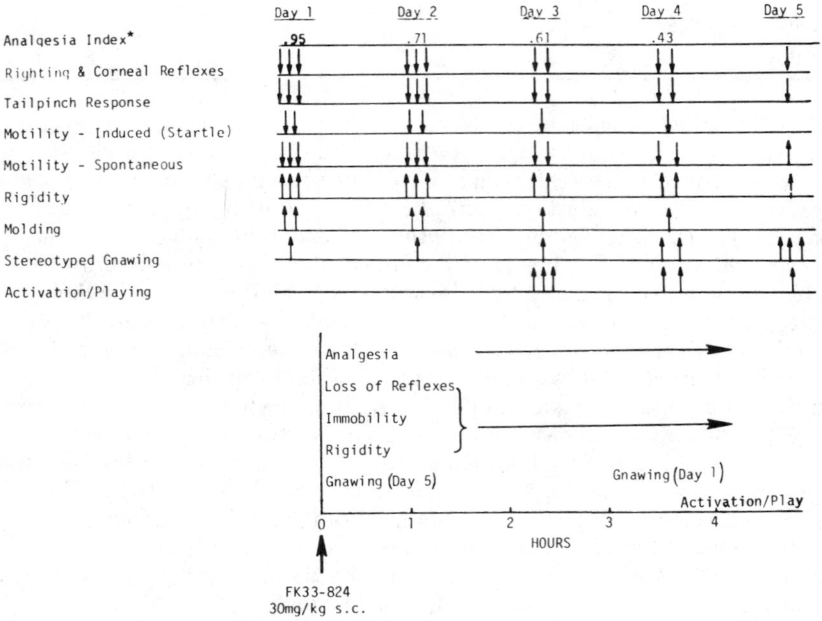

Figure 25.3 Behavioral effects of repeated daily administration of FK33–824, 30 mg/kg s.c., to the rat. *Analgesia index is derived from twice daily doses of FK33–824 (3.2 mg/kg s.c.) in a separate experiment (R. C. Hill, unpublished).

Behavioral Observations and Neuroendocrine Effects in the Monkey
The drug piperoxan has been used to provoke anxiety behaviors in the monkey (Gold and Redmond, 1977; Redmond *et al.*, 1977). Piperoxan is thought to stimulate the noradrenergic cells of the locus coeruleus by blockade of adrenergic autoreceptors (Gold and Redmond, 1977), and thus mimics the behavioral and biochemical effects of electrical stimulation of the noradrenergic locus coeruleus. Anxiety behavior is thought to be mediated via these central norepinephrine neurons. The behavior induced by piperoxan is a model for drug-induced anxiety, and thus also for testing potential anxiolytic effects of drugs.

FK33-824 was administered to female *M. arctoides* monkeys in a behavioral study paradigm described previously (Gold and Redmond, 1977; Redmond *et al.*, 1977). The monkeys had been chair-trained for one month and acclimated for another month to the test cubicle situation including i.v. infusion. FK33-824 was administered alone in doses of 0.01, 0.04 and 0.4 mg/kg i.v. In other experiments, piperoxan 1 mg/kg i.v. was administered first, and then 15 mniutes later, FK33-824 (0.04 or 0.4 mg/kg i.v.) was injected. Naloxone (0.04 mg/kg i.v.) was injected 15 min after the FK33-824. Serial blood samples were obtained from monkeys treated with FK33-824 alone for assay of PRL and GH.

FK33-824 (0.4 mg/kg i.v.) abolished normal resting behaviors such as eye turning, creating a somewhat placid monkey who could be more easily handled. Doses of 0.04 and 0.01 mg/kg i.v. had similar effects though the monkey seemed more alert than after 0.4 mg/kg i.v. All of these behavioral effects were reversed by naloxone (0.04 mg/kg i.v.).

Piperoxan raised the anxiety behavior score from a baseline of 5 to 20 (figure 25.4). Fifteen min later FK33-824 in doses of either 0.04 or 0.4 mg/kg

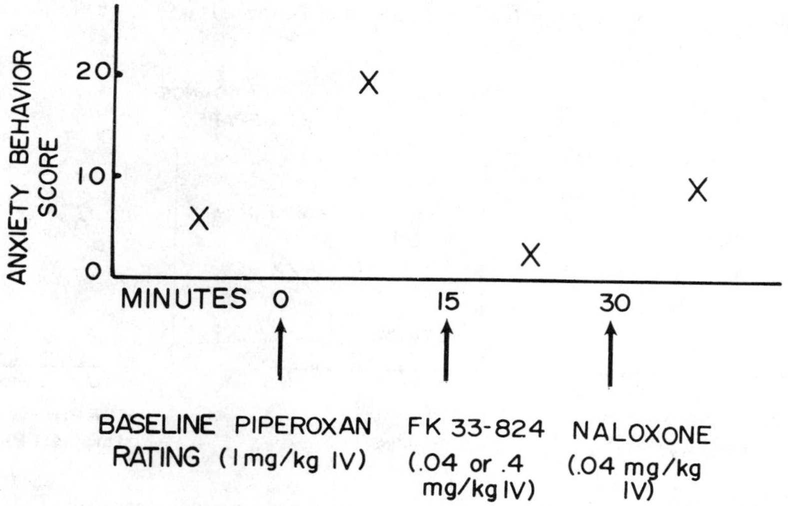

Figure 25.4 FK33-824 reversal of piperoxan-induced anxiety behaviors in the monkey.

i.v. reduced the anxiety score to below baseline. Naloxone (0.04 mg/kg i.v.) 15 min after the FK33–824 resulted in an increase of the anxiety score back above baseline to 9. The FK33-824-induced reduction in anxiety behavior was similar to that induced by morphine, but the naloxone reversal of the FK33–824 effect was more transient than the reversal of the morphine effect. These studies are reported in more detail elsewhere (Gold *et al.*, 1977).

FK33–824 showed an anxiolytic effect that may be mediated by an inhibition of central noradrenergic systems. There is other evidence also for an opiate-norepinephrine interaction (Eidelberg, 1976). It is of note that FK33–824 had an anxiolytic effect at doses of 0.04 and 0.01 mg/kg i.v., which are lower than the dose of 0.1 mg/kg i.v. required to obtain self-administration in monkeys (R. C. Hill, unpublished).

Serum prolactin was elevated from a baseline of 19.6 ± 1.6 ng/ml to 132 ± 16 ng/ml 45 min after injection of FK33–824 (0.4 mg/kg i.v.) in three male *M. arctoides* monkeys. This effect has been reported with opiates and is suggestive of inhibition of dopaminergic transmission that may be predictive of antipsychotic properties (Gold *et al.* 1977).

Conditioned Avoidance

Rats are trained in this paradigm to perform a task in order to avoid an aversive stimulus, usually an electric shock (Cook and Catania, 1964). If they do not perform the task and hence experience the shock, they then have the opportunity to escape from the shock. Traditionally, this paradigm has been used to distinguish sedative-hypnotic drugs from neuroleptics (figure 25.5). Sedative-hypnotics such as barbiturates will inhibit avoidance behavior, but only at high doses that nonspecifically inhibit all behavior, including escape behavior. Neuroleptics, such as chlorpromazine, in an intermediate dose range will inhibit avoidance behavior, while not effecting escape; that is, there is a selective loss

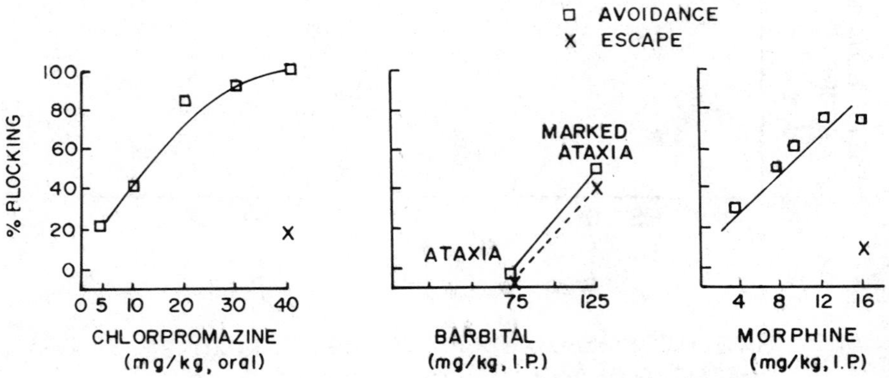

Figure 25.5 Effects of chlorpromazine, barbital, and morphine on conditioned avoidance and escape behavior in the rat (Cook and Weidley, 1957).

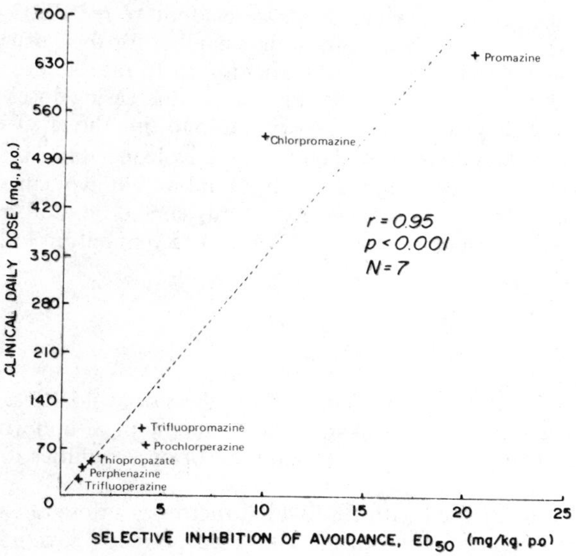

Figure 25.6 Correlation of potency of phenothiazines in selective inhibition of the conditioned avoidance response in rats, with clinical antipsychotic potency. (Cook and Catania, 1964).

of the avoidance response not explained simply by gross sedation. This effect correlates with antipsychotic effects (figure 25.6). Morphine, like the neuroleptics, inhibits avoidance but not escape in the dose range 10–20 mg/kg intraperitoneally (i.p. (Verhave *et al.*, 1959).

Methods.

Male Sprague-Dawley rats weighing 230–350 g had access to food and water *ad libitum.* A light-dark cycle of 24 hours was maintained and testing was done during light hours. The rats were trained in a conditioned avoidance task in shelf-jump avoidance chambers. Each trial consisted of three 10-s intervals. During the first 10 s the rat has the opportunity to jump from the wire grid floor on to a shelf. During the next 10 s shocks of 50–70 mA intensity and 0.4 ms duration are delivered every 2 s through the grid floor. During the next 10 s a wall moves out, pushing the rat off the shelf and onto the grid floor. The cycle then repeats. In each cycle the rat has the opportunity to avoid the shock by jumping onto the shelf before the shocks begin. If it does not, it then has the opportunity to escape the shocks once they begin by jumping onto the shelf. Fifty trials were done daily. By the second day the rats were avoiding in 98–100 per cent of the trials. They were given 5 days of avoidance training before drug effects were tested.

In the drug studies avoidance-trained rats were administered FK33–824 or chlorpromazine 30 min before being put in the chamber for their usual 50 trials. FK33–824 was injected in doses of 1–10 mg/kg i.p. to 16 rats; chlorpromazine in doses of 0.5 to 5 mg/kg i.p. to 10 rats. In each rat, increasing doses were administered every 2–3 days. On days between drug testing the rats were given the usual 50 trials and maintained 98–100 per cent avoidance criteria. In five of the rats, once the dose was determined which should inhibit avoidance but not escape, the rat was retested several days later at this same dose. Before this retest the rat was pretreated with naloxone (2 mg/kg s.c.) 15 min before FK33–824 injection.

Results

The data were tabulated each day in terms of numbers of avoidances, escapes, and no escapes. The percentage blockade of avoidances out of opportunities to avoid, and the percentage blockade of escapes out of opportunities to escape were calculated.

In 13 of the 16 rats treated with FK33–824, there was a dose range which inhibited avoidance behavior without inhibiting escape. There was, however, much individual variation in the dose required, and pooling the data obscured the effect. Data from individual animals demonstrating the selective inhibition of avoidance is presented in figures 25.7 and 25.8. The dose to inhibit avoidance

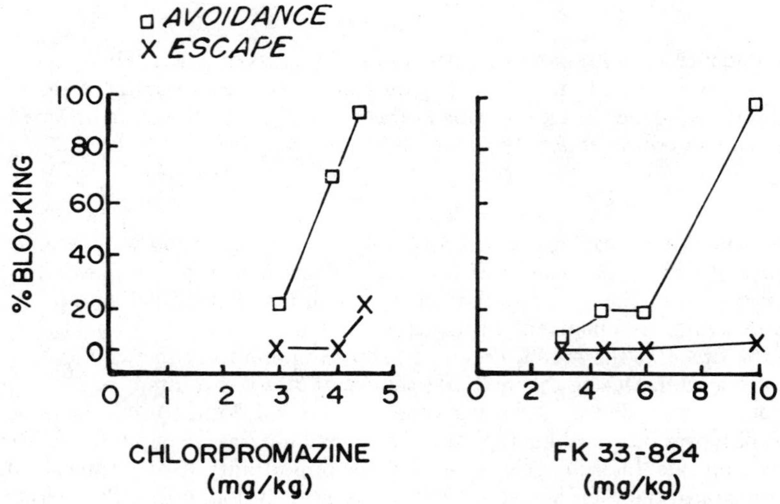

Figure 25.7 Examples of the inhibition of conditioned avoidance but not escape behavior by FK33–824 and chlorpromazine in the rat.

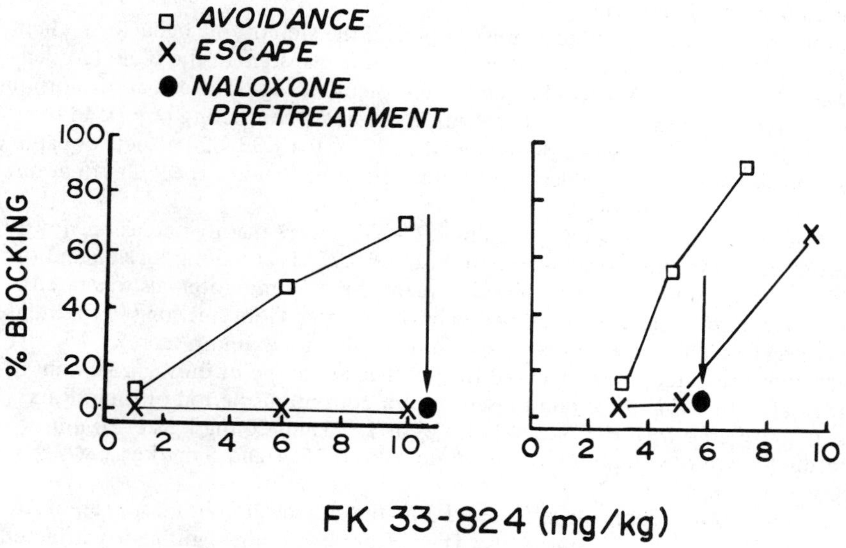

Figure 25.8 Examples of the blockade of FK33-824-induced inhibition of conditioned avoidance behavior by pretreatment with naloxone (2 mg/kg s.c.) in the rat.

selectively ranged from 4-10 mg/kg FK33-824 i.p. In general, doses above 10 mg/kg i.p. were grossly sedating and also inhibited escape behavior. The chlorpromazine-treated rats showed the same individual variation, with selective inhibition of avoidance at doses of 1-3 mg/kg i.p.

Pretreatment with naloxone totally abolished the FK33-824-induced selective blockade of avoidance (figure 25.8). Several days after the naloxone was used, the same dose of FK33-824 whose effect was blocked by naloxone was able to inhibit avoidance selectively when administered alone.

Discussion

The possible role of analgesia in FK33-824-induced inhibition of avoidance behavior must be considered when the behavior under study is the avoidance of a painful stimulus. However, the inhibition of avoidance is probably not completely explained by analgesia; the rats still escape from the shock, indicating that the shock is still aversive. The naloxone reversal of FK33-824-induced inhibition of avoidance cannot be explained by tolerance, because subsequent FK33-824 administrations in the same dose blocked avoidance.

The results show FK33-824 to have a neuroleptic-like profile on the conditioned avoidance paradigm. The ability of naloxone to block the FK33-824 effect reinforces the notion that this blockade of avoidance involves specific opiate receptors. This suggests the drug may have antipsychotic properties.

Apomorphine Stereotypy

Apomorphine is a dopamine agonist drug, and the stereotypic behavior it elicits in rats is thought to be mediated via the dopamine system in the brain (Anden *et al.*, 1967). Stereotypy is blocked by neuroleptic drugs. The effect of morphine on apomorphine stereotypy is less clear, there being conflicting reports in the literature (Lal, 1975; Scheel-Kruger *et al.*, 1977). If FK33–824 affects dopaminergic transmission, as the evidence indicates, then one would expect an effect on apomorphine stereotypy.

Male Sprague-Dawley rats weighing 200–250 g were maintained as previously noted. Apomorphine was injected in doses of 0.25, 1, and 5 mg/kg s.c., and the rats' behavior during each of the subsequent three 10-min intervals was rated on a five-point scale of stereotyped behavior ranging from sniffing (1) to intense gnawing (5). The three scores were summed, with a maximum score of 15. Behavior was rated on the basis of its presence at any point during a 10-min interval, rather than based on presence for a continuous period of time. Rats were pretreated with FK33–824 in doses of 1, 10 and 20 mg/kg s.c. 30 min before injection with apomorphine in doses of 0.25, 1 and 5 mg/kg s.c. ($N = 4$ for each group).

Apomorphine doses of 0.25, 1 and 5 mg/kg s.c. resulted in mean stereotypy scores of 9, 14 and 15 respectively. These scores were not significantly affected by pretreatment with FK33–824 in doses of 1, 10 or 20 mg/kg s.c.

There were difficulties in rating apomorphine stereotyped behavior in FK33–824-pretreated rats because of sedation. It was particularly difficult to know how to rate rats who were basically immobilized by the FK33–824 but had brief sporadic outbursts of stereotypy or 'slow motion' stereotypy, such as remaining frozen in a position such as jaws around the wire grid floor. In any event, no clear-cut potentiation or inhibition of stereotypy was noted.

Dopamine Metabolites in Monkey CSF

The CSF levels of the major DA metabolite HVA have been shown to reflect the rate of turnover of DA in the brain (reviewed in Tamarkin *et al.*, 1970). DA blocking drugs cause a compensatory increase in the activity of DA cells and an increase in CSF HVA in animals and man. If FK33–824 has similar effects to the neuroleptics, one might expect it to raise CSF HVA levels.

A 6 kg male Rhesus monkey with a permanent cannula in a lateral ventricle was injected with FK33–824 (0.4 mg/kg i.v.). CSF was collected automatically and continuously at the rate of about 0.75 ml/h, and assayed for HVA by a gas chromatographic-mass spectroscopic method (Gordon *et al.*, 1974). The HVA level in the ventricular CSF was 1680 ng/ml before administration of FK33–824 and did not change significantly in the following 8 hours (E. K. Gordon, M. Ebert, A. J. L., I. E., F. K. G., unpublished).

The lack of elevation of HVA at a dose that had an obvious calming effect is inconsistent with a neuroleptic-like dopamine blocking effect. It is also inconsistent with the PRL increase caused by FK33–824 in the monkey. The negative findings may be related to dose or failure to block HVA egress with probenecid. Data in the rat show increased DA metabolite accumulation after opiates (Lal,

1975) and FK33-824 (R. C. Hill, unpublished), though this was not found in humans chronically on the opiate methadone (Tamarkin *et al.*, 1970).

DISCUSSION AND CONCLUSIONS

FK33-824, in common with other opiate-like drugs, can be shown in a number of ways to inhibit dopamine systems, probably through indirect mechanisms. Some of our results, especially the selective inhibition of conditioned avoidance in the rat and elevation of PRL in the monkey are consistent with a neuroleptic-like profile for FK33-824. The akinetic state induced by high doses of FK33-824, although showing some similarity to that induced by neuroleptics, is also clearly different from a neuroleptic effect. To the extent that FK33-824 inhibits DA systems, it may be expected to have antipsychotic effects in man. Because its site and mechanism of action are not precisely known, the possibility exists that it might act different from known antipsychotic drugs. The anxiolytic effect in monkeys, which may be the result of inhibition of noradrenergic systems, suggests the possibility of anxiolytic effects in low doses in humans. Opiates have many properties different from neuroleptics, including mood-elevating effects, which FK33-824 may share. Most intriguing for psychiatrists is the possibility that FK33-824, as an enkephalin analogue, has properties different from those of known exogenous drugs.

To what extent the spectrum of action of FK33-824 is different from that of morphine is an interesting question. There is some suggestion from behavioral observations in rat that they differ. The discovery of multiple opiate receptors (Lord *et al.*, 1976) opens intriguing possibilities of finding opiate-like drugs which differ significantly from morphine.

In conclusion, evidence is accumulating that the endorphins have a role in a variety of CNS functions in animals and man. Laboratory and early clinical reports suggest that opiates and endorphins have effects on neuronal systems that regulate mood, thinking, and behavior. FK33-824 is a prototype of an endorphin-like drug which can be synthesized and administered to humans with relative ease and safety. We plan preliminary studies of FK33-824 in humans, both to characterize its clinical pharmacology and to follow up preliminary reports of efficacy of β-endorphin in some schizophrenic and depressed patients (Kline *et al.*, 1977). We plan to employ a double-blind design with an active placebo (nicotinic acid), measuring the effects of FK33-824 on mental status, pain perception, cognition and neuroendocrine status in psychiatric patients.

REFERENCES

Anden, N. E., Rubenson, A., Fuxe, K. and Hokfelt, T. (1967). *J. Pharm. Pharmac.*, **19**, 627–9
Bloom, F., Segal, D., Ling, N. and Guillemin, R. (1976). *Science*, **194**, 630–2
Browne, R. G. and Segal, D. S. (1977). *Soc. Neurosci. Abstr.*, **3**, 287
Cook, L. and Catania, A. C. (1964). *Fedn. Proc.*, **23**, 818–35
Cook, L. and Weidley, E. (1957). *Ann. N. Y. Acad. Sci.*, **66**, 740–52
Davis, G. C., Bunney, W. E., Jr, DeFraites, E. G., Kleinman, J. E., Post, R. M., VanKammen, D. P. and Wyatt, R. J. (1977). *Science*, **197**, 74–7

Eidelberg, E. (1976). *Prog. Neurobiol.*, **6**, 81–102
Gold, M. S., Donabedian, R. K., Dillard, J., Jr, Kleber, H. D., Riordan, D. E. and Slobetz, F. W. (1977). *Lancet*, **ii**, 398–9
Gold, M. S. and Redmond, D. E., Jr (1977). *Soc. Neurosci. Abstr.*, **3**, 250
Gordon, E. K., Oliver, J., Black, K. E. and Kopin, I. J. (1974). *Biochem. Med.*, **11**, 32–40
Graffenried, B. V., Pozo, E. D., Roubicek, J., Krebs, E., Pöldinger, W., Burmeister, P. and Kerp, L. (1978). *Nature*, **272**, 729–30
Gunne, L. M., Lindstrom, L. and Terenius, L. (1977). *J. Neural Transmission*, **40**, 13–9
Jacquet, Y. F. and Marks, N. (1976). *Science*, **194**, 632–5
Kline, N. S., Li, C. H., Lehmann, H. E., Lajtha, A., Laski, E. and Cooper, T. (1977). *Archs gen. Psychiat.*, **34**, 1111–3
Lal, H. (1975). *Life Sci.*, **17**, 483–95
Loh, H. H., Brase, D. A., Sampath-Khanna, S., Mar, J. B. and Way, E. L. (1976). *Nature*, **264**,567–8
Lord, J. A. H., Waterfield, A. A., Hughes, J., Kosterlitz, H. W. (1976). In *Opiates and Endogenous Opioid Peptides*, (ed. H. W. Kosterlitz), Elsevier/North-Holland Biomedical Press, Amsterdam, pp. 275–80
Pollard, H., Llorens-Cortis, C., Schwartz, J. C. (1977). *Nature*, **268**, 745–7
Redmond, D. E., Jr, Huang, Y. H. and Gold, M. S. (1977). *Soc. Neurosci. Abstracts*, **3**, 258
Roemer, D., Buescher, H. H., Hill, R. C., Pless, J. C., Bauer, Cardinaux, F., Closse, A., Hauser, D. and Huguenin, R. (1977). *Nature*, **268**, 547
Scheel-Kruger, J., Golembiowska, K. and Mogilnicka, E. (1977). *Psychopharmacology*, **53**, 55–63
Tamarkin, N. R., Goodwin, F. K., Axelrod, J. (1970). *Life Sci.*, **9**, 1397–408
Tseng, L. F., Loh, H. H. and Li, C. H., (1976). *Nature*, **263**, 239–40
Verhave, T., Owen, J. E. and Robbin, E. B. (1959). *J. Pharmac. exp. Ther.*, **125**, 248–51

26
Actions of opiate agonists and substance P on dorsal horn neurons of the cat

W. Zieglgänsberger and I. F. Tulloch
(Max-Planck-Institut für Psychiatrie,
Department of Neuropharmacology,
Kraepelinstrasse 2, 8000 Munich 40, G.F.R.)

There is evidence that narcotic analgesics can attenuate behavioral responses to nociceptive stimuli by direct actions on the spinal cord and by facilitation of descending supraspinal pathways which are probably serotonergic in nature (for review see Besson, 1976; Mayer, 1976; Yaksh and Rudy, 1977). Both systemically and locally applied opiate receptor agonists depressed the discharge activity of dorsal horn cells in the spinal cord of cats and rats and it might be assumed that such a depressant effect is the basic mechanism underlying the attenuation of, for example, segmentally mediated spinal reflexes (Besson *et al.*, 1973; Calvillo *et al.*, 1974; Davies and Dray, 1977; Dostrovsky and Pomeranz, 1973; Duggan *et al.*, 1976; Iwata and Sakai, 1971; Kitahata *et al.*, 1974; Le Bars *et al.*, 1975; Zieglgänsberger and Bayerl, 1976; Zieglgänsberger and Satoh, 1975). Recent investigations have shown that these dorsal horn neurons are located in a region containing a high density of opiate binding sites (Atweh and Kuhar, 1977; La Motte *et al.*, 1976; Pert *et al.*, 1975; for review see Snyder and Simantov, 1977; Frederickson *et al.*, 1977; Bloom, 1976) as well as strikingly high concentrations of enkephalin (Elde *et al.*, 1976; Simantov *et al.*, 1977) and substance P (Hökfelt *et al.*, 1975*a,b*). Therefore, attention had been focused on the dorsal horn since it may have a central role in both morphine and stimulation-produced analgesia.

The undecapeptide, substance P, may also serve as an excitatory neurotransmitter or neuromodulator in primary afferent fibers (Konishi and Otsuka, 1974*a*, *b*; Lembeck, 1953; Otsuka *et al.*, 1972). However, it is apparent from iontophoretic studies that substance P has a slow, but prolonged, excitatory effect on dorsal horn neurons which is inconsistent with the fast synaptic events evoked by primary afferent fiber stimulation (Henry *et al.*, 1975; Krnjevic and Morris, 1974; Krnjevic, 1977). In this respect L-glutamate, which has both a fast excitatory effect and a very efficient uptake system (see Curtis and Johnston, 1974) resembles more closely the transmitter in the primary afferent system.

In a previous study the actions of microelectrophoretically applied opiates on dorsal horn neurons and their interaction with electrophoretically applied L-glutamate was investigated (Zieglgänsberger and Bayerl, 1976). The aim of the present study was to investigate the action of the endogenous opiate receptor ligand, enkephalin, and its interaction with L-glutamate and substance P. Extra and intracellular recordings were performed in cells in laminae 1, 4, 5 and 6 of Rexed. We present evidence that phoretically applied opiate agonists cause a depression of both nociceptive and 'non-nociceptive' neurons. Furthermore, excitation induced by substance P is reduced by phoretically applied morphine and enkephalin. Preliminary evidence is presented that both pre and postsynaptic mechanisms are involved. Intracellular studies on the dorsal horn neurons revealed that substance P excitatory effects are mediated by an ionic mechanism clearly distinct from that activated by L-glutamate and that enkephalin depressed discharge activity without altering either the membrane resistance or the membrane potential.

METHODS

Experiments were performed in the lumbar segments of the spinal cord of 35 adult cats. Surgery was carried out after induction of anesthesia by sodium pentobarbitone (35 mg/kg, i.p.). Thereafter, during the later surgical stages and the recording, anesthesia was maintained by regular i.v. injections of the anesthetic. The animals and the recording were set up as described previously (Zieglgänsberger and Bayerl, 1976).

Multibarreled micropipettes were carefully aligned with either a glass-coated tungsten electrode (for extracellular recording) or an ultrafine glass micropipette (for intracellular recording) and then fixed together by means of a fast-setting epoxy resin (see inset in figure 26.3). The solutions used for microelectrophoresis were as follows: monosodium-L-glutamate (0.5 M; pH 8.0); morphine HCl (50 mM; pH 5.0); met-enkephalin (Serva) (12.5 mM; pH 5.5); synthetic substance P (Beckman) dissolved in 20 mM acetic acid to give a final concentration of 1.9 mM (pH 5.0–5.5); NaCl (1.0 M; pH 5.0) (used for current neutralization). All compounds, with the exception of L-glutamate, were applied by means of cationic currents; 'doses' are given in nA. The pipettes were always filled immediately before use, thus minimizing the peptide degradation (see Gozlam *et al.*, 1977). The electrodes were only used, once and then only rarely for periods longer than 5 hours in any experiment.

Cells were classified as lamina 1, 4, 5 and 6 (Rexed, 1952) as described by Wall (1967), Hillman and Wall (1969) and Christensen and Perl (1970), by studying their responsiveness to an array of different kinds of stimulation applied to their peripheral receptive fields (air puffs, gentle touch, joint movement and heavy mechanical stimulation, painful to the experimenters hand). Intracellularly recorded motoneurons from the ventral horn were identified by antidromic stimulation of the ventral root.

In a series of six animals, dorsal root potentials were recorded and excitability tests using Wall's technique (see Schmidt *et al.*, 1967; Jänig *et al.*, 1968) were performed on single fibers of the sural nerve. The opiate agonists and the antagonist naloxone were administered i.v. (2.0–2.9 mg/kg and 1.0 mg/kg, respectively) over a period of 20 min. All cats showed signs of central morphine actions, such as mydriasis and a slight drop in blood pressure which were reversed by naloxone within the first minute after the start of the infusion of the atagonist.

These pilot experiments, designed to test the effects of opiates on presynaptic mechanisms, were performed in collaboration with Dr Zimmermann and coworkers University of Heidelberg, and are part of a more detailed study.

RESULTS

Extra and intracellular recordings were made in the 6th and 7th lumbar segments, from 88 neurons recorded extracellularly and 28 neurons recorded intracellularly. The receptive fields of the neurons were predominantly located on the ipsilateral hindlimb, and the responsiveness of the cells to physiological input was tested both before and after the application of the compounds.

The main sample of neurons encountered were cells identified as lamina 5 cells (Hillman and Wall, 1968; Wall, 1967), a population of cells most probably involved in the transmission of painful stimuli. Cells located on the surface of the dorsal horn, in lamina 1, are also thought to play a part in nociception (Christensen and Perl, 1970). Cells in lamina 4 are activated preferentially by hair movement and they do not respond to an increasing pressure applied to their very restricted receptive fields. Lamina 6 cells are activated by joint movement and are, like lamina 4 cells, most unlikely to be involved in nociception. A most intriguing finding was that the effects of phoretically applied morphine, enkephalin and substance P, as well as glutamate, were consistent and reproducible on all neuronal types in the various laminae. A prerequisite for this was that the neurons were either spontaneously active (lamina 5 cells) or were adequately stimulated to fire repetitively as a consequence of applying phasic air puffs or joint movements with high repetition rates. Figure 26.1 illustrates the effect of enkephalin (100nA) on a spontaneously

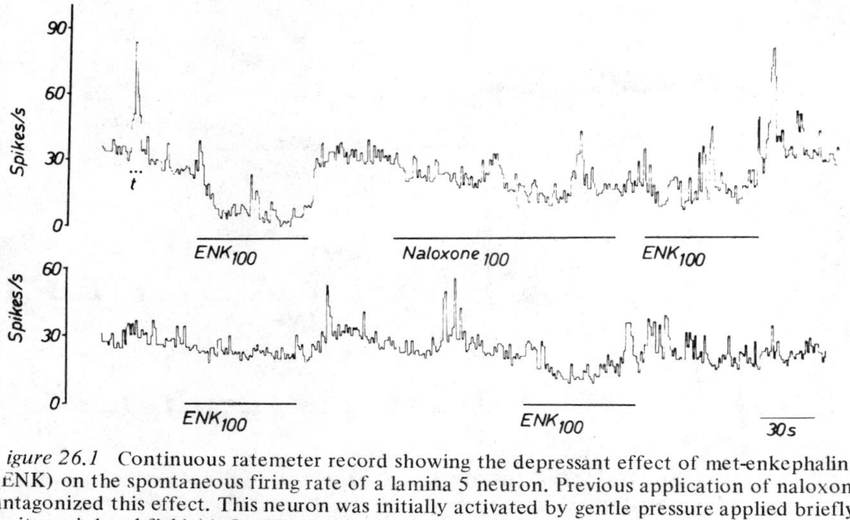

igure 26.1 Continuous ratemeter record showing the depressant effect of met-enkephalin (ENK) on the spontaneous firing rate of a lamina 5 neuron. Previous application of naloxone antagonized this effect. This neuron was initially activated by gentle pressure applied briefly to its peripheral field (t). In this and in subsequent figures the electrophoretic currents are indexed and expressed in nA (10^{-9} A). Total recovery of the depressant response after about 8 min.

active lamina 5 cell. The depressant effect of enkephalin is antagonized by previous application of naloxone (100 nA), thus indicating that stereospecific opiate receptors are involved as demonstrated previously (Zieglgänsberger and Bayerl, 1976). Recovery was complete after 450 s. In the majority of tests, enkephalin was applied in a dose range of 5–120 nA. In contrast to opiates, enkephalin did not interfere with the spike-generating mechanism (local anesthetic action) (Satoh *et al.*, 1976). In several cells the depressant effect diminished during the application of enkephalin and the neuron gradually increased its firing rate (Fry and Zieglgänsberger, 1977). Figure 26.2B illustrates the effect of enkephalin on a lamina 4 cell excited by phasic applications of L-glutamate (80 nA for 10 s at a time). Administration of enkephalin (50 nA) resulted, after about 20 s, in a marked decrease in the response to these chemically induced excitations. Complete recovery occurred within 120 s. Naloxone (100 nA) antagonized this 'anti-glutamate' effect of enkephalin.

The study of the interaction between the excitatory action of substance P and enkephalin was hampered by the occasional variable release of substance P from the micropipette. Substance P caused an increase in the firing rate of the cells within about 15 s after the start of its application and peaked approximately 5–20s after application ceased. A typical feature of this excitatory effect was the slow decay of the increased firing rate. Some neurons stayed excited for more than 2 min (see also intracellular recording in figure 26.3). The typical interaction between phoretically administered substance P (40 nA) and enkephalin (50 nA) in a lamina 5 cell is illustrated in figure 26.2A. This excitatory effect of substance P was antagonized for up to 10 min by enkephalin. Short pulses of L-glutamate applied in addition to substance P to quiescent neurons usually led to a more marked discharge of the neuron under study during the amino acid application. In spontaneously active neurons with high firing rates the responses to the amino

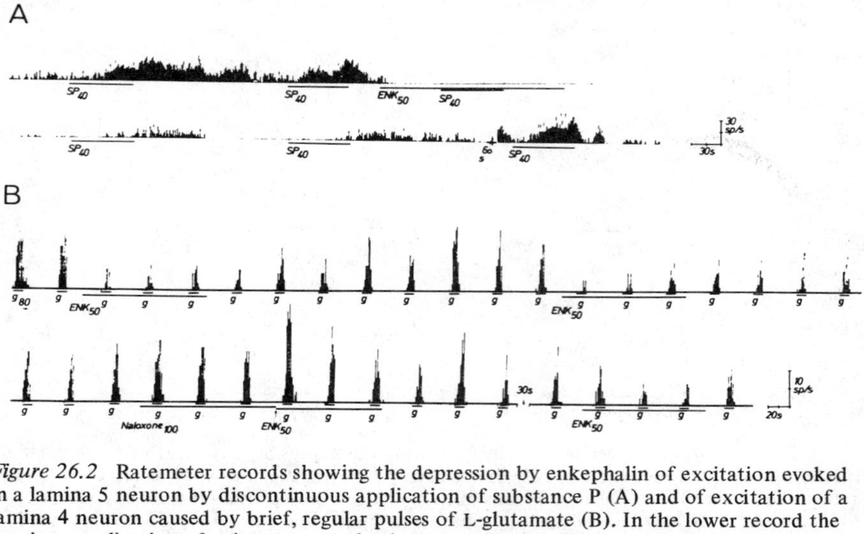

Figure 26.2 Ratemeter records showing the depression by enkephalin of excitation evoked in a lamina 5 neuron by discontinuous application of substance P (A) and of excitation of a lamina 4 neuron caused by brief, regular pulses of L-glutamate (B). In the lower record the previous application of naloxone completely antagonized the depressant effect of met-enkephalin (ENK). The applications of L-glutamate (80 nA) are indicated by short bars (g).

acid were occasionally reduced during the excitation induced by substance P.

Intracellular recordings were obtained from all types of neuron encountered in the extracellular study. The application of substance P caused a dose-related depolarization of most of these neurons with a time course comparable to that seen in the extracellular recordings (figure 26.3). Continuous measurement of the membrane resistance and current/voltage plots obtained during these depolarizations demonstrated that there was no obvious conductance change associated with this depolarization.

Applications of enkephalin at dosages which readily depressed spontaneous activity, as well as synaptically and chemically-induced firing were usually not accompanied by changes in membrane potential or membrane resistance. This finding is in agreement with previous results, which showed that phoretically administered opiates depressed the rate of rise of postsynaptic-excitatory-potentials (e.p.s.p's) without altering membrane polarization or resistance (Zieglgänsberger and Satoh, 1975).

Recent histological data suggest that axo–axonic synapses in the substantia gelatinosa might modulate the activity of primary afferent fibers by a presynaptic mechanism (Hökfelt *et al.*, 1977; Jessell and Iversen, 1977; Snyder and Simantov, 1977). A likely presynaptic location of at least some of the opiate receptors in the dorsal horn is indicated by the finding that dorsal rhizotomy results in about a 50 percent decrease of opiate binding sites in that region (LaMotte *et al.*, 1976). These data led us to investigate the effects of systemically applied opiates on presynaptic mechanisms. Therefore, dorsal root potentials and the excitability of single fibers in the sural nerve were investigated. Following the i.v. injection of 2.0–2.9 mg/kg of morphine or levorphanol, the dorsal root potentials were not detectably influenced. However, in the same animal sub-narcotic doses of pentobarbitone (10 mg/kg i.v.) had the effect on this response previously described

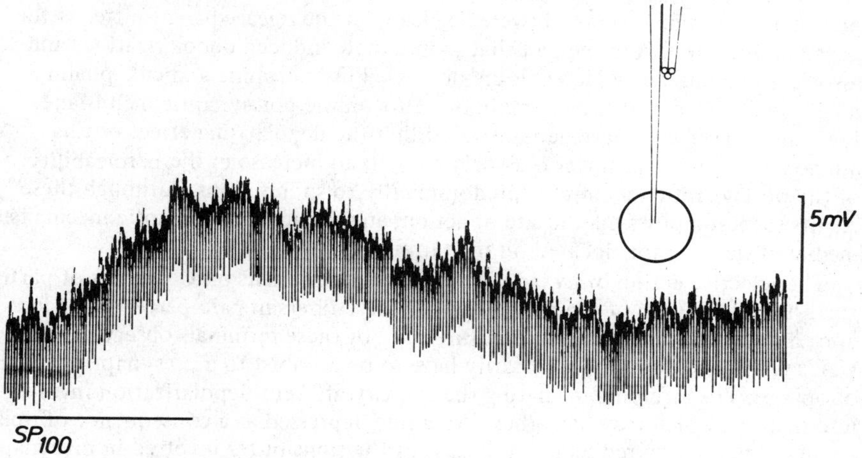

Figure 26.3 Depolarizing action of substance P on the membrane potential of a lamina 5 neuron. The regular hyperpolarizing deflections indicate the (intracellular) application of negative current pulses: 2 nA, 20 ms duration. Substance P was applied for 60 s and the voltage calibration is 5 mV.

(see Schmidt, 1977) The excitability tests showed a different effect on A-fibers and C-fibers. Only the threshold for the antidromic activation of C-fibers was increased, whereas the thresholds for A-delta and A-fibers were not detectably altered. The effect on C-fibers was naloxone-reversible.

DISCUSSION

We consistently found that all neuronal types in the dorsal horn were influenced by enkephalin, substance P or L-glutamate. Enkephalin, apart from depressing neurons in lamina 1, which are most likely involved in pain perception (Christensen and Perl, 1970), and those in lamina 5 which are known to be influenced by sensory information from both light and heavy mechanical stimulation, also had a depressant effect on neurons in laminae 4 and 6. Demonstration of the depressant effect of enkephalin on quiescent neurons in laminae 4 and 6 required the repeated adequate stimulation of these neurons by air puffs and joint movement, respectively. Data from our previous experiments suggest that the decrease in the rate of rise and amplitude of the e.p.s.p. are the most important factors in determining whether or not the synaptic transmission is markedly affected. Thus, spontaneously firing lamina 5 cells are activated by rather slow rising e.p.s.p.'s following stimulation of their receptive fields, whereas lamina 4 cells fire following fast rising e.p.s.p.'s evoked by gentle hair movement. Such responses. with high safety factors for synaptic transmission, as observed in lamina 4 cells, are not so readily suppressed by opiate agonists as those in other neurons, although the rise time of their e.p.s.p.'s is decreased to the same extent. This fact might also account for the finding that specific sensory functions involving few synapses are obviously not influenced to the same extent as functions, pain perception for example, which involve polysynaptic pathways. This reduction in the rate of rise of the e.p.s.p.'s of spinal neurons might be interpreted as a reduced release from presynaptic terminals or as a lowered efficacy of the released transmitter at the postsynaptic site. From the fact that L-glutamate-induced depolarizations and associated conductance increases are depressed by morphine and enkephalin it might be deduced that the interaction occurs on the postsynaptic membrane. Previous experiments have demonstrated that the depolarising effect of this amino acid neurotransmitter is associated with an increase in the permeability of the postsynaptic membrane, predominantly to sodium ions. Although these results suggest a postsynaptic site of action, an additional presynaptic mechanism mediated via receptors located on the terminals cannot be excluded.

The selective action of i.v. administered opiate agonists on C-fibers is of particular interest in view of the central role of these fibers in pain perception. However, an increase in the stimulation threshold of these terminals observed using Wall's technique does not necessarily have to be ascribed to a presynaptic action of opiates. The afferents mediating the primary afferent depolarization involve interneurons which may have their firing rate depressed as a consequence of opiate application, thereby reducing the release of the transmitter involved in presynaptic depolarization. Further experiments are needed to analyze this effect in more detail. It is still debatable whether descending influences projecting to both pre and postsynaptic sites in the spinal cord are important in the control of sensory perception, although very recent evidence does suggest that this could be the case (Basbaum *et al.*, 1976; Fields *et al.*, 1977).

The intracellular recordings have shown that the ionic mechanisms of the depolarizations induced by substance P and L-glutamate were quite distinct. In contrast to L-glutamate, substance P does not detectably alter the conductance

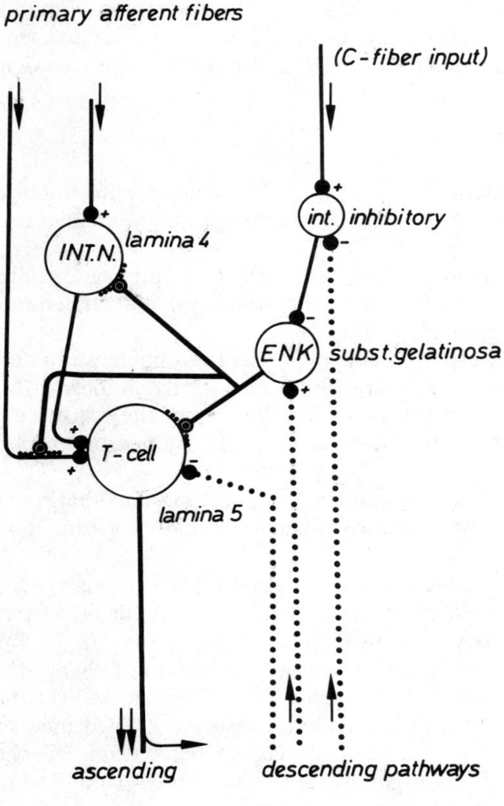

Figure 26.4 A proposed circuitry of an enkephalinergic modulatory system in the dorsal horn of the cat. This system may be considered as a coactivated switch mechanism which enables the animal to react quickly and efficiently to noxious stimulation. Heavy mechanical stimulation activates A-delta and C-fiber input which excites an inhibitory interneuron (int.), thereby depressing the spontaneous activity of enkephalinergic neurons in the substantia gelatinosa (Cervero *et al.*, 1977). A decrease in the firing rate of these neurons would result in a reduction of the tonic inhibitory influence (enkephalinergic) on taıget cells (T-cells, for example lamina 5 cells) which give rise to ascending tracts. These latter neurons are known to possess opiate receptors and also to be activated synaptically by primary afferent systems and interneurons (INT.N), for example lamina 4 cells. Thus, as a consequence of a reduction of enkephalinergic input the synaptic transmission through these cells is facilitated. Terminals originating from the enkephalinergic neurons may also exert a presynaptic modulatory influence on incoming sensory information (see Results section). The descending pathways shown may be involved in stimulus-induced analgesia and may exert inhibitory or excitatory influences on neurons in this circuitry.

of the neurons. In this instance it was not possible to differentiate pre from postsynaptic mechanisms as has been reported for L-glutamate, where it is known that postsynaptic Na^+ ions fluxes are blocked by the opiate agonists. From the close histological relation between enkephalin and substance P-containing nerve fibers and cell bodies in the dorsal horn of the spinal cord and other structures (Hökfelt *et al.*, 1977; Snyder and Simantov, 1977; Jessel and Iversen, 1977) it seems likely that the interaction between these two putative neurotransmitters may be involved in the control of primary sensory information, although we are still far from understanding the neuronal circuitry (see figure 26.4) and ionic mechanisms involved.

SUMMARY

Extra and intracellular recordings were obtained from dorsal horn neurons (laminae 1, 4, 5 and 6 of Rexed (1952)) of the lumbar segments of the spinal cord of cats.

Enkephalin, morphine, naloxone and the two putative excitatory neurotransmitters of primary afferent fiber systems, L-glutamate and substance P were applied microelectrophoretically.

The predominant effect of enkephalin and morphine was a depression of both the spontaneous and the synaptically or chemically-induced firing of cells in all the laminae studied, irrespective of whether or not they received nociceptive information. All these effects were antagonized by microiontophoretic application of naloxone.

Substance P was found to cause a slow, prolonged excitation of spontaneous firing rate and an enhancement of L-glutamate-induced firing in the majority of neurons studied.

Preliminary evidence is presented that both pre and postsynaptic mechanisms might be involved in the effects of systemically administered morphine and levorphanol on primary afferent fibers.

Intracellular studies showed that enkephalin did not change the membrane potential or membrane resistance. Substance P depolarized the majority of cells without markedly altering the membrane resistance. The time course of this depolarization was in good agreement with the excitation observed extracellularly. It is concluded that L-glutamate and substance p-induced depolarizations are mediated by different ionic mechanisms.

ACKNOWLEDGEMENT

I.F. Tulloch wishes to thank the Royal Society for financial support during the course of this work.

REFERENCES

Atweh, S. F. and Kuhar, M. J. (1977). *Brain. Res.*, **124**, 53–68.

Basbaum, A. I., Clanton, C. H. and Fields, H. L. (1976). *Proc. natn. Acad. Sci. U.S.A.*, **73**, 4685–8

Besson, J. M. and Le Bars, D. (1977). In *Factors affecting the action of narcotics*, International Symposium, Milan, 1977 (in press)

Besson, J. M., Wyon-Maillard, M. C., Benoist, J. M., Conseiller, C. and Hamann, K. F. (1973). *J. Pharmac. exp. Ther.*, **187**, 239–45
Bloom, F. E. (1976). *Ann. N. Y. Acad. Sci.*, **281**, 11-23
Calvillo, O., Henry, J. L. and Neuman, R. S. (1974). *Can. J. Physiol. Pharmac.*, **52**, 1207–11
Cervero, F., Molony, V. and Iggo, A. (1977). *Brain Res.*, **136**, 565–9
Christensen, B. N. and Perl, E. R. (1970). *J. Neurophysiol.*, **33**, 293–307
Curtis, D. R. and Johnston, G. A. R. (1974). *Rev. Physiol.*, **69**, 97–188
Davies, J. and Dray, A. (1977). In *Iontophoresis and Transmitter Mechanisms in the Mammalian central Nervous System* (Eds Ryal, R. W. and Kelly, J. S.). Elsevier/North-Holland Biomedical Press, Amsterdam
Dostrovsky, J. and Pomeranz, B. (1973). *Nature new Biol.*, **246**, 222–4
Duggan, A. W., Hall, J. G. and Headley, P. M. (1976). *Nature*, **264**, 456–8
Elde, R., Hökfelt, T., Johansson, O. and Terenius, L. (1976). *Neuroscience*, **1**, 349–57
Fields, H. L., Basbaum, A. I., Clanton, C. H. and Anderson, S. D. (1977). *Brain Res.*, **126**, 441–53
Frederickson, R. C. A. (1977). *Life Sci.*, **21**, 23–42
Fry, J. P., Zieglgänsberger, W. and Herz, A. (1977). In *Iontophoresis and Transmitter Mechanisms in the Mammalian Central Nervous System* (Eds Ryall, R. W. and Kelly, J. S.), Elsevier/North-Holland Biomedical Press, Amsterdam
Gozlam, H. Legal la Salle, Michelot, R. and Ben-Ari, Y. (1977). *Neurosci. Lett.*, **6**, 27–33
Henry, J. L., Krnjevic, K. and Morris, M. E. (1975). *Can. J. Physiol. Pharmac.*, **53**, 423–32
Hillman, P. and Wall, P. D. (1969). *Exp Brain Res.*, **9**, 284–306
Hökfelt, T., Kellerth, J. O., Nilsson, G. and Pernow, B. (1975*a*). *Science*, **190**, 889–90
Hökfelt, T., Kellerth, J. O., Nilsson, G. and Pernow, B. (1975*b*). *Brain Res.*, **100**, 235–52
Hökfelt, T., Ljungdahl, A., Terenius, L., Elde, R. and Nilsson, G. (1977). *Proc. natn. Acad. Sci. U.S.A.*, **74**, 3081–5
Iwata, N. and Sakai, Y. (1971). *Jap. J. Pharmac.*, **21**, 413–6
Jänig, W. , Schmidt, R. F. and Zimmermann, M. (1968). *Exp Brain Res.*, **6**, 116–29
Jessell, T. M. and Iversen, L. L. (1977). *Nature*, **268**, 549–51
Kitahata, L. M., Kosaka, Y., Taub, A., Bonikos, K. and Hoffert, M. (1974). *Anaesthesiology*, **41**, 39–47
Konishi, S. and Otsuka, M. (1974*a*). *Brain. Res.*, **65**, 397–410
Konishi, S. and Otsuka, M. (1974*b*). *Nature*, **252**, 734–5
Krnjevic, K. (1977). In *Substance P* (Ed. von Euler, U.S. and Pernow, B.). Raven Press, New York, pp. 217–30
Krnjevic K. and Morris, M. (1974). *Can. J. Physiol. Pharmac.*, **52**, 736–44
LaMotte, C., Pert, C. B. and Snyder, S. H. (1976). *Brain Res.*, **112**, 407–12
Le Bars, D., Menetrey, D., Conseiller, C. and Besson, J. M. (1975). *Brain Res.*, **98**, 261–77
Lembeck, F. N. (1953). *Naunyn-Schmiedeberg's Arch. Pharmac.*, **219**, 197–213
Mayer, D. J. and Price, D. D. (1976). *Pain*, **2**, 379–404
Otsuka, M., Konishi, S. and Takahashi, T. (1972). *Proc. Jap. Acad.*, **48**, 342–6
Pert, C. B., Kuhar, M. J. and Snyder, S. H. (1975). *Life Sci.*, **16**, 1849–54
Rexed, B. (1952). *J. comp. Neurol.*, **96**, 415–96
Satoh, M., Zieglgänsberger, W. and Herz, A. (1976). *Brain Res.*, **115**, 99–110
Schmidt, R. F., Senges, J. and Zimmermann, M. (1967). *Exp Brain Res.*, **3**, 220–33
Simantov, R., Kuhar, M. J., Uhl, G. R. and Snyder, S. (1977). *Proc. natn. Acad. Sci. U.S.A.*, **74**, 2167–71
Snyder, S. H. and Simantov, R. (1977). *J. Neurochem.*, **28**, 13–20
Wall, P. D. (1967). *J. Physiol., Lond.*, **188**, 403–23
Yaksh, T. L. and Rudy, T. A. (1977). *Pain*, **4**
Zieglgänsberger, W. and Bayerl, J. (1976). *Brain Res.*, **115**, 111–28
Zieglgänsberger, W. and Satoh, M. (1975). *Exp Brain Res.*, **23** Suppl., 444

27

Effects of endorphins on motor behavior, striatal dopaminergic activity and dopaminergic receptors

Jorge Perez-Cruet, Jan Volavka, Ashok Mallya, Sadat Baig
(Psychopharmacology and Psychophysiology Units,
Missouri Institute of Psychiatry, University of Missouri-Columbia,
5400 Arsenal Street, St Louis, Missouri 63139, U.S.A.)

The recent discoveries of endogenously produced opioid peptides in the brain (Hughes *et al.*, 1975; Hughes, 1975; Simantov and Snyder, 1975; Pasternak *et al.*, 1975; Terenius and Wahlström, 1975), have suggested that these opioid peptides may be involved in the pathogenesis of schizophrenia and other psychiatric illnesses. The endorphin hypothesis of schizophrenia was also supported by preliminary findings that the concentration of an opioid-like substance, that binds to opiate receptors, was raised in the cerebrospinal fluid of schizophrenics and that these elevated levels decreased to normal when the patients improved clinically (Terenius *et al.*, 1976).

There is evidence that endorphins exert profound behavioral effects in animals by producing catalepsy or analgesia (Bloom *et al.*, 1976; Tseng *et al.*, 1977, Izumi *et al.*, 1977), and that injections of β-endorphin in schizophrenic and depressed patients may have some therapeutic value (Kline *et al.*, 1977). Similarities between behavioral effects of endorphins and neuroleptics have been reported by Jacquet and Marks (1976), but recent experiments by Segal *et al.* (1977) cast doubt on the neuroleptic activity of β-endorphin. We present new evidence that β-endorphin injected intracerebrally increases striatal dopaminergic activity and blocks dopaminergic receptors.

EFFECTS OF β AND α-ENDORPHINS ON MOTOR BEHAVIOR, STRIATAL DOPAMINERGIC ACTIVITY AND DOPAMINERGIC RECEPTORS

β-endorphin injected i.c. produces marked catalepsy (Bloom *et al.*, 1976; Tseng *et al.*, 1977; Izumi *et al.*, 1977; Jacquet and Marks, 1977). The catalepsy produced by β-endorphin and other endogenous peptides, after i.c. injection is similar to that produced by drugs such as bulbocapnine an alkaloid with a chemical structure similar to opiates (Perez-Cruet, 1967).

It has been shown that methadone blocks dopaminergic receptors (Gessa *et al.* 1972), and that the catalepsy induced by methadone can be reversed by naloxone or apomorphine, but not by scopolamine (Sasame *et al.*, 1971, 1972). Methadone increases the synthesis of striatal dopamine and the production of striatal homovanillic acid (HVA), the main metabolite of dopamine. The fact that β-endorphin produces a profound catalepsy reversible by naloxone (Bloom *et al.*, 1976) indicates that the mechanism producing this catalepsy may be similar to that mediating the catalepsy produced by methadone.

Experiments were performed to determine whether β or α-endorphin alters dopaminergic activity and whether the dopaminergic receptors are also blocked. Serotonin and acetylcholine receptors were blocked with cinanserin, a potent serotonergic receptor blocker, and scopolamine, a cholinergic receptor blocker, respectively.

Sprague-Dawley rats weighing 300 g were used. All rats were housed individually and fed *ad libitum.* A group of rats was anesthetized with ether and 50 μg/rat of β-endorphin was injected i.v.t. according to the technique of Noble *et al.* (1967). The animals recovered from the ether anesthesia within 10 min. Another two groups of rats also anesthetized with ether were injected i.v.t. with either saline or α-endorphin. The i.v.t. injections were done in each lateral ventricle; a volume of 25 μl of solution was injected.

The behavior of the animals was observed in an open field or in the cages for periods ranging from 1 to 3 hours. Catalepsy was evaluated as described elsewhere (Sasame *et al.*, 1972) by placing the rat in an upright position with forelimbs touching the top of a rat cage, as shown in figure 27.1. The criteria for catalepsy were met when the rat maintained immobility and abnormal posture for more than 2 min.

The effects of endorphins on dopamine metabolism were studied by measuring the concentration of striatal HVA in rats receiving i.v.t. injections of saline, β or α-endorphin. Animals were killed by decapitation 1 hour after treatment and the brains were quickly removed and dissected. The basal ganglia from two rats were pooled and HVA was analyzed as described elsewhere (Perez-Cruet *et al.*, 1972).

In a third experiment rats received i.v.t. injections of β-endorphin in a dose of 50 to 100 μg/rat in order to produce a clear-cut cataleptic state as described previously. This endorphin catalepsy was treated with i.p. injections of naloxone (5 mg/kg), cinanserin (25 mg/kg), apomorphine (a dopamine agonist) (10 mg/kg) or scopolamine (5 mg/kg). The rats were observed for at least 2 hours after treatment with these drugs.

The results of i.v.t. injections of β and α-endorphins in the rat are summarized in Table 27.1. β-endorphin produced a marked catalepsy lasting at least 2 hours. Neither saline nor α-endorphin injected i.v.t. produced any evidence of catalepsy. These results are in agreement with the findings of Bloom *et al.* (1976) and others, that the i.c. injection of β-endorphin produces profound behavioral effects.

Table 27.2 shows the effects of α and β-endorphins after i.v.t. injection on the concentration of striatal HVA. A significant ($P < 0.001$) 59 per cent increase in

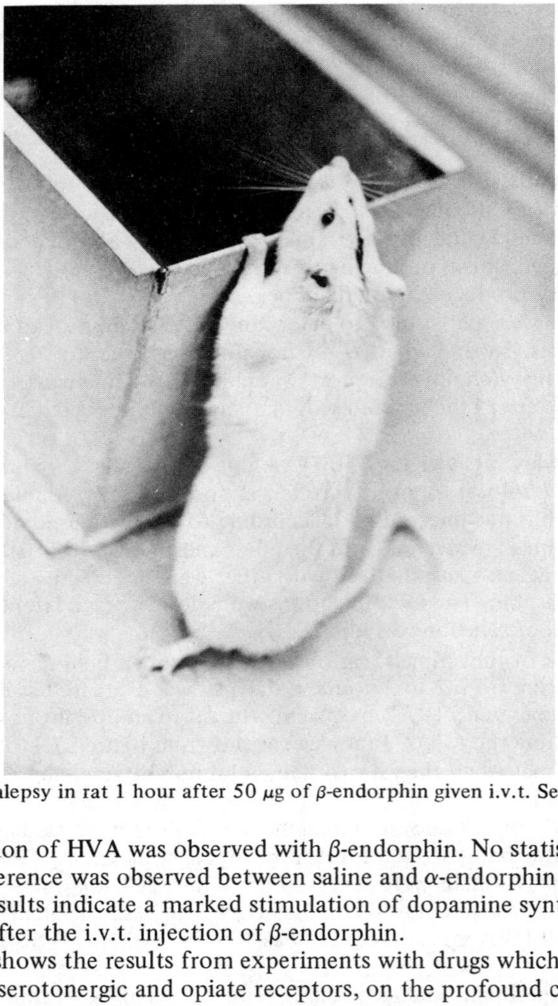

Figure 27.1 Catalepsy in rat 1 hour after 50 μg of β-endorphin given i.v.t. See text for explanation.

the concentration of HVA was observed with β-endorphin. No statistically significant difference was observed between saline and α-endorphin on striatal HVA. These results indicate a marked stimulation of dopamine synthesis in striatal tissue after the i.v.t. injection of β-endorphin.

Table 27.3 shows the results from experiments with drugs which intereact with dopaminergic, serotonergic and opiate receptors, on the profound catalepsy produced by β-endorphin; only naloxone and apomorphine blocked the catalepsy. Saline and scopolamine had no effect on the immobility state, but cinanserin prolonged and intensified the catalepsy. Rats treated with apomorphine, in addition to the blockade of the catalepsy, showed marked stereotype behavior such as chewing, as well as episodes of sudden jumping which we call the 'pop corn effect'.

DISCUSSION AND SUMMARY

If an actual relationship between endorphins and mental illnesses exists, it is possible that other approaches may be needed. The analytical measurement and quantitation of endorphins after opiate antagonist treatment in human cerebro-

Table 27.1 Catalepsy in rats after intraventricular injection of saline, β or α-endorphin

Condition	Dose	*N*	Time elapsed after injection 15 min	30 min	45 min	60 min
Saline	25 μl	6	0	0	0	0
β-Endorphin	50 μg	6	6	6	6	6
α-Endorphin	50 μg	6	0	0	0	0

Intraventricular injection was done bilaterally with a volume of 25 μl according to Noble *et al.* (1967).

Table 27.2 Effects of β and α-endorphins on concentration of HVA in corpora striata in rats

Condition	*N*	Striatal HVA (μg/g ± s.d.)
Saline	8	1.12 ± 0.30
β-Endorphin	6	1.78 ± 0.30*
α-Endorphin	4	0.91 ± 0.10 N.S.

Striatal HVA was determined from pools of basal ganglia from two rats. Rats were killed 1 h after i.v.t. injection. Data was analyzed using Student's *t* test.
$^*P < 0.001$
N.S., not significant.

Table 27.3 Effects of apomorphine, cinanserin, scopolamine, and naloxone on catalepsy induced by β-endorphin

Condition	Dose (mg/kg)	Fraction of cataleptic rats at various time intervals 15 min	30 min	60 min	120 min
Saline	None	6/6	6/6	6/6	6/6
Apomorphine	10 mg/kg	4/6	0/6	0/6	0/6
Cinanserin	25 mg/kg	6/6	6/6	6/6	6/6
Scopolamine	5 mg/kg	6/6	6/6	6/6	6/6
Naloxone	5 mg/kg	0/6	0/6	0/6	0/6

Rats were made cataleptic by injecting 50–100 μg β-endorphin i.v.t. Drugs were injected i.p. 30 min after the onset of catalepsy.

spinal fluid (CSF) may be useful. It is conceivable that the study of endorphin levels in CSF could help in the classification of psychological subtypes of schizophrenia.

The fact that naloxone blocks the catalepsy induced in rats by the i.v.t. injection of β-endorphin suggests that the endorphin catalepsy is mediated by opiate receptors. However, an additional interpretation is needed because we have found that β-endorphin also blocks dopaminergic receptors and apomorphine produces reversal of the endorphin catalepsy. The discovery that β-endorphin blocks dopaminergic receptors opens new vistas on the interaction between these peptides and monoamines. It is unlikely that serotonergic receptor mechanisms are involved in the reversal, since their blockade with cinanserin worsened the endorphin catalepsy. Since scopolamine did not have any effect on the catalepsy, it is unlikely that cholinergic mechanisms are involved.

It is possible that β-endorphin has some atypical neuroleptic activity produced by blocking dopaminergic receptors and stimulating opiate receptors. On the basis of these preliminary observations, it is possible to speculate that catalepsy due to β-endorphin is due to a dopamine receptor blockade coupled with a stimulation of the opiate receptor. We should like to propose that the catalepsy produced by opiates may be produced by stimulation of opiate receptors and blockade of catecholaminergic receptors.

REFERENCES

Bloom, F., Segal, D., Ling, N. and Guillemin, R. (1976). *Science*, **194**, 630

Gessa, G. L., DiChiara G., Tagliamonte, A. and Pérez-Cruet, J. (1972). *Proc. 5th Intern. Congr. Pharmacol.* (Free abstracts) San Francisco, p. 77

Hughes, J. (1975). *Brain Res.*, **88**, 295–308

Hughes, J., Smith, T. W., Kosterlitz, H. W., Fothergill, L. A., Morgan, B. A. and Morris, H. R. (1975). *Nature.* **258**, 577–9

Izumi, K., Motomatsu, T., Chretien, M., Butterworth, R. F., Lis, M., Seidah, N. and Barbeau, A. (1977). *Life Sci.*, **20**, 1149

Jacquet, Y. F. and Marks, N. (1976). *Science,* **198**, 411–4

Kline, N. S., Li, C. H., Lehmann, H. E., Lajtha, A., Laski, E. and Cooper, T. (1977). *Archs gen. Psychiat.*, **34**, 1111–3

Noble, E. E., Wurtman, J. and Axelrod, J. (1967). *Life Sci.*, **6**, 281–91

Pasternak, G. W., Goodman, R. and Snyder, S. H. (1975). *Life Sci.*, **16**, 1765

Pérez-Cruet, J., DiChiara, G., Gessa, G. L. (1972). *Experientia,* **28**, 926–7

Pérez-Cruet, J. (1967). *Proc 5th Int. Congr. Neuropharmacol.* (Ed. Brill, H.) Excerpta Medica, p. 912–7

Sasame, H. A., Pérez-Cruet, J., DiChiara, G., Tagliamonte, A., Tagliamonte, P. and Gessa, G. L. (1971). *Riv. di Farmacol. e Terap.*, **11**, 99–105

Sasame, H. A., Pérez-Cruet, J., DiChiara, G., Tagliamonte, A., Tagliamonte, P. and Gessa, G. L. (1972). *J. Neurochem.*, **19**, 1953–7

Segal, D. S., Browne, R. G., Bloom, F., Ling, N. and Guillemin, R. (1977). *Science*, **198**, 411–4

Simantov, R. and Snyder, S. H. (1975) *Proc. natn. Acad. Sci. U.S.A.*, **73**, 2515–9

Terenius, L. and Wahlström, A. (1975). *Acta physiol. scand.*, **94**, 74–81

Terenius, L., Wahlström, A., Lindstrom, E. and Widerlov E. (1976). *Neurosci. Lett.*, **3**, 157–62

Tseng, L. F., Loh, H. H., and Li, C. H. (1977). *Biochem. biophys. Res. Commun.*, **74**, 390

28
Characteristics of β-endorphin-induced behavioral activation and immobilization

David S. Segal, Ronald G. Browne, Amy Arnsten and David C. Derrington (Department of Psychiatry, School of Medicine, University of California, San Diego, La Jolla, California 92093, U.S.A.)
Floyd E. Bloom, Arthur V. Davis (Center for Behavioral Neurobiology, Salk Institute, San Diego, California 92112, U.S.A.)
Roger Guillemin and Nicholas Ling (Laboratory of Neuroendocrinology, Salk Institute, San Diego, California 92112 U.S.A.)

β-endorphin produces a broad spectrum of dose- and time-related behavioral effects, ranging from hyperactivity to rigid immobility (Bloom *et al.*, 1976; Segal *et al.*, 1977). Our efforts to characterize further these effects and to compare them with the behavioral actions of opiates are described below.

BEHAVIORAL ACTIVATING EFFECTS OF OPIATES AND OPIOID PEPTIDES

Biphasic alterations in locomotion induced by opiates and opioid peptides

Opiates

Rats have been shown to respond to opiates with a characteristic biphasic alteration in locomotor activity (Domino *et al.*, 1976). We have observed a similar response pattern after injection of methadone, etonitazene or morphine (table 28.1). For these studies, adult, male Wistar rats (350–400 g) were habituated to the experimental chambers for at least 24 hours before s.c. administration of the opiates. Locomotion in the form of crossovers and rearings was then monitored for 4 hours.

In comparison to the effects of saline, methadone at doses of 1.0 mg/kg or greater, significantly reduced crossovers and rearings for the first hour after injection and stimulated both measures of locomotion during the subsequent 3 hours. An initial depression and subsequent increase in locomotor activity

Table 28.1 Biphasic alterations in locomotion induced by opiates

			Hour 1		Hours 2–4	
Treatment (s.c.)	Dose	*N*	Crossovers	Rearings	Crossovers	Rearings
Saline	1.0 ml/kg	15	22 ± 2	14 ± 1	9 ± 2	2 ± 1
Methadone (mg/kg)	0.25	5	28 ± 9	18 ± 5	9 ± 3	3 ± 1
	0.5	5	41 ± 12	17 ± 3	28 ± 8***	6 ± 2
	1.0	11	13 ± 5	7 ± 2***	34 ± 10***	14 ± 4***
	2.5	5	1 ± 1***	1 ± 1***	45 ± 10***	15 ± 4***
Etonitazene (μg/kg)	0.5	5	29 ± 8	15 ± 2	11 ± 5	2 ± 1
	1.0	5	38 ± 13	14 ± 3	10 ± 5	3 ± 1
	2.5	10	16 ± 6	7 ± 2**	19 ± 6**	9 ± 4*
	5.0	5	5 ± 1***	3 ± 1***	39 ± 13***	14 ± 6***
Morphine (mg/kg)	1.0	5	17 ± 5	11 ± 4	26 ± 6***	11 ± 3***
	2.5	5	12 ± 2***	5 ± 2***	42 ± 5***	7 ± 2
	5.0	10	4 ± 1***	2 ± 1***	38 ± 8***	3 ± 1
	10.0	5	1 ***	0 ***	62 ± 9***	6 ± 1

Values are mean (± s.e.m.). Significant differences from control values are indicated, *$P < 0.05$, **$P < 0.02$, ***$P < 0.01$ (two-tailed *t*-test).

Table 28.2 Biphasic alterations in locomotion produced by β-endorphin and related substances

Treatment (i.v.t.)	Dose (μg/10 μl)	*N*	Hour 1		Hours 2–4	
			Crossovers	Rearings	Crossovers	Rearings
Saline	10.0 μl	12	55 ± 8	27 ± 5	16 ± 5	3 ± 1
β-Endorphin	1.0	5	46 ± 9	14 ± 5	53 ± 8***	8 ± 4
	2.5	10	27 ± 9*	6 ± 2***	93 ± 22***	19 ± 5***
	5.0	13	36 ± 12	3 ± 1***	140 ± 26***	32 ± 11*
D-Ala^2-Met^5.NH_2	10.0	4	67 ± 8	7 ± 5*	63 ± 15***	7 ± 4
D-Met^2-Pro^5.NH_2	1.0	4	10 ± 2**	0.5 ± 0.3***	113 ± 18***	8 ± 4

Values are mean (± s.e.m.). Significant differences from control values are indicated, *$P < 0.05$, **$P < 0.02$, ***$P < 0.01$ (two-tailed *t*-test).

Table 28.3 Effects of naloxone on β-endorphin-induced alterations in locomotion

Treatment	*N*	Hour 1		Hours 2–4	
		Crossovers	Rearings	Crossovers	Rearings
Saline	12	55 ± 8	27 ± 5	16 ± 5	3 ± 1
β-endorphin (2.5 μg/10 μl)	10	27 ± 9*	6 ± 2†	93 ± 22†	19 ± 5†
Naloxone (5 mg/kg, s.c.) + β-Endorphin (2.5 μg/10 μl)	5	62 ± 18	31 ± 12	26 ± 11	4 ± 2

Values are mean (± s.e.m.). Naloxone was injected s.c. 15 min before i.v.t. administration of β-endorphin.
Significant differences from control values are indicated: *$P < 0.05$, †$P < 0.01$ (two-tailed *t*-test).

Table 28.4 Rigidity induced by i.v.t. administration of opioid peptides

Treatment	Dose (μg/10 μl)	*N*	Rigidity 0–4	Righting reflex (10 s)	Vertical grid (0–3)
Saline	10 μl	13	0	+	0
β_p-Endorphin	2.5	4	0	–	0
	5.0	19	2.0 ± 0.2	–	Slides
	10.0	12	2.8 ± 0.3	–	Slides
	25.0	4	3.5 ± 0.5	–	Slides
	50.0	43	3.7 ± 0.1	–	Slides
	100.0	4	4.0	–	Slides
	150.0	3	4.0	–	Slides
	300.0	5	4.0	–	Slides
β_h-Endorphin	50.0	3	3.6 ± 0.3	–	Slides
D-Met^2-Pro^5.NH_2	25.0	3	4.0	–	Slides
D-Ala^2-Met^5.NH_2	50.0	5	1.6 ± 0.2	–	Slides

The rigidity score represents a composite measure derived from three tests: (1) stiffness, assessed during handling (scored 0–3); (2) trunk rigidity, based on the time (up to 4 s) that the animals remained in an upright posture when held above the knee joints of the hind limbs (scored 0–4); and (3) bridge test, a positive score assigned when the animal remained self-supporting for 10 s when placed across metal bookends. A minus righting reflex was designated when the rat stayed in a supine position for 10 s. The vertical grid was scored on a 0–3 scale, based on the time (up to 60 s) that the rat remained immobile on the grid. Values (expressed as mean ± s.e.m.) indicate peak effects after injection. β_p-synthetic porcine β-endorphin; β_h-synthetic human β-endorphin.

were also exhibited by rats injected with doses as low as 2.5 μg/kg of etonitazene or 2.5 mg/kg of morphine. With all three opiates increasing the dose resulted in a progressively greater and longer depression; locomotion during the stimulant phase also showed a dose-dependent increase in magnitude and duration. Both components of the response pattern were antagonized by naloxone, in agreement with the findings of Domino *et al.* (1976).

Opioid peptides

A similar biphasic pattern of locomotion resulted with i.v.t. infusion of β-endorphin, [D-Ala^2-Met^5]-enkephalinamide (D-Ala^2-Met^5.NH_2), or [D-Met^2-Pro^5]-enkephalinamide (D-Met^2-Pro^5.NH_2) (table 28.2). During the first hour after infusion of β-endorphin, locomotion (as reflected primarily in the rearing measure) was reduced in a dose-dependent manner. Similarly, 10 μg of D-Ala^2-Met^5.NH_2 produced a significant decrease in rearings during this initial interval, and 1 μg of D-Met^2-Pro^5.NH_2 markedly reduced both measures of locomotion. Videotape monitoring revealed that during the period of reduced activity the locomotion of many animals was interrupted by recurrent episodes of wet-dog shaking and immobility, the rats often remaining motionless in a standing or rearing position for up to 15-min intervals.

Following the depression of behavior, all three opioid peptides significantly enhanced locomotion during the second through fourth hours after infusion. We also found that biphasic behavioral effects resulted after s.c. administration with doses of D-Met^2-Pro^5.NH$_2$ as low as 2.5 mg/kg. Pretreatment with naloxone (5 mg/kg s.c.) antagonized both the depression and stimulation of locomotor activity produced by i.v.t. infusion of 2.5 μg β-endorphin (table 28.3).

With the higher doses of the opiates or opioid peptides the rigid immobility phase (table 28.4) is followed by a period of motor activation in which oral stereotypy is a prominent feature. Both the locomotion and stereotypy produced by 50 μg of β-endorphin i.v.t. or by 7.5 mg/kg of methadone s.c. were antagonized by injection with either haloperidol (0.5 mg/kg s.c.) or naloxone (0.1 mg/kg s.c.). These results suggest that opiates and opioid peptides may exert their behavioral activating effects through a common mechanism.

Opiate and opioid peptide-induced locomotion in mice

Opiates

In contrast to the biphasic effects in rats, many strains of mice have been shown to respond to systemic administration of opiates, over a wide range of doses, with enhanced locomotor activity (Kuschinsky and Hornykiewicz, 1974; Shuster *et al.*, 1975; Brase *et al.*, 1977). Similarly, we have found that mice exhibit a dose-related increase in locomotion after i.v. injection of morphine, methadone or etonitazene. For these studies, male Swiss-Webster mice (25–35 g) were habituated to the experimental chambers for 1 hour before injection. Locomotor activity was significantly enhanced after injection with doses as low as 5 mg/kg morphine, 5 mg/kg methadone or 10 μg/kg etonitazene (figure 28.1). The increased activity appeared within 1 min after injection and was characterized by perseverative running close to the walls of the chamber. In addition, mice responded to all three opiates with tail elevations. Both these actions were prevented by naloxone. Figure 28.2 shows that pretreatment with naloxone (5 mg/kg s.c.) blocked the locomotor activating effects of methadone (5 mg/kg i.v.).

Opioid Peptides

Some evidence indicates that i.v. administration of β-endorphin produces behavioral effects in experimental animals and humans (Tseng *et al.*, 1976; Kline *et al.*, 1977). Therefore, we examined the response of mice to β-endorphin and D-Met^2-Pro^5.NH$_2$ to determine whether these peptides induce an opiate-like enhancement of motility. As with the opiates, i.v. injection of D-Met^2-Pro^5.NH$_2$ resulted in a dose-related increase in stereotyped locomotion (figure 28.3); D-Met^2-Pro^5.NH$_2$ also elicited tail erections. In contrast to the effects of the opiates and D-Met^2-Pro^5.NH$_2$, behavioral activation was not observed with injection of β-endorphin. Mice treated with the lower doses of β-endorphin (5 and 10 mg/kg) were indistinguishable from saline controls with respect to both locomotor activity and general appearance. With the highest dose tested (20 mg/kg) locomotion was significantly reduced. Therefore, after systemic administration, β-endorphin may not accumulate in the brain in amounts sufficient to produce opiate-like changes in locomotion. However, the similarity in the responses induced

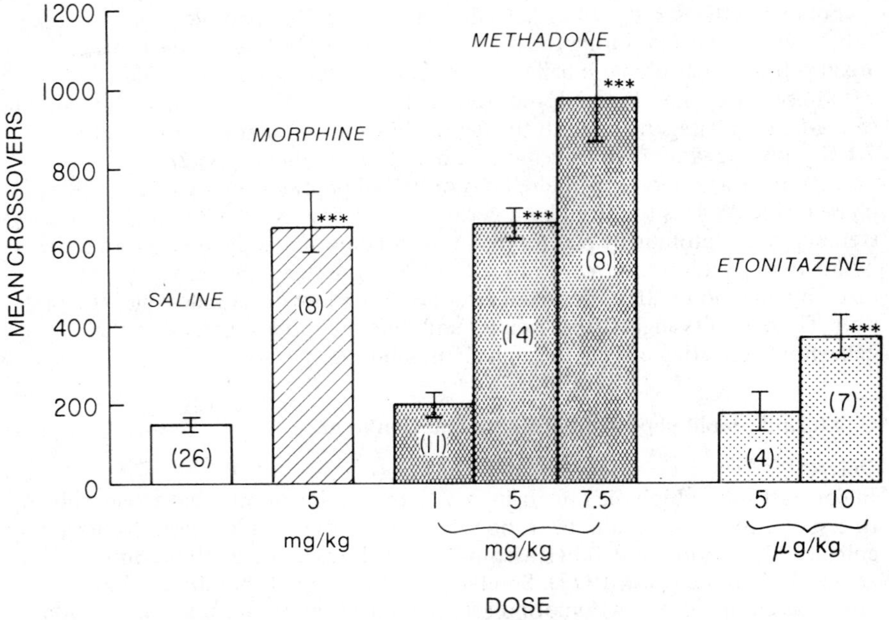

Figure 28.1 Mean crossovers ± s.e.m. during the first hour after i.v. injection of isotonic saline or opiates in mice; ( ) = N. Significant differences from control values are indicated: $*P < 0.05$, $**P < 0.02$, $***P < 0.01$ (two-tailed t-test).

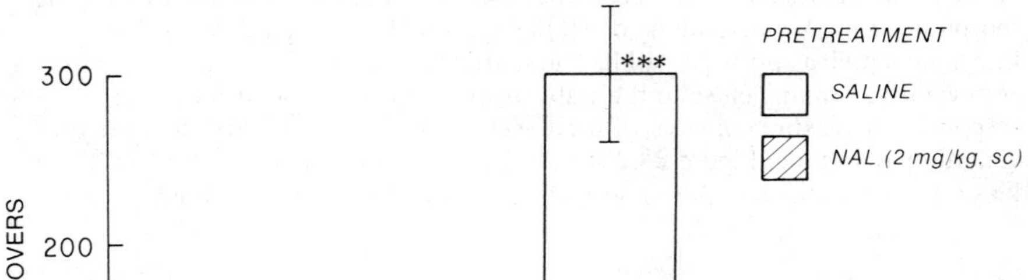

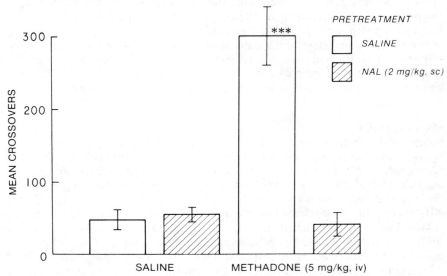

Figure 28.2 Mean crossovers ± s.e.m. during the first hour after i.v. injection of either isotonic saline or methadone (5 mg/kg). Mice were previously injected (2 min) with either naloxone (NAL) (2 mg/kg s.c.) or isotonic saline; N = at least four animals in each group. Significant differences from control values are indicated: $*P < 0.05$, $**P < 0.02$, $***P < 0.01$ (two-tailed t-test).

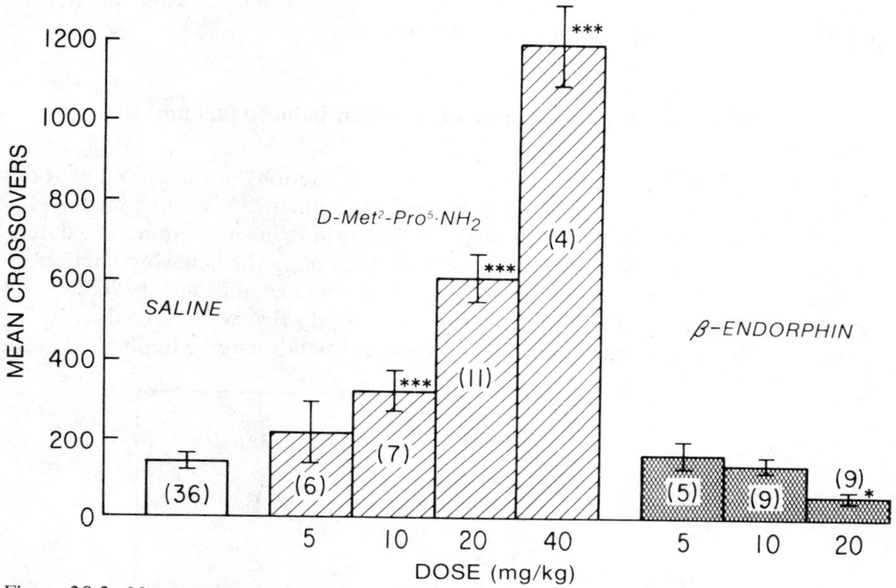

Figure 28.3 Mean crossovers ± s.e.m. during the first hour after i.v. injection of either isotonic saline or opioid peptides in mice; ( ) = N. Significant differences from control values are indicated: $^*P < 0.05$, $^{**}P < 0.02$, $^{***}P < 0.01$ (two-tailed t-test).

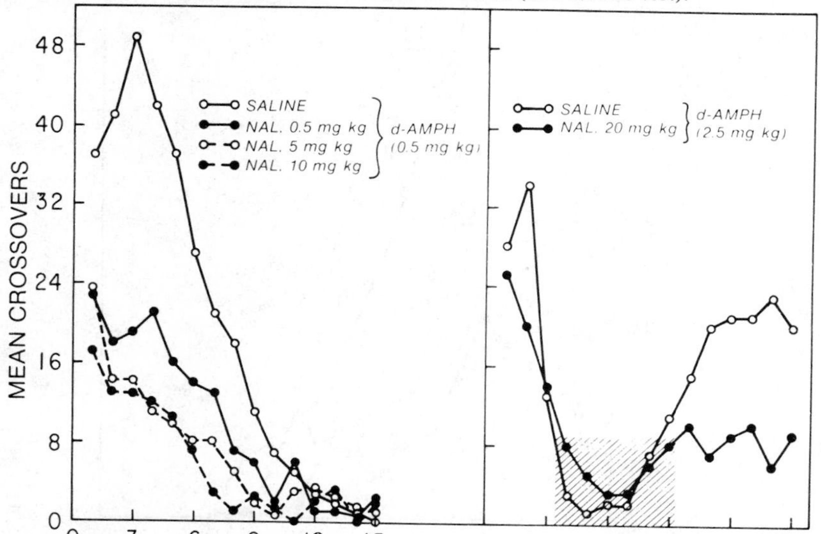

Figure 28.4 Mean crossovers ± s.e.m. during successive 12-min intervals following s.c. injection of d-amphetamine (d-AMPH) (0.5 mg/kg, left panel or 2.5 mg/kg, right panel). Rats were previously injected (2 min) with either isotonic saline or naloxone (NAL); N = at least five animals in each group. The shaded area indicates the presence of focused stereotypy during which most animals do not display crossovers or rearings.

by the opiates and D-Met^2-Pro^5 . NH_2 further indicates that the same underlying mechanism may subserve their behavioral effects.

Effects of naloxone on spontaneous and stimulant-induced locomotor activity

The ability of naloxone to antagonize many of the actions of the opioid peptides suggests that this opiate antagonist may similarly influence behaviors mediated by endogenous opioids. In fact, numerous studies have been attempted to determine the functional role of these peptides by examining the behavioral actions of naloxone (Jacob *et al.*, 1974; Lal *et al.*, 1976; Pomeranz and Chiu, 1976; Frederickson *et al.*, 1977). The alterations in motility that we observed with the opioid peptides suggest that the endogenous opioids may be implicated in the

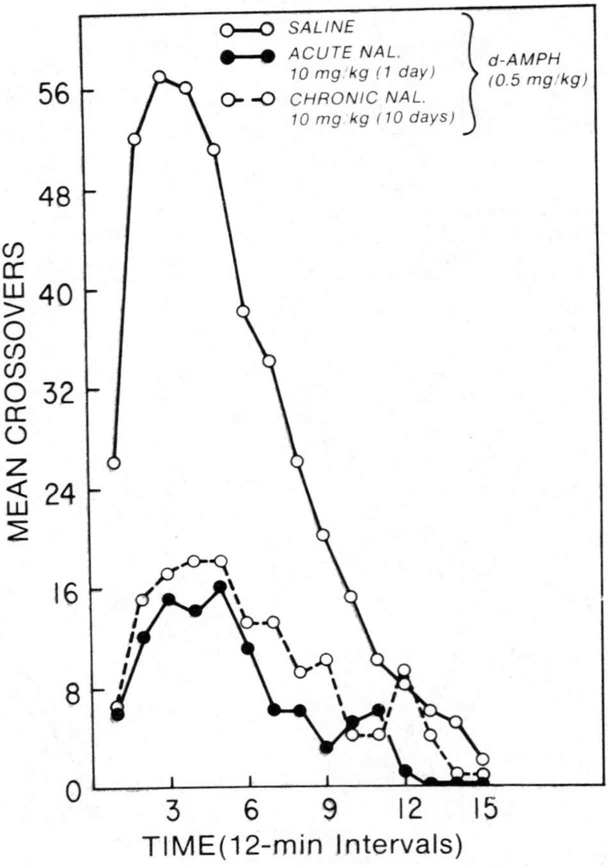

Figure 28.5 Effects of single or repeated administration of naloxone (NAL) (10 mg/kg s.c.) on locomotion induced by amphetamine (d-AMPH) (0.5 mg/kg s.c.); N = at least five animals in each group.

regulation of behavioral arousal. Therefore, to test this possibility further, we examined the effects of naloxone on spontaneous and stimulant-induced activity in rats.

Stimulant-induced hyperactivity
Holtzman (1974) reported that naloxone, at doses of 3 mg/kg or greater, reduced the locomotor activation produced by some, but not all, doses of amphetamine in the rat; the naloxone antagonism was not dose-related. Our results showed that naloxone at doses as low as 0.5 mg/kg reduced the enhanced locomotion produced by 0.5 mg/kg of *d*-amphetamine (figure 28.4, left panel); tolerance did not develop to this suppressive effect after 10 daily injections of 10 mg/kg of naloxone (figure 28.5). The locomotor effects of 2.5 mg/kg of *d*-amphetamine were also antagonized by naloxone; however, pretreatment with naloxone at doses as high as 20 mg/kg did not appear significantly to alter stereotypy (figure 28.4, right panel). Naloxone had comparable effects on the response to methylphenidate: locomotor activation induced by doses of 5 and 25 mg/kg methylphenidate was significantly reduced, whereas stereotypy appeared to be unaffected (figure 28.6).

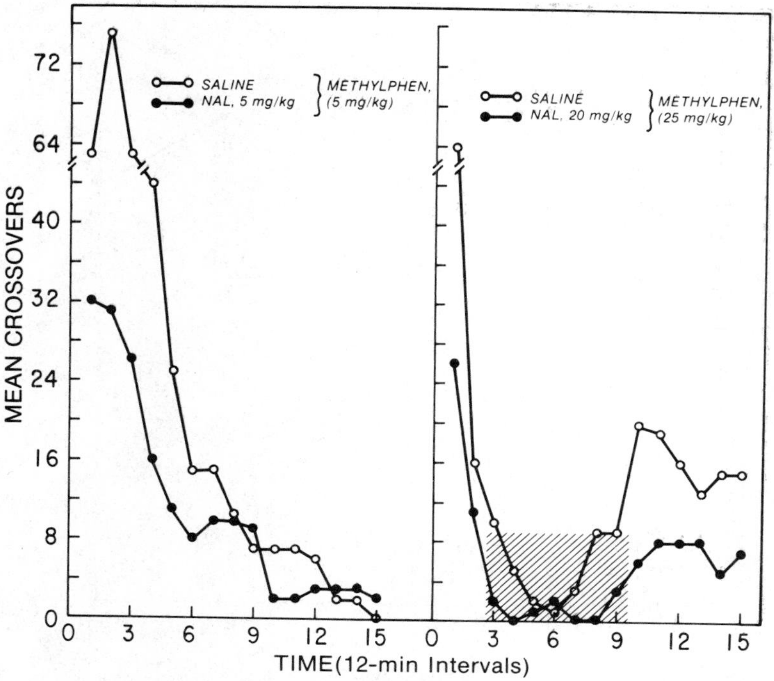

Figure 28.6 Locomotor activity (mean ± s.e.m.) during successive 12-min intervals after injection of methylphenidate (5 mg/kg, left panel or 25 mg/kg, right panel). Rats previously received (2 min) either isotonic saline or naloxone (NAL); N = at least five animals in each group. The shaded area indicates the presence of focused stereotypy during which most animals do not display crossovers or rearings.

Spontaneous activity
Doses of naloxone as high as 20 mg/kg did not alter significantly locomotion in rats that were habituated to the experimental chambers. In contrast, the activity of non-habituated rats was reduced by doses of naloxone as low as 0.5 mg/kg (figure 28.7). These results suggested that investigatory behaviors, which occur primarily during the initial exposure to a novel environment, might be selectively altered by naloxone.

Therefore, we further examined the effects of naloxone with the use of a multi-compartment experimental chamber (31 x 31 x 22") (Arnsten and Segal, manuscript in preparation, 1977). Each of the nine compartments (10 x 10 inches) contains two wire mesh stimuli, one suspended from the ceiling and the other recessed in the floor. Rats were placed singly in the chamber 15 min after injection with either saline or naloxone (5 mg/kg); locomotion (compartment

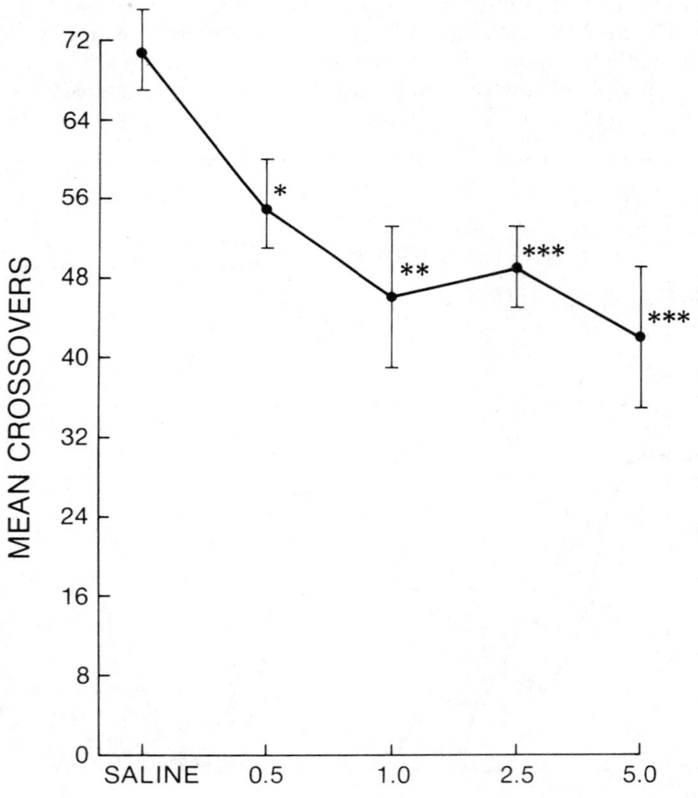

Figure 28.7 Dose–response effects of naloxone in rats that were not previously habituated to the activity chambers. Points represent mean locomotion (± s.e.m.) during the first hour after injection; N = at least five animals in each group. Significant differences from control values are indicated: $*P < 0.05$, $**P < 0.02$, $***P < 0.01$ (two-tailed t-test).

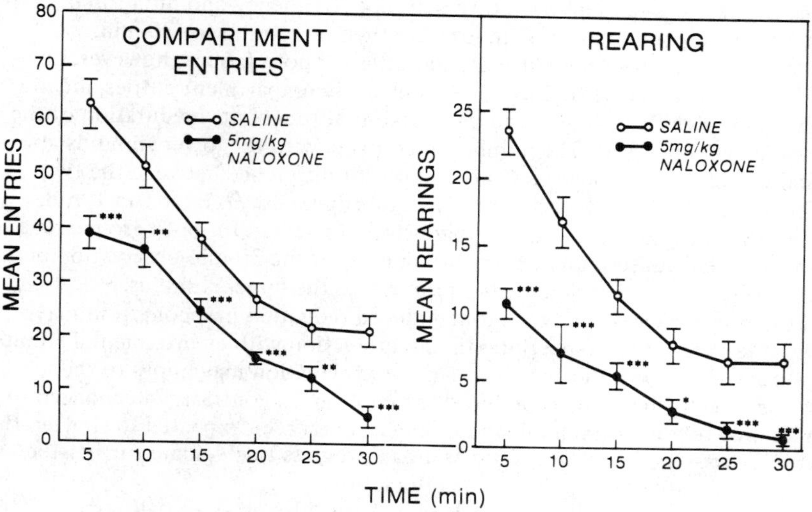

Figure 28.8 Mean compartment entries ± s.e.m. (left panel) and rearings ± s.e.m. (right panel) during successive 5-min intervals. Rats were placed in the experimental chambers 15 min following subcutaneous injection of either isotonic saline or naloxone (5 mg/kg); N = ten animals in each group. Significant differences from control values are indicated: $*P < 0.05$, $**P < 0.02$, $***P < 0.01$ (two-tailed t-test).

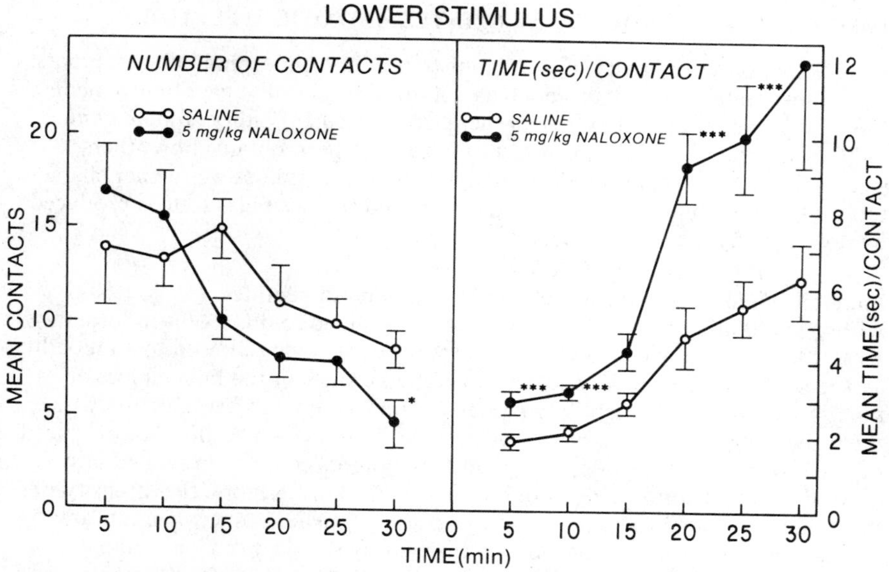

Figure 28.9 Effect of naloxone on the number of stimulus contacts (left panel) and time spent per stimulus contact (right panel); N = seven rats per group. Points indicate means ± s.e.m. during successive 5-min intervals 15 min after subcutaneous injection of either isotonic saline or naloxone (5 mg/kg). Significant differences from control values are indicated: $*P < 0.05$, $**P < 0.02$, $***P < 0.01$ (two-tailed t-test).

entries and rearings) and investigatory behavior (frequency and duration of contact with the upper and lower stimuli) were then monitored for 30 min.

Locomotor activity declined at similar rates for both groups; however, in accord with our previous findings, the number of compartment entries and rearings were significantly reduced by naloxone throughout the duration of the test session (figure 28.8). The number of contacts with the lower stimulus also gradually declined, although the only significant difference between the two groups occurred during the last 5-min interval (figure 28.9). In contrast, time spent per stimulus contact, which progressively increased for both groups, was significantly enhanced by naloxone during most of the 30-min observation period. Similar effects were observed for the response to the upper stimulus.

These results suggest that naloxone-induced reduction in locomotion may result, at least in part, from a potentiated interaction with environmental stimuli. Preliminary evidence indicates that a similar explanation may apply to the naloxone effects on stimulant-induced locomotion. In contrast, an enhanced interaction with environmental stimuli might, in fact, be expected to shorten the onset of stereotyped behavior. Studies are in progress to elucidate further the nature of the naloxone–amphetamine interaction.

In conclusion our results show that opioid peptides produce naloxone-reversible alterations in motility which closely resemble the effects of opiates. Furthermore, the opiate antagonist naloxone reduces spontaneous and stimulant-induced locomotion. These findings are consistent with a role for endogenous opioids in the regulation of behavioral activity.

IMMOBILIZATION INDUCED BY OPIATES AND OPIOID PEPTIDES

In addition to hyperactivity, i.v.t. administration of β-endorphin induces, in rats, a profound state of immobilization characterized by the absence of movement, loss of righting reflex and extreme generalized muscular rigidity (Bloom *et al.*, 1976; Segal *et al.*, 1977). Similar results have since been obtained by others (Izumi *et al.*, 1977; Tseng *et al.*, 1977). In subsequent studies we further characterized the immobility syndrome and have found that a similar state is produced by opiates and other opioid peptides.

Immobility induced by β-endorphin and other opioid peptides

Within 15-30 min after injection, most rats responded to doses of β-endorphin greater than 2.5 μg with a brief period of wet-dog shaking followed by immobility and general muscular rigidity accompanied by stiffness of the tail and loss of the righting reflex. The rigidity persisted for up to 6 hours after injection with the highest dose (300 μg). During the period of rigidity (especially that produced by the lower doses of β-endorphin, 5 and 10 μg), rats could be provoked into moving by mild auditory, visual or tactile stimuli. Furthermore, the intensity of the rigidity appeared to be reduced during tests at night, a time when rats are normally active. These results indicate that during the rigidity phase animals were capable of coordinated motor activity and that the behavioral immobility may have been partially due to an impaired ability to initiate voluntary movement. A similar profile of effects was produced by D-Met^2-Pro^5.NH_2 (25 μg) and D-Ala^2-Met^5.NH_2 (50 μg) (table 28.4).

Rats injected with β-endorphin or other opioid peptides would quickly climb off a vertical grid before and after the period of rigidity and typically would slide or fall off the grid during the rigidity phase. In contrast, rats that received haloperidol tightly grasped the grid and remained stationary for relatively long periods of time (table 28.5).

Table 28.5 Haloperidol-induced immobility

Treatment	Dose (mg/kg)	*N*	Rigidity (0–4)	Righting reflex (10 s)	Vertical grid (0–3)
Saline	1 ml/kg	10	0	+	0
Haloperidol	0.5	12	0	+	1.8 ± 0.3
	1.0	12	0	+	2.9 ± 0.1
	2.0	15	0	+	2.6 ± 0.2
	4.0	10	0	+	2.5 ± 0.2
	8.0	15	0	+	2.3 ± 0.2
	12.0	6	0	+	2.6 ± 0.2

The values, representing the peak effects, were derived using the assessment procedures described in table 28.4. Note that unlike the effects of β-endorphin, no dose of haloperidol produced rigidity or loss of the righting reflex. Instead, animals injected with haloperidol displayed a hunched posture, abducted limbs, vocalized when touched, and frequently urinated when placed on the vertical grid.

Table 28.6 Opiate-induced immobility: subcutaneous administration

Treatment	Dose	*N*	Rigidity (0–4)	Righting reflex (10 s)
Saline	1 ml/kg	13	0	+
Morphine (mg/kg)	5.0	18	0	+
	7.5	11	0.7 ± 0.2	+–
	10.0	18	1.9 ± 0.3	–
	20.0	10	3.5 ± 0.2	–
Methadone (mg/kg)	1.0	10	0	+
	2.5	17	0	+
	5.0	21	2.5 ± 0.6	–
	7.5	20	3.6 ± 0.2	–
	10.0	11	3.9 ± 0.1	–
Etonitazene (μg/kg)	1.0	8	0	+
	5.0	11	2.1 ± 0.4	+–
	10.0	11	3.7 ± 0.2	–
	20.0	4	4.0	–

Subcutaneous injection of morphine, methadone, and etonitazene resulted in rigidity and accompanying loss of righting (+–, rats remained supine for at least 5s but were capable of self-righting within 10 s).

Opiate-induced immobility

Subcutaneous administration

The opiates morphine, methadone and etonitazene produced a dose and time-related pattern of effects which closely resembled the β-endorphin-induced immobility syndrome (table 28.6). However, in contrast to the effect of the opioid peptides and etonitazene, animals injected with low doses of morphine or methadone exhibited a positive response on the vertical grid test.

Intraventricular administration

Intraventricular injection of morphine or etonitazene produced effects which were comparable to those resulting from their systemic administration (table 28.7). Rigidity occurred rapidly after injection of etonitazene and, in fact, rats frequently became maximally rigid before the removal of the i.v.t. infusion needle. Interestingly, i.v.t. and s.c. administration of etonitazene produced similar dose–response effects (tables 28.6 and 28.7). Thus, for example, injection with 5 μg of etonitazene by either route produced the same magnitude of rigidity. Because it is strongly lipophilic, etonitazene may be rapidly absorbed from the ventricles into the blood stream and subsequently be redistributed throughout the brain (Herz and Teschemacher, 1971). The failure of i.v.t. injected methadone to produce rigidity may be explained on the basis of dispositional factors, such as

(1) an active methadone metabolite may be formed peripherally but not centrally (Lemberger and Rubin, 1976)
(2) there is insufficient diffusion of methadone from the ventricles
(3) higher brain levels of methadone can be achieved after s.c. injection than after i.v.t. administration of sub-lethal doses.

Table 28.7 Intraventricular administration of morphine and etonitazene produced dose-related increases in rigidity and loss of the righting reflex

Treatment	Dose (μg/10 μl)	*N*	Rigitidy (0–4)	Righting reflex (10 s)
Saline	10 μl	13	0	+
Morphine	25.0	3	0	+–
	50.0	4	1.2 ± 0.6	–
	100.0	5	2.4 ± 0.4	–
Methadone	25–200	16	0	+
Etonitazene	0.5	2	0	+
	1.0	10	1.5 ± 0.6	+–
	2.0	2	3.5 ± 0.5	–
	5.0	10	3.2 ± 0.3	–
	10.0	6	4.0	–

Comparison of β-endorphin and opiate-induced immobility: pharmacological interactions

Rigidity resulting from injection of β-endorphin or methadone could be rapidly reversed by naloxone administered s.c. (0.1 mg/kg) or i.v.t. (0.5 μg/10 μl) (table 28.8). In contrast, the effects of haloperidol were unaltered by doses of naloxone as high as 2 mg/kg. Rats made rigid with β-endorphin (50 μg) and later injected with haloperidol (2 mg/kg) became flaccid; rigidity produced by methadone (7.5 mg/kg) was significantly reduced by haloperidol (4 mg/kg). In rats rendered flaccid by the combined treatment of β-endorphin and haloperidol, naloxone (2 mg/kg) administration resulted in the emergence of the typical haloperidol effects (table 28.8). Thus, naloxone, by selectively antagonizing the action of β-endorphin, unmasked the behavioral pattern induced by haloperidol.

β-Endorphin-induced immobility: neuroanatomical substrates

Doses of β-endorphin or D-Met^2-Pro^5.NH_2 that produced rigid immobility when injected (i.v.t.) did not elicit this syndrome after bilateral injection into the caudate, globus pallidus or amygdala (table 28.9). However, administration of β-endorphin into the ventromedial region of the periaqueductal gray (PAG) produced a behavioral profile identical in most respects to that observed after i.v.t. administration (table 28.9). Moderate rigidity (2.2 ± 0.2) was achieved with β-endorphin (8 μ in 1 ml) 30 min after injection into the PAG. During the rigidity period the righting reflex was lost and rats slid or fell off the vertical grid. All these actions were reversed within minutes after s.c. injection of naloxone (2 mg/kg). Furthermore, as with i.v.t. administration, most rats became flaccid after injection of haloperidol (2 mg/kg). Nevertheless, injections of β-endorphin into the ventromedial PAG did not produce rigidity as intense as that resulting from ventricular administration (table 28.4). Therefore, although the ventromedial region of the PAG may be implicated in the β-endorphin-induced rigidity syndrome, additional sites activated by ventricular administration of β-endorphin may also be involved. Those rats (n = 6) found to have cannula placements in the lateral or dorsal aspects of the PAG displayed marginal or no effects after injection of β-endorphin over the same dose range; however, morphine (10 μg in 1 μl) induced intensely violent responsivity in those animals with dorsolateral PAG placements. Explosive motor activity and convulsions were also observed following 200 μg of morphine administered i.v.t.

In contrast to the effects produced by β-endorphin, extreme muscular rigidity was induced by injection of etonitazene into the caudate, globus pallidus or PAG. Injections of etonitazene into the amygdala resulted in a milder form of immobility which resembled the effects observed after s.c. or i.v.t. administration with doses of etonitazene which do not produce rigidity. Injections of naloxone (2–10 μg) into the caudate, globus pallidus, amygdala or PAG reversed the rigidity induced by methadone (7.5 mg/kg s.c.). The effectiveness of etonitazene and naloxone after their injection into widely divergent sites may be attributable to the high lipid solubility of these drugs, which are rapidly absorbed into the circulatory system after i.c. injection and thus distributed throughout the CNS (Herz and Teschemacher, 1971).

Table 28.8 Comparison of β-endorphin and opiate-induced immobility: pharmacological interactions

Pretreatment	Treatment	N	Rigidity (0–4)	Righting reflex (10 s)	Vertical grid (0–3)
None	Naloxone (2 mg/kg)	4	0	+	0
None	β-Endorphin (50 μg/10 μl)	43	3.7 ± 0.1	–	Slides
β-Endorphin (50 μg/10 μl)	Naloxone (0.1–2.0 mg/kg)	15	0	+	0
None	Methadone (7.5 mg/kg)	20	3.6 ± 0.2	–	Slides
Methadone (7.5 mg/kg)	Naloxone (0.1–2.0 mg/kg)	10	0	+	0
Methadone (7.5 mg/kg)	Naloxone (0.5 μg/10 μl)	3	0	+	0
None	Haloperidol (2 mg/kg)	15	0	+	2.6 ± 0.2
β-Endorphin (50 μg/10 μl)	Haloperidol (2 mg/kg)	14	Flaccid	–	Slides
β-Endorphin (50 μg/10 μl) + Haloperidol (2 mg/kg)	Naloxone (2 mg/kg)	7	0	+	2.1 ± 0.5
Methadone (7.5 mg/kg)	Haloperidol (4 mg/kg)	6	1.3 ± 0.5*	–	Slides

Successive injections were made at 1-hour intervals; $^*P < 0.01$.

Table 28.9 Opioid-induced immobility: neuroanatomical substrates

Site (coordinates)	Treatment	Dose (μg/side)	N	Rigidity (0–4)	Righting reflex (10 s)
Caudate	Saline	1 μl	6	0	+
AP 7.5– 8.9	β-Endorphin	1.0–10.0	17	0	+
ML ± 2.5–±3.0	D-Met^2 Pro^5.NH$_2$	16.0	8	0	–
DV + 0.5	Etonitazene	1.0	7	1.9 ± 0.7	–
		2.0	13	3.7 ± 0.2	–
Globus pallidus	Saline	0.5 μl	5	0	+
Ap 6.3	β-Endorphin	10.0	6	0	+
ML ±2.7	D-Met^2 Pro^5.NH$_2$	5.0	2	0	+
DV –0.5	Etonitazene	2.0	2	4.0	–
Amygdala	Saline	0.5 μl	10	0	+
AP 4.9	β-Endorphin	1.0–15.0	16	0	+
ML ±2.6– ±4.0	D-Met^2 Pro^5.NH$_2$	10.0	2	0	+
DV –2.4––3.0	Etonitazene	0.1–1.0	14	0	+
PAG (unilateral)	Saline	0.5–1.0 μl	4	0	+
AP 0.3	β-Endorphin	8.0	9	2.2 ± 0.2	–
ML 0.0	Etonitazene	2.0	2	4.0	–
DV –0.5					

For localized injections, the rats were stereotaxically implanted with a stainless steel cannula (21 ga) (Coordinates refer to Konig and Klippel, 1963). Injections and behavioral testing took place more than 1 week after surgery. The injections were administered over a 1-min interval followed by an additional 1 min delay before removal of the 27 gauge injection needle which extended at least 2 mm beyond the guide cannula. Cánnula placements were identified by injection of methylene blue dye (0.5–1.0 μl) and 80 μm sections were examined throughout the extent of dye spread. The latency to onset of etonitazene-induced rigidity was consistently longer after localized injection (3–5 min) compared with i.v.t. administration (0.5–2 min).

In conclusion our results indicate that β-endorphin produces a broad spectrum of behaviors ranging from locomotor activation to extreme muscular rigidity. These behavioral effects, similar to those produced by the opiates and other opioid peptides, appear to be mediated through the activation of opiate receptors in the brain. Thus, the endogenous opioid peptides may play an important part in the regulation of behavior.

ACKNOWLEDGEMENTS

This research was supported in part by PHS Grant DA-01568-02; D.S.S. is the recipient of Research Scientist Award MH70183-05; R.G.B. is the recipient of a postdoctoral fellowship provided by PHS Grant AA-07129-02; D.C.D. was supported by PHS Grant GM-07198.

REFERENCES

Bloom, F., Segal, D. S., Ling, N. and Guillemin, R. (1976). *Science,* **194**, 630–2

Brase, D. A., Loh, H. H. and Way, E. L. (1977). *J. Pharmac. exp. Ther.,* **201**, 368–74

Domino, E. F., Vasko, M. R. and Wilson, A. M. (1976). In *Tissue Responses to Addictive Drugs*, (eds D. H. Ford and D. H. Clouet), Spectrum Publications, New York

Frederickson, R. C. A., Burgis, V. and Edwards, J. D. (1977). *Science,* **198**, 756–8

Herz, A. and Teschemacher, H.-J. (1971). In *Advances in Drug Research* (eds N. J. Harper and A. B. Simmonds), **6**, Academic Press, New York

Holtzman, S. G. (1974). *J. Pharmac. exp. Ther.,* **189**, 51–60

Izumi, K., Motomatsu, T., Chretien, M., Butterworth, R. F., Lis, M. and Seidah, A. (1977). *Life Sci.,* **20**, 1149–56

Jacob, J. J., Tremblay, E. C. and Colombiel, M. C. (1974). *Psychopharmacologia, Berl.,* **37**, 217–23

Kline, N. S., Li, C. H., Lehmann, H. E. , Lajtha, A., Laski, E. and Cooper, T. (1977). *Archs gen. Psychiat.,* **34**, 1111–3

Kuschinsky, K. and Hornykiewicz, O. (1974). *Eur. J. Pharmac.,* **26**, 41–50

Lal, H., Miksic, S. and Smith, N. (1976). *Life Sci.,* **18**, 971–6

Lemberger, L. and Rubin, A. (1976). *Physiologic Disposition of Drugs of Abuse,* Spectrum Publications, New York

Pomeranz, B. and Chiu, D. (1976). *Life Sci.,* **19**, 1757–62

Segal, D. S., Browne, R. G., Bloom, F., Ling, N. and Guillemin, R. (1977). *Science,* **198**, 411–14

Shuster, L., Webster, G. W., Yu, G. and Eleftheriou, B. E. (1975). *Psychopharmacologia, Berl.,* **42**, 249–54

Tseng, L. F., Loh, H. H. and Li, C. H. (1976). *Nature,* **263**, 239–40

Tseng, L. F., Loh, H. H. and Li, C. H. (1977). *Biochem. biophys. Res. Commun.,* **74**, 390–6

29
Morphine: exogenous endorphin?

Yasuko F. Jacquet (New York State Institute for Neurochemistry, Ward's Island, New York City, New York 10035, U.S.A.)

There is now increasing evidence that the multiple pharmacological actions of morphine are mediated by different sites in the central nervous system (CNS). For example, the periaqueductal gray (PAG) is now known to mediate the analgesic action of morphine (Jacquet and Lajtha, 1976), as well as the explosive motor behavior (EMB) observed following local morphine administration (Jacquet and Lajtha, 1974). Some morphine abstinence signs such as wet-dog shakes, teeth chattering, and so on, were found to be mediated by sites adjacent to the lateral ventricle (Herz, 1972), and body temperature changes induced by morphine were found to be mediated by hypothalamic sites (Lotti, 1973). However, other characteristic morphine effects such as opiate immobility have not yet been localized to any specific CNS site.

Recently, Jacquet *et al.* (1977) reported that unnatural (+)-morphine injected in the PAG resulted in EMB but not analgesia, while natural (–)-morphine at this site resulted in both effects. In parallel *in vitro* assays, such as the electrically-stimulated guinea pig ileum, rat brain homogenate binding, and the inhibition of adenylate cyclase in neuroblastoma × glioma hybrid cell homogenates, it was found that (+)-morphine had minimal activity. These results suggested the existence of at least 2 classes of opiate receptor, one ('Type 1') that is stereospecific and is sensitive to naloxone, and the other ('Type 2') that is not stereospecific and is not sensitive to naloxone. It was suggested that some CNS sites of high opiate binding with no identifiable physiological function may in fact have a 'silent' function, that is, to inhibit or dampen the hyperexcitatory effects of morphine at other CNS sites, such as the PAG (which mediates EMB). Precipitated abstinence may be due to the selective stimulation by morphine of Type 2 opiate receptors following the removal of the inhibitory influence of Type 1 opiate receptors by naloxone blockade. Thus, opiate withdrawal was suggested to be due to the *presence* of morphine rather than its *absence* at certain CNS sites.

Intracerebral injections of miniscule amounts (1.2 nmol) of β-endorphin, the recently-discovered opioid peptide (corresponding to amino-acid sequence 61–91 of β-lipotropin) were found to result in episodes of profound and prolonged sedation, catatonia and analgesia, and these effects were fully reversible by naloxone (Jacquet and Marks, 1976). These results suggested that the physiological role of this endogenously-occurring peptide may be to function as endogenous morphine, or as the brain's 'own morphine.' We have suggested, however, that β-endorphin may be the endogenous ligand only for Type 1 but not for Type 2 opiate receptors, and that the physiological function of β-endorphin is to mediate effects which overlap with, but are not fully identical to those typically seen following the administration of morphine (see table 29.1). (We have, in fact, suggested that β-endorphin may be an endogenous neuroleptic antipsychotogen. However, this does not necessarily imply that the pharmacological profile of β-endorphin should exactly parallel that of any known synthetic neuroleptic.) Here we attempt to delineate further the separate roles of the two opiate receptors.

Table 29.1 Physiological functions of opiate receptors

Type 1 (β-endorphin) (naloxone-sensitive)	Type 2 (?) (naloxone-insensitive)
Analgesia	EMB
Catatonia	Other abstinence effects
Sedation	Convulsions and toxicity
Respiratory depression	
Inhibition of Type 2	

The basic approach consisted of injecting opiates directly into the brains of unrestrained drug-naive rats, either into the lateral ventricle from where Type 2 opiate receptors may be reached, since adjacent sites are known to mediate some of the opiate abstinence signs (Herz, 1972), or into the PAG, a CNS site already known to mediate morphine analgesia and EMB. We aimed to avoid the blood-brain barrier (BBB) since morphine crosses the BBB poorly (for example, it has been estimated that less than 1 per cent of the systemically-administered morphine reaches the CNS.).

Rats were implanted with a single i.c. cannula at least 5 days before an experiment, and were habituated to the injection procedure for 3 days before an actual injection. The lateral ventricle coordinates (using a horizontal head position with bregma and lamda at the same horizontal plane) were: 0.6 mm posterior to bregma, 1.2 mm lateral to the midline, and 5.0 mm below the surface of the skull. The PAG coordinates were (with horizontal head position): 1.0 mm anterior to lamda, 0.75 mm lateral to the midline, and 6.0 mm below the surface of the skull. The intracerebroventricular (i.v.t.) cannula was a 23-gauge stainless steel (SS) needle, filed to a predetermined length and beveled at a 45° angle at the tip, while the injection needle was a 30-gauge stainless steel needle with a beveled tip which extended 1 mm beyond the guide cannula tip. The PAG guide cannulae were a pair of 30-gauge SS needles beveled at the tips, and mounted in parallel on a single pedestal with a 1.5–2.0 mm separation, while the injection cannula was a 35-gauge SS needle which extended 2 mm beyond the guide cannula tip.

Intraventricular injection
In preliminary work, we were surprised to find that wet-dog shakes, rearing on the hind legs ('exploration'), sneezing, grooming, and to a less extent, teeth chatter, which are regarded as signs of opioid abstinence behavior in rats, occurred not only following 50 μg of morphine sulfate (the threshold dose) administered i.v.t., but also following i.v.t. saline, and even following empty i.v.t. injections. These behaviors apparently occur non-specifically in response to any disturbance in the cerebral ventricles, or any slight stress (for example, brief restraint for the i.v.t. injection). The only behavior which we found to occur specifically in response to the i.v.t. administration of morphine was EMB. Unfortunately, the dose level required for this behavior was very close to the lethal dose resulting in convulsions and death.

Figure 29.1 shows that 250 μg of morphine sulfate administered i.v.t. resulted in EMB in 38 per cent of the rats, and in 31 per cent of these animals, led to convulsions and death. However, the same dose (250 μg) of morphine injected in a few animals with misplaced guide cannulae (not situated in the lateral ventricle) resulted in a variety of behavioral effects, but never in EMB, convulsions or death, confirming that the EMB and toxic effects of morphine are specific to a given CNS site which is accessible from the ventricular system.

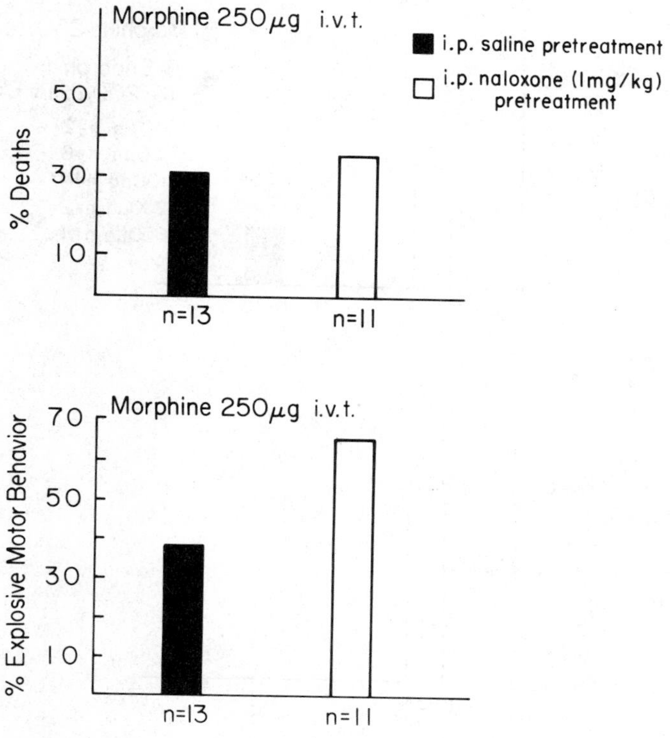

Figure 29.1 Percentage deaths and EMB as a function of saline versus naloxone pretreatment given i.p. 2 min previously.

Figure 29.1 (lower graph) also shows that pretreatment with naloxone given intraperitoneally (i.p.) resulted in a significant increase in the occurrence of EMB compared to saline pretreated controls (from 38 to 64 per cent) following i.v.t. morphine (250 μg). A slight, but non-significant increase in the toxicity was also observed in this naloxone-pretreated group compared to saline-pretreated controls (from 31 to 36 per cent) (figure 29.1, upper graph). Thus, naloxone pretreatment did not protect the animals from the toxic effects of i.v.t. morphine, but on the contrary, had a potentiating effect.

Table 29.2 shows that pretreatment with systemic morphine (30 mg/kg, 30 min before the i.v.t. morphine) resulted in blocking the occurrence of EMB but not of analgesia. Conversely, naloxone pretreatment (1 mg/kg, 2 min before the i.v.t. morphine) blocked analgesia but not EMB. A combination of the two pretreatments, that is, i.p. morphine at 30 mg/kg given 30 min before, and i.p. naloxone at 1 mg/kg given 2 min before the i.v.t. morphine (250 μg) resulted in the occurrence of EMB but not of analgesia.

These results suggest that systemically-administered morphine activates both Types 1 and 2 opiate receptors, and that Type 1 normally inhibits Type 2, but naloxone blocks only Type 1, thus releasing Type 2 from its inhibitory influence, resulting in EMB and other 'abstinence' phenomena.

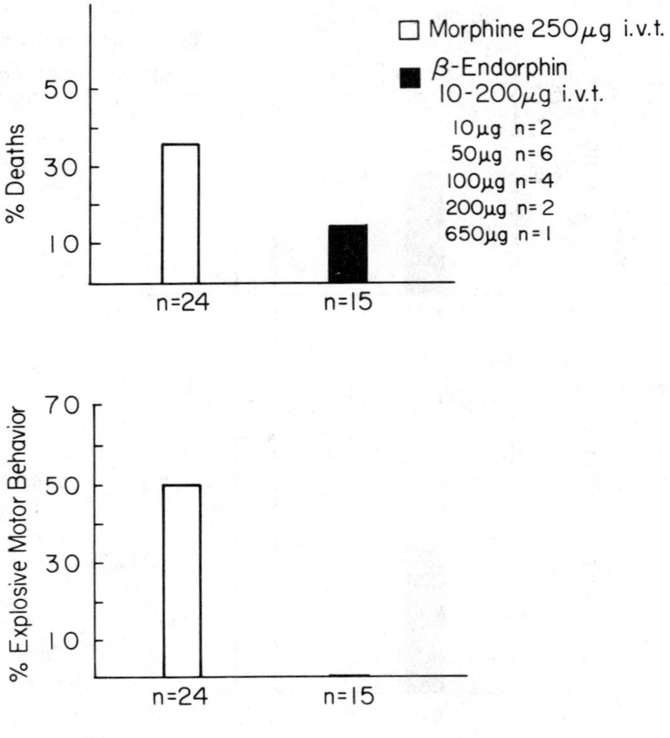

Figure 29.2 Percentage deaths and EMB as a function of morphine or β-endorphin given i.v.t.

Table 29.2 Effects of pretreatment with morphine and naloxone on EMB and analgesia induced by morphine

Pretreatment	Treatment	Effect	
		EMB	Analgesia
A. Morphine 30 mg/kg i.p. (0.5 h previously)	Morphine 250 μg i.v.t.	–	+
B. Naloxone 1 mg/kg i.p. (2 min previously)	Morphine 250 μg i.v.t.	+	–
A + B. (Combination of above)	Morphine 250 μg i.v.t.	+	–
A. Morphine 30 mg/kg i.p. (0.5 h previously)	Morphine 10 μg PAG	–	+
B. Naloxone 1 mg/kg i.p. (2 min previously)	Morphine 10 μg PAG	+	–

Table 29.3 Intracerebroventricular injection

	β-Endorphin		Morphine	
	10, 50, 100 μg	200, 650 μg	50 μg	250 μg
Analgesia	+	+	±	+
Catatonia	+	+	–	–
Body temperature drop (°C)	+	+	–	± (–1° – +2°)
Sedation	+	±	–	–
Distress vocalization	–	–	–	+
EMB	–	–	–	+
Death	–	+	–	+
		(Respiratory depression)		(Convulsions)

β-endorphin administered i.v.t. in doses ranging from 10, 50, 100, 200 to 650 μg (in 10-μl volumes) never resulted in EMB (figure 29.2). Toxicity was observed only at the 200 μg level and above, and occurred following a gradually increasing respiratory depression coupled with bronchial congestion, whereas the toxicity resulting from 250 μg of morphine given i.v.t. was due to violent convulsions. Some behavioral excitation was observed following the higher β-endorphin doses (200 and 650 μg) given i.v.t., but never the distress vocalizations and EMB observed following 250 μg of morphine given i.v.t. Moreover, when 200 μg of β-endorphin was injected in an animal with a misplaced cannula (not located in the lateral ventricle), some excitatory effects were observed, but not analgesia and catatonia, confirming that these latter effects were due to the interaction of β-endorphin at specific CNS sites. Board-like rigidity was never observed at any of these dose levels. Instead, the catatonia consisted of a waxy flexibility wherein it was possible to 'mold' the passive rat in any position which it would then hold for long periods. However, following 650 μg of β-endorphin given i.v.t., flaccidity rather than muscular rigidity ensued. A summary of the effects observed following the i.v.t. administrations of β-endorphin and of morphine is shown in table 29.3.

PAG injection studies

We previously reported (Jacquet and Lajtha, 1974) that an i.c. injection of morphine in the PAG of rats resulted in two behavioral events which occurred dose-depend-

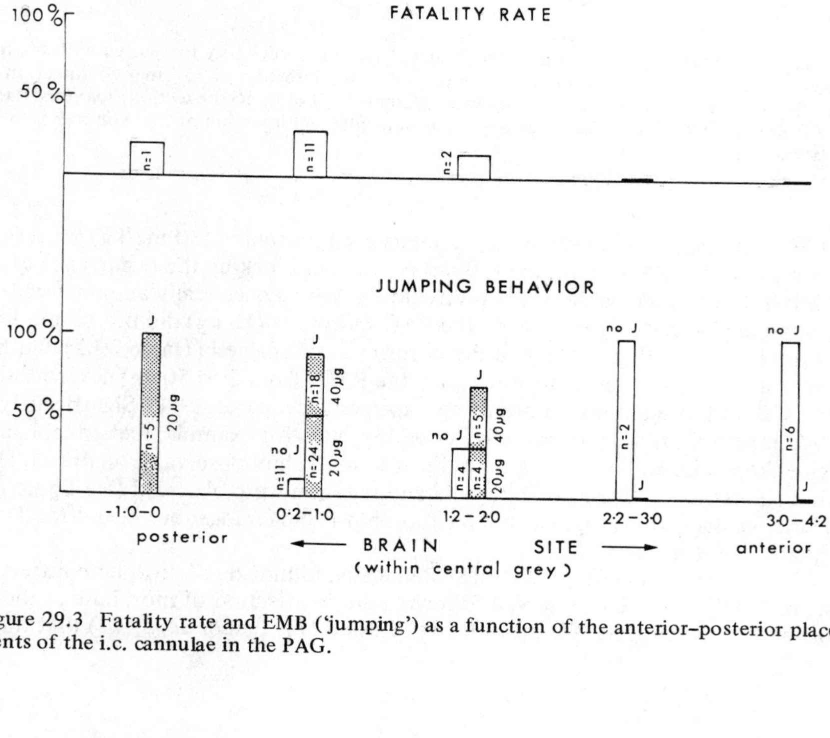

Figure 29.3 Fatality rate and EMB ('jumping') as a function of the anterior–posterior placements of the i.c. cannulae in the PAG.

ently: (1) analgesia, and (2) EMB (hyperreactivity to previously neutral stimuli), consisting of high repetitive jumps accompanied by distress vocalizations. This EMB is indistinguishable from the behavior seen following precipitated abstinence in rats treated with high doses of opiates. Figure 29.3 shows that the CNS site for this behavior was the caudal portion of the midbrain PAG. We have observed, however, that an undamaged PAG is necessary for the expression of this behavior. When the PAG was lesioned unintentionally by large-gauge injection needles, or following a large injection volume or overly rapid infusion (see figure 29.4), EMB did not occur following morphine injection in the PAG.

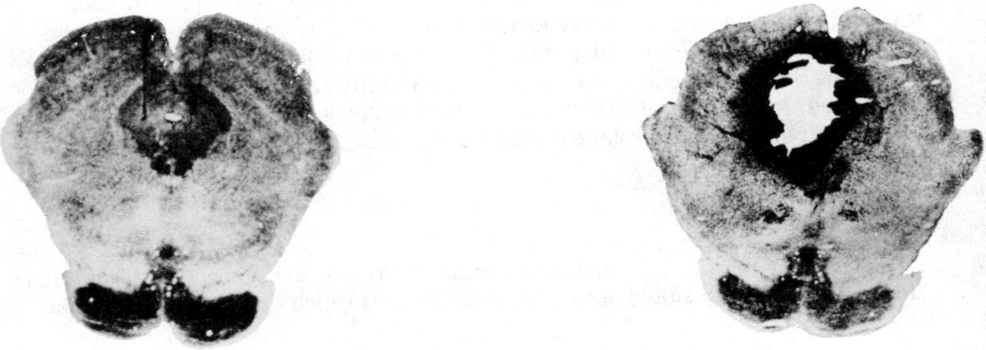

Figure 29.4 Histological section of the brains of two rats previously implanted with bilateral PAG cannulae. Left section: minimal damage following insertion of 35-gauge SS injection needle and injection of 0.5 μl volumes into bilateral PAG sites. Right section: maximal damage following insertion of 35-gauge SS injection needle and injection of 2 μl volumes into bilateral PAG sites.

Pretreatment with systemically-administered morphine (30 mg/kg) given 0.5 h previous to the PAG morphine (10 μg) resulted in blocking the occurrence of EMB but not of analgesia, while pretreatment with systemically administered naloxone (1 mg/kg) 2 min before the PAG morphine (10 μg) did not block the occurrence of EMB but blocked the occurrence of analgesia (table 29.2). On the other hand, β-endorphin injections into the PAG (from 2 to 50 μg) never resulted in EMB, but in sedation, catatonia and analgesia (see table 29.4). Significantly, PAG injections of high doses of other endorphins, for example, met-enkephalin, leu-enkephalin, and α-endorphin, never resulted in any observable analgesia, although attenuated forms of catatonia and sedation were observed (see figure 29.5). These results further suggest that β-endorphin is the endogenous ligand for Type 1 opiate receptor.

The pharmacological profile of systemically-administered morphine differs significantly from that observed following direct injection of morphine in the PAG or the lateral ventricle. We previously suggested (Jacquet *et al.*, 1977) that this may be due to the interaction of morphine with two different classes of opiate receptor, the function of one being to inhibit the behavioral expression of the excitatory effects of the other. Our present results suggest that β-endorphin is the endogenous ligand for Type 1 opiate receptor, but that it probably does not interact directly with Type 2 opiate receptor. Thus, β-endorphin and morphine share overlapping, but *not identical,* physiological functions.

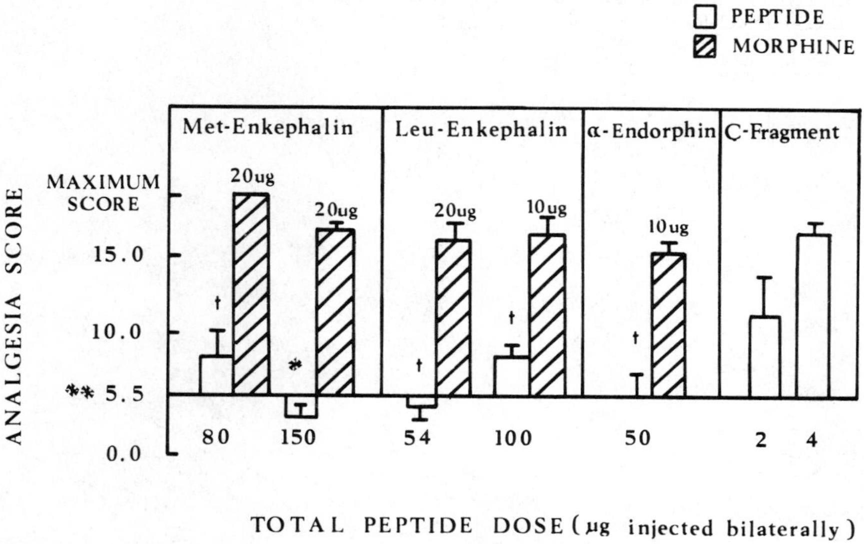

Figure 29.5 Mean analgesia scores following i.c. injection of peptides (open bars) or morphine (hatched bars) into the PAG of rats. Each peptide was injected in 1–2 μl vehicle, 0.5 to 1.0 μl being injected into each bilateral PAG site. The morphine dose was either 10 or 20 μg. The effects of 2 and 4 μg of the C-fragment (β-endorphin) resulted in an analgesic response comparable to 10 and 20 μg of morphine sulfate.

Table 29.4 Periaqueductal gray injection

	β-Endorphin (4 μg)	Morphine (10 μg)
Analgesia	+	+
Catatonia	+	–
Sedation	+	–
Distress vocalization	–	+
EMB	–	+

REFERENCES

Herz, A. (1972). In *Pharmacology and the Future of Man. Proc. 5th Int. Congr. Pharmacology*, San Francisco, Karger, Basel, pp. 125–39
Jacquet, Y. F. and Lajtha, A. (1974). *Science,* **185**, 1055–7
Jacquet, Y. F. and Lajtha, A. (1976). *Brain Res.,* **103**, 501–13
Jacquet, Y. F. and Marks, N. (1976). *Science,* **194**, 632–5
Jacquet, Y. F., Klee, W. A., Rice, K. C., Iijima, I. and Minamikawa, J. (1977). *Science,* **198**, 842–5
Lotti, V. J. (1973). In *The Pharmacology of Thermoregulation. Symp.* San Francisco, Karger, Basel pp. 382–94

30
Effects of endorphins and their analogues on prolactin and growth hormone secretion

F. Labrie, A. Dupont, L. Cusan, J. C. Lissitzky, J. Lepine, V. Raymond and D. H. Coy (Laboratory of Molecular Endocrinology, Le Centre Hospitalier de l'Université Laval, Quebec G1V 4G2, Canada)

Following reports of the presence of endogenous opiate activity in brain (Hughes, 1975; Pasternak *et al.*, 1975; Terenius *et al.*, 1975), the pentapeptide Tyr–Gly–Gly–Phe–Met (met-enkephalin) has been isolated from porcine (Hughes *et al.*, 1975) and calf (Simantov *et al.*, 1976) brain. The sequence of this peptide is the same as the N-terminus of the C-fragment (β-LPH$_{61-91}$), also called β-lipotropin, first isolated from sheep pituitaries (Li *et al.*, 1965). Both met-enkephalin and β-endorphin have potent morphine-like activity (Chang *et al.*, 1976; Hughes *et al.*, 1975; Li *et al.*, 1976*a*) and bind to the opiate receptor (Chang *et al.*, 1976; Li *et al.*, 1976*b*; Morin *et al.*, 1976).

The possibility was thus raised that met-enkephalin and β-endorphin, beside their well-known analgesic potency (Belluzi *et al.*, 1976; Bradbury *et al.*, 1976; Pert, 1977) and activity as behavior modulators (Bloom *et al.*, 1976) could be involved in the neuroendocrine control of prolactin (PRL) and growth hormone (GH) secretion. The present paper describes the stimulatory effect of met-enkephalin, β-endorphin and their analogues on PRL and GH release in the rat after i.v.t. injection and show that met-enkephalin analogues resistant to enzymatic degradation have a markedly increased GH and PRL-releasing activity.

RESULTS AND DISCUSSION

As illustrated in figure 30.1A, the i.v.t. injection of 0.5 to 25 μg of β-endorphin (β-LPH$_{61-91}$) led to a rapid and important stimulation of PRL release in unanesthetized freely-moving rats. With the 0.5 μg dose, a significant rise was measured 5 min after injection of the peptide and a maximal stimulation (approximately seven-fold) was measured after 10 min with a slow return toward basal plasma

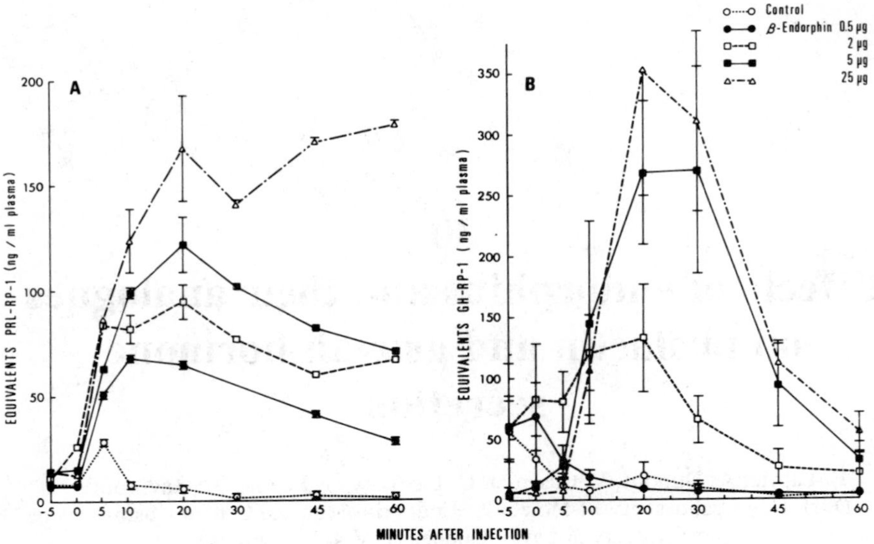

Figure 30.1 Effect of increasing doses of β-endorphin on plasma PRL (A) and GH (B) levels in the rat. Male rats bearing i.v.t. and intrajugular cannulae were injected i.v. with 0.2 ml of sheep somatostatin antiserum 5 min before the i.v.t. injection of the indicated amounts of synthetic β-endorphin. Prolactin and GH concentrations were measured at the indicated time intervals after administration of β-endorphin to 8–10 animals per group. Data are presented as mean ± S.E.M. (Dupont *et al.*, 1977).

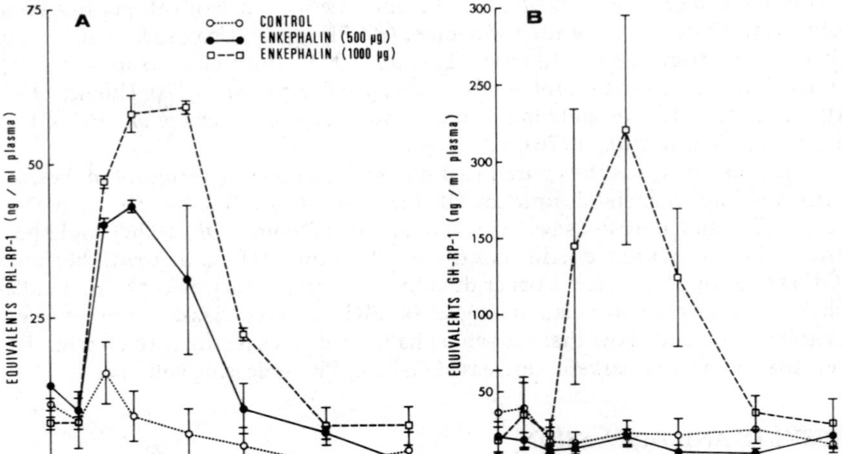

Figure 30.2 Effect of 0.5 or 1.0 mg of met-enkephalin on plasma PRL (A) and GH (B) levels in the rat. The experiment was performed as described in figure 30.1 (Dupont *et al.*, 1977).

hormone levels at later time intervals. The higher doses of β-endorphin (2, 5 and 25 μg) led to a progressive increase of PRL release, a 30- to 60-fold increase being measured between 20 and 60 min after injection of 25 μg of the peptide.

Although inactive at 0.5 μg, doses of 2 μg and higher of β-endorphin led to a significant stimulation of plasma GH release. With the 2 μg dose, a 6 to 10-fold stimulation of the plasma GH concentration was measured 10 and 20 min after injection of β-endorphin, with a progressive decrease toward basal levels reached at 45 min. The two higher doses (5 and 25 μg) of β-endorphin led to a maximal 20 to 30-fold stimulation of plasma GH levels measured 20 and 30 min after injection of the peptide.

As shown in figure 30.2, met-enkephalin, the NH_2-terminal pentapeptide of β-endorphin, was much less potent than β-endorphin to stimulate PRL and GH release. In fact, at the 500 and 1000 μg doses, met-enkephalin led to approximately 4 and 6-fold increases of plasma PRL levels, respectively. Maximal stimulation was measured 5 to 20 min after injection of the pentapeptide with a rapid return to basal levels between 30 and 45 min. It can be seen in figure 30.2B that stimulation of GH release was observed only at the 1000 μg dose, thus indicating again a greater sensitivity of the PRL than GH responses to the opioid peptide. Specificity of the stimulatory effect of β-endorphin on PRL and GH release was indicated by reversal of the inhibitory effect by concomitant administration of naloxone.

The present data demonstrate clearly that β-endorphin administered i.v.t. can be a potent stimulus of PRL and GH release in the rat, while the activity of met-enkephalin is much lower. As calculated from the areas under the plasma GH response curves, β-endorphin is, on a molar basis, approximately 2000 times more potent than met-enkephalin. β-Endorphin and met-enkephalin have also been found to display markedly different potencies in various other bioassays.

Despite its much higher biological activity demonstrated in most assays, β-endorphin shows a binding affinity for the opiate receptor approximately three times lower than met-enkephalin (table 30.1) when binding studies are performed at 0 °C under conditions which minimize enzymatic degradation. It is thus likely that the markedly lower biological activity of met-enkephalin after injection is due to a higher resistance of β-endorphin to enzymatic degradation.

In search of opiate peptide analogues with increased activity, it occurred to us that substitution of D-amino acids into the peptide chain might offer a fruitful approach. This has certainly been the case for two hypothalamic hormones, luteinizing hormone-releasing hormone (LHRH) and somatostatin. In fact, substitution of D-amino acids in position 6 of the decapeptide led to peptides with much greater potency and duration of action (Coy *et al.*, 1976*a*; Monahan *et al.*, 1973) while replacement of the tryptophan residue at position 8 in somatostatin by its D-isomer enhanced the GH-release inhibiting activity of the molecule approximately eight-fold (Rivier *et al.*, 1975). Thus, replacement of glycine in position 2 of met-enkephalin by D-amino acids might be expected to yield analogues with increased activities.

While the minimal effective dose of met-enkephalin on GH and PRL release after i.v.t. injection in the rat is approximately 500 μg (Figure 30.2), it can be seen in figure 30.3 that [D-Ala^2, Met^5]-enkephalin had a maximal stimulatory effect on PRL and GH release at the doses of 50 and 150 μg, respectively.

Table 30.1 Relative affinity of met-enkephalin, endorphins and their analogues for the brain opiate receptor

Substance	Percent displacing ability
Met-enkephalin	100
[D-Tyr^1, Met^5]-enkephalin	<1
[D-Ala^2, Met^5]-enkephalin	120
[D-Ala^2, Met^5]-enkephalin-NH_2	150
N-acetyl-[D-Ala^2, Met^5]-enkephalin-NH_2	<1
[D-Ala^2, D-Leu^5, Met^5]-enkephalin	30
[β-Ala^2, Met^5]-enkephalin	1
[Ser^2, Met^5]-enkephalin	10
[D-Leu^2, Met^5]-enkephalin	<1
[D-Phe^2, Met^5]-enkephalin	<1
[D-Ala^3, Met^5]-enkephalin	10
[D-Phe^4, Met^5]-enkephalin	<1
[D-Met^5]-enkephalin	10
Met-enkephalin ethylamide	120
β-Endorphin	30
[D-Ala^2]-β-endorphin	30
α-Endorphin	3
[D-Ala^2]-α-endorphin	3
γ-Endorphin	3
[D-Ala^2]-γ-endorphin	3
β-LPH	<1

The relative affinities were calculated from the concentrations of the various peptides giving 50 percent displacement of [^3H] met-enkephalin binding to rat brain membranes. Incubations were performed at 0–4 °C as described (Morin *et al.*, 1977) to minimize enzymatic degradation.

The present data show that substitution of the glycine residue of met-enkephalin by D-alanine leads to a dramatic increase of the GH and PRL releasing potency of the peptide. In fact, comparison of figures 30.1 and 30.3 indicates that [D-Ala^2, Met^5]-enkephalin given by i.v.t. injection is 1000 to 2000 times more potent than met-enkephalin itself.

Substitution of the C-terminal glycine-amide residue in the LHRH molecule by ethylamide had led to an analogue 10 to 15 times more potent than the natural hormone (Fujino *et al.*, 1972). It was interesting to see that addition of the ethylamide group at the COOH-terminus of met-enkephalin markedly increased its GH and PRL-releasing activity (Cusan *et al.*, 1977). In fact, while maximal stimulation of PRL and GH release was obtained with [D-Ala^2, Met^5]-enkephalin at the 300 μg dose, a similar effect was obtained with 62.5 μg of [D-Ala^2, Met^5]-enkephalinamide, a peptide at least 5000 times more potent than met-enkephalin in this assay.

It is interesting to observe in figure 30.4 that coupling of two molecules of [D-Ala^2, Met^5]-enkephalin at the α and ε amino groups of Lys-NH_2 led to a mole-

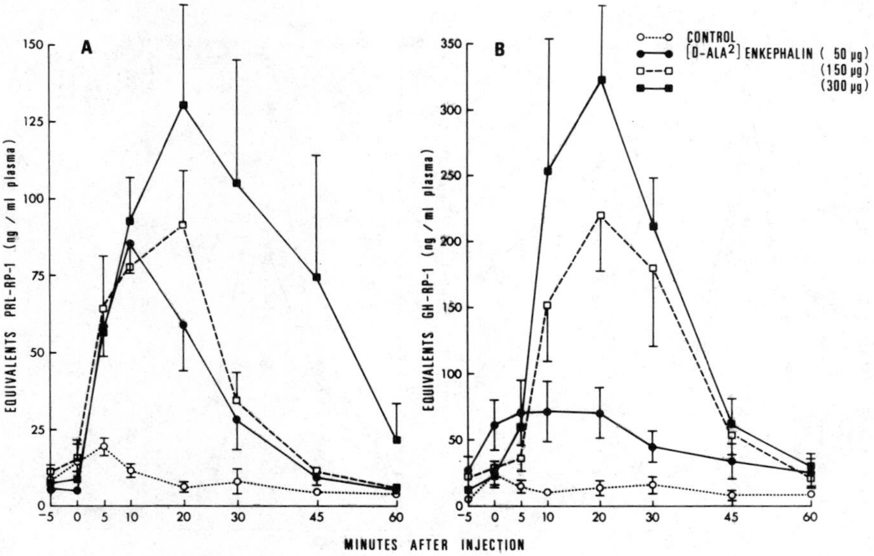

Figure 30.3 Effect of increasing doses of [D-Ala^2, Met^5]-enkephalin on plasma PRL (A) and GH (B) levels in the rat. The experiment was performed as described in figure 30.1 (Cusan *et al.*, 1977).

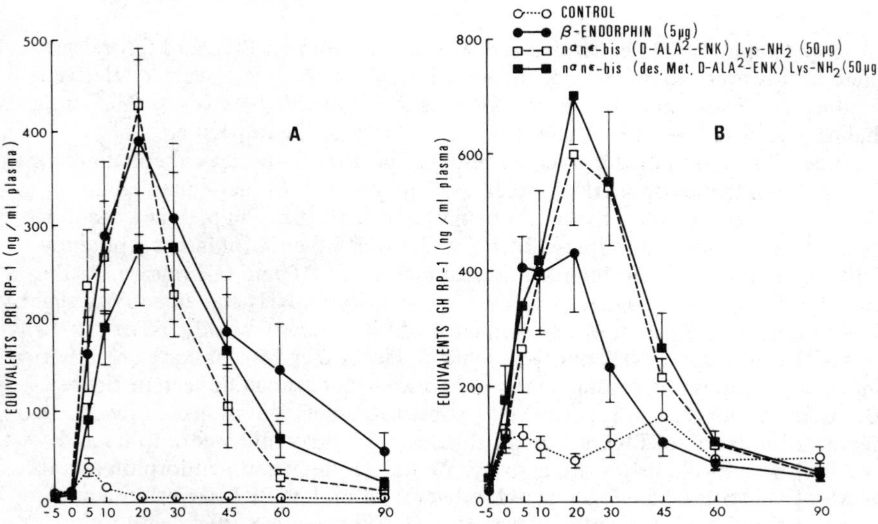

Figure 30.4 Effect of n$^{\alpha}$n$^{\epsilon}$*bis*-[D-Ala^2-enkephalin] Lys-NH$_2$ (50 μg), n$^{\alpha}$n$^{\epsilon}$*bis* [desMet, D-Ala^2-enkephalin] Lys-NH$_2$ (50 μg) and β-endorphin (5 μg) injected i.v.t. on plasma PRL (A) and GH (B) levels in the rat. The experiment was performed as described in figure 30.1.

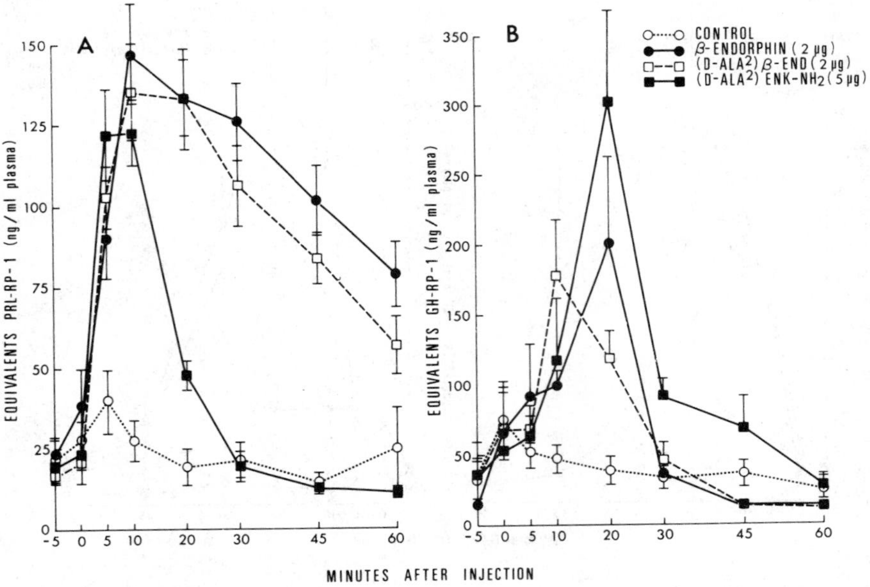

Figure 30.5 Effect of i.v.t. injection of 2 μg of β-endorphin, 2 μg of [D-Ala^2]-β-endorphin or 5 μg of [D-Ala^2, Met^5]-enkephalinamide on plasma PRL (A) and GH (B) levels in the rat. The experiment was performed as described in figure 30.1.

cule approximately 20 per cent as active as β-endorphin on PRL and GH release. There is, however, no increase of the duration of action of the peptide relative to β-endorphin. Removal of the methionine residue ($n^{\alpha}n^{\epsilon}$*bis* [desMet, D-Ala^2-enkephalin] Lys-NH_2) had no influence on the activity of the molecule.

Since substitution of the glycine residue at position 2 of met-enkephalin by a D-alanine residue led to marked increase of the potency of met-enkephalin, it was of interest to study the effect of similar substitutions in β, α, and γ-endorphins. It can be noticed in figure 30.5 that [D-Ala^2]-β-endorphin has a potency similar to that of β-endorphin itself as stimulator of PRL and GH release. As illustrated in figure 30.6, [D-Leu^{17}, D-Lys^{29}]-β-endorphin-NH_2 has an activity slightly higher than β-endorphin itself as stimulator of PRL release, while [D-Thr^6, D-Leu^{17}, D-Lys^{29}]-β-endorphin-NH_2 and [parachloro, Phe^4]-β-endorphin have an activity almost superimposable to that of the parent molecule. It can be seen in figure 30.7 that β-endorphin and its [D-Ala^2] substituted analogues injected i.v. led to a marked stimulation of PRL release at the dose of 2 mg while γ-endorphin and [D-Ala^2]-γ-endorphin show no activity. We have found that γ-endorphin and its [D-Ala^2] substituted analogue could, however, stimulate PRL secretion when injected i.c. although the potency was at least 100 times less than β-endorphin (data not shown).

Since the present and our previous observations on the stimulatory effect of met-enkephalin, β-endorphin and their analogues were performed in animals where circulating somatostatin was neutralized by excess somatostatin antiserum, it is likely that the observed increased GH release is due to stimulated release of GH-

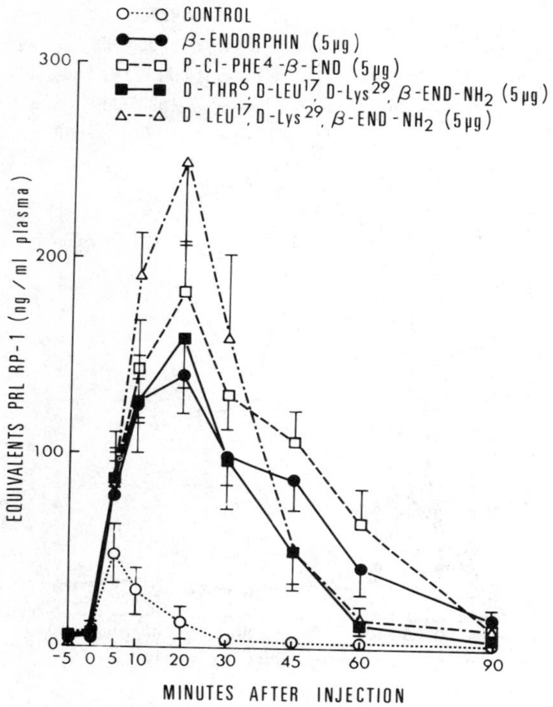

Figure 30.6 Effects of i.v.t. injection of 5 μg of β-endorphin (●), P-Cl-Phe[4]-β-endorphin (□), D-Thr[6], D-Leu[17], D-Lys[29]-β-endorphin-NH_2 (■) or D-Leu[17], D-Lys[29], β-endorphin-NH_2 (△) on plasma PRL levels in the rat. (○) Control. The experiment was performed in conscious freely-moving adult male animals as described in figure 30.1.

releasing activity (GHRH) from the hypothalamus.

Increasing evidence suggests a physiological role of dopamine as inhibitor of PRL secretion (MacLeod *et al.*, 1974; Schally *et al.*, 1976). It is thus likely that opiates and opioid peptides exert at least part of their marked stimulatory effect on PRL release through inhibition of dopamine release from nerve endings in the external layer of the median eminence. This is supported by the findings that β-endorphin can inhibit dopamine release from caudate nucleus *in vitro* (Loh *et al.*, 1976).

The present data show that met-enkephalin analogues have been obtained which have an activity comparable to that of β-endorphin as stimulators of GH and PRL release after i.v.t. injection and should be useful tools for studying the physiological role of endogenous opiate peptides, not only as analgesics (Pert *et al.*, 1976) and behavioral modulators (Bloom *et al.*, 1976) but also in the control of neuroendocrine functions. β-Endorphin and its [D-Ala[2]] substituted analogue were also found to be active by i.v. injection on PRL secretion. The present model could also be very useful for precise evaluation of the biological activity of endogenous and synthetic opiate-like substances.

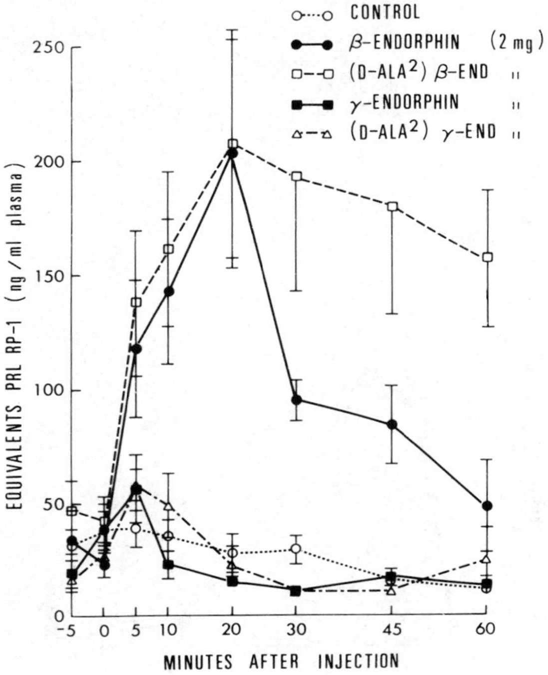

Figure 30.7 Effect of i.v. injection of 2 mg of β-endorphin (●), [D-Ala²]-β-endorphin (□), γ-endorphin (■) or [D-Ala²]-γ-endorphin (△) on plasma PRL levels in the rat. (○), Control. Unanesthetized and freely-moving male rats bearing intrajugular cannulae were used.

REFERENCES

Belluzi, J. D., Grant, N., Garsky, V., Sarantakis, D., Wise, C. D. and Stein, L. (1976). *Nature,* **260**, 625–6

Bradbury, A. F., Smyth, P. G. and Snell, C. R. (1976). *Nature,* **260**, 793–805

Bloom, F., Segal, D., Ling, N. and Guillemin, R. (1976). *Nature,* **194**, 630–6

Chang, J. K., Fong, B. T. W., Pert, A. and Pert, C. B. (1976). *Life Sci.,* **18**, 1473–82.

Coy, D. H., Kastin, A. J., Schally, A. V., Morin, O., Caron, M. G., Labrie, F., Walker, J. M., Fertel, R., Berntson, G. G. and Sandman, C. A. (1976*a*). *Biochem. biophys. Res. Commun.* **73**, 632–8

Coy, D. H., Vilchez-Martinez, J. A., Coy, E. J. and Schally, A. V. (1976*b*). *J. med. Chem.,* **19**, 423–8

Cusan, L., Dupont, A., Kledzik, G. S. and Labrie, F. (1977). *Nature,* **268**, 544–6

Dupont, A., Cusan, L., Labrie, F., Coy, D. H. and Li, C. H. (1977). *Biochem. biophys. Res. Commun.,* **75**, 76–82

Fujino, M., Kobayashi, S., Obayashi, M., Shinagawa, S., Fukuka, T., Kitada, C., Nayayama, R., Yamazaki, I., White, W. F. and Rippel, R. H. (1972). *Biochem. biophys. Res. Commun.,* **49**, 863–9

Hughes, J. (1975). *Brain Res.,* **88**, 295–308

Hughes, J., Smith, T. W., Kosterlitz, H. W., Fothergill, L. A., Morgan, B. A. and Morris, H. R. (1975). *Nature,* **258**, 577–9

Li, C. H. and Chung, D. (1976). *Proc. natn. Acad. Sci. U.S.A.,* 73, 1145–8

Li, C. H., Lemaire, S., Yamashiro, D. and Doneen, B. A. (1976). *Biochem. biophys. Res. Commun.*, **71**, 19–21
Loh, H. H., Tseng, L. F., Wei, I. and Li, C. H. (1976*a*). *Proc. natn. Acad. Sci. U.S.A.*, **73**, 2895–8
Loh, H. H., Braxe, D. A., Dampath-Khanna, S., Mar, J. B. and Way, E. L. (1976*b*). *Nature*, **264**, 567–8
MacLeod, R. M. and Lehmeyer, J. E. (1974). *Endocrinology*, **94**, 1077–85
Morin, O., Caron, M. G., De Léan, A. and Labrie, F. (1976). *Biochem. biophys. Res. Commun.*, **73**, 940–6
Monahan, M. W., Amoss, M. S., Anderson, H. A. and Vale, W. (1973). *Biochemistry*, **12**, 4616–20
Pasternak, G. W., Goodman, R. and Snyder, S. H. (1975). *Life Sci.* **16**, 1765–9
Pert, C. B., Pert, A., Chang, J. K. and Fong, B. T. W. (1976). *Science*, **194**, 330–2
Pert, A. (1977). In *Opiates and Opioid Peptides*, (eds H. Kosterlitz, S. Archer, E. J. Simon and A. Goldstein), Elsevier Publishing Co., Amsterdam, pp. 87–94
Rivier, J., Brown, M. and Vale, W. (1975). *Biochem. biophys. Res. Commun.*, **65**, 746–51
Schally, A. V., Dupont, A., Arimura, A., Takahara, J., Redding, T. W., Clemens, J. and Shaar, C. (1976). *Acta endocrin.*, **82**, 1–14
Simantov, R. and Snyder, S. H. (1976). *Proc. natn. Acad. Sci. U.S.A.*, **73**, 2515–9
Terenius, L. and Wahlström, A. (1975). *Acta physiol. scand.*, **94**, 74–81

31

Effect of enkephalin on sensory neurons in cell culture: inhibition of substance P release and reduction of inward calcium currents

Anne W. Mudge, Susan E. Leeman and Gerald D. Fischbach (Department of Physiology, Laboratory of Human Reproduction and Reproductive Biology, and Department of Pharmacology, Harvard Medical School
Boston, Massachusetts, 02115, U.S.A.)

The two peptides substance P and β-enkephalin are associated anatomically in many areas of the nervous system that are related to pain and analgesia. For example, β-enkephalin is present in interneurons in the dorsal horn of the spinal cord; substance P is present in unmyelinated C-fiber sensory nerves which have terminals in the same regions of the spinal cord as the enkephalin terminals (Hökfelt *et al.*, 1977). A third peptide, somatostatin, is also present in a separate population of C-fibers (Hökfelt *et al.*, 1976).

Several indirect lines of evidence suggest that enkephalin-containing nerve terminals may act on primary afferent neurons to regulate transmission in the nociceptive pathway. Iontophoresis of β-enkephalin into lamina II of the cat spinal cord depresses units in laminae IV-V that respond to noxious stimuli (Duggan *et al.*, 1976). Substance P excites this same type of unit (Henry, 1976). It has also been shown that there is a high density of opiate receptors in the dorsal horn (Lamotte *et al.*, 1976). Since the density of opiate receptors decreases markedly following dorsal rhizotomy, Lamotte *et al.* suggested that some opiate receptors may be located presynaptically on the endings of primary afferent neurons.

There are many reports that morphinomimetic drugs can inhibit the release of transmitter compounds (Paton, 1957; Kosterlitz and Hughes, 1975; Starke, 1977; Loh *et al.*, 1976). Of particular relevance is the report by Jessell and Iversen (1977) who showed that morphine or [D-Ala^2]-enkephalinamide can block the potassium-evoked release of substance P from a slice preparation of the rat trigeminal nerve nucleus. They suggested that the site of action of enkephalin is on the terminals of the substance P-containing neurons.

We thought it would be advantageous to study the effects of β-enkephalin on substance P-containing sensory neurons in dispersed cell culture in the absence of any spinal cord neurons. In such a system the neurons are easily accessible to biochemical manipulations and the cell bodies can be penetrated with intracellular electrodes. We found that in our cultures the sensory neurons contain substance P and that they can release this peptide when depolarized by potassium. We therefore investigated the effect of enkephalin on the neurons, both on the release of substance P and on their electrophysiological properties.

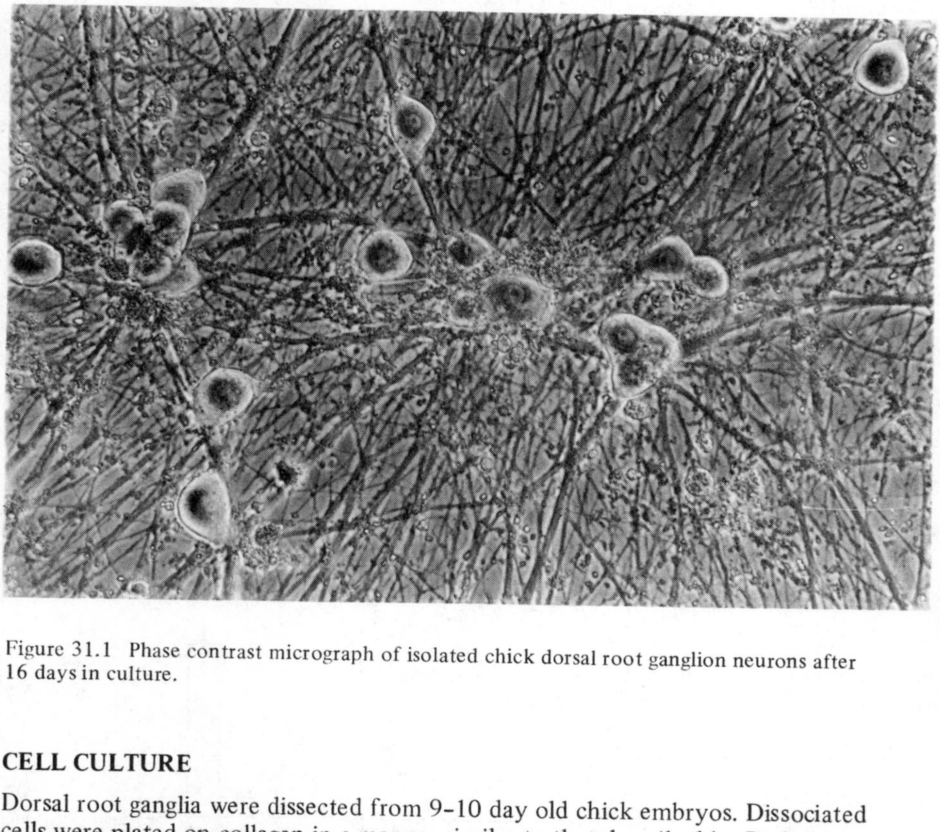

Figure 31.1 Phase contrast micrograph of isolated chick dorsal root ganglion neurons after 16 days in culture.

CELL CULTURE

Dorsal root ganglia were dissected from 9–10 day old chick embryos. Dissociated cells were plated on collagen in a manner similar to that described by Dichter and Fischbach (1977), but with the addition of Methocel (Dow Chemical Co.) and nerve growth factor (Varon *et al.*, 1967) to the growth medium. Cytosine arabinoside was added for the first 3 days of culture; this drug kills dividing cells so that there are few if any fibroblasts, glia or other non-neuronal cell types present (Fischbach, 1972).

Figure 31.1 shows a representative field from a typical plate of sensory neurons after 16 days in culture. The cell bodies are round and phase bright with a prominent nucleus and nucleolus. The dish at this time is covered with a dense network of neuronal processes.

Using sensitive and specific RIA (Mroz *et al.*, 1977; Patel *et al.*, 1975) we have found that, as is the case *in vivo,* such neurons in culture contain substance P and also somatostatin in easily measurable amounts. A 60 mm dish, after 2 weeks in culture, contains about 2.5 pmol of substance P and about 1 pmol of somatostatin (Mudge *et al.*, 1977; Mudge *et al.*, 1978).

RELEASE OF SUBSTANCE P

Potassium-evoked release

The neurons were incubated either in salt solutions containing the usual composition of electrolytes or in solutions where the potassium concentration was increased to depolarize the cells. At the end of the experiment, the neurons were extracted and assayed. The histogram in figure 31.2 shows the amount of substance P present in the medium at the end of successive 5 min incubations. The amount released is expressed as a percentage of the total substance P present at each time point assuming no net synthesis or degradation. There was little substance P released into the control (6 mM K^+) medium. However, when the neurons were depolarized in medium containing 120 mM potassium about 4 percent of the substance P was released. The neurons responded to repeated depolarizations.

We have partially characterized the immunoreactive material present in the cells and in the medium. On Sephadex G-25, the single peak of substance P immunoreactivity cochromatographed with synthetic substance P. Recovery was better than 90 percent. Furthermore, on cation-exchange chromatography using sulfopropyl-Sephadex both the cell extract and the released material were eluted by the same conditions as was synthetic substance P.

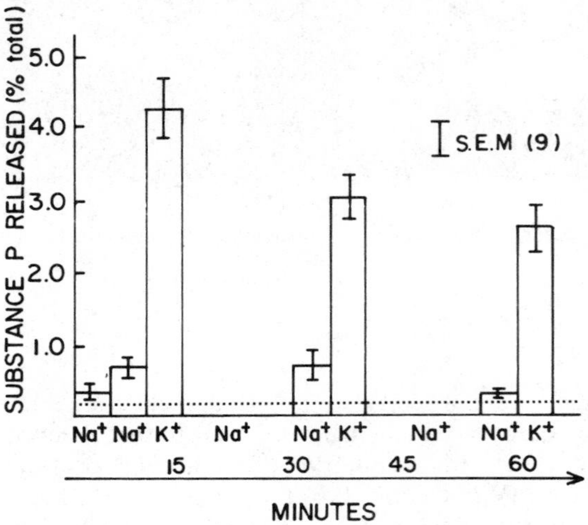

Figure 31.2 Successive 5-min incubations of cultured neurons in HEPES-buffered salt solutions containing either the usual cation concentration indicated as Na^+ (Na^+ 130 mM; K^+ 6 mM; Ca^{2+} 1.8 mM; Mg^{2+} 0.8 mM) or high K^+ concentration–K^+ (Na^+ 17 mM; K^+ 119 mM; Ca^{2+} 1.8 mM; Mg^{2+} 0.8 mM). The amount of peptide present in the solution at the end of each 5-min incubation is expressed as per cent total of the peptide present in the cells. The dashed line gives the limit of detection of the assay. DAEA, [D-Ala^2]-enkephalinamide. (See also Figures 31.3 and 31.4.)

Calcium dependence

Calcium influx into the nerve terminal is required for the release of neurotransmitters (Katz and Miledi, 1967; Rubin, 1970). Cobalt is known to block competitively calcium influx (Hagiwara and Takahashi, 1967; Baker *et al.*, 1973). If cobalt was added to the bathing medium there was no release of substance P in response to potassium depolarization, as shown in figure 31.3. However, after the cobalt was removed the neurons released substance P in response to the depolarization. This indicates that the release is calcium dependent. The calcium dependence of substance P release was studied in further detail; increasing the calcium concentration in the medium from 0 to 5.4 mM increased the release of substance P (Mudge *et al.*, 1978).

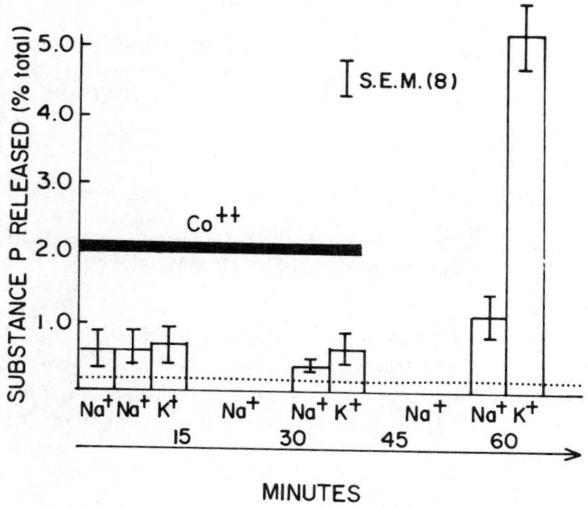

Figure 31.3 Same as figure 31.2 except that 5 mM Co^{2+} was added to all solutions for the first 40 min of incubations. The Ca^{2+} concentration was lowered to 0.2 mM and Mg^{2+} was omitted when Co^{2+} was present.

EFFECT OF [D-ALA^2]-ENKEPHALINAMIDE ON SUBSTANCE P RELEASE

The first bar in figure 31.4 shows the percentage of substance P released from control neurons after 5 min of depolarization in 30 mM potassium. [D-Ala^2]-enkephalinamide at 10^{-5} M markedly inhibited the potassium-evoked release of substance P. There was no inhibition of the release if naloxone was simultaneously added with the enkephalin. There was less inhibition of substance P release by 10^{-6} M [D-Ala^2]-enkephalinamide. The neurons are depolarized about 40 mV in 30 mM potassium. At greater depolarizations (higher potassium concentrations) the inhibition by [D-Ala^2]-enkephalinamide is not as marked.

This result is in general agreement with that reported by Jessell and Iversen (1977) who showed that 3×10^{-6} M [D-Ala^2]-enkephalinamide could block

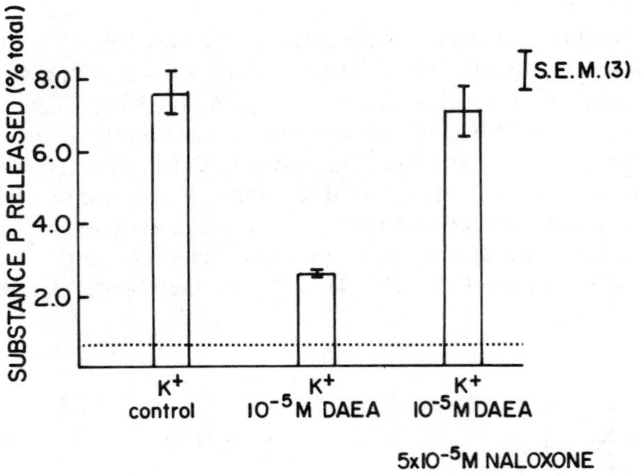

Figure 31.4 Release of substance P from sibling cultures during depolarization for 5 min. All three groups were depolarized by 30 mM potassium; the second group was depolarized in the presence of 10^{-5} M [D-Ala^2]-enkephalinamide the third group was depolarized in the presence of 10^{-5} M [D-Ala^2]-enkephalinamide plus 5×10^{-5} M naloxone.

potassium-evoked release of substance P from perfused slices of the substantia gelatinosa of the trigeminal nerve. Our experiments support the suggestion that the site of action of enkephalin is directly on the terminals of the substance P-containing sensory neurons since primary sensory neurons were the only cells present in the cultures.

ELECTROPHYSIOLOGICAL PROPERTIES OF SENSORY NEURONS

Three possibilities for the inhibitory action of β-enkephalin on substance P release are that: (1) β-enkephalin causes a conductance change in the neuronal membrane and thus prevents potassium from depolarizing the membrane; or (2) β-enkephalin uncouples the relationship between depolarization and the calcium influx which is required for release; or (3) β-enkephalin uncouples the relationship between calcium influx and the release process.

The action potential recorded in the cell body of cultured sensory neurons is in part mediated by inward calcium current (Dichter and Fischbach, 1977). There are similar voltage-sensitive calcium channels in several other types of neurons (Hagiwara, 1975) and it has been suggested that these somatic calcium channels may share common properties with the channels present in nerve terminals (Stinnakre and Tauc, 1973). Therefore the calcium channels in the sensory neuron cell bodies may serve as models for the channels present in nerve terminals which result in the calcium influx necessary for transmitter release. We have studied the effect of β-enkephalin on these channels.

The nature of the action potential in sensory neurons

Figure 31.5 shows action potentials recorded from a dorsal root ganglion neuron (A) and from a spinal cord neuron (B) in culture. In the dorsal root ganglion neuron there is an initial fast rising phase which is followed by a plateau region during the repolarization phase. In contrast, the spinal cord neuron does not have a plateau. The inward current during the first phase of the sensory-neuron action potential is carried by sodium ions and can be blocked by tetrodotoxin (TTX). The active response which remains in the presence of TTX is dependent on calcium and can be blocked by cobalt. Thus the action potential is a mixed sodium and calcium action potential, with the plateau region due to an inward calcium current (Dichter and Fischbach, 1977).

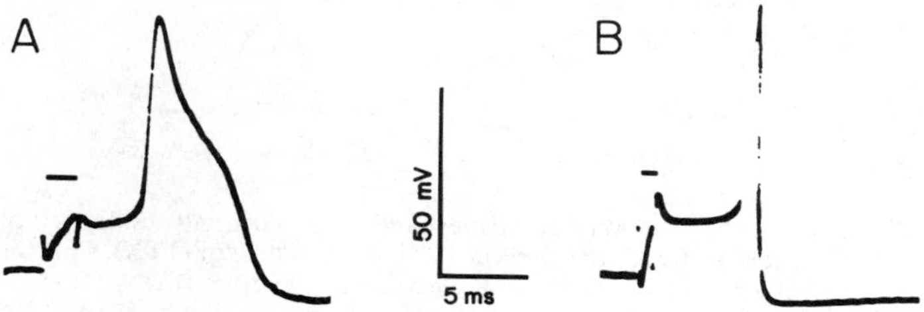

Figure 31.5 A, dorsal root ganglion neuron and B, spinal cord neuron action potentials evoked in balanced salt solutions. The membrane potential of both cells was –53 mV. Calibration bar, 50 mV, 5 ms.

Effect of [D-Ala^2]-enkephalinamide on the calcium component of the action potential

In the presence of barium which passes through the calcium channels and also blocks the delayed outward (repolarizing) potassium current, the action potential is prolonged. Figure 31.6A shows a 'barium spike' which is almost 1 s in duration. When 10^{-5} M [D-Ala^2]-enkephalinamide was applied to the cell soma by pressure ejection from a nearby micropipette (1-5 μm diameter), the duration of the action potential was immediately and dramatically reduced. The action potential returned to almost control duration by about 1 min after the ejection of the drug.

In the experiment shown in figure 31.6B, the action potential was evoked in the presence of TTX. This trace shows that in addition to reducing the duration of the action potential, [D-Ala^2]-enkephalinamide also decreased the amplitude and the rate of rise of the spike. Thus [D-Ala^2]-enkephalinamide apparently decreases the duration and the magnitude of the inward calcium current. Similar results were obtained when recording in normal calcium-containing solutions without barium. Complete dose-response curves have not yet been done, but 10^{-7}M β-enkephalin is also effective in reducing the duration of the spike.

The effect of β-enkephalin on the duration of the calcium current was antagonized by naloxone. We have used two micropipettes to eject either β-enkephalin alone or a solution containing both enkephalin and naloxone in equimolar concen-

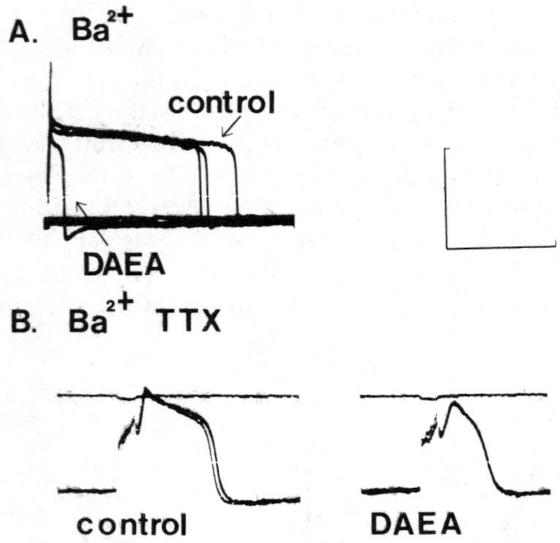

Figure 31.6 Sensory neuron action potential evoked in balanced salt solutions with the addition of A, 5 mM barium and B, 5 mM barium 10^{-7} M tetrodotoxin (TTX). Control indicates several action potentials evoked before the application of the drug. DAEA ([D-Ala^2]-enkephalinamide) indicates the action potential following the application of [D-Ala^2]-enkephalinamide to the cell soma membrane. Calibration for A, 60 mV, 300 ms; B, 60 mV, 30 ms.

trations. In all cases, a neuron which responded to the application of enkephalin showed no response to the application of enkephalin plus naloxone.

We saw no change in the resting membrane potential and no change in the input resistance of the membrane following the β-enkephalin application.

SUMMARY

These results show that β-enkephalin acts directly on sensory neurons in culture to inhibit substance P release. Enkephalin can also decrease the inward calcium current of the action potential in these neurons. It is therefore likely that the inhibition of substance P release is due to the inhibition of the calcium influx which is necessary for release.

Unlike other inhibitory neurotransmitters that have been described, enkephalin did not alter the passive membrane properties of the target neurons. It may instead directly modify the voltage-sensitive calcium channel.

Thus the ability of β-enkephalin to inhibit transmission in the nociceptive pathway may in part be due to a mechanism which decreases the entry of calcium into nerve terminals, thereby decreasing the release of substance P and possibly of other compounds.

REFERENCES

Baker, P. F., Meves, H. and Ridgeway, E. B. (1973). *J. Physiol., Lond.*, **231**, 511–26
Dichter, M. A. and Fischbach, G. D. (1977). *J. Physiol., Lond.*, **267**, 281–98
Duggan, A. W., Hall, J. G. and Headley, P. M. (1976). *Nature*, **264**, 456–8

Fischbach, G. D. (1972). *Dev Biol.*, **28**, 407–29
Hagiwara, S. (1975). In *Membranes. Vol. 3. Lipid Bilayers and Biological Membranes: Dynamic Properties,* (Ed. G. Eisenman) Marcel Dekker, New York
Hagiwara, S. and Takahashi, K. (1967). *J. gen. Physiol.*, **50**, 583–601.
Henry, J. L. (1976). *Brain Res.*, **114**, 439–51
Hökfelt, T., Elde, R., Johansson, O., Luft, R., Nilsson, G. and Arimura, A. (1976). *Neuroscience,* **1**, 131–6
Hökfelt, T., Ljungdahl, Å., Terenius, L., Elde, R. and Nilsson, G. (1977). *Proc. natn. Acad. Sci. U.S.A.*, **74**, 3081–5
Jessell, T. M. and Iversen, L. L. (1977). *Nature,* **268**, 549–51.
Katz, B. and Miledi, R. (1969). *J. Physiol., Lond.*, **203**, 689–706
Kosterlitz, H. W. and Hughes, J., (1975). *Life Sci.*, **17**, 91–6
Lamotte, C., Pert, C. B. and Snyder, S. H. (1976). *Brain Res.*, **112**, 407–12
Loh, H. H., Brase, D. A., Sampath-Khanna, S., Mar, J. B., Way, E. L. and Li, C. H. (1976). *Nature,* **264**, 567–8
Mroz, E. A., Brownstein, M. J. and Leeman, S. E. (1977). In *Substance P,* (eds U.S. von Euler and B. Pernow). Raven Press, New York
Mudge, A. W., Fischbach, G. D. and Leeman, S. E. (1977). *Abstracts, Society for Neuroscience,* 7th *Annual Meeting,* p.410
Mudge, A. W., Leeman, S. E. and Fischbach, G. D. (1978). *Proc. natn. Acad. Sci. U.S.A.*
Patel, Y. C., Weir, G. C. and Reichlin, S. (1975). *Program of 57th Annual Meeting of the Endocrine Society,* p. 127
Paton, W. D. M. (1957). *Br. J. Pharmac.*, **12**, 119–27
Rubin, R. P. (1970). *Pharmac. Rev.*, **22**, 389–427
Starke, K. (1977). *Rev. Physiol. Biochem. Pharmac.*, 77, 1–124
Stinnakre, J. and Tauc, L. (1973). *Nature,* **242**, 113–5
Varon, S., Nomura, J. and Shooter, E. M. (1967). *Biochemistry,* **7**, 2202–9

32

Evidence for tonic activity of enkephalins in brain and development of systemically active analogues with clinical potential

Robert C. A. Frederickson and Edward L. Smithwick, Jr (The Lilly Research Laboratories, Eli Lilly and Company, Indianapolis, Indiana 46206, U.S.A.)

The origin and physiological role of the various brain endorphins (Hughes, 1975; Terenius and Wahlström, 1975; Goldstein, 1975) remains an intriguing question. In particular, the elucidation of the source, manner of synthesis and specific functions of the brain pentapeptides, [Met^5]-enkephalin and [Leu^5]-enkephalin, provides an exciting challenge to investigators in the field. There is considerable evidence that these endogenous brain peptides are neurotransmitters or neuromodulators in various brain areas (see for example, Frederickson, 1977). They are present in these areas together with stereospecific receptors and immunohistochemical studies have shown that they are localized in nerve terminals and cell bodies. They affect the firing rate of neurons in these particular brain areas by an action on specific receptors and there is a highly effective system in brain for their inactivation.

We will present evidence for tonic activity of the brain's enkephalinergic systems which is compatible with a physiological role in brain for these interesting small peptides. Indeed, if these substances do have a physiological role, then analogues modified to reach the receptors in brain after systemic administration should have the appropriate pharmacology. We have tested this prediction and found support for it as well as an indication of clinical utility for these unique substances. We have concentrated on the pentapeptides since these moieties seem to be extremely potent when degradation is not a problem and provide significant advantages for a synthetic program compared to the larger endorphins.

METHODS

Synthesis and characterization of peptides

Peptides were prepared by classical solution methodology. The general approach involved the dicyclohexylcarbodiimidehydroxybenzotriazole–mediated coupling of an N^{α}-Boc-protected N-terminal tripeptide with the desired C-terminal dipeptide amide or ester. All intermediates were crystalized or preparatively chromatographed on silica-gel to give pure compounds with correct (±3 per cent) amino acid analysis, elemental analysis (±0.3 per cent), and thin-layer homogeneity in several solvent systems. All final peptide products were purified when necessary by chromatography on DEAE–Sephadex A-25 in 1 per cent pyridine: 0.05 per cent acetic acid aqueous buffer. Characterization included, in addition to the methods used for blocked intermediates, h.p.l.c. on C_{18} reverse-phase silica (effluent monitoring at 210 and 280 nm).

Determination of serum growth hormone and prolactin

Immature (29-day-old) Sprague-Dawley derived female rats were used. The concentrations of serum growth hormone (GH) and prolactin (PRL) were determined by RIA (Birge *et al.*, 1967; Niswender *et al.*, 1969; Shaar *et al.*, 1977). Physiological saline or test drugs were administered to the rats by s.c. injection and 20 min later the rats were decapitated. Blood samples were collected from all rats and sera were obtained by centrifugation at 1600 *g* for 20 min at 4 °C.

Analgesic tests

The hot plate test (Eddy and Leimbach, 1953; Frederickson *et al.*, 1976*b*, 1977) utilized an apparatus with an electrically heated, thermostatically controlled metal plate (Technilab Instruments, Mod 475). A Plexiglass cylinder, 12 inches (30 cm) high and 4.75 inches (12 cm) inner diameter, was used to confine the animals to a defined surface of the hot plate. The hot plate was maintained at 52 °C for the studies reported here. The time in seconds from contact with the plate until a hind-paw lick occurred was recorded as the response latency. The latency until an escape jump occurred was also recorded. Each mouse was used only once. Rat tail heat and mouse writhing tests were also used to test analgesia. These tests are described elsewhere (Frederickson and Smits, 1973; Smits and Myers, 1974). Drugs were administered either s.c., i.v., or i.v.t. Hamilton microsyringes bearing 27-gauge needles with stops at 2.5 mm from the needle tip were utilized for i.v.t. administration (Frederickson *et al.*, 1976*b*).

Physical dependence

Male Sprague-Dawley rats (90–100 g at start of experiment, Harlan Industries) were used to assess primary dependence liability of opioids. The rats were injected s.c. four times daily for 14 days with either saline or an opioid drug (morphine, meperidine, pentazocine, codeine or enkephalin analogue) with doses increasing gradually from 10 mg/kg to 160 mg/kg per injection. The degree of dependence developed was assessed at days 4, 7, 10 and 14 by challenge with naloxone and scoring of the resulting withdrawal signs. This withdrawal scoring technique has been previously described (Frederickson and Smits, 1973; Frederickson, 1975; Frederickson *et al.*, 1976*a*).

Similar studies were also done with mice using the naloxone- induced jumping response to measure withdrawal severity. Mice were treated four times daily with saline or opioid drug for either 3 days or 5 days. Jumps were counted after challenge with naloxone at 100 mg/kg, s.c.

Mouse vas deferens

Single vasa deferentia (MVD) from mature mice (Cox, 30–40 g) were suspended in 3 ml of modified Krebs' solution (Henderson *et al.*, 1972) aerated with 95 per cent O_2–5 per cent CO_2 and maintained at 37 °C. The twitch induced by field stimulation (0.15 Hz, 1 ms, 40 V) was recorded on a polygraph (Grass Model 78) via an isometric transducer (Grass FTO3C). Drugs were added to the bath in 20–30 μl aliquots with Hamilton syringes. Dose-response curves were constructed by cumulative addition of appropriate amounts of drug to the bath. Comparison of relative agonist potency was made on the basis of IC_{50} values (concentration causing a depression of 50 per cent of the electrically evoked contraction). The peptides were compared to normorphine as a standard of reference (Frederickson *et al.*, 1976*b*, *c*).

Measurement of enkephalin levels

Mice (Cox Standard, Harlan 23–27 g) were killed by microwave irradiation for 3 s in a Litton oven with focused wavepath. Whole brain minus cerebellum and spinal cord was removed and stored (–20 °C) until extraction and assay of enkephalins the following day. Brains were homogenized in pairs in 25 ml of 0.1 N HCl and centrifuged at 20 000*g* for 10 min in a Sorvall superspeed automatic refrigerated centrifuge (RC2-B). Enkephalins were extracted from the samples with Amberlite XAD-2 according to the procedure of Smith *et al.* (1976). The total opioid activity in each sample was assayed with the MVD as described previously (Henderson *et al.*, 1972; Frederickson *et al.*, 1976*c*) except that synthetic [Met^5]-enkephalin was used as standard instead of normorphine. The inhibitory actions of all extracts after XAD-2 chromatography were completely reversed by naloxone (0.3–1 μM).

D-Amphetamine and L-DOPA-induced jumping in mice

Male Cox Standard Mice (23–27 g) were injected s.c. with D-amphetamine at 2 mg/kg followed 15 min later by a s.c. injection of saline or test drug plus L-DOPA at 200 or 300 mg/kg, i.p. The mice were then placed inside an acrylic cylinder (12 inches (30 cm) high and 4.75 inches (12 cm) inner diameter) and jumps were counted for a 30 min period beginning 10 min after they were placed in the cylinder. This is a slight modification of a test originally described by Lal *et al.* (1975) and Lal (1976).

RESULTS

Basic studies

Evidence for tonic activity in neuroendocrine regulation
The partially metabolically protected analogues of the enkephalins, [D-Ala²-Met⁵]-enkephalinamide and [D-Ala²-Leu⁵]-enkephalinamide, as well as morphine sulfate, at doses of 1, 3 and 10 mg/kg s.c. caused significant dose-dependent elevations of serum GH and PRL (Shaar *et al.*, 1977). These effects could be antagonized by naloxone in a dose-dependent fashion (figures 32.1 and 32.2). Naloxone's antagonistic effects peaked at a dose of 0.2 mg/kg, s.c. Naloxone was more effective at antagonizing morphine than either of the peptides since the dose–response curve versus morphine was to the left of those versus the opioid peptides (figures 32.1 and 32.2). A tonic physiological effect of endogenous peptides to facilitate the release of GH and PRL would demand an inhibitory effect of naloxone itself on basal hormone release. Indeed we did observe such a phenomenon, and the dose–response curve of the inhibitory effect of naloxone alone was coincident with its curve for antagonism of the opioid peptides (figures 32.1 and 32.2). This is suggestive that naloxone's inhibitory effect is due to antagonism of endogenous opioids and supports the concept of tonic physiological activity of such systems. We have earlier provided evidence that this activity is in the CNS and not at the level of the pituitary (Shaar *et al.*, 1977).

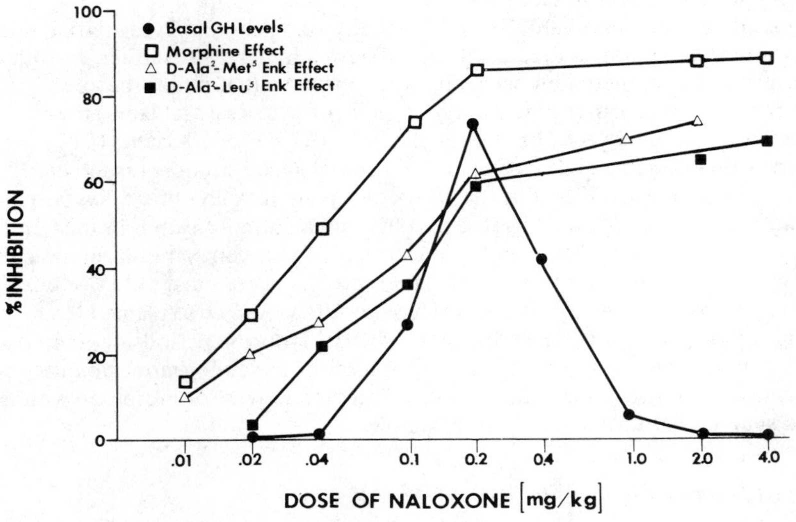

Figure 32.1 Dose–response curves of inhibitory effects of naloxone hydrochloride on basal growth hormone concentrations and on the stimulatory effects of morphine sulfate, [D-Ala², Met]⁵-enkephalinamide and [D-Ala², Leu⁵]-enkephalinamide (from Shaar *et al.*, 1977).

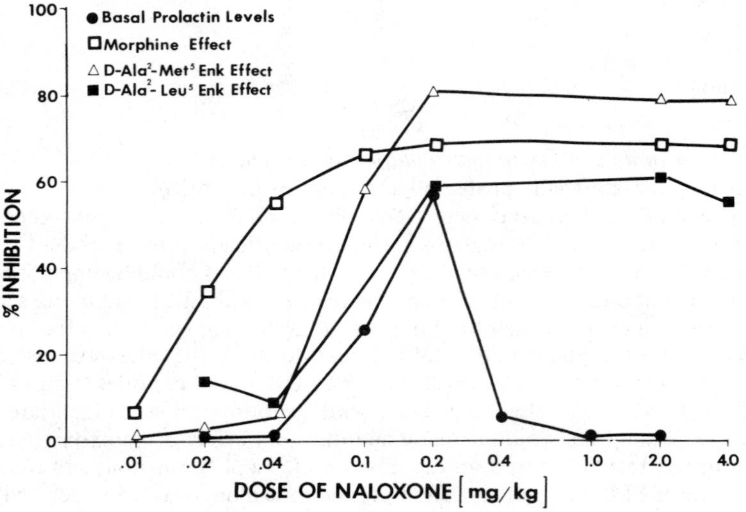

Figure 32.2 Dose-response curves of inhibitory effects of naloxone hydrochloride on basal prolactin concentrations and on the stimulatory effects of morphine sulfate, [D-Ala^2, Met^5]-enkephalinamide and [D-Ala^2, Leu^5]-enkephalinamide (from Shaar *et al.*, 1977).

Evidence for endogenous opioid activity regulating nociception

The opioid peptides are likely also to have a physiological role in regulating nociception. In this event naloxone itself should have a hyperalgesic effect. In spite of earlier controversy, there now seems to be a consensus that under the appropriate conditions naloxone can produce a hyperalgesic effect as several laboratories (Frederickson *et al.*, 1976*b*; Frederickson *et al.*, 1977; Frederickson, 1977; Grevert and Goldstein, 1977) have now confirmed Jacob's report (Jacob *et al.*, 1974) of a hyperalgesic effect in the mouse hot plate test. In our studies (Frederickson *et al.*, 1977) utilizing this test we observed a diurnal rhythm in the control latencies to the jump response and in the effects of naloxone and morphine on these latencies (figure 32.3). Naloxone and morphine were most effective during the times of highest control latencies. These results would be explained by a diurnal rhythm in activity of endogenous opioids. Thus the periods of greater activity of naloxone would be due to antagonism of the endogenous opioids when their activity was highest and the periods of greater activity of morphine would be due to synergism with the endogenous opioids.

Levels of brain opioid peptides

We observed levels of total opioid peptide activity in mouse brain to be 50–100 ng (met-enkephalin equivalent) per brain. The total levels of opioid activity in mouse brain were occasionally higher at 1500 h when jump latencies were near maximum than at 0800 h when these latencies were near minimum but we did not detect any evidence of a diurnal rhythm in this measure.

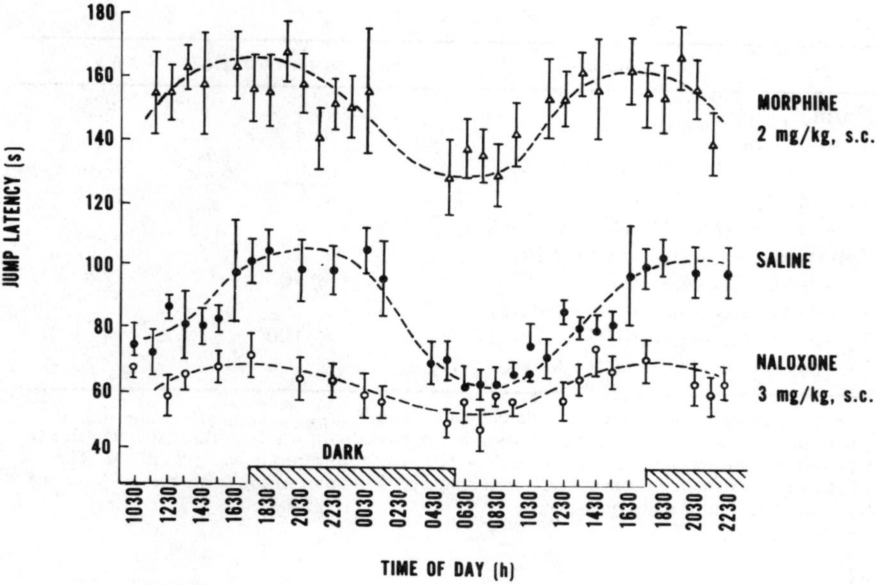

Figure 32.3 Diurnal rhythm in latencies to the jump response on the mouse hot plate maintained at 52 °C. Closed circles refer to animals treated with saline, subcutaneously, 15 minutes before testing. Open circles refer to animals treated with naloxone at 3 mg/kg, subcutaneously, 15 min before testing. Open triangles refer to animals treated with morphine at 2 mg/kg, subcutaneously, 30 min before testing. The latencies (mean ± s.e., N = 10 to 100) in seconds are plotted as a function of the time of day. The datum points at each $\frac{1}{2}$ hour are the means of values collected over a 1-hour period. For example, the points plotted at 0930 h are the means of measurements made from 0900 h to 1000 h. Lights were off during the time period marked by the hatched bars. Several points are repeated beyond 24 hours in order to better illustrate the rhythm (from Frederickson *et al.*, 1977).

Study of enkephalin analogues

Mouse vas deferens data

In order to develop systemically active analogues it was necessary first to provide compounds with high activity at the receptor then to modify these to provide protection from degradation. The MVD preparation was utilized to develop structure-activity relationships without interference from pharmacokinetic factors. Some of these data have been already published (Frederickson *et al.*, 1976*b*; Frederickson, 1977). Further data showing the activity of some of the protected analogues compared to normorphine and the natural peptides are summarized in table 32.1.

The replacement of Gly^2 with D-Ala^2 provides protection from cleavage by peptidases from the N-terminal while N-methylation at the peptide link at position 5 provides protection at the C-terminal. It is interesting and fortunate that these modifications do not interfere with binding to the receptor but indeed even result in increased receptor activity. Evidence that these modified peptides still utilize the same receptors as the natural materials is provided by determination of pA_2 values for naloxone versus the different analogues.

Table 32.1 Mouse vas deferens data

Compound	Molar potency ratio	pA_2
Normorphine	1	8.2
β-Endorphin	0.7	
Tyr–Gly–Gly–Phe–Met–COOH	20.0	7.6
Tyr–Gly–Gly–Phe–Met–$CONH_2$	9	
Tyr–Gly–Gly–Phe–Leu–$CONH_2$	5	
Tyr–D-Ala–Gly–Phe–Leu–$CONH_2$	33	
Tyr–D-Ala–Gly–Phe–Met–$CONH_2$	50	7.5
Tyr–D-Ala–Gly–Phe–D-Met–$CONH_2$	7	
Tyr–D-Ala–Gly–Phe–*N*(CH_3)Leu–$CONH_2$	100	
Tyr–D-Ala–Gly–Phe–*N*(CH_3)Met–$CONH_2$	100	7.6

The molar potency ratios were calculated as the ratio IC_{50} normorphine/IC_{50} compound where the IC_{50} refers to the concentration in the tissue bath which inhibits the electrically stimulated contractions by 50 per cent. The IC_{50} for normorphine was 3×10^{-7} M. The pA_2 values were derived from linear regression analysis of the plot of log (dose ratio −1) versus log concentration of naloxone.

Analgesic data–intraventricular injection

The mouse hot plate test was utilized to assess the activity of the various peptides compared to morphine on analgesic receptors in brain. In these studies the compounds were administered directly into the lateral ventricles in order to bypass the blood-brain barrier (BBB). The results of these studies are summarized in table 32.2. These data show that the protected [Met^5]-enkephalin analogue, Tyr–D-Ala-Gly-Phe-*N*(CH_3)Met-$CONH_2$, for example, was 100 times more potent than morphine and 25-30 000 times as potent as the natural peptide when administered directly into the brain.

The effects of the enkephalin analogues in both the MVD assay and the hot plate test were completely antagonizable by naloxone, although this required 3 to 10 times as much naloxone as to comparatively antagonize morphine or normorphine.

Analgesic data–subcutaneous injection

The above data show that the protected enkephalin analogues are highly active analgesics when they can reach the appropriate receptors. To examine the extent to which they cross the BBB we tested them in the mouse hot plate, mouse writhing and rat tail heat tests for analgesia after s.c. injection. Dose-response curves comparing the effects of morphine and Tyr–D-Ala–Gly–Phe–*N*(CH_3)Met–$CONH_2$ in the mouse hot plate test are shown in figures 32.4 and 32.5. Clearly this analogue of enkephalin can produce considerable analgesia even after systemic administration. This compound also showed potent analgesic activity in the mouse writhing test and to a somewhat lesser degree in the rat tail heat test. The relative analgesic potency of several narcotic analgesics and several enkephalin analogues in the mouse hot plate and mouse writhing tests is shown in table 32.3. The time course of analgesic activity of Tyr–D-Ala–Gly–Phe–*N*(CH_3)Met–$CONH_2$ is shorter

Table 32.2 Mouse hot plate data

Compound	Molar potency ratio $\frac{ED_{50}\ \text{Morphine}}{ED_{50}\ \text{Compound}}$
Morphine	1
β-Endorphin	16.2
*Tyr-Gly-Gly-Phe-Met-COOH	0.003
*Tyr-Gly-Gly-Phe-Met-$CONH_2$	0.004
Tyr-D-Ala-Gly-Phe-Leu-$CONH_2$	1.23
Tyr-D-Ala-Gly-Phe-Met-$CONH_2$	0.43
Tyr-D-Ala-Gly-Phe-D-Met-$CONH_2$	16.6
Tyr-D-Ala-Gly-Phe-*N*(CH_3)Leu-$CONH_2$	55
Tyr-D-Ala-Gly-Phe-*N*(CH_3)Met-$CONH_2$	100

Tests were run at 15 min after i.v.t. administration of the compounds except for the two starred materials which were run at 3 min. These peptides had no effect at 15 min. The data presented are for the hind paw lick response for which morphine's ED_{50} was 0.25 μg per mouse.

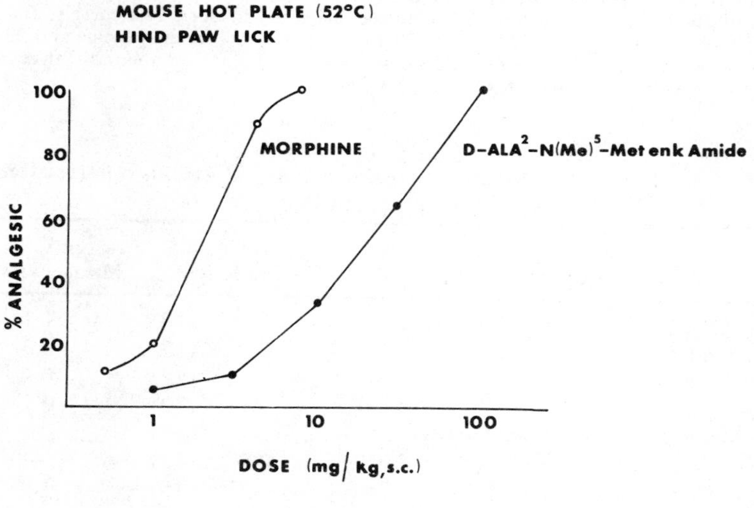

Figure 32.4 Dose-response curves of analgesic activity of morphine and Tyr-D-Ala-Gly-Phe-*N*(CH_3) Met-$CONH_2$ in the mouse hot plate test. These curves represent the effects on the hind paw lick response. The effects of morphine were tested at 30 min after injection while the effects of the peptide were tested at 15 min after injection. Percentage analgesia was determined as the proportion of test animals with response latencies greater than the control latency + 2 s.d.

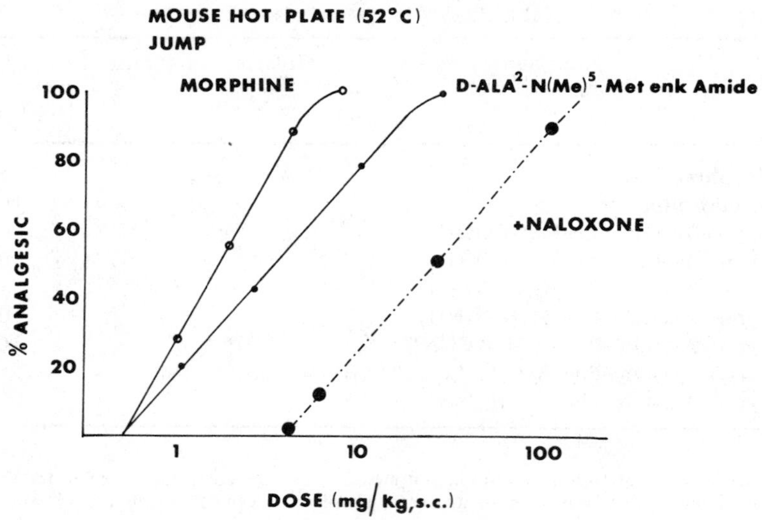

Figure 32.5 Dose-response curves of analgesic activity of morphine and Tyr-D-Ala-Gly-Phe-$N(CH_3)$ Met-$CONH_2$ in the mouse hot plate test. These curves represent the effects on the jump response. The effects of morphine were tested at 30 min after injection and of the peptide at 15 min after injection. The dotted line is the dose-response curve to the peptide together with naloxone which was injected immediately before the peptide at 0.03 mg/kg, s.c. Percentage analgesia was determined as the proportion of test animals with response latencies greater than the control latency + 2 s.d.

Table 32.3 Relative analgesic activity of various opioids after subcutaneous injection.

Compound	Mouse hot plate test		Mouse writhing test	
Morphine	1	(30)	1	(30)
Meperidine	0.8	(15)	0.3	(10)
Pentazocine	0.2	(15)	0.4	(15)
Codeine	0.1	(30)	0.1	(15)
Tyr–D-Ala–Gly–Phe–D-Met–$CONH_2$	<0.1	(15)	–	
Tyr–D-Ala–Gly–Phe–$N(CH_3)$Leu–$CONH_2$	0.2	(15)	–	
Tyr–D-Ala–Gly–Phe–$N(CH_3)$Met–$CONH_2$	0.3	(15)	1.5	(20)

The data are expressed as molar potency ratios (ED_{50} morphine/ED_{50} compound) compared to morphine. The ED_{50} values for morphine were 2 mg/kg for the hot plate and 1 mg/kg for the writhing test. The ratios were corrected for relative molecular weights. The numbers in brackets refer to the time in minutes after injection when the tests were run and represent approximate times for peak effect.

than that of morphine but very similar to the duration of activity of equianalgesic doses of meperidine or pentazocine. A comparison of the time courses of morphine, meperidine and Tyr-D-Ala-Gly-Phe-*N*(CH_3)Met-$CONH_2$ in the mouse writhing test is shown in figure 32.6.

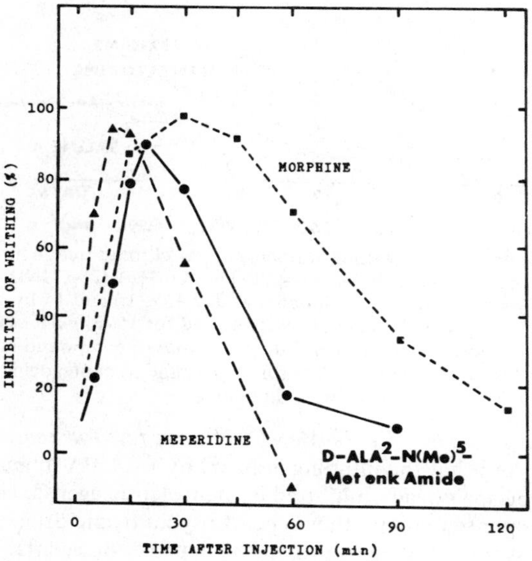

Figure 32.6 Time course of analgesic effects of morphine, meperidine and Tyr-D-Ala-Gly-Phe-*N*(CH_3) Met-$CONH_2$ in the mouse writhing test. Morphine was tested at 2 mg/kg, s.c., meperidine at 8 mg/kg, s.c. and the peptide at 8 mg/kg, s.c.

Physical dependence liability

The relative capacity of Tyr-D-Ala-Gly-Phe-*N*(CH_3)Met-$CONH_2$ to produce physical dependence was compared with that of morphine, meperidine, pentazocine and codeine in mice and rats. The rats were treated chronically with each of the drugs for 14 days as described in Methods and the withdrawal scores obtained on each of the test days after injection of naloxone are shown in figure 32.7. In this experiment morphine produced a high level of dependence, and meperidine and pentazocine an intermediate level of dependence. The enkephalin analogue resembled saline in this test. In a second test the enkephalin analogue did produce some withdrawal compared to saline control but this was much less than that produced by codeine. Similar results were obtained in the mouse jumping test. Chronic treatment with the enkephalin analogue for 3 days resulted in no withdrawal jumping after naloxone while the group treated for 5 days showed a small amount of jumping which was less than that produced by morphine, meperidine, pentazocine, codeine or *d*-propoxyphene. No tolerance in the mouse writhing test was seen for the enkephalin analogue after such chronic treatment while we were able to demonstrate tolerance to morphine and pentazocine with identical treatment.

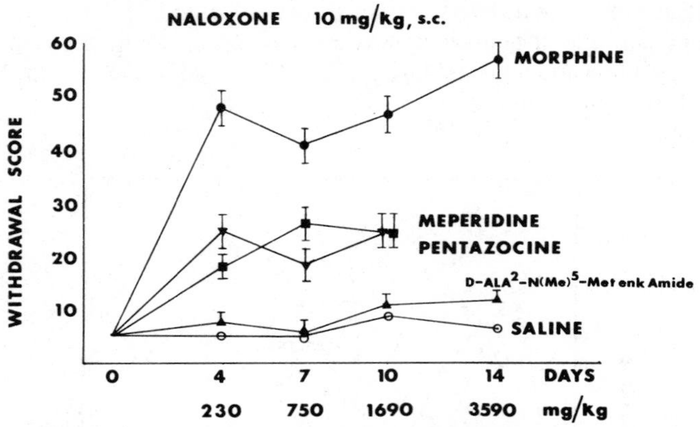

Figure 32.7 Naloxone precipitated withdrawal scores after chronic treatment of rats with morphine, meperidine, pentazocine, Tyr–D-Ala–Gly–Phe–*N*(CH_3)Met–$CONH_2$ or saline as described in Methods. Withdrawal was precipitated at day 4, 7, 10 and 14 by the injection of naloxone at 10 mg/kg, s.c. Withdrawal signs were scored for 15 min after injection of naloxone. The numbers below the abscissa give the total dose of compound in mg/kg administered by each time of testing. There is no data for meperidine or pentazocine after day 10 since the rats died after further treatment with these drugs.

*Effect of Tyr–*D*-Ala–Gly–Phe–N(CH_3)Met–$CONH_2$ in test for neuroleptic activity*

Lal (1976) has reported that the jumping induced by L-DOPA in amphetamine-treated mice is rather specifically inhibited by neuroleptic agents. He observed no inhibition of this response by any other type of psychotropic drug except morphine, which was less potent, however, than the neuroleptic agents. The enkephalin analogue was active in this test. It inhibited the jumping with an ED_{50} of 7.4 mg/kg, s.c. as shown in figure 32.8. Thus it is roughly equipotent with clozapine (Lal, 1976) on a molar basis.

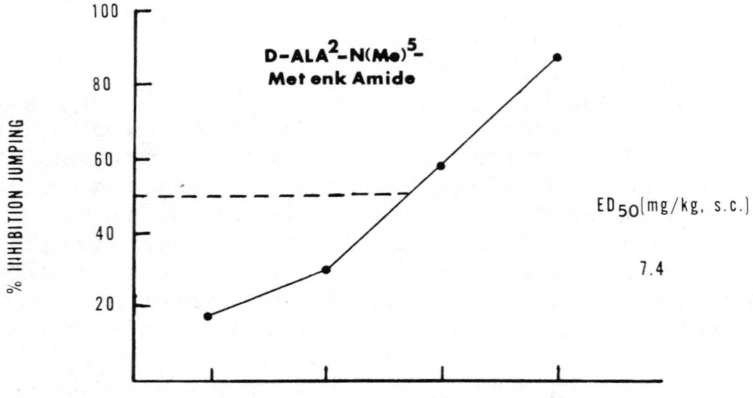

Figure 32.8 Dose–response curve of inhibitory effect of Tyr–D-Ala–Gly–Phe–*N*(CH_3)Met–$CONH_2$ on jumping induced in mice by D-amphetamine plus L-DOPA. This test is described in the methods section. The enkephalin analogue was injected 15 min before testing. The ED_{50} in this test was 7.4 mg/kg, s.c. *N*, 6–12 mice per point.

DISCUSSION

We have presented evidence for tonic activity of the brain's opioid peptide systems which is compatible with a physiological role in brain for these substances. Analogues of the natural peptides which have been modified to protect them from cleavage of the Tyr–Gly peptide bond act in the CNS to cause a release of GH and PRL. The opioid antagonist, naloxone, has direct actions in the opiate-naive animal to inhibit the release of these hormones. The dose–response curve for this effect is superimposable on that for its antagonism of the releasing effects of the exogenously administered opioid peptides but to the right of that for antagonism of the releasing effects of morphine.

Naloxone also has hyperalgesic activity in opiate-naive animals. We have observed a diurnal rhythm in this effect of naloxone which seemed to be secondary to a diurnal rhythm in the baseline latency or sensitivity to noxious stimuli. We interpreted these results as possibly due to a diurnal rhythm in activity of endogenous opioids such that the periods of greater activity of naloxone would be due to antagonism of the endogenous opioids when their activity was highest. Measurement of levels of total opioid activity in whole mouse brain at different times of day provided no evidence of diurnal rhythm in this parameter. The rhythm, however, might occur for only one of the several opioid peptides, in only selected brain areas and/or be seen only in the turnover or activity rather than the levels of the substance. Evidence for turnover of the endogenous peptides could be provided by measuring the incorporation of labeled amino acids. Clouet and Ratner (1976) earlier reported the incorporation of [^{3}H] glycine into enkephalin. We are presently utilizing RIA techniques to measure specific levels of met-enkephalin and leu-enkephalin and studying the incorporation of [^{3}H] tyrosine to measure turnover of these peptides. These studies look promising and should provide further insight into the nature and mechanism of the endogenous rhythm which could offer strong evidence for a physiological role for opioid peptides in the regulation of nociception.

We felt that if the opioid peptides in brain were indeed endogenous transmitter substances with specific physiological roles, then analogues with adequate metabolic stability to reach receptors in the brain after systemic administration should possess the appropriate pharmacology reflecting these physiological roles. This, of course, would be true only if the modifications did not alter the receptor specificity of the natural compound.

We utilized the MVD preparation to work out the structure–activity relationships of the enkephalins as the first step in drug design and used this test also as a first screen for appropriate receptor activity for the modified analogues. Fortunately the replacement of Gly^2 with D-Ala^2 to provide metabolic protection at the N-terminal conferred increased potency on the vas deferens receptor and *N*-methylating the peptide bond between Phe^4 and Met^5 to protect the C-terminal increased potency even further. Confirmation that these modified enkephalins were acting at the same receptor sites as the natural peptides was provided by determination of the pA_2 of naloxone versus these compounds compared to its pA_2 value versus the natural substance. The pA_2 values were identical.

Examination of the analgesic activity of these compounds after i.v.t. administration was utilized to assess whether the synthetic peptides also acted on the appropriate receptors in brain. The natural peptides produce only very fleeting analgesia after injection of huge quantities (50–200 μg) into the lateral ventricles. There is apparently a highly effective enzyme system in brain for inactivation of these natural substances. The synthetic analogues, however, were extremely potent when injected directly into brain. Tyr-D-Ala-Gly-Phe-*N*(CH_3) Met-$CONH_2$ was at least 100 times as potent on a molar basis as morphine and almost 30 000 times more potent than met-enkephalin itself by this route. This enkephalin analogue was active in several analgesic tests after subcutaneous administration. It was intermediate in potency between that of morphine or meperidine and that of codeine, pentazocine or *d*-propoxyphene. Its duration of analgesic activity was equivalent to that of meperidine or pentazocine. It produced very little primary dependence after chronic treatment in rodents, having less dependence liability in these tests than morphine, meperidine, pentazocine, codeine or *d*-propoxyphene. It was also less potent than all these drugs in suppressing withdrawal jumping in morphine-dependent mice and was much less toxic upon chronic treatment. There have been reports that β-endorphin and the enkephalins will produce physical dependence on chronic i.v.t. perfusion (for example Wei and Loh, 1976). While the analogue discussed here can induce physical dependence, it seems to be far less liable to produce dependence, relative to its analgesic activity, when it is administered systemically.

There have been several reports implicating endorphins in schizophrenia although the data are limited and controversial and the role of these peptides in the etiology or amelioration of this disease is not clear (Terenius *et al.*, 1976; Gunne *et al.*, 1977; Volavka *et al.*, 1977; Davis *et al.*, 1977; Kline *et al.*, 1977). Many of these studies are discussed elsewhere in this volume. The data presented here on enkephalin analogues have shown that the systemically active compound, Tyr-D-Ala-Gly-Phe-*N*(CH_3)Met-$CONH_2$, is active in an animal test purported to be responsive rather specifically to antipsychotic agents (Lal, 1976). This modified opioid peptide is equally active in this test, on a molar basis, as clozapine, a known antipsychotic agent with a diminished propensity to produce extrapyramidal side-effects. There seems to be a real potential for development of analogues of the small opioid peptides with potent and specific clinical utility but this remains to be critically tested in man. The small peptides seem to have significant advantages over the larger endorphins in this regard since pharmacological activity seems clearly to reside in the smaller fragment which is much easier and more economical to synthesize.

The clinical potential of the modified opioid peptides remains to be realized but we feel that the data presented here provide support for an important physiological role for the small opioid peptides.

ACKNOWLEDGMENTS

We wish to thank Dr S. E. Smits, Dr C. J. Shaar, R. Shuman, V. Burgis, C. E. Harrell and J. D. Edwards for their contribution to the work reported here and L. Witter for assistance in preparation of this manuscript.

REFERENCES

Birge, C. A., Peeke, G. T., Mariz, I. K. and Daughaday, W. H. (1967). *Endocrinology,* **81**, 195–9

Clouet, D. H. and Ratner, M. (1976). *In* Opiates and Endogenous Opioid Peptides, (ed. H. W. Kosterlitz) Elsevier/North-Holland Biomedical Press, Amsterdam, pp. 71–78

Davis, G. C., Bunney, W. E., Jr, DeFraites, E. G., Kleinman, J. E., Van Kammen, D. P., Post, R. M. and Wyatt, R. J. (1977). *Science,* **197**, 74–7

Eddy, N. B. and Leimbach, D. (1953). *J. Pharmac. exp. Ther.,* **107**, 385–93

Frederickson, R. C. A. (1975). *Nature,* **257**, 131–2

Frederickson, R. C. A. (1977). *Life Sci.,* **21**, 23–42

Frederickson, R. C. A., Burgis, V. and Edwards, J. D. (1977). *Science,* **198**, 756–8

Frederickson, R. C. A., Hewes, C. R. and Aiken, J. W. (1976*a*). *J. Pharmac. exp. Ther.,* **199**, 375–84

Frederickson, R. C. A., Nickander, R., Smithwick, E. L., Shuman, R. and Norris, F. H. (1976*b*). In Opiates and Endogenous Opioid Peptides, (ed. H. W. Kosterlitz). Elsevier/North-Holland Biomedical Press, Amsterdam, pp. 239–46

Frederickson, R. C. A., Schirmer, E. W., Grinnan, E. L., Harrell, C. E. and Hewes, C. R. (1976*c*). *Life Sci.,* **19**, 1181–90

Frederickson, R. C. A., and Smits, S. E. (1973). *Res. Commun. Chem. Path. Pharmac.,* **5**, 867–70

Goldstein, A. (1975). *Brain Sci.,* **193**, 1081–6

Grevert, P. and Goldstein, A. (1977). *Psychopharmacology,* **53**, 111–13

Gunne, L. M., Lindstrom, L. and Terenius, L. (1977). *J. Neural Transmission,* **40**, 13–19

Henderson, G., Hughes, J. and Kosterlitz, H. W. (1972). *Br. J. Pharmac.,* **46**, 764–6

Hughes, J. (1975). *Brain Res.,* **88**, 295–308.

Jacob, J. J., Tremblay, E. C. and Colombel, M. C. (1974). *Psychopharmacologia,* **37**, 217–23

Kline, N. S., Li, C. H., Lehmann, H. E., Lajtha, A., Laski, E. and Cooper, T. (1977). *Arch. gen. Psychiat.,* **34**, 1111–3

Lal, H. (1976). *Neuropharmacology,* **15**, 669–71

Lal, H., Colpaert, F. C. and Laduron, P. (1975). *Eur. J. Pharmac.,* **30**, 113–6

Niswender, G. D., Chen, C. L., Midgley, A. R. Jr., Meites, J. and Ellis, S. (1969). *Proc. Soc. exp. Biol. Med.,* **130**, 793–7

Shaar, C. J., Frederickson, R. C. A., Dininger, N. B. and Jackson, L. (1977). *Life Sci.,* **21**, 853–60

Smith, T. W., Hughes, J., Kosterlitz, H. W. and Sosa, R. P. (1976). In Opiates and Endogenous Opioid Peptides, (ed. H. W. Kosterlitz). Elsevier/North-Holland Biomedical Press, Amsterdam, pp. 57–62

Smits, S. E. and Myers, M. B. (1974). *Res. Commun. Chem. Path. Pharmac.,* **7**, 651–62

Terenius, L. and Wahlström, A. (1975). *Acta physiol. scand.,* **94**, 74–81

Terenius, L., Wahlström, A., Lindstrom, L. and Widerlöv, E. (1976). *Neurosci. Lett.,* **3**, 157–62

Volavka, J., Mallya, A., Baig, S. and Perez-Cruet, J. (1977). *Science,* **196**, 1227–8

Wei, E. and Loh, H. (1976). *Science,* **193**, 1262–3

33
Differential binding properties of some opiates and opioid peptides

Ian Creese, Steven R. Childers, Rabi Simantov and Solomon H. Snyder
(Departments of Pharmacology and Experimental Therapeutics and Psychiatry and Behavioral Sciences, Johns Hopkins University School of Medicine, Baltimore, Maryland 21205, U.S.A.)

The opioid peptide enkephalins were discovered as endogenous substances in the brain which mimic effects of morphine pharmacologically at presumed receptor sites in smooth muscle systems (Hughes, 1975) and compete for [^{3}H] opiate binding to opiate receptor sites in brain membranes (Terenius and Wahlstrom, 1975; Pasternak *et al.*, 1975*a*). Accordingly, these opiate receptor sites which bind opiates with high affinity and in proportion to their pharmacological activity (Snyder, 1975) presumably serve physiologically to interact with endogenous opioid peptides. In the brain the quantitatively predominant opioid peptides are the two pentapeptides met and leu-enkephalin while lower concentrations of a 39-amino acid opioid peptide β-endorphin may also presumably interact with opiate receptors. However, since the localization of enkephalin throughout the brain corresponds more closely with that of opiate receptors than does localization of β-endorphin (Simantov *et al.*, 1977; Rossier *et al.*, 1977), it is likely that the majority of opiate receptors in the brain normally interact with enkephalins rather than β-endorphin.

Whereas most opiates are small molecules consisting of 3–5 fused rings, enkephalin is a highly flexible molecule containing five amino acids. It is thus surprising, at first sight, that both series of compounds might interact with the same receptor. Consideration of their similar pharmacological profiles and the dependence of opioid peptide activity on the amino-terminal tyrosine (corresponding to the 'tyramine' moiety 'A' ring common to many potent opiates (figure 33.1)) (Terenius *et al.*, 1976; Chang *et al.*, 1976; Day *et al.*, 1976; Ling and Guillemin, 1976; Schiller *et al.*, 1977) suggests a similar mode of action for the two series (Feinberg *et al.*, 1976; Bradbury *et al.*, 1976; Horn and Rodgers, 1977; Schiller *et al.*, 1977). However, in spite of such structural and pharmacological similarities amongst opiates such as morphine, ketocyclazocine and other benzomorphans, subtle

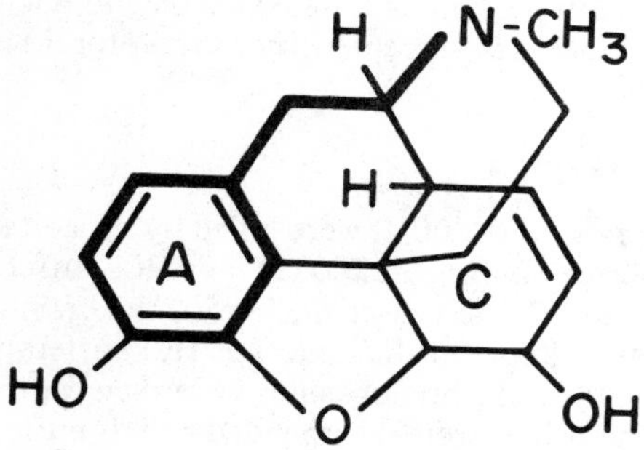

Figure 33.1 Morphine: the 'tyramine' moiety common to many opiates and the opioid peptides is outlined, by the heavy rule.

differences in their pharmacological profiles in the spinal dog, and more importantly, their inability to substitute for morphine in some instances, has led Martin to propose that there is a heterogeneity among opiate receptors (Martin *et al.*, 1976). Kosterlitz has reached a similar conclusion from comparisons of certain benzomorphan's activities in the guinea pig ileum (GPI) and mouse vas deferens (MVD) and their antagonism by naloxone (Lord *et al.*, 1977). Such data provide a precedence for the hypothesis that enkephalin and some opiates may not interact with the same receptor sites. In initial studies, [^{3}H] enkephalin binding sites were shown to differ from those of [^{3}H] opiates in terms of the relative potencies of some drugs (Birdsall *et al.*, 1976; Lord *et al.*, 1976; Simantov and Snyder, 1976). Whether or not this indicated that enkephalins and opiates bind to different receptor sites was not clear as so few opiates had been studied.

The enkephalins are 'pure' agonists in terms of their opiate-like effects upon smooth muscle systems (Hughes, 1975; Lord *et al.*, 1977) and their ability to elicit analgesia (Beluzzi *et al.*, 1976; Chang *et al.*, 1976; Büscher *et al.*, 1976; Pert *et al.*, 1976; Walker *et al.*, 1977). Interactions of opiate agonists and antagonists with opiate receptor sites can be differentiated by the influence of sodium ions (Pert *et al.*, 1973; Simon *et al.*, 1975). Low concentrations of sodium selectively diminish the potencies of opiate agonists in competing for receptor sites while not reducing the binding of pure antagonists. Drugs with mixed agonist–antagonist properties are affected in an intermediate fashion (Pert and Snyder, 1974). Opiate agonists vary fourfold in sensitivity to sodium's reducing their apparent affinity for receptor sites. For instance, the pure opiate agonists levorphanol and etorphine become about 12 times less potent in competing for [^{3}H] naloxone binding in the presence of 100 mM sodium while the corresponding value for the agonists dihydromorphine and normorphine is 50-fold (Pert and Snyder, 1974). The pharmacological significance of this difference in the effect of sodium is unclear. Since mixed agonist–antagonist opiates with a relatively lesser addictive potential have 'sodium ratios' somewhat lower than those of conventional opiate agonists, it is conceivable that pure opiate agonists with relatively lower sodium ratios might have lower addictive propensities than other opiates.

In the present paper we describe the relative influences of various opiates on receptor binding of [^{3}H] met-enkephalin and other [^{3}H] opiates. Differences among drugs in their relative affinities for enkephalin and opiate binding sites are shown to relate to differences in susceptibility to receptor interaction perturbation by sodium.

MATERIALS AND METHODS

Male Sprague-Dawley rats (150–200 g) were killed by decapitation and the brains rapidly removed and placed in ice-cold 0.05 M Tris HCl buffer, pH 7.7 at 25 °C. For routine binding assays (Pasternak *et al.*, 1975*b*) the brain minus cerebellum was homogenized in 40 volumes of the same Tris HCl buffer using a Brinkmann Polytron (setting = 5, 20 s). The homogenates were then centrifuged at 4 °C for 10 min at 49 000 *g*. The pellets were resuspended in Tris buffer (about 10 mg tissue/ml), incubated for 40 min at 37°C, centrifuged at 4°C for 10 min, resuspended in the same buffer (10 mg original brain tissue/ml) and used for binding studies.

The standard binding experiments were performed at 25 °C for 40 min. Reaction mixtures (final volume 2 ml) contained tissue suspension, unlabeled drug and one of the following radioactive compounds: [^{3}H] naloxone, 1.1 nM (20 Ci/mmol), [^{3}H] dihydromorphine, 0.7 nM (45 Ci/mmol), [^{3}H] met-enkephalin, 1.3 nM (17.4 Ci/mmol, New England Nuclear Corporation), [^{3}H] etorphine, 0.42 nM (30 Ci/mmol) or [^{3}H] diprenorphine, 0.54 nM (25 Ci/mmol). Bacitracin (50 μg/ml) was added to all assays containing enkephalins.

RESULTS AND DISCUSSION

As observed previously (Simantov and Snyder, 1976) the relative potencies of some drugs differ in competing for [^{3}H] met-enkephalin and some [^{3}H] opiate binding sites in the absence of sodium (table 33.1). All drugs examined, whether agonists, antagonists, mixed agonist–antagonists or opioid peptides, display similar affinities in competing for binding sites labeled by [^{3}H] dihydromorphine and [^{3}H] naloxone. However, some drugs, such as morphine, dihydromorphine, normorphine, oxymorphone and fentanyl (among agonists) are 19–55 times more potent in competing for [^{3}H] dihydromorphine or [^{3}H] naloxone than for [^{3}H] met-enkephalin binding. In contrast, etorphine, levorphanol, phenazocine and the opioid peptides have more similar affinities for [^{3}H] met-enkephalin, [^{3}H] naloxone and [^{3}H] dihydromorphine binding sites. Among this latter group of opiates and opioid peptides the largest discrepancy between affinity for met-enkephalin and dihydromorphine binding occurs for levorphanol and β-endorphin which are nine and sixfold more potent in competing for dihydromorphine than enkephalin binding. Among matching pairs of opiate antagonists and agonists, the antagonists, in general, have higher affinity for [^{3}H] met-enkephalin than [^{3}H] dihydromorphine or [^{3}H] naloxone binding sites. Drug potencies in competing for [^{3}H] etorphine and [^{3}H] diprenorphine are intermediate between their influences on [^{3}H] met-enkephalin and [^{3}H] dihydromorphine or [^{3}H] naloxone binding.

Earlier we observed that opiate agonists and antagonists differ markedly in the extent to which sodium would reduce their potency in competing for [^{3}H] naloxone binding sites. Amongst pure opiate agonists there was a fourfold variation in sensitivity of receptor binding to sodium (Pert and Snyder, 1974). In table 33.2

Table 33.1 K_i values (nM) of opiates determined from competition with various [^{3}H] ligands

Drug			K_i (nM) [^{3}H] ligand		
	DHM	M-ENK	ET	DPN	NAL
Naloxone (NAL)	1.5	6.6	2.5	0.8	0.5
Diprenorphine (DPN)	0.2	0.9	0.2	0.1	0.2
Levallorphan	0.3	1.0	0.3	0.4	0.3
Cyclazocine	0.2	0.6	0.3	0.3	0.2
Nalorphine	0.5	4.7	1.9	1.0	0.5
Pentazocine	12	25	20	6.4	6.4
Phenazocine	0.3	0.8	0.6	0.5	0.2
Levorphanol	0.2	1.7	0.4	0.5	0.3
Etorphine (ET)	0.2	0.4	0.1	0.8	0.1
Morphine	1.5	29	8.9	4.5	1.3
Dihydromorphine (DHM)	0.5	26	2.5	1.4	0.9
Normorphine	2.5	47	13	9.7	5.3
Oxymorphone	0.6	23	3.1	4.2	0.5
Fentanyl	0.6	33	3.4	4.0	0.4
[Met^5]-Enkepahlin (M-ENK)	4.3	2.0	2.9	2.4	3.0
[Leu^5]-Enkephalin	12	6.2	9.4	7.8	7.4
[D-Ala^2]-Enkephalin	6.3	4.7	1.2	2.8	5.3
α-Endorphin	21	18	23	11	21
β-Endorphin	0.3	1.8	0.4	0.4	0.8

IC_{50} values from one to three determinations against each [^{3}H] ligand were determined from log-probit plots and converted to K_i values according to the Cheng–Prusoff equation. The concentrations of the [^{3}H] ligands were DHM, 0.70 nM; M-ENK, 1.3 nM; ET, 0.42 nM; DPN, 0.54 nM; NAL, 1.1 nM.

opiates and opioid peptide agents are divided into groups on the basis of the extent to which sodium reduces their potencies in competing for [^{3}H] naloxone binding. As observed previously sodium ratios for antagonists are quite low. Pure antagonists such as naloxone and diprenorphine display the same potencies in the presence or absence of sodium and hence have a sodium ratio of one. Antagonists with some agonist activity have sodium ratios of two or three. Agonists are subdivided into group A, with sodium ratios of 30 or more and group B with sodium ratios of less than 30. All the opioid peptides display sodium ratios less than 30.

The division of opiate agonists into groups on the basis of their sodium ratios corresponds well to their division into groups on the basis of relative affinities for met-enkephalin and dihydromorphine binding sites. Drugs in group A, with higher sodium ratios, also display higher ratios of K_i values for met-enkephalin and dihydromorphine binding. The opiate antagonists behave more like group B than group A agonists. All are less potent in competing for met-enkephalin than [^{3}H] dihydromorphine binding, with 2–10-fold lower potencies in reducing enkephalin and dihydromorphine binding.

Table 33.2 Comparison of relative affinities of opiates for [^{3}H]-enkephalin and [^{3}H] dihydromorphine binding with their 'sodium ratios'

Drug	'Sodium ratio'	K_i [^{3}H] met-enkephalin / K_i [^{3}H]-dihydromorphine	
Agonists			
Oxymorphone	30	38	
Fentanyl	35	55	
Morphine	37	19	Group A
Normorphine	47	19	
Dihydromorphine	47	52	
[Met^5]-enkephalin	6	0.5	
Etorphine	12	2	
Phenazocine	13	3	
Levorphanol	15	9	Group B
β-Endorphin	17	6	
[Leu^5]-Enkephalin	19	0.5	
[D-Ala^2]-Enkephalin	26	0.8	
Antagonists			
Naloxone	1	4	
Diprenorphine	1	5	
Levallorphan	2	3	
Cyclazocine	2	3	
Pentazocine	3	2	
Nalorphine	3	9	

The 'sodium ratio' for each drug was determined from its IC_{50} in displacing [^{3}H] naloxone binding in the presence of 100 mM NaCl divided by its IC_{50} in displacing [^{3}H] naloxone binding in the absence of added sodium as detailed in Pert and Snyder, (1974). The value for β-endorphin is taken from Pert *et al.*, (1977).

How might one account for the differential effects of opiates upon [^{3}H] enkephalin and [^{3}H] opiate binding, differences which qualitatively parallel the variations in sodium ratios for these drugs? One possibility is to assume that opiate agonists in groups A and B bind to distinct opiate receptors, with drugs in group B binding to true 'enkephalin receptors' while drugs in group A bind to a distinct 'opiate specific' receptor. Such a conclusion is not consistent with the considerable pharmacological similarities between drugs in groups A and B. Moreover it does not fit with the finding that the numbers and distribution of enkephalin and opiate binding sites are similar and that opiates and enkephalins display mutual competition in their bindings.

An alternative possibility to that of separate opiate and enkephalin receptors is that enkephalin, being a flexible peptide containing five amino acids, binds to multiple sites on the opiate receptor. Previous structure–activity analyses have concluded that opiates themselves have a minimum two distinct points of attachment (Beckett and Casey, 1954; Portoghese, 1966; Bentley and Lewis. 1973; Feinberg *et al.*, 1976). We have previously hypothesized that opiate agonists and antagonists bind to the same receptor but that sodium ions are able to control allosterically the availability of a site(s) that favors the binding of the antagonist *N*-substituent while lowering affinity for agonists (Snyder, 1975). However, the gradation of sodium effects amongst different opiate agonists suggests the presence of yet another binding site which influences overall receptor affinity. Thus certain opiates, such as those in group B, may bind to most or all of these sites to which enkephalin binds, while drugs in group A may bind to fewer. Group A agonists compete with [^{3}H] met-enkephalin binding with shallow displacement curves (figure 33.2). The low affinity components of these drugs in competing for [^{3}H] met-enkephalin binding might represent the weak influences of these drugs upon binding sites for which group B opiates and the opioid peptides have much higher affinity than do the group A drugs.

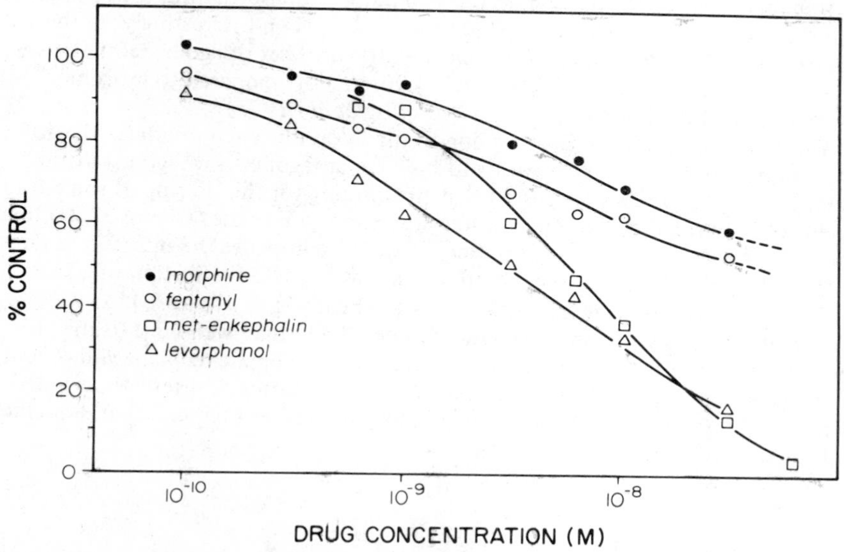

Figure 33.2 Displacement curves of [^{3}H] met-enkephalin binding by morphine, fentanyl, met-enkephalin and levorphanol. Data are from a single experiment. Higher concentrations of all drugs (not shown) will displace all stereospecific [^{3}H] met-enkephalin binding.

What differences between group A and group B opiate agonists might explain their differential affinities for enkephalin binding sites? Drugs in groups A and B all possess the tyramine structure of a phenolic ring A and similar *N*-substituents. However, they display differences in ring C. Morphine, normorphine, oxymorphone, and fentanyl possess hydroxyl or keto groupings at the corresponding locus in ring C or its equivalent position in fentanyl. Such relatively hydrophilic substituents are lacking in the ring C structures of the group B opiate agonists. Accordingly ring C or its equivalent (in phenazocine) tends to be relatively more hydrophobic in group B agonists.

Several groups have examined the preferred conformation of enkephalin in crystal (Garby-Jaureguiberry *et al.*, 1976) or in solution (Jones *et al.*, 1976; Rogues *et al.*, 1976) or by molecular calculations and modeling (Schiller *et al.*, 1977). If one superimposes opiate structure upon the apparently preferred conformation of enkephalin, with a β_1-bend resulting from a hydrogen bond between methionine and glycine (2), ring C substituents correspond to the placement of the methyl group of the methionine side chain. The importance of this hydrophobic character of methionine in binding to the opiate receptor is evident in structure-activity relationships of enkephalin analogues in which substitutions which increase the hydrophobic character of this amino acid also increase affinity for receptor binding (Römer *et al.*, 1977). This extra lipophilic binding site for enkephalin and group B opiates might be expected to reduce the dissociation rate of enkephalin from the receptor and, as predicted, enkephalin does have about a three-fold lower dissociation rate constant than dihydromorphine (group A) which we hypothesize is unable to bind at this site (Simantov *et al.*, 1978). [^{3}H] Etorphine which presumably binds to this lipophilic site also has about a sevenfold slower dissociation rate than dihydromorphine (Simantov *et al.*, 1978). Interestingly, in the GPI, *in vitro*, Kosterlitz has shown that the rate of offset of agonist activity was about eightfold slower for etorphine and levorphanol compared to morphine, normorphine and dihydromorphine (Kosterlitz *et al.*, 1975).

This hypothesis implies that binding to the lipophilic site modulates the ability of sodium to transform the receptor to the high antagonist–low agonist affinity state. We have previously suggested that the binding for the 'F' ring of some other potent opiates (of the oripavine and tetrahydrothebaine series (figure 33.3)) to a lipophilic site in the vicinity of the ring 'C' site also impedes the interconversion of the receptor to the antagonist binding state as *N*-allyl substitution of these agonists does not result in antagonist activity (Feinberg *et al.*, 1976). As we suggested previously the phenylalanine of enkephalin may well bind to this 'F' ring binding site. Thus, differential potencies of some opiate agonists and opioid peptides at the opiate receptor may be explicable in terms of interactions with different binding sites on the same macromolecule rather than on separate opiate and enkephalin receptors.

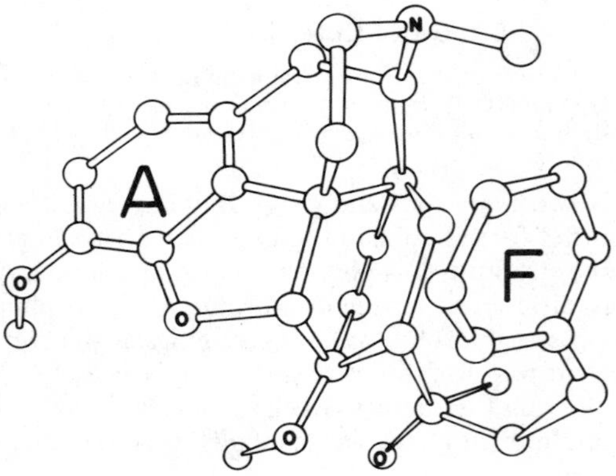

Figure 33.3 Structure of 7-[1-phenyl-3-hydroxybutyl-3-] endoethenotetrahydrothebaine; a potent opiate, showing an orientation of ring F which may correspond to the position of the phenylalanine residue in enkephalin (from Feinberg *et al.*, 1976).

It should be noted that since the binding interactions of opiates may involve a number of sites on the same receptor and 'induced fit' may be occurring in the displacement of some ligands by others (as seen in the high affinity of opioid peptides for [^{3}H] met-enkephalin binding) it may not be correct to apply simple kinetic analyses in the calculation of K_i values from IC_{50} data as has been done here. However the relative potency of drugs at different [^{3}H] ligand binding sites has not been distorted by this transformation.

ACKNOWLEDGEMENTS

We thank Adele Snowman for technical assistance and Pam Morgan for manuscript preparation. Supported by USPHS grants DA-00266, DA 01645 and DA 05328 to I.C.

REFERENCES

Beckett, A. H. and Casey, A. F. (1954). *J. med. Chem.*, **18**, 619–21

Bentley, K. W. and Lewis, J. W. (1973). In *Agonist and Antagonist Actions of Narcotic Analgesic Drugs,* (eds H. W. Kosterlitz, D. H. Clouet, J. E. Villareal). University Park Press, Baltimore, pp. 7–16

Beluzzi, J. D., Grant, N., Garsky, V., Sarantakes, D., Wise, C. D. and Stein, L. (1976). *Nature,* **260,** 625–6

Birdsall, N. I. M., Hulme, E. C., Bradbury, A. F., Smyth, D. G. and Snell, C. R. (1976). In *Opiates and Endogenous Opioid Peptides* (ed H. W. Kosterlitz). North-Holland, Amsterdam, pp. 19–26

Bradbury, A. F., Smyth, D. G. and Snell, C. R. (1976). *Nature*, **260**, 160–6

Büscher, H. H., Hill, R. C., Römer, D., Cardinaux, F., Closse, A., Hauser, D. and Pless, J. (1976). *Nature,* **261,** 423–4

Chang, J. K., Fong, B. T. W., Pert, A. and Pert, C. B. (1976). *Life Sci.,* **18,** 1473–82

Day, A. R., Liyán , M., Dewey, W. L., Harris, L. S., Radding, J. A. and Freer, R. J. (1976). *Res. Commun. chem. Path. Pharmac.*, **14,** 597–603

Feinberg, A. P., Creese, I. and Snyder, S. H. (1976). *Proc. natn. Acad. Sci. U.S.A.,* **73,** 4215–19

Garbay-Jaureguiberry, C., Rogues, B. P., Oberlin, R., Anteunis, M. and Lala, A. K. (1976). *Biochem. biophys. Res. Commun.* **71**, 558–603

Horn, A. S. and Rodgers, J. R. (1977). *J. Pharm. Pharmac.,* **29,** 257–65

Hughes, J. T. (1975). *Brain Res.,* **88,** 295–308

Jones, C. R., Gibbons, W. A. and Garsky, V. (1976). *Nature,* **262,** 779–82

Kosterlitz, H. W., Leslie, F. M. and Waterfield, A. A. (1975). *Eur. J. Pharmac.,* **32,** 10–16

Ling, N. and Guillemin, R. (1976). *Proc. natn. Acad. Sci. U.S.A.,* **73,** 3308–10

Lord, J. A. H., Waterfield, A. A., Hughes, J. and Kosterlitz, H. W. (1976). In *Opiates and Endogenous Opioid Peptides,* (ed. H. W. Kosterlitz). North-Holland, Amsterdam, pp. 275–80

Lord, J. A. H., Waterfield, A. A., Hughes, J. and Kosterlitz, H. W. (1977). *Nature,* **267,** 495–9

Martin, W. R., Eades, C. G., Thompson, J. A., Huppler, R. E. and Gilbert, P. E. (1976). *J. Pharmac. expl Ther.,* **197,** 517–22

Pasternak, G. W., Goodman, R. and Snyder, S. H. (1975*a*). *Life Sci.,* **16,** 1765–9

Pasternak, G. W., Wilson, H. A. and Snyder, S. H. (1975*b*). Molec. Pharmac., **11,** 478–84

Pert, C. B., Pasternak, G. W. and Snyder, S. H. (1973). *Science,* **182,** 1359–61

Pert, C. B. and Snyder, S. H. (1974). *Molec. Pharmac.,* **10,** 868–79

Pert, C. B., Pert, A., Chang, J. K. and Tiang, B. (1976). *Science,* **194,** 330–2

Pert, C. B., Bowie, D. L., Pert, A., Morell, J. L. and Gross, E. (1977). *Nature,* **269,** 73–5

Portoghese, P. S. (1966). *J. Pharm. Sci.,* **55,** 865–87

Romer, D., Pless, J., Bauer, W., Cardinaux, F., Closse, A., Hauser, D. and Huguenin, R. (1977). *Nature,* **268,** 547–9

Rogues, B. P., Garbay-Jaureguiberry, C., Oberlin, R., Anteunis, M. and Lala, A. K. (1976). *Nature,* **262,** 778–9

Rossier, J., Bayan, A., Vargo, T. M., Ling, N., Guillemin, R. and Bloom, F. (1977). *Life Sci.,* **21,** 847–52

Schiller, P. W., Yam, C. F. and Lis, M. (1977). *Biochemistry,* **16,** 1831–8

Simantov, R. and Snyder, S. H. (1976). In *Opiates and Endogenous Opioid Peptides,* (ed. H. W. Kosterlitz). North-Holland, Amsterdam, pp, 41–8

Simantov, R., Childers, S. R. and Snyder, S. H. (1977). *Brain Res.,* **135,** 358–67

Simantov, R., Childers, S. R. and Snyder, S. H. (1978). *Eur. J. Pharmac.,* (in press)

Simon, E. J., Hiller, J. M., Groth, J. and Edelman, I. (1975). *J. Pharmac. exp Ther.,* **192,** 531–7

Snyder, S. H. (1975). *Nature,* **257,** 185–9

Terenius, L. and Wahlström, A. (1974). *Life Sci.,* **16,** 1759–64

Terenius, L., Wahlström, A., Lindeberg, G., Karlsson, S. and Ragnarsson, Y. (1976). *Biochem. biophys. Res. Commun.,* **71,** 175–82

Walker, J. M., Bernston, G. G., Sandman, C. A., Coy, D. H., Schally, A. V. and Kastin, A. J. (1977). *Science,* **196,** 85–7

34
Brain endorphins: possible mediators of pleasurable states

Larry Stein and James D. Belluzzi (Wyeth Laboratories PO Box 8299
Philadelphia, Pennsylvania 19101, U.S.A.)

> . . . each seizure was preceded by an inexpressibly voluptuous feeling . . . . For a few moments, I experience such happiness as is impossible under ordinary conditions, and of which other people can have no notion. I feel complete harmony in myself and in the world, and this feeling is so strong and sweet that for several seconds of such bliss one would give ten years of one's life, indeed, perhaps one's whole life.
>
> Fyodor Dostoevsky

Present conceptions (Kosterlitz and Hughes, 1975; Akil and Liebeskind, 1975; Snyder, 1975) of endorphins as natural analgesic substances for regulation of the response to pain are probably correct (Belluzzi *et al.,* 1976), but these formulations are too narrow to accommodate the role postulated for these peptides in mental disease (Bloom *et al.,* 1976; Terenius *et al.,* 1976). We propose here a broadening of the functions attributed to endorphins—along lines previously suggested (Goldstein, 1976; Byck, 1976; Belluzzi and Stein, 1977*a*)—to include the regulation of affective states and appetitive drives. More precisely, we suggest that endorphins may serve as transmitters or modulators in neuronal systems for the mediation of pleasure and reward. The possibility that reward dysfunction is an etiological factor in affective disorders and schizophrenia has been considered elsewhere (Stein, 1962; Stein and Wise, 1971).

How can one test the hypothesis that endorphins or enkephalins are involved in reward function? First, by use of drug self-administration procedures, one can ask whether rats will work for enkephalin injections delivered directly into the ventricles of their own brains. Secondly, by use of brain stimulation procedures, one can ask whether electrical activation of enkephalin-rich brain regions will serve as a reward in self-stimulation experiments. And thirdly, by use of an appropriate learning test, one can ask whether enkephalin injections share the property of natural rewards in promoting long-term memory formation (Belluzzi and Stein, 1977*b*).

ENKEPHALIN SELF-ADMINISTRATION

Rats implanted with permanently-indwelling i.v.t. cannulae had continuous access during a single 66 hour test to one of the drug solutions shown in figure 34.1. Each lever-press response delivered 1 μl of fluid to the brain in 0.9 s. Each rat was tested once and had access to only one solution. No lever-press training was given; rats were merely placed in the Skinner box with food and water available for the 66 hour session. Rates of self-administration were significantly higher for the enkephalins and morphine (but not the structurally related tetrapeptide, Tyr–Gly–Gly–Phe) than for Ringer's solution (figure 34.1). The order of preference for the peptides when tested at either 1 or 10 μg per injection was leu-enkephalin > met-enkephalin > Tyr–Gly–Gly–Phe. Massive doses of leu-enkephalin in particular were taken by the best responders, despite the possibility of tissue damage or other adverse affects that might have been produced by the passage of large volumes of fluids through the brain ventricles.

It was also observed that the 1 μg dose of both pentapeptides caused more rapid learning of self-administration behavior than the 10 μg dose, but the 10 μg dose generated a more sustained performance level. Thus, the 1 μg dose of leu-enkephalin was self-administered at a higher rate than the 10 μg dose during the first 24 hours, but the 10 μg dose yielded a higher rate after prolonged exposure to the peptide (table 34.1). These results can be explained if tolerance develops to

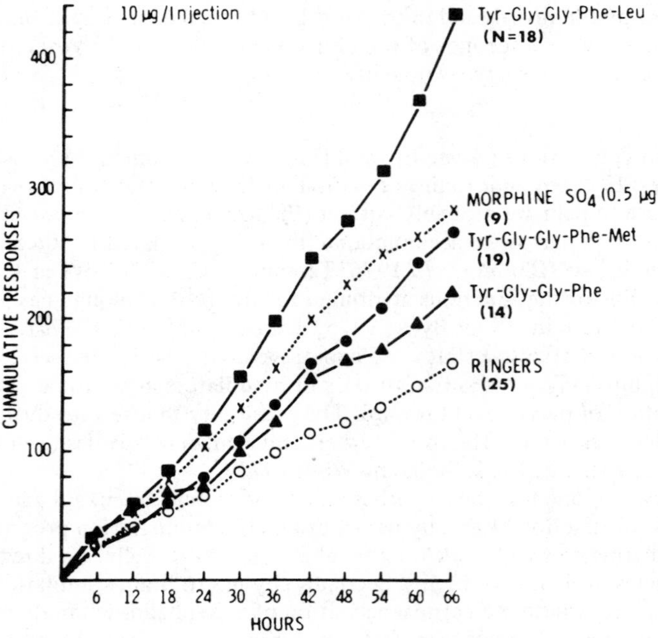

Figure 34.1 Intraventricular self-administration of opiate peptides (10 μg per injection) and morphine (0.5 μg per injection). Curves show mean number of self-injections cumulated at successive 6-hour intervals over the entire 66-hour test. Number of rats per group indicated in parentheses.

Table 34.1 Evidence of tolerance in leu-enkephalin self-administration

Drug	No. of rats	Dose (μg)	Self-administration rate mean ± s.e.m.	
			First 24 h	Final 24 h
Ringer's	25	–	64.0 ± 10.7	54.7 ± 11.3
Leu-enkephalin	6	1	141.7 ± 29.8*	99.7 ± 36.8
	18	10	116.6 ± 43.2	186.9 ± 56.4†

*Significantly different from Ringer's solution, $p < 0.005$
†$p < 0.025$

leu-enkephalin's reinforcing action, as it does to morphine's. Before the development of tolerance, 1 μg per injection of the peptide provides satisfactory reinforcement while 10 μg represents an overdose; and after tolerance develops, the 10 μg dose is more nearly optimal while 1 μg represents an underdose.

In related experiments, substance P was offered as a reward for self-administration behavior. In the case of this peptide, behavioral suppression rather than facilitation was regularly observed over a wide range of i.v.t. doses (figure 34.2). These results are generally consistent with the opposite pattern of biological effects typically displayed by opioid peptides and substance P (von Euler and Pernow, 1976), and further suggest a possible role for substance P in the mediation of behavioral punishment.

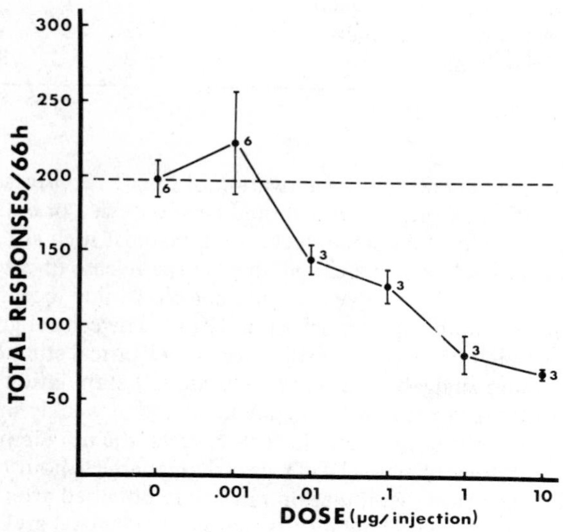

Figure 34.2 Substance P fails to support self-administration behavior, and in fact suppresses response rates over a wide range of intraventricular doses. See text for methods. Number of rats tested at each dose level indicated on curve.

SELF-STIMULATION OF ENKEPHALIN-RICH BRAIN SITES

Avid self-administration of leu-enkephalin supports the idea that opioid peptides may serve as reward transmitters. If this conjecture were true, reward should be produced not only by administration of exogenous enkephalin, but also by release of endogenous peptide following electrical activation of enkephalin-containing neurons in the brain. Behavioral (Stein *et al.*, 1977; Stein, 1978) and immunohistochemical (Elde *et al.*, 1976) observations may be consistent with this prediction. Sites that yield high rates of self-stimulation and those that contain dense networks of enkephalin-like immunoreactivity often overlap in precisely the same brain regions (table 34.2). According to our hypothesis, self-stimulation of these regions would depend at least in part on the electrically-induced release of enkephalin and the consequent activation of opiate 'reward' receptors. However, brain regions rich in enkephalin also contain high concentrations of catecholamines (Versteeg *et al.*, 1976), substances previously shown to be involved in self-stimulation (Stein *et al.*, 1977). Hence, it is possible that the release of catecholamines rather than the release of enkephalins is responsible for the brain stimulation reward.

Table 34.2 Catecholamine levels in enkephalin-rich self-stimulation sites

Site	pg/μg protein	
	NE	DA
Midbrain central grey, ventral part	24.5	3.9
Substantia nigra, zona compacta	11.7	5.4
Bed nucleus of stria terminalis	27.2	19.1
Nucleus accumbens	9.3	87.2

From Versteeg *et al.* (1976)

If self-stimulation depends on the activation of opiate receptors by electrically-released enkephalin, then the behavior should be suppressed or extinguished following administration of an opiate receptor antagonist such as naloxone. On the other hand, if reward behavior depended only on the release of catecholamines, then naloxone should be ineffective and only catecholamine receptor blockers or synthesis inhibitors should suppress self-stimulation. The central grey region was selected for initial pharmacological testing because electrical stimulation of this site induces profound analgesia as well as high-rate self-stimulation (Mayer *et al.*, 1971). Different doses of naloxone were administered at weekly intervals immediately before the behavioral test, and, in further tests, the noradrenaline synthesis inhibitor diethyldithiocarbamate (DDC) was administered 1 hour before the test. Dose-related decreases in self-stimulation rates were obtained after administration of both agents (figure 34.3). These results suggest that central grey self-stimulation depends on the activation of both enkephalin-containing and noradrenaline-containing neurons. Studies on i.v. self-administration of morphine similarly suggest that noradrenergic mechanisms are involved in opiate reinforcement (Davis *et al.*, 1975; Pozuelo and Kerr, 1972).

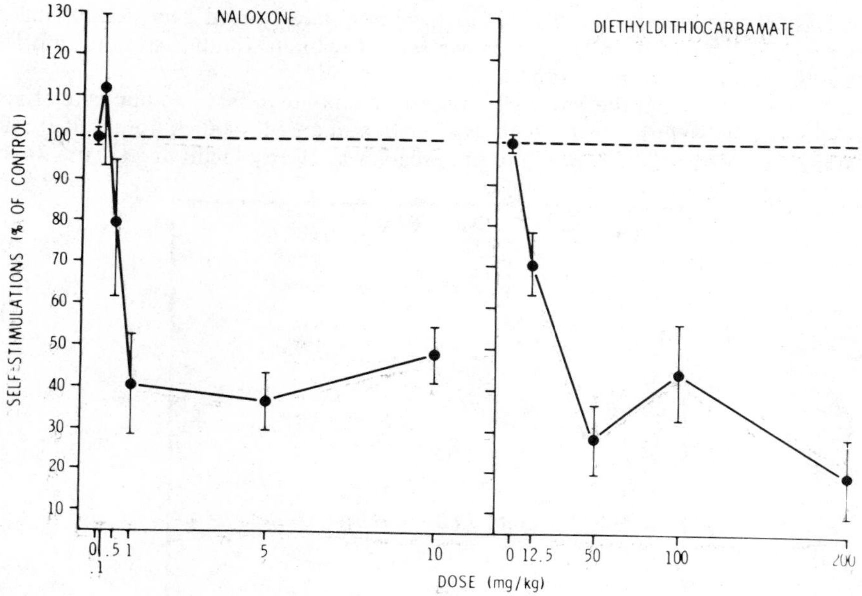

Figure 34.3 Dose-related suppression of central grey self-stimulation following s.c. administration of the opiate antagonist naloxone or the dopamine-β-hydroxylase inhibitor diethyldithiocarbamate. Each data point is the mean of 3–8 observations. Bars indicate standard errors. From Belluzzi and Stein (1977).

It is possible, however, that the suppression of central grey self-stimulation by naloxone was due to some non-specific effect of the drug rather than to an effect on reward processes. Direct observation did not reveal any obvious sedative or debilitating effects of even large doses of naloxone, but it is conceivable that the behavior could have been non-specifically suppressed in some non-obvious way.

To evaluate this possibility, rats were trained on a dual component brain-stimulation program in a 2-lever Skinner box. The program was made up of self-stimulation and escape components, which were alternated every 5 min (Hoebel and Thompson, 1969). In the first component, the rats worked at one lever on a normal self-stimulation schedule; the escape lever was inoperative. In the second component, the same brain stimulus was delivered automatically once every second; at many electrode sites, such forced stimulation is aversive and animals will work to escape it. During this period the self-stimulation lever was inoperative, but activation of the escape lever terminated the trains of forced stimulation for 5 s. In practice, escape rates are relatively low because of the predominantly positive nature of electrode sites that yield self-stimulation. How will performance on this schedule be affected by naloxone? If the drug produces a nonspecific debilitation, then lever-press behavior in both self-stimulation and stimulation-escape components should obviously be suppressed. On the other hand, if naloxone selectively antagonizes a rewarding aspect of the stimulation, self-stimulation behavior again should be suppressed but escape responding should be facilitated.

This is because blockade or partial blockade of opiate 'reward' receptors by naloxone would increase the relative aversiveness of the brain stimulus and thus motivate the animal to escape it more frequently.

As predicted from the reward hypothesis, naloxone in fact had opposite effects on the two behaviors. Thirty minutes after treatment with a high dose, self-stimulation was substantially suppressed but escape was clearly facilitated (figure 34.4).

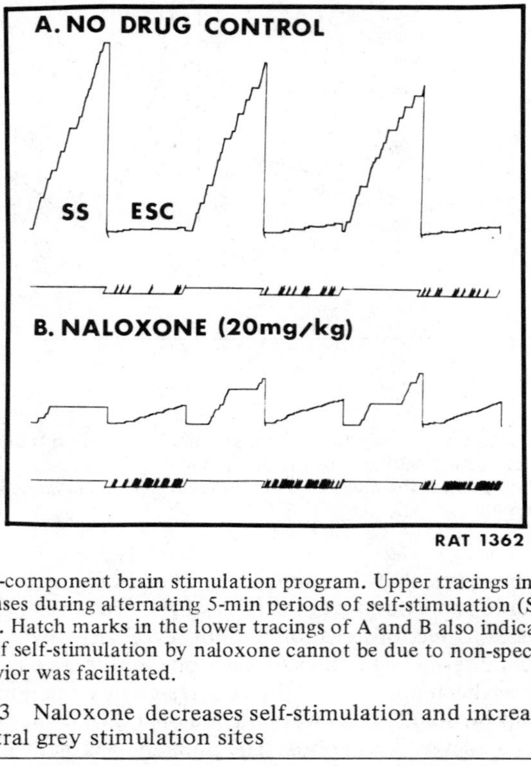

Figure 34.4 Two-component brain stimulation program. Upper tracings in A and B show cumulative responses during alternating 5-min periods of self-stimulation (SS) and stimulation-escape (ESC). Hatch marks in the lower tracings of A and B also indicate escape responses. Suppression of self-stimulation by naloxone cannot be due to non-specific debilitation since escape behavior was facilitated.

Table 34.3 Naloxone decreases self-stimulation and increases escape from central grey stimulation sites

Rat number	Naloxone dose (mg/kg)	Response rate (% of control)	
		Self-stimulation	Escape
1362	10	98.7	111.4
1424	10	91.0	113.6
1366	10	55.8	158.3
1423	10	32.6	17.8
1424	20	91.6	205.9
1362	20	21.2	356.4
1423	20	0.2	258.6
1424	40	0.1	12.4
1423	40	0.1	223.5

A similar result was obtained in three more cases (table 34.3). These results are consistent with the idea that naloxone specifically reduces brain stimulation reward and fail to support the hypothesis that the effects of the drug were merely due to sedation or debilitation. Interestingly, higher doses of naloxone were needed to suppress self-stimulation in the 2 component test than in conventional self-stimulation (compare table 34.3 and figure 34.3). Conceivably, endorphins released by the forced stimulation in the 2 component test can antagonize naloxone's suppressant action.

The effects of naloxone on self-stimulation at a number of other rewarding brain sites have also been studied. The septal region is of particular interest since Hökfelt and his colleagues (1977) find a well-defined group of enkephalin-immunoreactive cell bodies in this region. As in the case of central grey self-stimulation, naloxone and DDC treatments produced dose-related decreases in septal self-stimulation (figure 34.5). However, septal self-stimulation seemed to be less sensitive to DDC than central grey self-stimulation, although the naloxone sensitivities of the two sites were similar. The naloxone sensitivities of three additional sites are reported in table 34.4. Of all self-stimulation sites tested so far, substantia nigra has proved most sensitive to naloxone suppression.

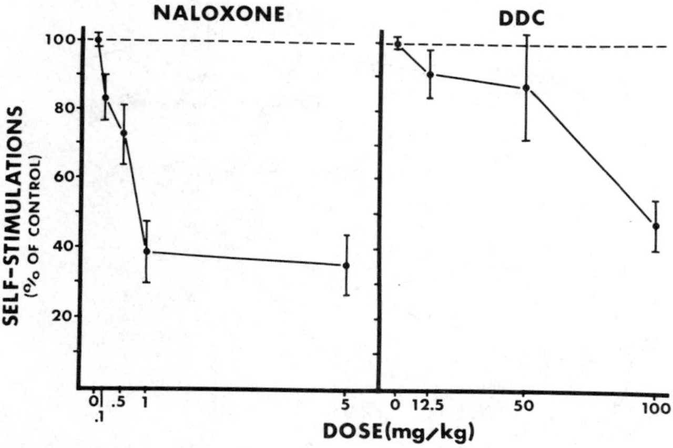

Figure 34.5 Dose-related suppression of septal self-stimulation following subcutaneous administration of naloxone or DDC. Each data point is the mean of 3–5 observations. Bars indicate standard errors.

A strong demonstration that self-stimulation may depend on enkephalin release would be identification of new self-stimulation sites on the basis of enkephalin mapping. Since the brain has been closely mapped for self-stimulation, demonstration of a new reward site would not be trivial. Most regions of thalamus do not support self-stimulation and they also contain little enkephalin. However, one region of thalamus, the nucleus paratenialis, is reported by Elde *et al.* (1976) to yield a high enkephalin immunoreactivity. As predicted, five probes in or near the nucleus paratenialis in fact supported a respectable rate of self-stimulation (figure 34.6). Furthermore, the behavior was suppressed in a dose-related fashion by naloxone (figure 34.7).

Table 34.4 Naloxone-induced suppression of self-stimulation in several brain regions

Electrode site	No. of rats	Dose for 50% suppression* (mg/kg) mean ± s.e.m.
Medial forebrain bundle (MFB)	16	5.83 ± 1.66
Locus coeruleus	10	3.33 ± 2.08
Substantia nigra	10	0.48 ± 0.13†

*Subcutaneous injections of naloxone (dose range: 0.04–20 mg/kg) were administered immediately before the daily 1-h self-stimulation session. Drug rate was computed as a percentage of the mean of the previous two control sessions. Stimulation intensity set just above reward threshold.
†$P < 0.02$ v MFB group

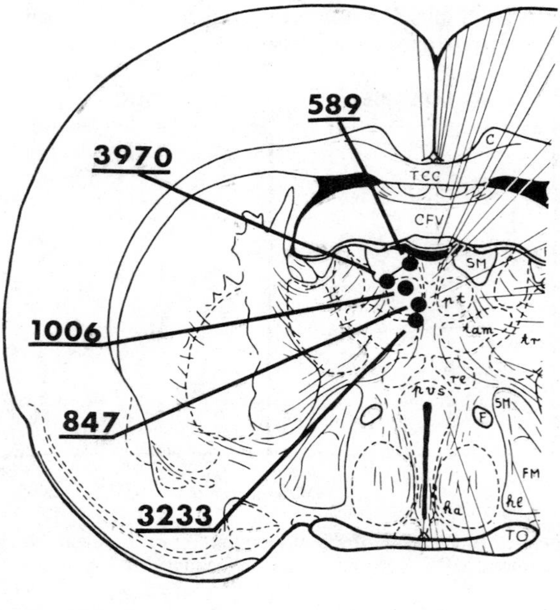

Figure 34.6 Location of five electrode tips in or near the nucleus paratenialis. Numbers indicate the maximum hourly self-stimulation rate obtained for each of the placements. Brain section drawing and stereotactic level after König and Klippel (1963).

The globus pallidus yields profuse and intense enkephalin immunofluorescence, perhaps the most intense in the brain (Elde *et al.*, 1976; Simantov *et al.*, 1977). Since, to the best of our knowledge, self-stimulation has not yet been localized in the globus pallidus, this structure provides an ideal test of the enkephalin reward hypothesis. Eight probes in or near the globus pallidus yielded maximum self-

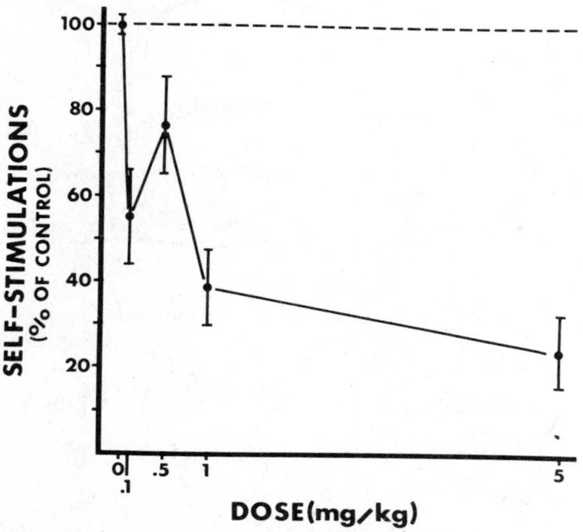

Figure 34.7 Dose-related suppression of nucleus paratenialis self-stimulation following s.c. administration of naloxone. Each data point is the mean of 4–5 observations. Bars indicate standard errors.

stimulation rates of 1000 responses per hour or more (figure 34.8). Reward effects seem highly localized in this region since two electrodes in the internal capsule (just medial to the globus pallidus) supported much lower response rates. It may be no coincidence that Keene (1975) has found single units in medial globus pallidus whose discharge rates are controlled by rewarding and punishing inputs. Rewarding stimulation of the medial forebrain bundle increased the firing rates of these pallidal neurons, whereas escape-eliciting midbrain reticular formation stimulation decreased them (figure 34.9). Since the pallidal units alone exhibited this precise relationship to reward and punishment (units in medial thalamus uniquely exhibited an opposite pattern), Keene concluded that the globus pallidus may have a significant role in the neural coding of positive affect.

ENKEPHALIN FACILITATION OF LONG-TERM MEMORY

The important role of reinforcement in learning and long-term memory formation, although controversial at the level of theory, cannot be disputed at the practical level. Accordingly, enkephalin and morphine treatments were administered immediately following training in a single-trial learning task in an attempt to facilitate long-term retention of the learned response. Rats with permanently-indwelling i.v.t. cannulae received a mildly painful foot shock after stepping down from a shelf to a grid floor (Stein *et al.*, 1975). Different groups received i.v.t. injections either immediately or 15 min after the shock, as indicated in table 34.5. Three days later, long-term memory of the shock (as reflected by long step-down times) was measured in a retention test. Significant facilitation of the learned response was observed in the groups given immediate post-shock treatments of met-enkephalin or morphine. Two further observations suggest that these effects of

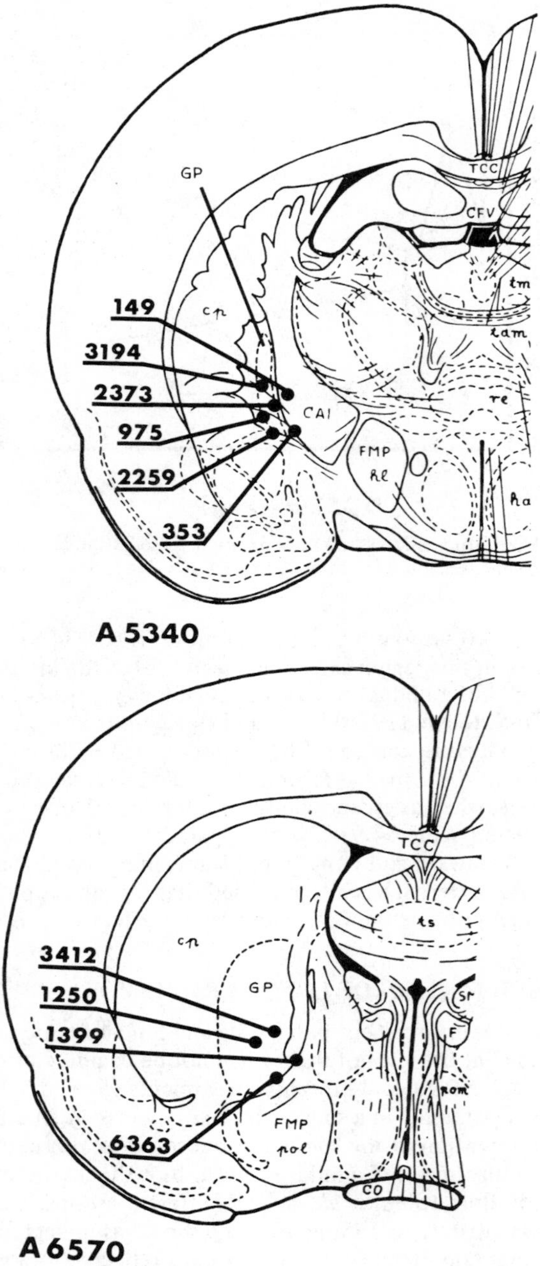

Figure 34.8 Location of eight electrode tips in or near the globus pallidus. Numbers indicate the maximum hourly self-stimulation rate obtained for each of the placements. Brain section drawings and stereotactic levels after König and Klippel (1963).

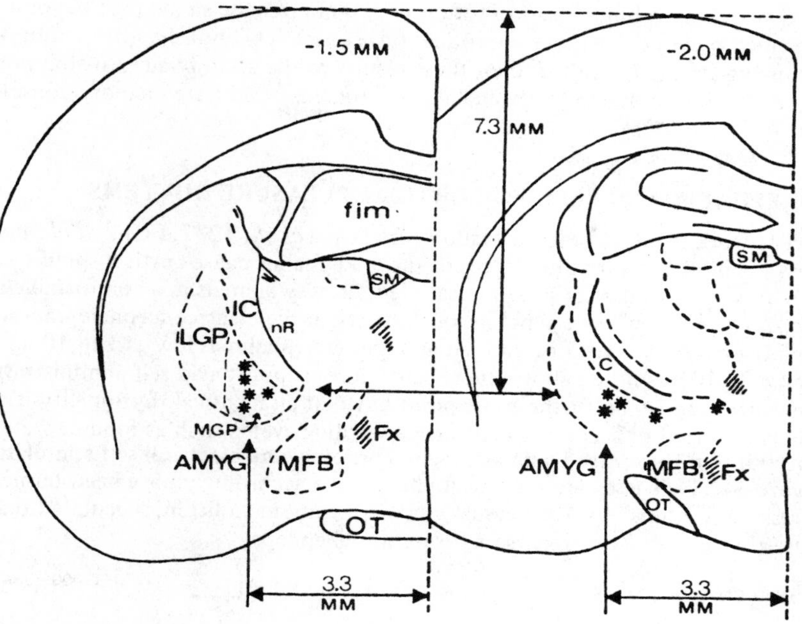

Figure 34.9 Location of units (asterisks) in globus pallidus on which long lasting medial forebrain bundle-evoked excitation and reticular-evoked inhibition converged. Compare locations of these 'affect-coding' units with those of self-stimulation probes in figure 34.8. Abbreviations: fim, hippocampal fimbria; SM, stria medullaris; IC, internal capsule; LGP, lateral pallidum; MGP, medial pallidum; nR, nucleus reticularis; AMYG, amygdala; MFB, medial forebrain bundle; Fx, fornix; OT, optic tract. From Keene (1975).

Table 34.5 Effects of post-training morphine or enkephalin injections on the formation of long-term memory

Treatment	Dose (μg)	No. of rats	Step-down time (s) mean ± s.e.m.
Ringer's	–	17	36.23 ± 9.37
Morphine	20	19	78.24 ± 12.14*
Morphine (shock withheld)	20	8	5.75 ± 0.94†
Morphine (15 min delay)	20	7	39.50 ± 23.70
Leu-enkephalin	200	8	47.04 ± 19.71
Met-enkephalin	200	10	114.25 ± 27.74*

*$P < 0.02$ *v* Ringer's
†$P < 0.001$ *v* morphine

the opiates on retention were in fact due to an enhanced memory of the shock. First, if the shock was withheld on the training day (so that there could be no memory of it) the morphine treatments were ineffective (table 34.5). Secondly, delaying the morphine injection for only 15 min after the shock (but beyond the presumed period of memory consolidation) completely abolished its memory-enhancing effect. Taken together, these results would seem to suggest that post-trial activation of opiate (enkephalin) receptors may facilitate memory consolidation.

ENKEPHALIN AND ELECTROCORTICAL PLEASURE RHYTHMS

Recent work from Liebeskind's laboratory (Urca *et al.*, 1977; Frenk *et al.*, in press) demonstrates that low doses of the enkephalins cause cortical spindle activity similar to that observed in satiated, drowsy animals in a comfortable and safe situation. Slow wave synchronous activity in the electroencephalogram was reliably evoked by i.v.t. doses of leu and met-enkephalin as low as 1 to 10 μg (figure 34.10); as noted above, these same doses support avid self-administration behavior. Frenk *et al.* furthermore point out that an identical rhythmicity is widely reported to accompany 'diverse rewarding events such as food or water consumption in deprived animals, vaginal probing, and electrical self-stimulation' (figure 34.11). These electrocortical phenomena accordingly have been termed "pleasure rhythms" by Myslobodsky (1976), who, in addition, speculated that these rhythms may be precursors for petit mal epilepsy.

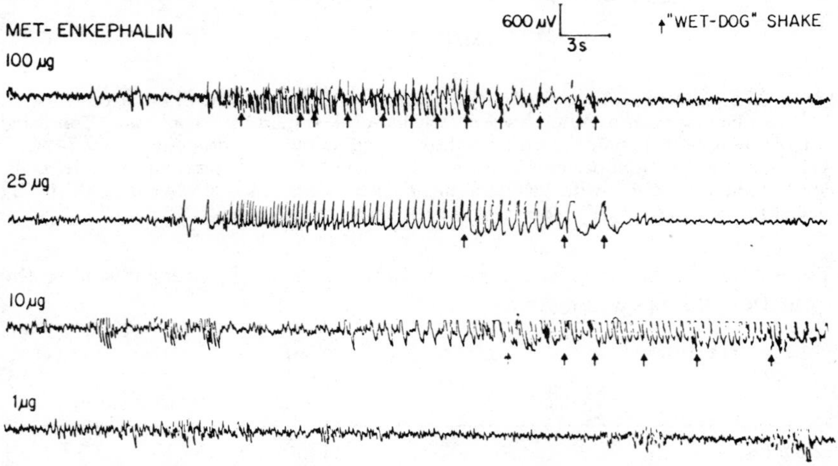

Figure 34.10 Electrocortical spindles induced by i.v.t.-administered met-enkephalin in four different rats. The electroencephalogram, recorded between frontal and occipital leads, starts 40 s after enkephalin injections. According to Bloom (this volume), similar effects, including wet-dog shaking, are observed after i.v.t. administration of β-endorphin. After Frenk *et al.* (in press).

All these observations are consistent with the present hypothesis that enkephalin systems normally may mediate states of pleasure and reward. Furthermore, as Frenk *et al.* (in press) ingeniously suggest, in certain disease conditions such as epilepsy, enkephalin-induced hypersynchrony may develop into actual seizures. Emotional disturbances are a frequent concomitant of epilepsy and often constitute part of the aura of the onset of the seizure. Extraordinary feelings of joy and

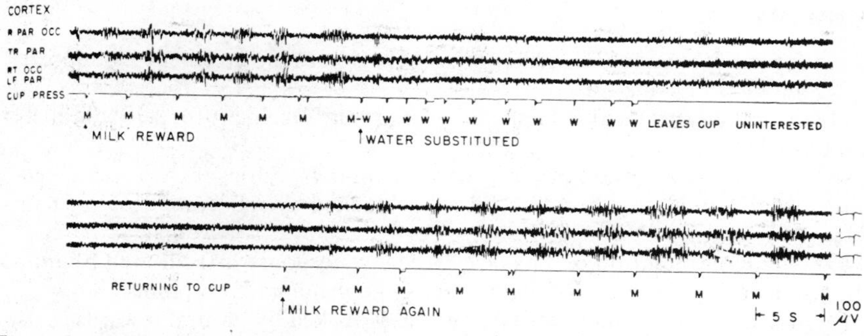

Figure 34.11 Cortical spindles in the electroencephalogram of a trained, hungry cat regularly follow operant responses and consumption of a milk-broth reward. When water is substituted for the milk reward, the spindles disappear and the EEG pattern exhibits only low voltage, high frequency activity. When milk again is made available, operant behavior is reinstated and the postreinforcement reward rhythms quickly reappear. From Clemente *et al.* (1964).

satisfaction have been described during electrical stimulation of an enkephalin-rich area in the amygdala of a patient suffering from psychomotor automatisms and episodes of violence (figure 34.12) and in the moments preceding the fits experienced by Fyodor Dostoevsky.

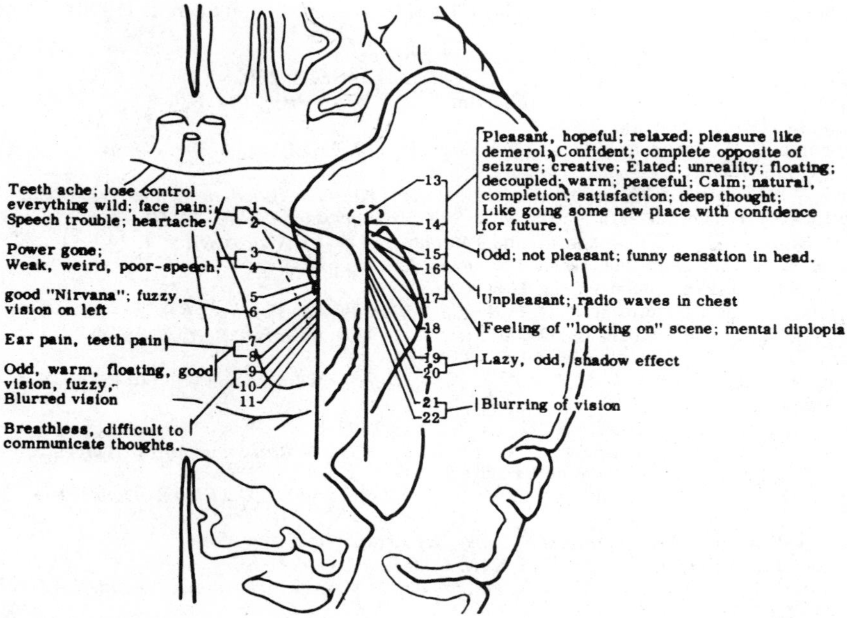

Figure 34.12 Verbal reports of a 33-year-old epileptic and violence-prone man in response to electrical stimulation of different points in the amygdalar complex. Pleasurable sensations lasting minutes to hours after cessation of stimulation were localized at a particular site. Although the reports are subjective, it is interesting that the positive feelings were described as opiate-like–'pleasure like demerol'. From Mark *et al.* (1972).

SUMMARY

A role for enkephalin in the mediation of behavioral reinforcement is supported by several lines of evidence

(1) central injections of enkephalin serve as reinforcement for self-administration behavior;

(2) electrical stimulation of many enkephalin-rich regions serve as reinforcement for self-stimulation behavior, which is blocked by moderate doses of naloxone;

(3) long-term retention of a passive avoidance response is facilitated by immediate post-learning injections of methionine-enkephalin and morphine;

(4) electrocortical spindle activity typically evoked by natural rewards is also evoked by central injections of enkephalin.

ACKNOWLEDGEMENT

The careful technical assistance of William J. Carmint, Herman Morris and Alfred T. Shropshire is gratefully acknowledged.

REFERENCES

Akil, H. and Liebeskind, J. C. (1975). *Brain Res.*, **94**, 279–96

Belluzzi, J. D., Grant, N., Garsky, V., Sarantakis, D., Wise, C. D. and Stein, L. (1976). *Nature*, **260**, 625–6

Belluzzi, J. D. and Stein, L. (1977*a*). *Nature*, **266**, 556–8

Belluzzi, J. D. and Stein, L. (1977*b*). *Soc. Neurosci. Abstr.*, **3**, 230

Bloom, F., Segal, D., Ling, N. and Guillemin, R. (1976). *Science*, **194**, 630–2

Byck, R. (1976). *Lancet*, **ii**, 72–3

Clemente, C. D., Sterman, M. B. and Wyrwicka, W. (1964). *Electroenceph. clin. Neurophysiol.*, **16**, 355–65

Davis, W. M., Smith, S. G. and Khalsa, J. H. (1975). *Pharmac. Biochem. Behav.*, **3**, 477–84

Dostoevsky, F. cited in Yarmolinsky, A. (1934). *Dostoevsky: A Life*, 132–59

Elde, R., Hökfelt, T., Johansson, O. and Terenius, L. (1976). *Neuroscience*, **1**, 349–51

Frenk, H., Urca, G. and Liebeskind, J. C. *Brain Res.* (in press)

Goldstein, A. (1976). *Science*, **193**, 1081–6

Hoebel, B. G. and Thompson, R. D. (1969). *J. comp. physiol. Psychol.*, **68**, 536–43

Hökfelt, T., Elde, R., Johansson, O. and Stein, L. (1977). *Neurosci. Lett.*, **5**, 25–31

Keene, J. J. (1975). *Expl Neurol.*, **49**, 97–114

König, J. F. R. and Klippel, R. A. (1963). *The Rat Brain.* Williams and Wilkins, Baltimore, Maryland

Kosterlitz, H. W. and Hughes, J. (1975). *Life Sci.*, **17**, 91–6

Mark, V. H., Ervin, F. R. and Sweet, W. H. (1972). In *The Neurobiology of the Amygdala*, (ed. B. E. Eleftheriou) Plenum Press, New York

Mayer, D. J., Wolfe, T. L., Akil, H., Carder, B. and Leibeskind, J. C. (1971). *Science*, **174**, 1351–4

Myslobodsky, M. (1976). *Petit Mal Epilepsy*, Academic Press, New York

Pozuelo. J. and Kerr, F. W. L. (1972). *Mayo Clin. Proc.*, **47**, 621–8

Simantov, R., Kuhar, M. J., Uhl, G. R. and Snyder, S. H. (1977). *Proc. natn. Acad. Sci. U.S.A.*, **74**, 2167–71

Snyder, S. H. (1975). *Nature*, **257**, 185–9

Stein, L. (1962). In *Recent Advances in Biological Psychiatry*, (ed. J. Wortis) Vol. 4, Plenum Press, New York

Stein, L. (1978). In *Psychopharmacology: A Generation of Progress*, (eds M. A. Lipton, A. DiMascio and K. F. Killam) Raven Press, New York

Stein, L., Belluzzi, J. D. and Wise, C. D. (1975). *Brain Res.*, **84**, 329–35
Stein, L., Belluzzi, J. D. and Wise, C. D. (1977). In *Handbook of Psychopharmacology*, (eds L. L. Iversen, S. D. Iversen and S. H. Snyder) Vol 8, Plenum Press, New York
Stein, L. and Wise, C. D. (1971). *Science*, **171**, 1032–6
Terenius, L., Wahlström, A., Lindstrom, L. and Widerlov, E. (1976). *Neurosci. Lett.*, **3**, 157–62
Urca, G., Frenk, H., Liebeskind, J. C. and Taylor, A. N. (1977). *Science*, **197**, 83–6
Versteeg, D. H. G., Van Der Gugten, J., DeJong, W. and Palkovits, M. (1976). *Brain Res.*, **113**, 563–74
von Euler, U. S. and Pernow, B. (1976). *Nobel Symposium 37: Substance P*, Raven Press, New York

Section Two
Endorphin Antagonists

35
Use of narcotic antagonists to study the role of endorphins in normal and psychiatric patients

Glenn C. Davis, William E. Bunney, Jr, Monte S. Buchsbaum, E. Gerald DeFraites, Wallace Duncan, J. Christian Gillin, Daniel P. van Kammen, Joel Kleinman, Dennis L. Murphy, Robert M. Post, Victor Reus and Richard J. Wyatt
(National Institute of Mental Health, Bethesda, Maryland 20014, U.S.A.)

This chapter reviews our studies of the effects of narcotic antagonists on sleep, respiration and pain, and on the symptoms of certain psychiatric illnesses. The recent discoveries of endogenous polypeptides that bind to opiate receptors in brain (Hughes *et al.*, 1975; Teschemacher *et al.*, 1975) have stimulated a search for the physiological role of these opioid substances. The pharmacological effects of opiate alkaloids provide the best available model for the effects of endorphins. Thus, since morphine and its congeners affect mood, pain appreciation, sleep, respiration, and release of pituitary hormones, these physiological functions are prime candidates for endorphin activity.

The possible functions of endorphins in man are being shown in various ways. The direct administration of endorphins to man is one approach. As toxicological studies of endorphins in animals are incomplete, there have been only a few trials in humans (Kline *et al.*, 1977). On the basis of the hypothesis that endorphins may function as neurotransmitters or neurohormones, and that the resting level of endorphins may be low, attempts have been made to stimulate the release of endorphins by a variety of techniques, including experimental pain, stress, sexual activity and implanted electrodes. The measurement of endogenous opioids in urine, plasma and CSF by RIA and radioreceptor assay is a third strategy. At present the use of narcotic antagonists is the most popular strategy for elucidating endorphin function.

Narcotic antagonists reverse or block the effect of narcotic analgesics *in vivo* and *in vitro*. Many compounds have been synthesized which reverse narcotic effects, but only a few have 'pure' antagonist properties. Two such 'pure' narcotic antagonists are used clinically: *N*-allyl-noroxymorphone (naloxone) and EN-1639A (naltrexone). Naloxone is administered parenterally and has a plasma half-life of 64 min (Ngai *et al.*, 1976). Naltrexone is administered orally and has antagonist activity for 72 hours (Martin *et al.*, 1973). Just as these narcotic antagonists reverse the effects of opiates, they have also been found effectively to reverse the effects of endorphins in animals (Bloom *et al.*, 1976; Bruni *et al.*, 1977; Meyerson and Terenius, 1977; Tseng *et al.*, 1976; Meglio *et al.*, 1977). Thus, if endorphins regulate aspects of neurophysiological function, pure narcotic antagonists administered to man should alter such function. Most studies in man used low doses of naloxone (0.4–0.8 mg) comparable to doses administered clinically to reverse narcotic overdoses and to precipitate abstinence. In our acute studies we have progressively increased the amount of naloxone administered to the 30 mg range. Naloxone has been administered to man without adverse effects in dosages of up to 90 mg/day for up to 2 weeks (Martin, 1967).

Participation by all subjects and patients in the studies reported was voluntary and all gave informed consent.

SLEEP

The acute administration of morphine and heroin decreases the number and duration of rapid eye movement (REM) sleep periods and increases sleep correlates of arousal (such as alpha waves, muscle tension, non-REM light sleep) in man (Lewis *et al.*, 1970; Kay *et al.*, 1969). Chronic administration of morphine also produces

Table 35.1 Sleep variable data reported for naloxone and placebo nights*

	Placebo	Naloxone
Total recording period	442	433
Total sleep time	383	374
Non-REM time	297	284
REM time	86	92
Sleep latency	39	46
REM latency	90	89
Intermittent awake time	15	8
REM density	1.5	1.4
Stage 1	12	12
Stage 2	220	225
Stage 3	33	29
Stage 4	15	15
Total delta sleep	48	44
Delta sleep %	12.8	10.5
REM %	22.8	24.0
Sleep efficiency %	86.8	86.3
Stage 1 %	3.1	3.3
Stage 2 %	57.4	60.4
Stage 3 %	8.8	7.6
Stage 4 %	3.9	4.0
Number of REM periods	3.2	3.3

*All data are reported in minutes unless otherwise noted. Each value is the mean of six subjects.

increases in arousal and decreases in REM duration, though partial tolerance develops to these effects (Kay, 1975). These sleep effects contrast with the sleepiness produced by opiates. Because of these sleep effects of narcotic analgesics and the recent suggestion that endogenous opiate-like substances play a part in sleep (King *et al.*, 1976), naloxone effects on sleep were studied (Davis *et al.*, 1977*b*).

Six healthy, young male volunteer inpatients at the National Institute of Mental Health were adapted to a sleep laboratory environment for one night and then, on two subsequent nights, received naloxone or placebo i.v. in a randomized design. Three subjects received naloxone in a single 2.0 mg i.v. bolus, 30 min after onset of Stage II sleep. Three subsequent subjects received 0.4 mg of naloxone, also beginning 30 min after onset of Stage II, and then received 0.4 mg as a bolus every hour for 4 hours. Two dose administration schedules were utilized to maximize the chances of a sleep effect. All-night sleep recordings were obtained with electroencephalogram (EEG), electrooculogram (EOG), and submental electromyogram (EMG). Sleep records were scored blindly according to conventional criteria (Rechtschaffen and Kales, 1968).

No significant differences in sleep parameters were found by paired *t*-test (table 35.1). Additionally, no changes in REM cycle, length, and duration of REM periods were observed.

If endorphins act in a manner physiologically similar to opiates, naloxone should be expected to produce an increase in the number and duration of REM periods and a decrease in sleep correlates of arousal. These data fail to support this hypothesis.

RESPIRATION

Opiate alkaloids have a profound suppressant effect on respiratory rate (Goodman and Gillman, 1965). In fact, death in narcotic overdoses is frequently due to respiratory arrest as a result of respiratory suppression. Thus, if endorphins have a tonic suppressant role in regulation of respiration, the administration of naloxone should increase respiratory rate.

Three volunteers, while participating in the sleep experiment, had their respiratory rate measured during sleep by nasal thermistor. These subjects received 0.4 mg of naloxone 30 min after the onset of Stage II sleep and then hourly for 4 hours. Respiratory rates were determined for 1 min intervals for every 10-min segment of sleep and separated into two groups to analyze respiratory rates separately for REM and non-REM periods. Naloxone had no effect on respiratory rate during sleep (figure 35.1).

PAIN

In view of the prominent analgesic effects of opiates, the regulation of pain perception is a prime candidate for a physiological function of endorphins. Endorphins micro-injected into the periaqueductal grey matter of rats induce analgesia which is reversed by naloxone (Pert, 1976). Studies in rats (Frederickson *et al.*, 1977; Jacob *et al.*, 1974; Frederickson *et al.*, 1976) and one early study in man (Lasagna, 1965) have suggested slight hyperalgesic effects of naloxone. However, several studies in man (El-Sobky *et al.*, 1976; Grevert and Goldstein, 1977) failed

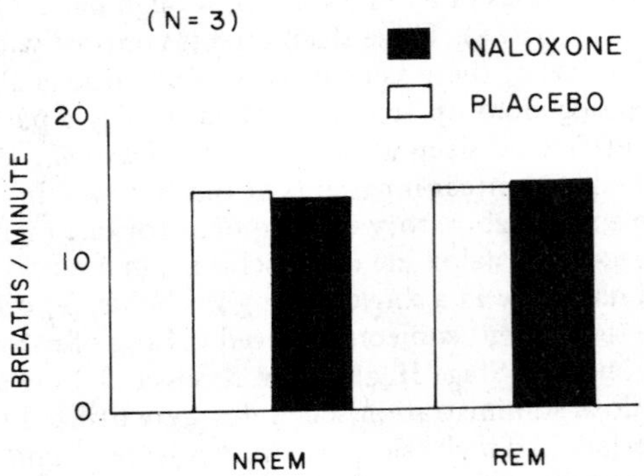

Figure 35.1 Lack of effect of naloxone on respiratory rate during sleep. NREM, non-rapid-eye-movement sleep; REM, rapid-eye-movement sleep.

to demonstrate hyperalgesic effects of naloxone. In our study 2 mg of naloxone had a hyperalgesic effect in pain-tolerant subjects (Buchsbaum *et al.*, 1977).

Normal adult volunteers (10 male, 11 female; mean age 20 years) participated in three similar experimental sessions. Each session consisted of two psychophysiological pain rating tests. The initial session was for familiarization and no drug was given. On the following two sessions, the subjects either received an i.v. injection of 2.0 mg (0.4 mg/ml) naloxone or an equal volume of saline in a random order and in double-blind fashion. Experimental procedures began 5 min after injection and lasted 20 min. All procedures involved single shocks administered to the left forearm by a computer-controlled constant current stimulator with a Tursky electrode. Subjects received three shocks at each 1 mA increment from 1 to 31 mA for a total of 93 shocks in random sequence at 2.5-s intervals. Subjects rated each shock in one of four categories: noticeable, distinct, unpleasant or very unpleasant. The number of unpleasant and very unpleasant responses were added and designated 'pain counts'. Subjects were divided into pain-sensitive and pain-insensitive groups on the basis of whether their pain sensitivity levels on the familiarization day fell above or below the mean of subjects used in two previous pain studies (Sitaram *et al.*, 1977; Lavine *et al.*, 1976).

Individuals defined as pain insensitive showed naloxone hyperalgesia. They judged a higher number of the 93 stimuli as unpleasant and very unpleasant after naloxone administration (figure 35.2). In contrast, pain sensitive individuals judged fewer of the stimuli unpleasant or very unpleasant after naloxone administration, thus becoming more pain tolerant (figure 35.2). Individuals with relatively higher levels of endorphins might be thought to be relatively pain tolerant and thus more naloxone responsive. If these factors were the only source of individual variation, however, one might have expected to see only the pain-insensitive group respond to naloxone rather than the bidirectional effects observed. Lasagna (1965) noted a biphasic quality of naloxone response, with 2 mg apparently causing analgesia but higher doses having hyperalgesic effects. Relevant to this finding of increased pain tolerance with naloxone in pain-sensitive subjects, Leybin *et al.* (1976) found an unexpected hyperalgesic effect of the endogenous opiate, met-enkephalin, in rats. Bidirectional effects may reflect individual differences in func-

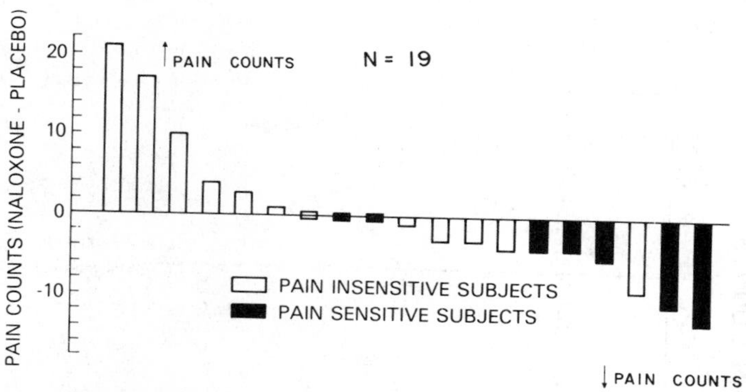

Figure 35.2 Differential pain response to naloxone in pain-sensitive and pain-insensitive subjects. Subjects were divided into pain-insensitive and pain-sensitive groups on the basis of a sensitivity measure derived from signal detection analysis during a separate pre-drug trial session. Pain counts (unpleasant plus very unpleasant subjective ratings) are illustrated as the difference between naloxone and placebo days for each individual studied. Positive differences thus indicate more stimuli rated as unpleasant and very unpleasant on naloxone than on placebo. Note that no pain-sensitive subject became more sensitive on naloxone while most pain-insensitive individuals did (groups significantly different by *t* test on individual difference scores, $P < 0.05$).

tional activity of complementary pain modulation systems rather than a dose-dependent effect at receptor sites. A primary analgesic action of endogenous opiate-like substances similar to the actions of exogenous opiates, is not clearly supported by our data. The bidirectional effects observed here and elsewhere suggest a modulatory rather than strictly analgesic role for endorphins. Nonetheless, our finding of naloxone effects on pain response supports the hypothesis that endogenous opiate-like substances have a physiological role in pain regulation.

PAIN EVALUATION IN AFFECTIVE ILLNESS

In the last section, we reported that endorphins may have a role in modulating sensitivity to pain. We initiated a study of pain perception in affective illness (Davis *et al.,* 1978).

Patients hospitalized on the clinical research wards at the National Institute of Mental Health with a diagnosis of primary affective illness participated in the somatosensory procedure previously described to study pain appreciation in normal subjects. All patients in this study were experiencing a depressive or manic episode at the time of testing and had been drug free for at least 2 weeks. Seventy-three affectively ill patients and 48 age and sex matched controls were included in this study. Figure 35.3 demonstrates the differences in pain appreciation among normal, depressed and manic individuals. There is a statistically significant decrease in pain sensitivity among all depressed patients and normal controls. Manic patients also show decreased pain sensitivity but this did not achieve statistical significance due to the small number of subjects tested and the large variance in individual response. It should be noted that 17 per cent of the depressed individuals fell outside of two standard deviations of our normal subjects in the direction of pain tolerance.

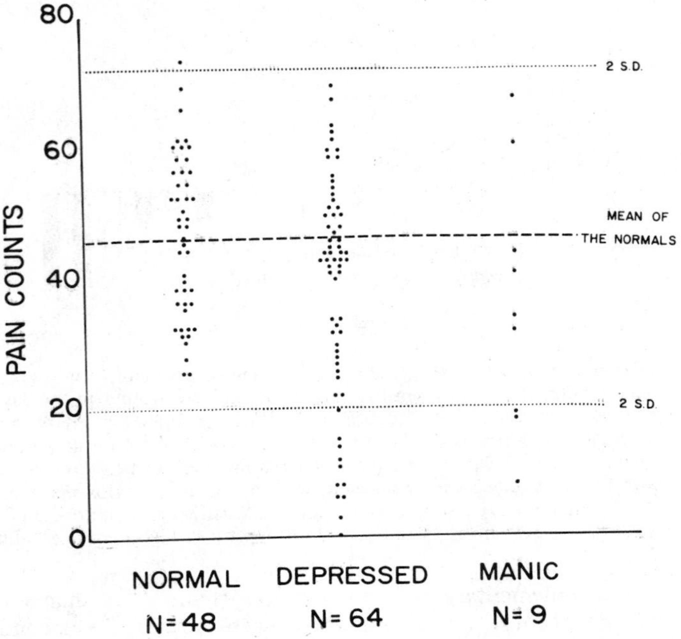

Figure 35.3 Decreased pain sensitivity in affective illness. The 'pain count' (unpleasant plus very unpleasant subjective ratings) for each normal, depressed, and manic patient studied with a psychophysical pain rating procedure is plotted in this scattergram. Dotted lines indicate 2 s.d. from the mean of the normal group. Depressed patients were significantly more pain tolerant than normals ($P < 0.05$ by unpaired t test).

This study is consistent with findings of Hemphill *et al.* (1952), Hall and Stride (1954), Merskey (1965) and von Knorring (1975): depressed patients are more tolerant than normal subjects to experimental pain stimuli. Is it possible that endogenous opiate-like substances play a part in this relative analgesia or pain tolerance? It appears from figure 35.3 that there is a subgroup of depressed patients who experience relatively less pain than normal individuals. It would be interesting to determine, in future investigations, whether this subgroup of patients would become more pain sensitive after naloxone administration. Do these depressed, pain-tolerant patients have an elevated level of endorphins? In support of this notion, Terenius *et al.* (1976) found that an endorphin fraction of CSF in bipolar patients was elevated. Thus, the pain procedure may have identified an interesting subgroup of affectively ill patients for future investigation.

SCHIZOPHRENIA

Reports of psychotomimetic actions of narcotics and certain narcotic antagonists have led to the suggestion that some behavioral disorders may be associated with an excess of endorphins in the CNS. A link between psychotic behavior and endorphins has been suggested by the resemblance of behavioral states induced by endorphins in rats to human catatonia and to neuroleptic-induced catalepsy

(Bloom *et al.*, 1976; Jacquet and Marks, 1976). In one study, the investigators reported that neuroleptic treatment of the symptoms of schizophrenia decreased the level of an endorphin fraction of CSF (Terenius *et al.*, 1976). Perhaps the most provocative suggestion is the recent report that naloxone reduces or even eliminates temporarily the auditory hallucinations of chronic schizophrenics (Gunne *et al.*, 1977). Although Davis *et al.*, (1977*a*), Volavka *et al.*, (1977), Kurland *et al.*, (1977) and Janowsky *et al.*, (1977) were unable to replicate Gunne *et al.'s* (1977) findings, Emrich *et al.*, (1977) has recently reported an antipsychotic action of 4 mg of naloxone.

In our study (Davis *et al.*, 1977*b*), patients participating were all seriously ill inpatients diagnosed as schizophrenic by the research diagnostic criteria of Spitzer *et al.* (1975). Naloxone or a matched volume of physiological saline was injected i.v. in a randomized double-blind fashion. Although dosages of 0.4 mg of naloxone were used for the most part, dosages up to 10 mg were administered. The following items were rated on a severity scale of 1 to 7 (not present to severe): hallucinations, mannerisms and posturing, conceptual disorganization, unusual thought content, psychosis, and the mood variables of depression, elation and dysphoria. These variables were chosen in order to evaluate possible antipsychotic effects of naloxone. Blind ratings were performed before, and 1, 2 and 3 hours after each injection. In addition, each patient was interviewed for 15 min before and 15 min immediately after each injection. Verbal reports of the patient and clinical impressions of physician observers were systematically recorded during interviews. Patients completed both a self-rating form, which included mood and thought content items, and a questionnaire concerning side effects. Most patients were tested in a drug-free state while others were tested while on standard neuroleptic maintenance therapy to replicate the study conditions of Gunne *et al.* (1977).

No overall clinical improvement in the schizophrenic group was noted during the placebo or naloxone day (table 35.2). Of the eight items studied, only 'unusual thought content' demonstrated a statistically significant improvement at 1 hour ($p < 0.04$, two-tailed sign test) when the placebo and naloxone days were compared. Although 10 of 14 patients had a slight improvement in symptoms when eight rating measures were combined, this was not statistically significant. It should be noted that the change scores themselves are quite small. Fifty-eight per cent of all scores did not change from baseline to the 1 hour rating after injection and another 30 per cent changed by only one unit. Of the 14 schizophrenic patients in this study, 8 reported auditory hallucinations on both the placebo and active compound or had obvious behavioral signs of hallucinations. In contrast to the previous report (Gunne *et al.*, 1977) auditory hallucinations were not altered after naloxone injection. The finding of improvement in 'unusual thought content' is puzzling. This item is a global measure of unusual, bizarre, or psychotic verbal productions of the patients. Other measures of psychosis in schizophrenia, such as 'conceptual disorganization', failed to demonstrate improvement. The finding of catatonia in animals given endorphins, and its reversal by naloxone (Bloom *et al.*, 1976) is interesting. However, in our study, 'mannerisms and posturing', behaviors which have some similarity in man to these motor effects in animals, failed to improve.

To date, two schizophrenic patients have received a clinical trial of naltrexone, the longer acting, orally administered, pure narcotic antagonist. The first patient

Table 35.2 Change in behavior ratings of schizophrenic patients during the first hour after infusion of naloxone (N) or placebo (P).

Patient	Halluci-nations		Mannerisms and posturing		Conceptual disorgan-ization		Unusual thought content*		Psychosis		Depressive mood		Elation		Dysphoric affect	
	P	N	P	N	P	N	P	N	P	N	P	N	P	N	P	N
W.J.	−1	0	1	1	5	5	−2	1	0	0	−3	2	1	2	−3	0
H.M.	0	0	−1	0	−1	0	−2	0	−1	0	−1	−1	0	0	0	0
A.D.	−1	0	1	0	1	−1	−2	0	0	0	0	0	−1	0	−1	0
P.M.	−2	−1	0	0	−1	0	0	3	1	−1	1	2	0	2	1	0
G.D.	0	0	−1	0	0	0	1	0	0	−1	0	0	0	0	0	0
M.R.	0	0	0	−2	0	−1	−1	0	0	0	0	0	0	0	0	0
N.R.	0	0	1	0	0	0	0	1	0	1	0	0	0	0	0	2
B.H.	0	0	−1	−2	0	−1	0	−2	−1	−1	0	0	1	−1	−1	−3
T.E.	0	0	0	0	0	0	0	0	0	0	−1	0	0	0	−1	0
Q.C.	2	0	1	−1	0	0	−1	1	0	−1	1	0	0	0	1	1
R.D.	0	0	−1	0	0	1	0	2	0	1	−1	−1	1	2	2	1
D.W.	0	0	0	0	0	0	0	0	0	0	−2	1	1	0	−1	0
H.B.M.	0	0	0	1	0	0	0	2	0	0	1	0	0	0	0	0
G.H.	0	0	−1	−1	0	1	−1	0	0	1	0	2	−1	−1	−1	1
Totals	−2	−1	−1	−4	4	4	−8	8	−1	−1	−5	5	2	4	−4	2

*$P < 0.04$, two-tailed sign test

Items were rated on a severity scale of from 1 (not present) to 7 (severe). Ratings for the first hour were subtracted from baseline ratings made before the infusions, and the signs were changed in order for positive numbers to reflect improvements as seen in diminished symptoms.

who received naltrexone in doses up to 200 mg/day for 14 days failed to show evidence of behavioral change. However, a second patient receiving doses up to 300 mg/day of naltrexone for 25 days showed an improvement in his psychosis ratings. When naltrexone was discontinued, psychosis rating increased. Thus, preliminary studies are inconclusive and further investigation is required.

CATATONIA

The link between catatonic illness and endorphins has already been suggested by the resemblance of behavioral states induced by opiates and endorphins in rats to human catatonia and to neuroleptic-induced catalepsy (Bloom *et al.*, 1976; Jacquet and Marks, 1976; Guillemin *et al.*, 1977). The catatonia in animals given endorphins is reversed by naloxone (Bloom *et al.*, 1976). Although 'mannerisms and posturing' failed to improve among the 14 schizophrenic patients studied, further testing of naloxone in patients with catatonia or other neuromuscular symptoms was warranted. One patient with prominent catatonic symptoms was given 10 mg of naloxone s.c. Motor retardation in this patient improved somewhat on the day of naloxone injection as compared with the day of placebo injection, but more subjects require testing and repeated drug trials should be utilized to document an effect of naloxone on catatonic symptoms.

AFFECTIVE ILLNESS

Depression

In one study linking opiates to mood disorders, cyclazocine, a mixed narcotic agonist–antagonist, had a clinical antidepressant action (Fink *et al.*, 1970). Patients with a diagnosis of primary affective illness, depressed state, were studied under the procedures previously reported for schizophrenic patients (Davis *et al.*, 1977*a*). Naloxone, in doses ranging from 0.4 to 6 mg, failed to affect the depressed mood of affectively ill patients (table 35.3).

Mania

A number of theoretical reasons exist for suggesting that endorphins may play a role in mania. Opiates produce euphoria which is similar to the euphoria associated with mania. Carroll and Sharp (1972) and Dhasmana *et al.* (1972) have reported that the behavior of morphinized cats may provide a model of mania. Some manic patients experience markedly less pain in response to experimental stimuli than normal subjects (Davis *et al.*, 1978), which would be compatible with altered endorphin levels. It has been observed that some manic patients undergoing major surgical operations require little or no analgesia. Increased psychomotor activity, another characteristic of mania, can be produced in animals with low doses of morphine.

Manic patients hospitalized in the clinical research units of the NIMH were studied in a fashion similar to depressed and schizophrenic patients (Davis *et al.*, 1977*a*). Table 35.4 reports the effects of naloxone in dosages from 2 mg to 30 mg on the symptoms of mania. One patient, followed on a longitudinal basis, received

Table 35.3 Study of patients given naloxone during depressive episodes

Patient	Study condition	Dose of naloxone	Effect on depression (naloxone compared with placebo)
Y.N.			
1	Double blind, placebo controlled	0.4 mg	No change
2	Double blind, placebo controlled	0.8 mg	No change
3	Double blind, placebo controlled	1.2 mg	No change
T.E.			
1	Single blind, placebo controlled	0.8 mg	No change
2	Single blind, placebo controlled	2.0 mg	Slight improvement
3	Single blind, placebo controlled	3.2 mg	No change
D.C.			
1	Double blind	2.0 mg	Slight worsening*
2	Double blind	4.0 mg	No change
3	Double blind	6.0 mg	No change
C.G.			
1	Double blind, placebo controlled	2.0 mg	No change

*No placebo control.
10 trials, 0.4–6.0 mg naloxone, 8/10 trials no change.

Table 35.4 Study of naloxone during hypomanic and manic episodes

Patient	Diagnosis	Study condition	Dose of naloxone	Effect on mania
M.W.	Hypomanic	Double blind, placebo controlled	0.8 mg	No change
K.D.	Hypomanic	Double blind, placebo controlled	6.0 mg	No change
T.W.	Manic	Double blind	4.0 mg	No change*
B.B.	Manic	Double blind, placebo controlled	10.0 mg (3) 20.0 mg (2) 30.0 mg (1)	"Improved"

*No placebo control

nine injections of naloxone or placebo. After each injection she was evaluated for 3 hours. After each of 20–30 mg naloxone doses, the patient reported that her 'thoughts were slow', that she had difficulty 'finding words', and 'it's as if a blanket is pulled over my mind'. Reports of subjective experience occurred in one of three 10 mg dosage trials but did not occur in three placebo trials. Thus, the 20–30 mg parenteral dose of naloxone appeared to produce a consistent subjective effect in this patient. Examination of the observer behavioral ratings also suggested an antimanic effect, but was not statistically significant. Further studies of the effects of high doses of naloxone in mania are indicated.

DISCUSSION

Utilization of the narcotic antagonist strategy for the investigation of endorphin function has provided evidence suggesting that endorphins play a part in the regulation of pain appreciation though they do not function solely as 'endogenous analgesics'. Naloxone failed to alter respiratory rate or sleep parameters in volunteers.

The results of our clinical studies are equivocal. At low dosages of naloxone, no clinical improvement in schizophrenia or affective illness occurred. While a small but significant effect on 'unusual thought content' was demonstrated, it was accompanied by no other indications of improvement in psychosis. The finding of a reduction in the pressure of thoughts and speech in one manic patient administered higher dosages of naloxone is provocative but will require further testing of manic patients to confirm. Equally suggestive are the two case reports: improvement of psychosis in a schizophrenic patient on chronic naltrexone and possible improvement in a catatonic patient administered naloxone.

The major drawback of the studies accomplished to date is the uncertainty as to what dose of an antagonist such as naloxone, should be adequate to alter endorphin function. The initial dose guidelines used were based on the dose of naloxone required to reverse coma brought about by narcotic overdoses, to precipitate abstinence, or to block opiate effects by pretreatment with naloxone. As these actions are pharmacological, not physiological, it is difficult to predict a dosage of naloxone that would alter the proposed physiological effects of endorphins. Lord *et al.* (1977) have demonstrated that the dose of naloxone required to reverse narcotic effects in a physiological preparation such as mouse vas deferens is substantially smaller than that required to reverse the identical effects brought about by endorphins. Reversing endogenous polypeptide actions in the CNS may require large doses of antagonist. New strategies to predict a maximum naloxone dosage are needed.

The brief duration of naloxone action is a potential problem of the antagonist strategy. If tonic antagonism of endorphinergic systems is required to alter function, perhaps longer-acting antagonists such as naltrexone, must be more widely used.

We suggested at the beginning of this chapter that the effects of opiates provide a model for the effects of endorphins. So, too, might we be misled by this approach. Instead of searching for several functions for endorphins, perhaps endorphins serve a physiological process that underlies seemingly independent behaviors. For example, let us speculate that endorphins mediate an important aspect of attention or arousal and thus influence mood, pain, and other cognitive functions. One study (Gritz *et al.*, 1976) of naltrexone in post-addicts suggests such an effect on attention. If endorphins play a part in attentional mechanisms, one would predict that an alteration of endorphins could affect schizophrenia and affective illness, as well as pain appreciation. Abnormal attentional mechanisms have been demonstrated in schizophrenia and depression.

The recent finding (Guillemin *et al.*, 1977) that β-endorphin is contained in a larger prohormone which includes the sequence of ACTH, and that the release of both hormones occurs simultaneously, is both physiologically and clinically provocative. ACTH has a diurnal rhythm. Pain sensitivity has also been shown to have diurnal variability (Frederickson *et al.*, 1977). Furthermore, affective illness is associated with changes in the rhythm of cortisol. If ACTH and β-endorphin release are linked, some of the symptoms of affective illness may be a consequence of β-endorphin.

SUMMARY

In our studies on the effects of narcotic antagonists in man, no clearcut improvement in symptoms could be demonstrated in schizophrenic, depressed or manic patient groups. Several individual case studies are reported that suggest improvement in schizophrenia, catatonia and mania, but more subjects need to be studied in order to document improvements. Repeated administrations of antagonist and placebo should be used to evaluate single cases. Naloxone did not alter sleep parameters or sleeping respiratory rate in normal subjects. Pain-tolerant normal subjects became more sensitive to stimuli after naloxone administration, while pain-sensitive subjects became more tolerant. This finding suggests that endorphins play a part in pain appreciation in man. Various methodological problems presented by this indirect approach to the study of endorphins in man are discussed.

REFERENCES

Bloom, F., Segal, D., Ling, N. and Guillemin, R. (1976). *Science,* **194**, 630–2

Bruni, J. F., vonVught, D., Marchall, S. and Meites, J. (1977). *Life Sci.,* **21**, 461–6

Buchsbaum, M. S., Davis, G. C. and Bunney, W. E., Jr (1977). *Nature,* **270**, 620–2

Carroll, B. J. and Sharp, P. T. (1972). *Psychopharmacologia* (Suppl.) **26**, 10

Davis, G. C., Bunney, W. E., Jr, DeFraites, E. G., Kleinman, J. E., van Kammen, D. P., Post, R. M. and Wyatt, R. J. (1977*a*). *Science,* **197**, 74–7

Davis, G. C., Duncan, W. C., Gillin, J. C. and Bunney, W. E., Jr (1977*b*). *Commun. Psychopharmac.,* **1**, 489–92

Davis, G. C., Buchsbaum, M. and Bunney, W. E., Jr (1978). Presented at Annual Meeting, American Psychiatric Association, Atlanta, Georgia

Dhasmana, K. M., Dixit, K. S., Jaju, B. P. and Gupta, M. L. (1972). *Psychopharmacologia* (Berl.), **24**, 380–3

El-Sobky, A., Dostrovsky, J. D. and Wall, P. D. (1976). *Nature,* **263**, 783–4

Emrich, H. M., Cording, C., Piree, S., Kolling, A., v.Zerssen, D. and Herz, A. (1977). *Pharmakopsychiatry,* **10**, 265–70

Fink, M., Simeon, J., Itil, T. M. and Freedman, A. M. (1970). *Clin. Pharmac. Ther.,* **11**, 41–8

Frederickson, R. C. A., Schirmer, E. W., Grinnan, E. L., Harrell, C. W. and Hewes, C. R. (1976). *Life Sci.,* **19**, 1181–4

Frederickson, R. C. A., Burgia, V. and Edwards, J. D. (1977). *Science,* **198**, 756–8.

Goodman, L. S. and Gillman, A. (1965). In *The Pharmacological Basis of Therapeutics,* 3rd edition, Macmillan Co., New York, pp. 249–73

Grevert, P. and Goldstein, A. (1977). *Proc. natn. Acad. Sci. U.S.A.*, **74**, 1291–4
Gritz, E. R., Shiffman, S. M., Jarvik, M. E., Schlesinger, J. and Charuvastra, V. C. (1976). *Clin. Pharmac. Ther.*, **19**, 773–6
Guillemin, R., Vargo, T., Rossier, J., Minick, S., Ling, N., Rivier, C., Vale, W. and Bloom, F. (1977). *Science*, **197**, 1367–9
Gunne, L. -M., Lindstrom, L. and Terenius, L. (1977). *J. Neural. Transmission*, **40**, 13–9
Hall, K. R. L. and Stride, E. (1954). *Br. J. med. Psychol.*, **27**, 48–60
Hemphill, R. E., Hall, K. R. L. and Crookes, G. G. (1952). *J. Mental Sci.*, **98**, 433–40
Hughes, J., Smith, T., Morgan, B. and Fothergill, L. (1975). *Life Sci.*, **16**, 1753–8
Jacob, J. J., Tremblay, E. C. and Colombel, M. C. (1974). *Psychopharmacologia (Berl.)*, **37**, 217–23
Jacquet, Y. and Marks, N. (1976). *Science*, **194**, 632–5
Janowsky, D. S., Segal, D. S., Bloom, F., Abrams, A. and Guillemin, R. (1977). *Am. J. Psychiat.*, **134**, 926–7
Kay, D. C. (1975). *Psychopharmacologia (Berl.)*, **44**, 117–24
Kay, D. C., Eisenstein, R. B. and Jasinski, D. R. (1969). *Psychopharmacologia (Berl.)*, **14**, 404–16
King, C. D., Masserano, J. M., Codd, E., Santos, N. and Byrne, W. (1976). Presented at the 16th Annual Meeting, Association for the Psychophysiological Study of Sleep, Cincinnati, Ohio
Kline, N. S., Li, C. H., Lehmann, H. E., Lajtha, A., Laski, E. and Cooper, T. (1977). *Arch. gen. Psychiat.*, **34**, 1111–13
Kurland, A. A., McCabe, O. L., Hanlon, T. E. and Sullivan, D. (1977). *Am. J. Psychiat.*, **134** 1408–10
Lasagna, L. (1965). *Proc. R. Soc. Med.*, **58**, 978–83
Lavine, R., Buchsbaum, M. S. and Poncy, M. (1976). *Psychophysiology*, **13**, 140–8
Lewis, S. A., Oswald, I., Evans, J. I., Akindale, M. O. and Tompsett, S. L. (1970). *Electroencephalogr. Clin. Neurophysiol.*, **28**, 374–81
Leybin, L., Pinsky, C., LaBella, F. S., Havlicek, F. and Rezek, M. (1976). *Nature*, **264**, 458–9
Lord, J. A. H., Waterfield, A. A., Hughes, J. and Kosterlitz, H. W. (1977). *Nature*, **267**, 495–9
Martin, W. R. (1967). *Pharmac. Rev.*, **19**, 463–521
Martin, W. R., Jasinski, D. R. and Mansky, P. A. (1973). *Arch. gen. Psychiat.*, **28**, 784–91
Meglio, M., Hosobuchi, Y., Loh, H. H., Adams, J. E. and Li, C. H. (1977). *Proc. natn. Acad. Sci. U.S.A.*, **74**, 774–6
Mersky, H. (1965). *J. psychiat. Res.*, **8**, 405–19
Meyerson, B. J. and Terenius, L. (1977). *Eur. J. Pharmac.*, **42**, 191–2
Ngai, S. H., Berkowitz, B. A., Young, J. O., Hempstead, J. and Spector, S. (1976). *Anesthesiology*, **44**, 398–403
Pert, A. (1976). In *Opiates and Endogenous Opioid Peptides*, Elsevier, North Holland/New York, pp. 87–94
Rechtschaffen, A. and Kales, A. (1968). *A Manual of Standardized Terminology*, NIH Publ. No. 204, U.S. Govt Printing Office, Washington, D.C.
Sitaram, N., Buchsbaum, M. and Gillin, J. C. (1977). *Eur. J. Pharmac.*, **42**, 285–90
Spitzer, R. L., Endicott, J. and Robbins, E. (1975). *Am. J. Psychiat.*, **32**, 1186–92
Terenius, L., Wahlström, A., Lindstrom, L., and Widerlov, E. (1976). *Neurosci. Lett.*, **3**, 157–62
Teschemacher, H., Opheim, K. E., Cox, B. M. and Goldstein, A. (1975). *Life Sci.*, **16**, 1771–6
Tseng, L. F., Loh, H. H. and Li, C. H. (1976). *Proc. natn. Acad. Sci. U.S.A.*, **73**, 4187–9
Volavka, J., Mallya, A., Baig, S., and Perez-Cruet, J. (1977). *Science*, **196**, 1227–8
von Knorring, L. (1975). Umea University Medical Dissertations, Umea.

36
Behavioral effects of naloxone and LSD

Jorge Perez-Cruet, Jan Volavka, Ashok Mallya, Sadat Baig, and Arthur Toga
(Psychopharmacology and Psychophysiology Units,
Missouri Institute of Psychiatry, University of Missouri-Columbia,
5400 Arsenal Street, St Louis, Missouri 63139, U.S.A.)

The etiology of schizophrenia is still unknown. A clinical single-blind investigation has shown that naloxone, a known pure opiate antagonist, given i.v. in small doses (0.4 mg), reversed hallucinatory behavior in schizophrenic patients (Gunne *et al.*, 1977). This interesting study suggested that opiate-like mechanisms may be involved in schizophrenia.

In the search to confirm Gunne *et al.*'s (1977) findings, and to explore the possible role of endorphins in schizophrenia, we have done a double-blind, placebo-controlled, clinical study with injections of naloxone in chronic schizophrenics showing hallucinations and unusual thought content (Volavka *et al.*, 1977). We could not duplicate Gunne *et al.*'s findings. Results similar to ours were reported somewhat later by Davis *et al.* (1977), but in their study they observed some significant improvement in the unusual thought content of the patients after treatment with naloxone. Several other investigators have reported no effects of naloxone (Janowsky *et al.*, 1977; Kurland *et al.*, 1977) or of naltrexone, a long acting opiate antagonist (Mielke and Gallant, 1977), on the hallucinatory behavior or global ratings of schizophrenics. Emrich *et al.* (1977), using a dose of 4.0 mg of naloxone, i.v., have not been able to confirm the initial studies of Gunne *et al.* (1977), but they did observe indications of an antipsychotic action of naloxone in schizophrenics within 2 to 7 hours after the injection of the antagonist. So far, it can be concluded that there is no clear-cut evidence that naloxone reverses hallucinatory behavior or improves global ratings in chronic schizophrenics.

This chapter presents a detailed account of our clinical data on the effects of naloxone in chronic schizophrenics as well as novel experiments on the behavioral effects of naloxone on an experimental psychosis caused by lysergic acid diethylamide (LSD) and on a fixed ratio operant behavior.

CLINICAL STUDIES

Seven hospitalized patients with a diagnosis of schizophrenia (one male and six females) fulfilling the research diagnostic criteria for schizophrenia (Feighner *et*

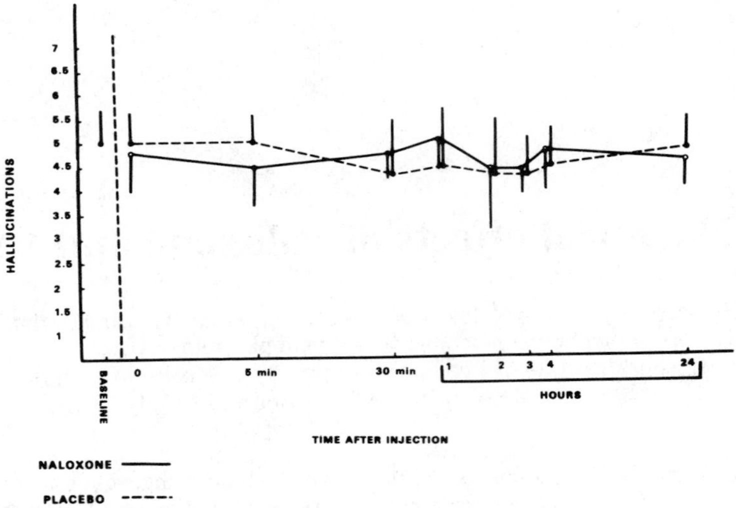

Figure 36.1 Effect of 0.4 mg of naloxone given i.v. and of saline placebo on hallucinations. Each point represents the average of six patients ± s.d. The baseline measure represents the average of three interviews held in a period of 1 week. Hallucinations were graded on a scale of 7, from absent (0) to extremely severe (7).

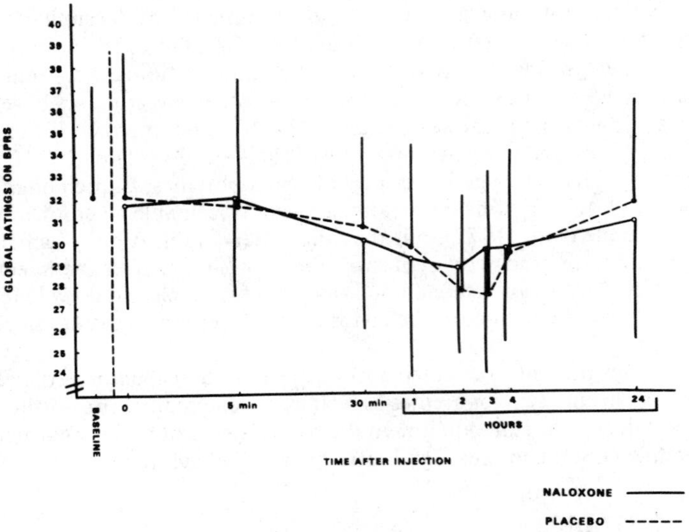

Figure 36.2 Effects of 0.4 mg naloxone i.v. and placebo on the global BPRS scores excluding the score 'hallucinatory behavior'. Each point is the average of seven patients ± s.d.

al., 1972), and having frequent auditory hallucinations, were our subjects. The age range was 24 to 50 years and the duration of illness varied from 4 to 30 years. Four patients were diagnosed as having paranoid schizophrenia and three as having chronic undifferentiated type. All patients were receiving antipsychotic medication before and during the experimental period. All subjects participated voluntarily with informed consent.

The methods of psychiatric evaluation have been described elsewhere (Volavka *et al.*, 1977). The Brief Psychiatric Rating Scale (BPRS) (Overall and Gorham, 1962) was administered by two psychiatrists and all interviews were videotaped. The BPRS evaluations were done immediately before each injection and then 5 min, 30 min, 1, 2, 3, 4, and 24 hours after the injection of naloxone or placebo. Each patient received at least one injection of placebo or naloxone on a double-blind basis. The injections were given 24 to 72 hours apart, at the same time of the day, in a randomized order. Since the dose of naloxone used by Gunne *et al.* (1977) was 0.4 mg, doses of 0.4 and 1.2 mg, i.v., were used. The potency of naloxone was tested in rats challenged with morphine at various doses (10, 20 and 30 mg/kg); the same solution of naloxone (0.4 mg per injection) used in the patients was effective in antagonizing the catalepsy induced in rats by morphine.

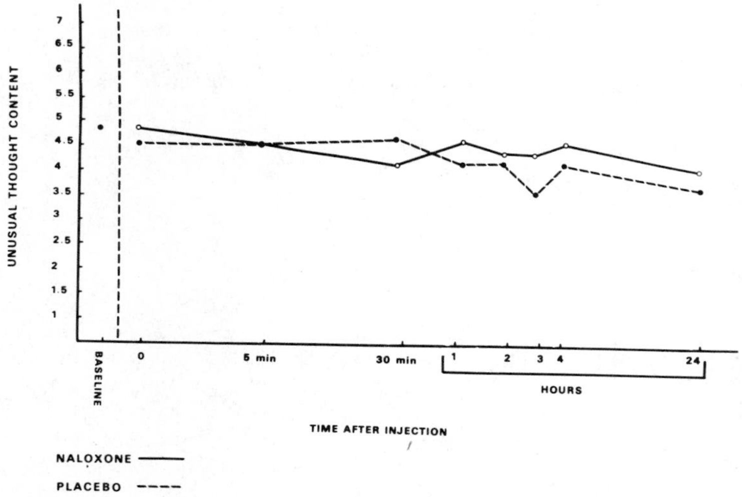

Figure 36.3 The effect of naloxone (0.4 mg, i.v.) on the score item 'unusual thought content'. Baseline and time periods same as in figure 36.1. Each point represents the average of seven patients.

The negative results of naloxone on hallucinations and global ratings are shown in figures 36.1 and 36.2.

Since Davis *et al.* (1977) have reported a reduction of the scores of 'unusual thought content' after an injection of naloxone, we have reviewed our own data on this item. Figure 36.3 shows no effects of i.v. injections of 0.4 mg of naloxone on 'unusual thought content' in our chronic schizophrenic patients.

One of the patients appeared initially to respond to 0.4 mg of naloxone by a reduction of psychopathology. To explore the consistency of this effect and the dose-response relationship, this patient was retested with various doses of naloxone. The results of the injection of various doses of naloxone on hallucinatory

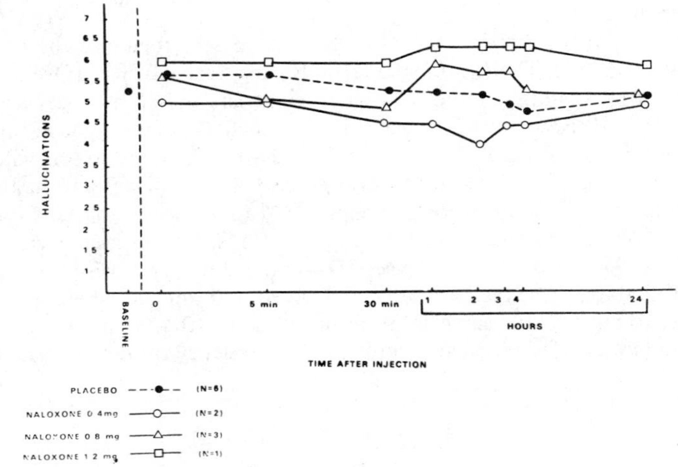

Figure 36.4 Effect of various doses of naloxone (0.4 mg, 0.8 mg and 1.2 mg given i.v.) on hallucinations in a single patient. *N* represents the number of trials at a given dose. Baseline and time periods same as in figure 36.1.

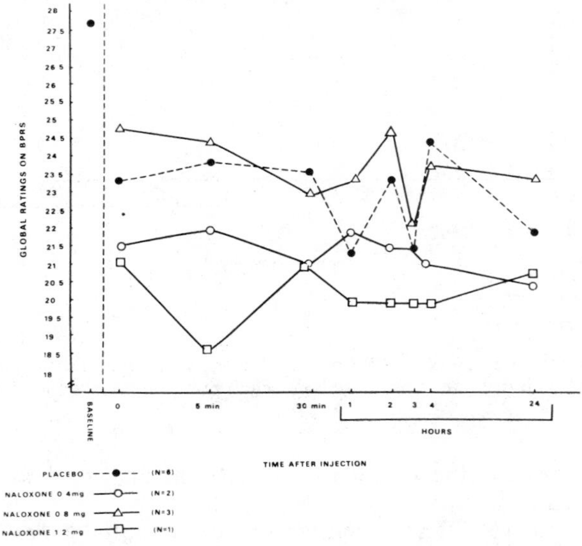

Figure 36.5 Effect of various doses of naloxone (0.4 mg, 0.8 mg and 1.2 mg, given i.v.) on global BPRS scores in a single patient. *N* represents the number of trials at a given dose. This is the same patient as in figure 36.4.

behavior are shown in figure 36.4. No statistically significant difference was observed in hallucinatory behavior after the injection of various doses of naloxone. Figure 36.5 shows no significant effect of various doses of naloxone on global rating from the BPRS scores. These results show that naloxone given i.v. at various doses ranging from 0.4 to 1.2 mg did not alter the hallucinatory behavior, the unusual thought content or the global rating of schizophrenic patients.

EFFECTS OF NALOXONE AND LSD IN CATS

It has been shown previously that naloxone has pronounced suppressant effects on operant behavior schedules reinforced with food in rats, and naloxone also interacts with the stimulant effects of d-amphetamine on operant lever pressing under conditions of continuous avoidance schedules (Holtzman and Jewett, 1973; Holtzman, 1974). No published studies are available to us on the effects of naloxone on fixed ratio schedules to food in cats, and on the interactions between naloxone and hallucinogenic drugs such as LSD.

A total of 10 cats were trained in sound-attenuated experimental chambers with multiple fixed ratio (FR) schedules (described in detail elsewhere (Ferster and Skinner, 1957)) for a period of 6 months. The animals were then trained on a FR-10 (the animal has to press a lever 10 times before he gets a food reinforcement) for an additional period of 2 months. After the animals had stable operant behavior, in order to determine the effects of handling during i.p. injections of drugs, the cats received several saline injections, given at different weekly intervals. All operant behavior was recorded in cumulative recorders and with a PDP 8 computer.

Naloxone in doses of 0.15, 0.8, 1.0, and 5.0 mg/kg, was given i.p. to determine its effects on an FR-10 operant schedule. The dose–response curves for naloxone on operant behavior were compared with similar dose–response curves for naltrexone. The effects of these antagonists on operant behavior were tested for at least 1 hour after injection. With naltrexone, the effects were also tested 48 hours after injection. LSD was injected i.p. at doses of 25 and 50 μg/kg, and its effects on operant behavior were tested for at least 1 hour after injection. In the third group of experiments, the naloxone and LSD treatments were combined. The following two combinations were studied: 25 μg/kg of LSD and 0.15 mg/kg of naloxone: 50 μg/kg of LSD and 5.0 mg/kg of naloxone. In addition, observations were made of the gross behavior of cats after LSD alone, naloxone alone, or the combination of drugs. Bizarre behaviors after LSD were recorded on videotape.

Statistical evaluation of the data on animal experiments was done by analysis of variance (ANOVA) and Student's *t* test (two-tailed).

The results of the separate and combined administration of naloxone and LSD on operant behavior are illustrated in figure 36.6. Naloxone (0.15 mg/kg) and LSD (25 μg/kg) separately produced a statistically significant ($P < 0.001$) increment in lever pressing behavior on an FR-10. Naloxone and LSD at the high doses of 5.0 mg/kg and 50 μg/kg, respectively, produced a significant ($P < 0.001$) obliteration of operant behavior. However, the combination of a low dose of naloxone (0.15 mg/kg) and a low dose of LSD (25 μg/kg) produced a pattern of operant responding similar to that observed after the injection of saline; the

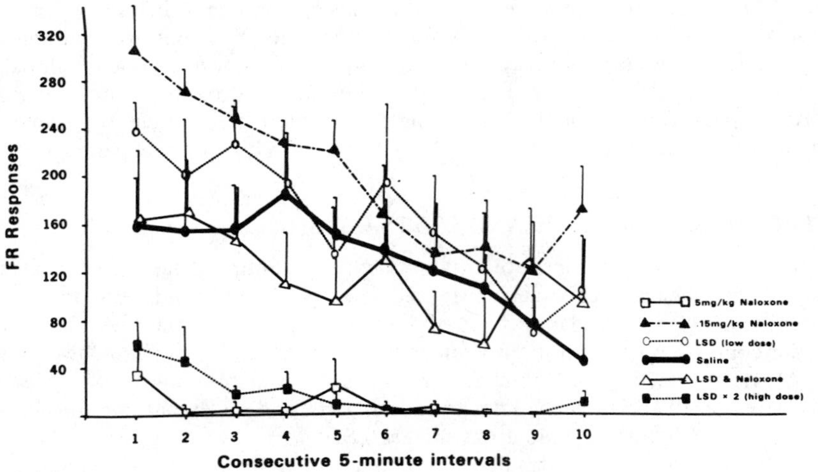

Figure 36.6 Effect of various i.p. doses of naloxone alone, LSD alone, and combined dose of LSD (25 μg/kg) and naloxone (0.15 mg/kg) on FR operant responses. Each point is the mean ± s.d. of five cats during 10 consecutive 5-min periods.

operant responding under the later combinations is shown in figure 36.7. Since both drugs individually produce an increase in lever pressing operant behavior at low doses and an obliteration of this same behavior at high doses, it is likely that this combined effect is due to a synergistic action. On the other hand, the synergistic action of the combination of naloxone and LSD cannot explain the partial blockade by naloxone of bizarre behaviors produced by LSD, such as abortive grooming, limb flicking, and disoriented circling, which were observed outside the operant situation. Therefore, it is likely that naloxone has synergistic and antagonistic properties at varying dose levels.

Figure 36.8 illustrates the overall averages of two half-periods during a 1 hour operant session. The analysis of the effects of drugs during the first and second half-periods was done because the FR-10 operant behavior decreased with satiation. During the first and second half-periods of the session, in spite of the reduction of operant responding due to satiation, naloxone (0.15 mg/kg) still produced significant enhancement of operant behavior, whereas the high dose obliterated the behavior.

In order to find out what dose of naloxone reversed the effects on operant behavior from an increase in operant output to a decrease, a dose-response curve of naloxone was obtained. The results of these experiments are summarized in figure 36.9. The reversal occurred at about a dose of 0.4–0.8 mg/kg, indicating a possible interaction of naloxone with the operant behavior that is dependent on dose levels.

The preliminary findings in cat experiments, that naloxone has a synergistic action with LSD, suggest a possible common receptor site for LSD and naloxone; they also suggest an interaction between LSD and endorphins. It seems likely that this receptor site, where LSD and naloxone interact, involves opiate receptors

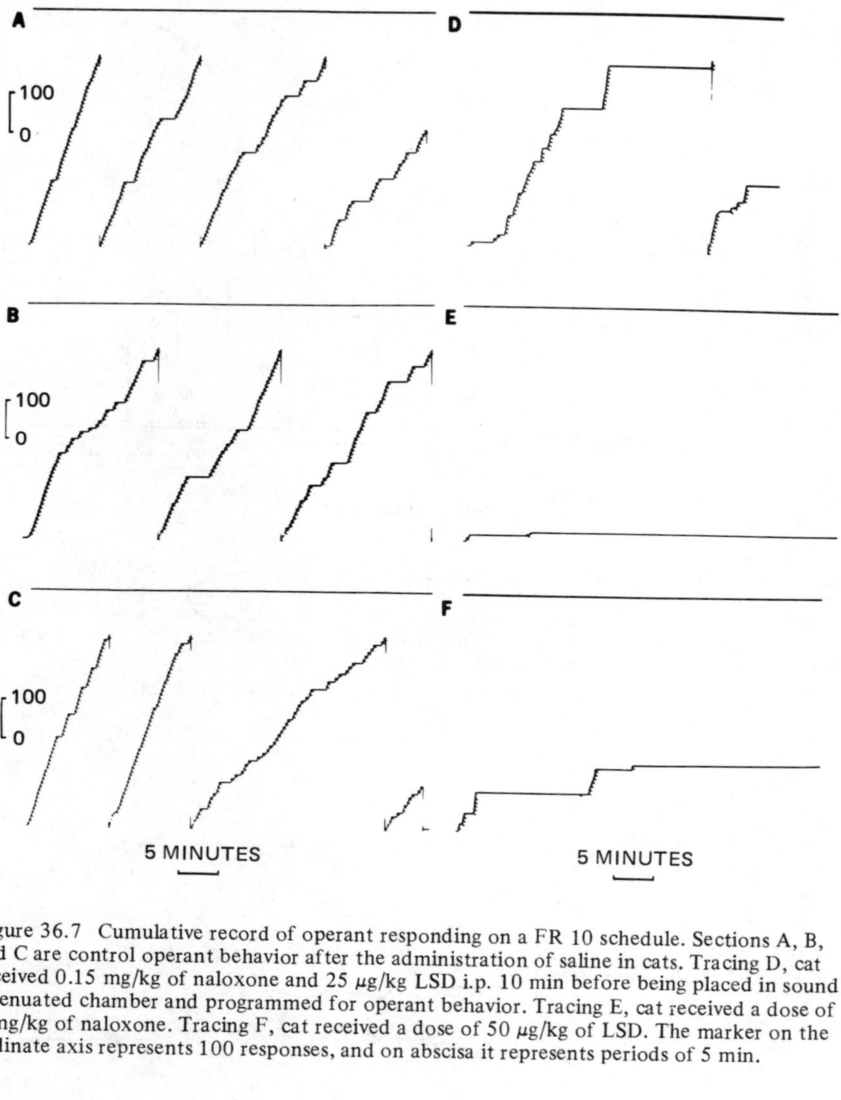

Figure 36.7 Cumulative record of operant responding on a FR 10 schedule. Sections A, B, and C are control operant behavior after the administration of saline in cats. Tracing D, cat received 0.15 mg/kg of naloxone and 25 μg/kg LSD i.p. 10 min before being placed in sound attenuated chamber and programmed for operant behavior. Tracing E, cat received a dose of 5 mg/kg of naloxone. Tracing F, cat received a dose of 50 μg/kg of LSD. The marker on the ordinate axis represents 100 responses, and on abscisa it represents periods of 5 min.

and endorphins. The fact that a very low dose of naloxone and LSD stimulates operant behavior whereas high doses of these drugs block this same behavior, suggests that these drugs are acting at similar receptor sites. Previously it has been shown that naloxone also acts synergistically with chlorpromazine (McMillan, 1971), and also with amphetamine (Holtzman and Jewett, 1973; Holtzman, 1974). Chlorpromazine is known to block dopaminergic receptors; amphetamine can act by stimulating release of dopamine, or by affecting the uptake of monoamines into the neuron, or by inhibiting monoamine oxidase. The combination of

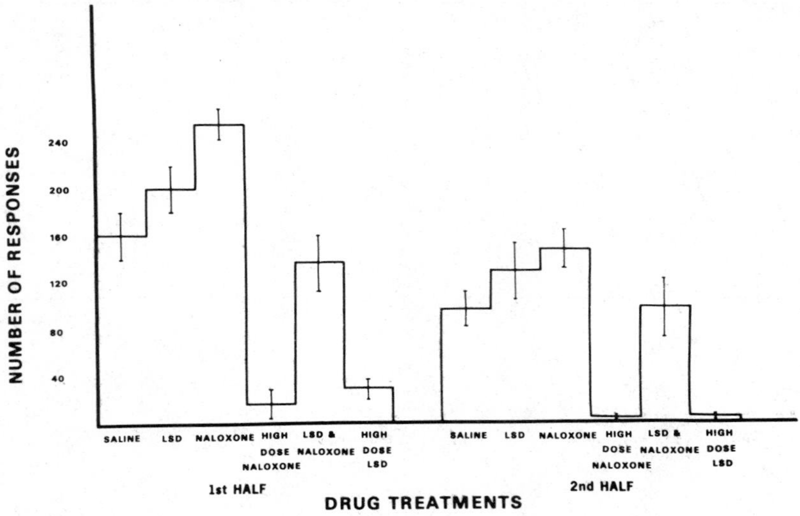

Figure 36.8 The effects of various intraperitoneal doses of naloxone alone, LSD alone, and combination of naloxone and LSD treatments. Number of operant (FR 10) responses on the vertical. The observations of operant behavior are displayed separately for the first 30 min after the injection of drugs and for the second 30 min after the injection (1st half, 2nd half). Each bar represents the mean ± s.d. from five cats.

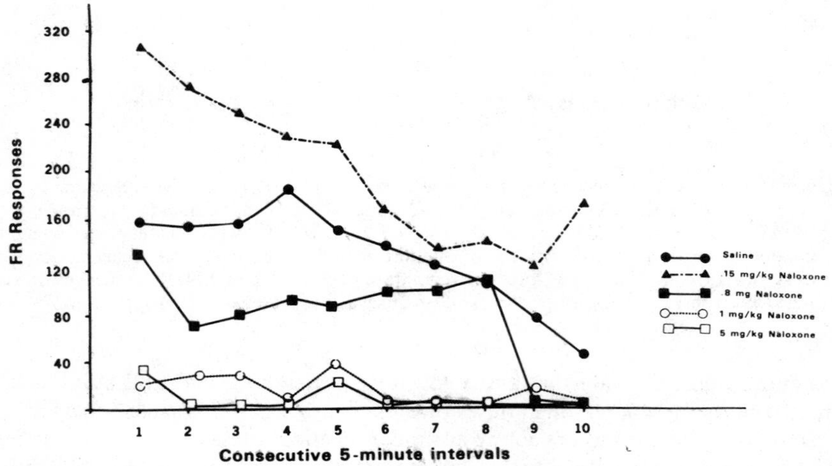

Figure 36.9 Dose-response curves for various doses of naloxone on operant FR responses over a period of 50 min. Each value is the average of five cats. Note that the responses after the low i.p. dose of naloxone (0.15 mg/kg) are above saline controls.

naloxone and LSD in small doses has not elicited the bizarre behavior (for example, abortive grooming, limb flicking, and circling behavior) produced by LSD alone. This fact, that naloxone can block effects of LSD in cats, suggests that naloxone might block the toxic psychosis elicited by LSD in humans.

DISCUSSION AND SUMMARY

Our initial report that naloxone does not improve hallucinations or global ratings in chronic schizophrenia has been subsequently confirmed by others (Davis *et al.*, 1977; Janowsky *et al.*, 1977; Kurland *et al.*, 1977). It is unlikely that endorphins are triggering hallucinations in the chronic schizophrenic patients with persistent hallucinations as in our patients. The overwhelming clinical evidence from double-blind studies by four independent groups showing negative results with naloxone and not confirming Gunne *et al.* (1977) seems ample evidence that it is unlikely that hallucinations are affected by the relative low doses of naloxone used by Gunne *et al.* (1977). It will be necessary to increase the dose of naloxone to higher levels in order to determine whether naloxone is beneficial in schizophrenia; double-blind clinical investigations using 4 mg of naloxone have shown positive results (Emrich *et al.*, 1977). However, Davis *et al.* (1977) have used up to 10 mg of naloxone with negative results. The hypothesis that a long acting antagonist such as naltrexone may be beneficial has so far not received support (Mielke and Gallant, 1977), but more rigorous studies using higher doses of naltrexone are needed. Our studies suggest that naloxone antagonizes LSD effects in cats and it also has profound effects on operant behavior.

REFERENCES

Davis, G. C., Bunney, W. E., DeFraites, E. G., Kleinman, J. E., van Kammen, D. P., Post, R. M. and Wyatt, R. J. (1977). *Science*, **197**, 74–7

Emrich, H. M., Cording, C., Pirée, S., Kolling, A., v. Zerssen, D. and Herz, A. (1977). *Pharmakopsychiatrie.*, **10**, 265–70

Feighner, J. P., Robins, E., Guze, S. B., Woodruff, R. A., Winokur, G. and Muñoz, R. (1972). *Archs gen. Psychiat.*, **26**, 57–63

Ferster, C. B. and Skinner, B. F. (1957). *Schedules of reinforcement.* Appleton–Century-Crofts, New York

Gunne, L. J., Lindstrom, L. and Terenius, L. (1977). *J. Neural Transmission,* **40**, 13–20

Holtzman, S. and Jewett, R. E. (1973). *J. Pharmac. exp. Ther.*, **187**, 380–90

Holtzman, S. G. (1974). *J. Pharmac. expl. Ther.*, **189**, 51–60

Janowsky, D. S., Segal, D. S., Abrams, A., Bloom, F. and Guillemin, R. (1977). *Psychopharmacology,* **53**, 295–97

Kurland, A., McCabe, L. O., Hanlon, T. and Sullivan, D. (1977). *Am. J. Psychiatry*, 134, 1408–10

McMillan, D. E. (1971). *Psychopharmacologia,* **19**, 128–33

Mielke, D. and Gallant, D. M. (1977). *Am. J. Psychiatry,* **134**, 1430–31

Overall, J. E. and Gorham, D. R. (1962). *Psychol. Rep.*, **10**, 799–812

Volavka, J., Mallya, A., Baig, S. and Pérez-Cruet, J. (1977). *Science*, 196, 1227–28

37
Participation of endorphins in the regulation of pituitary function

A. Guidotti and L. Grandison
(Laboratory of Preclinical Pharmacology, National Institute of Mental Health, Saint Elizabeths Hospital, Washington, D.C. 20032, U.S.A.)

Long before the discovery of endogenous opiate peptides, pharmacologists and neuroendocrinologists knew that there were several points of interaction between opiate drugs and endocrine systems. Narcotic analgesics, including morphine, are known to alter ACTH, GH (Gold and Ganong, 1967; George, 1971), prolactin (PRL) (Ojeda *et al.*, 1974; Martin *et al.*, 1975) and LH (Barraclough and Sawyer, 1955) release. Loss of sexual desire, abnormal menses, infertility and spontaneous abortion are frequently observed in addicted patients (George, 1971; Hollister, 1973). Lately, the isolation and identification of endogenous opiate peptides in the brain of all mammalian species studied (Cox *et al.*, 1976; Terenius and Wahlström, 1975; Hughes *et al.*, 1975; Pasternak *et al.*, 1975) and the synthesis of an impressive series of derivatives of these peptides with hormone releasing action (Lien *et al.*, 1976; Shaar *et al.*, 1977; Cusan *et al.*, 1977) have contributed several lines of indirect evidence suggesting that these endogenous opiate-like peptides may have physiological roles in the control of neuroendocrine function.

High concentrations of enkephalin pentapeptides (Fratta *et al.*, 1977; Elde *et al.*, 1977), β-endorphin (Rossier *et al.*, 1977) and stereospecific opiate receptor binding sites (Simantov *et al.*, 1976) have been found in the hypothalamus. Furthermore, β-endorphin-immunoreactive neurons have been identified between the dorso-lateral and arcuate nucleus and in the proximity of the anterior and lateral basal hypothalamus (Bloom *et al.*, 1977). Ample evidence indicates that the basal medial hypothalamus acts as a final common pathway for the integration of neuronal activity affecting pituitary secretion. Therefore, we have hypothesized that information arriving at the median eminence from other hypothalamic areas or from distant brain regions could be conveyed at least in part by the release of β-endorphin within the hypothalamus. To test this hypothesis, we have examined the *in vivo* and *in vitro* effect of morphine, β-endorphin (two opiate agonists) and naltrexone (a specific opiate receptor antagonist) on the release of PRL, LH, GH and TSH in basal conditions and after different stimuli. We have obtained data which are compatible with the proposal that intrahypothalamic, endogenous opiate-like peptides participate in the regulation of anterior pituitary hormone secretion.

HYPOTHALAMIC OPIATE RECEPTOR STIMULATION AND HORMONE RELEASE

It has been reported that intraventricular (i.v.t.) injection of β-endorphin, like enkephalins or morphine, induces PRL and GH release (Rivier *et al.*, 1977; Cusan *et al.*, 1977). Undoubtedly, this observation has great pharmacological significance but does not indicate whether endogenous opioid ligands interact with opioid receptors in the hypothalamus to control pituitary function. To gain some insight as to whether the hypothalamic endorphins modulate neuroendocrine functions, we injected β-endorphin directly into the ventral-medial hypothalamus or gave morphine systemically to rats with a deafferentated hypothalamus. In table 37.1,

Table 37.1 Effect of intrahypothalamic β-endorphin injection on hormone release from anterior pituitary

Intrahypothalamic treatment	Naltrexone 1 mg/kg, i.p.	PRL ng/ml	GH ng/ml	LH ng/ml	TSH μg/ml
Saline	–	12 ± 2.5	98 ± 28	150 ± 22	0.94 ± 0.18
	+	6 ± 1.2*	45 ± 10*	228 ± 21*	1.02 ± 0.16
β-Endorphin 1 μg	–	32 ± 3.8*	235 ± 40*	72 ± 9.8*	0.75 ± 0.15
	+	14 ± 3.5	92 ± 32	134 ± 28	0.90 ± 0.22

Rats (150–180 g) with chronic implanted guide cannulae were used. β-endorphin (1 μg) or saline was injected in the medial-based hypothalamus (4.5 mm A-P, 0.5 L, 8.3 D-V; Konig and Klippel, 1967) in a volume of 1 μl in 2 min. Naltrexone or 0.85 per cent NaCl was given 10 min before β-endorphin injection. Blood was collected by decapitation 20 min after the intrahypothalamic injection. Cannula position was verified histologically. PRL, GH, TSH were measured in normal male rats. LH was measured in OVX estrogen-primed (5 μg/day for 5 days) rats. The hormone concentration was measured using the NIAMD radioimmunoassay kit provided by NIAMD-NIH Pituitary Hormone Program. Each value is the mean ± s.e. of 6–8 determinations.
*$P < 0.05$ when compared with saline-treated rats.

we show that 1 μg of β-endorphin injected in the basal-medial hypothalamus of unanesthetized rats implanted with a chronic cannula significantly increased PRL and GH release in intact male rats and decreased LH release in ovariectomized female rats, but did not alter serum TSH concentrations.

Ten micrograms of α-endorphin did not significantly change PRL, GH and TSH release (not shown). Naltrexone (1 mg/kg, i.p.) blocked all these effects of intrahypothalamic β-endorphin. Morphine sulfate, given systemically, stimulated PRL release in male rats that had the medial-basal hypothalamus surgically isolated from the rest of the brain (see table 37.2). No changes in the serum TSH concentration were noted.

Table 37.2 Effect of morphine and naltrexone on serum PRL and TSH levels of rats with deafferention of the hypothalamus

Intraperitoneal treatment	Intact PRL ng/ml	Intact TSH μg/ml	Hypothalamic deafferention PRL ng/ml	Hypothalamic deafferention TSH μg/ml
Saline	18 ± 2.8	0.94 ± 0.18	22 ± 3.1	1.0 ± 0.22
Morphine SO_4 15 mg/kg	48 ± 7.5*	0.92 ± 0.25	50 ± 9.5*	0.98 ± 0.28
Naltrexone 1 mg/kg	8.4 ± 3*	–	8.7 ± 3*	–

Male rats (200–220 g) were used 7 days after hypothalamic deafferentation (Halasz and Pupp, 1965). Morphine was injected 40 min and naltrexone 30 min, before the cardiac puncture. Blood samples were collected under light ether anesthesia. Each value is the mean ± s.e. of six experiments.

EVIDENCE FOR A PHYSIOLOGICAL ROLE FOR HYPOTHALAMIC ENDORPHINS

As shown in figure 37.1, naltrexone significantly decreased PRL release when injected systemically in male rats. Maximal effects were observed with 1 mg of naltrexone by about 1 hour following its administration. The effect of naltrexone lasted for more than 3 hours and the blockade of PRL release was even more impressive in ovariectomized estrogen-primed rats. In these animals, doses of naltrexone as small as 0.25 mg/kg produced within 1 hour, a 50 per cent decrease

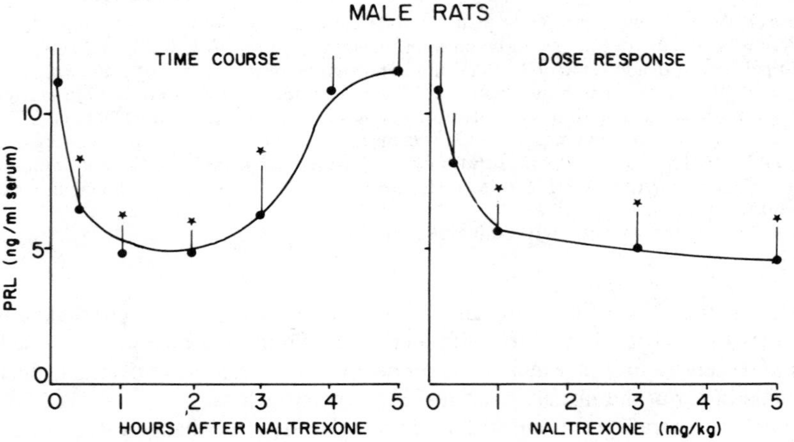

Figure 37.1 Male rats (Sprague-Dawley) of 180–220 g were killed by decapitation. For the dose–response curve the animals were killed 30 min after naltrexone. PRL, prolactin measured with the rat prolactin RIA kit provided by the NIAMD-NIH Pituitary Hormone Program. Each value is the mean ± s.e. of 8–10 rats.
*$P < 0.05$ when compared with control groups.

of serum PRL levels (Grandison and Guidotti, 1977*a*). As reported in table 37.1, naltrexone also decreased serum GH and increased serum LH concentration but did not influence serum TSH. These effects of naltrexone were opposite to those observed after intrahypothalamic injection of β-endorphin.

Systemically administered naltrexone may alter the production and release of PRL by interfering with the endorphin system at any of several brain levels. To establish the site at which naltrexone acted to change the PRL release, we studied: the direct action on isolated pituitary glands, the effect after intrahypothalamic injection, and the effect in rats with a deafferentated hypothalamus. Naltrexone, in concentrations up to 10^{-4} M failed to decrease PRL release from isolated pituitary glands. In contrast, it produced a marked decrease in serum PRL levels when injected in doses of 25 μg intrahypothalamically (table 37.3) in intact rats or in doses of 1 mg/kg, i.p., in rats with a deafferentated hypothalamus (table 37.2).

Table 37.3 Effect of intrahypothalamic injection of naltrexone on serum PRL

Intrahypothalamic treatment	PRL ng/ml serum
Saline (1 μl)	29.3 ± 3.9
Naltrexone (25 μg in 1 μl)	6.7 ± 1.2*

Saline or naltrexone were injected in the medial-basal hypothalamus 20 min before blood collection. Each value is the mean ± s.e. of six rats.
*$P < 0.05$ when compared with saline-injected rats.

From these results, we have inferred that the action of naltrexone on hormone release can be mediated by a blockade of opiate receptors in the hypothalamus and also that hypothalamic opiate receptor ligands participate tonically in the control of hormone secretion under physiological conditions.

In recent experiments, we have shown that naltrexone prevented the increase of PRL release induced by foot shock (Grandison and Guidotti, 1977*a*). These results suggest that in addition to tonic control, endogenous opiate receptor ligands may mediate some of the adaptive sensory and emotional responses to stress; a contention in line with reports which associate alteration of endogenous opiate-like systems with some behavioral disorders (Terenius *et al.*, 1976; Gunne, 1977).

INTERACTION BETWEEN DOPAMINE, GABA AND OPIATE RECEPTOR SYSTEMS IN THE CONTROL OF PRL RELEASE

The hypothalamus contains agents that can stimulate and inhibit PRL release. Under most conditions, the overriding influence of the hypothalamus is inhibitory. Two putative neurotransmitter substances have been suggested to be the physiological inhibitory agents. These are dopamine (DA) (Mueller *et al.*, 1976) and γ-amino-

Table 37.4 Effect of naltrexone and pargyline on haloperidol, reserpine and morphine-induced PRL release

Treatment	Saline	Naltrexone	Pargyline
		PRL (ng/ml serum)	
Saline	11 ± 2.5	6.1 ± 0.5*	5.2 ± 0.6*
Haloperidol (0.25 mg/kg, i.p.)	68 ± 7.9*	55 ± 4.3*	–
Reserpine (2 mg/kg, i.p.)	44 ± 3.0*	45 ± 6.0*	–
Morphine SO_4 (15 mg/kg, i.p.)	52 ± 6.5*	15 ± 4.2	48 ± 6.0*

Haloperidol and morphine were injected 45 min before killing. Reserpine was injected 6 h before. Blood samples were collected after decapitation 30 min after naltrexone (1 mg/kg, i.p.) or 45 min after pargyline (50 mg/kg, i.p.). Each value is the mean ± s.e. of 7–9 rats.
$*P < 0.05$ when compared with controls receiving saline.

butyric acid (GABA) (Schally *et al.*, 1977). Therefore, it became important to understand whether opiate-induced PRL release involves an action on DA or GABA neurons.

As a model to study the interactions with DA neurons we injected naltrexone into animals in which the DA receptor function was blocked by haloperidol (a DA receptor blocker) or reserpine (a drug which depletes hypothalamic DA content). Both drugs produced a marked increase in the level of serum PRL. Naltrexone failed to reduce PRL in haloperidol or reserpine treated rats (see table 37.4). Furthermore, morphine increased PRL release in rats injected with pargyline, a treatment (see table 37.4) which is known to increase hypothalamic catecholamine content and decrease the serum PRL levels in both normal (Chen *et al.*, 1977) and reserpine-treated rats.

Table 37.5 Effect of muscimol and β-endorphin-induced PRL release

	Saline	Morphine
	PRL (ng/ml serum)	
Intraventricular injection		
Saline (5 μl)	14 ± 3	51 ± 6*
Muscimol (250 μg)	15 ± 5	72 ± 9*
Intrahypothalamic injection		
Saline (1 μl)	22 ± 3	63 ± 9*
Muscimol (250 μg)	28 ± 4	85 ± 10*

Morphine SO_4 (15 mg/kg, i.p.) was injected 10 min before the i.v.t. injection of muscimol. Muscimol was injected 20 min before killing. Each value is the mean ± s.e. of six rats.
$*P < 0.05$ when compared with saline-treated rats.

To study the interaction with the GABA receptor system, morphine was injected together with muscimol (a powerful GABA receptor agonist). In these experiments, muscimol was administered either i.v.t. or intrahypothalamically to avoid indirect peripheral effects. As shown in table 37.5, stimulation of GABA receptors by muscimol failed to alter the response to morphine. The dose of muscimol used in these experiments was sufficient to produce marked behavioral effects (that is, increase of food intake) (Grandison and Guidotti, 1977*b*) to counteract the action of 450 mg isoniazid per kg, i.p. and to increase cyclic AMP content of the anterior pituitary (unpublished observation).

The results of these experiments suggest that endogenous opiate ligands contro PRL release by an intrahypothalamic mechanism which perhaps is independent o DA or GABA inhibition. However, these experiments do not exclude the possibility that another PRL release-inhibiting factor (PIF) on which opiates act, represents the final pathway regulating hormone release. Indeed, considering the anatomical disposition of the hypothalamic endorphin-containing-neurons and the lack of a direct PRL releasing action of β-endorphin or enkephalin when directly applied to pituitary halves *in vitro* (Rivier *et al.*, 1977), it is possible that β-endorphin neurons and the tuberoinfundibular tract regulate PRL release according to an arrangement in which the two systems act in series.

CONCLUSION

Our data show that the stimulation of intrahypothalamic opioid receptors by β-endorphin and morphine generates a sustained change in the release of GH, PRL and LH release. Naltrexone can block the action of intrahypothalamic injection of β-endorphin and by itself, naltrexone injected systemically or intrahypothalamically produces effects opposite to that of β-endorphin.

In most experimental situations, the absence of any direct action of opiate antagonists has been taken as an argument against any tonic role of endorphins. The only evidence which shows that opiate antagonists do modify central processes mediated by endorphins is the capacity of naloxone to lower pain threshold under appropriate conditions in animals and man (Akil *et al.*, 1976; Jacobs *et al.*, 1974).

The data reported in this chapter, together with the report on the histoimmunochemical localization of the β-endorphin-containing-neurons in the hypothalamus, suggest that endogenous opiate-like peptides in the hypothalamus are involved in the physiological regulation of hormone release from the anterior pituitary. In our opinion, this is the first direct evidence for a tonic role of endogenous opiate ligands in the nervous system.

The proposed relationship between endogenous opiate systems and regulation of hormone release raises very interesting possibilities for interpreting some of the proposed behavioral consequences of opiate receptor medication. If environmental stimuli or behavioral responses control the secretion of all or some pituitary hormones through β-endorphin or enkephalins, it is also possible that hormones may influence behavior through long, short or ultra-short feedback loops. Recently, we have obtained evidence that morphine also induces a marked rise in serum PRL in rats treated chronically with morphine pellets. These results agree with the clinical observations showing that narcotic analgesics produce symptoms of endocrine dysfunction in addicted patients (George *et al.*, 1971; Kreek, 1973). Therefore, acute and chronic use of opiate agonists and antagonists should open interesting possibilities for an understanding of the role of endorphins in mental health research.

REFERENCES

Akil, H., Mayer, D. J. and Liebeskind, J. C. (1976). *Science*, **191**, 961–2

Barraclough, C. A. and Sawyer, C. H. (1955). *Endocrinology*, **57**, 329–37

Bloom, F. E., Rossier, J., Battenberg, E. L. F., Bajon, A., French, E., Henriksen, S. J., Siggins, G. R., Segal, D., Browne, R., Ling, N. and Guillemin, R. (1977). In *Advances in Biochemical Psychopharmacology*, (eds. E. Costa, and M. Trabucchi), Vol. **18**, Raven Press, New York, pp. 89–109

Chen, H. T., Simpkins, J. W., Mueller, G. P. and Meites, J. (1977). *Life Sci.* **21**, 533–42

Cox, B. M., Goldstein, A. and Li, C. H. (1976). *Proc. natn. Acad. Sci. U.S.A.*, **73**, 1821–3

Cusan, L., Dupont, A., Kledzik, G. S., Labrie, F., Coy, D. H. and Schally, A. V. (1977). *Nature*, **268**, 544–7

Elde, R., Hökfelt, T., Johansson, O. and Terenius, L. (1976). *Neuroscience*, **1**, 349–51

Fratta, W., Yang, H-Y. T., Hong, J. and Costa, E. (1977). *Nature*, **268**, 452–4

George, R. (1971). In *Narcotic Drugs, Biochemical Pharmacology*, (ed. D. Clouet). Plenum Press, New York, pp. 283–99

Gold, E. M. and Ganong, W. F. (1967). In *Neuroendocrinology*, (eds. L. Martini and W. F. Ganong), Vol. **II**, Academic Press, New York, pp. 377–437

Grandison, L. and Guidotti, A. (1977*a*). *Nature*, **240**, 357–9

Grandison, L. and Guidotti, A. (1977*b*). *Neuropharmacology*, **16**, 533–6

Gunne, L. M., Lindström, L. and Terenius, L. (1977). *J. Neural. Transmission*, **40**, 13–9

Halasz, B. and Pupp, L. (1965). *Endocrinology*, **77**, 553–62

Hollister, L. E. (1973). *Prog. Brain Res.*, **39**, 373–81

Hughes, J., Smith, T. W., Kosterlitz, H. W., Fothergill, L. A., Morgan, B. A. and Morris, H. R. (1975). *Nature*, **258**, 577–9

Jacobs, J. J., Tremblay, E. C. and Colombel, M. C. (1974). *Psychopharmacology*, **37**, 217–23

König, J. F. R. and Klippel, R. A. (1967). *The Rat Brain*, Krieger Publishing Co., Basel

Kreek, M. J. (1973). *J. Am. Med. Ass.*, **223**, 665–8

Lien, E. L., Fewichel, R. L., Garsky, U., Sarantakis, D. and Grant, W. H. (1970). *Life Sci.*, **19**, 837–40

Martin, J. P., Audent, J. and Saunders, A. (1975). *Endocrinology*, **96**, 839–47

Mueller, G. P., Simpkins, J., Meites, J. and Moore, K. E. (1976). *Neuroendocrinology*, **20**, 121–35

Ojeda, S. R., Harms, P. G. and McCann, S. M. (1974). *Endocrinology*, **96**, 1695–703

Rivier, C., Vale, W., Ling, N., Brown, M. and Guillemin, R. (1977). *Endocrinology*, **100**, 238–41

Rossier, J., Vargo, T. M., Minick, S. M., Ling, N., Bloom, F. E. and Guillemin, R. (1977). *Proc. natn. Acad. Sci. U.S.A.*, **74**, 5162–5

Schally, A. V., Redding, T. W., Arimura, A., Dupont, A. and Linthicum, G. L. (1977). *Endocrinology*, **100**, 681–91

Shaar, C. J., Frederickson, R. C. A., Dininger, N. B. and Jackson, L. (1977). *Life Sci.*, **21**, 853–60

Pasternak, G. W., Goodman, R. and Snyder, S. H. (1975). *Life Sci.*, **16**, 1765–9

Simantov, R., Kuhar, M. J., Pasternak, G. W. and Snyder, S. H. (1976). *Brain Res.*, **106**, 189–97

Terenius, L. and Wahlström, A. (1975). *Life Sci.*, **16**, 1759–64

Terenius, L., Wahlström, A., Lindström, L. and Widerlöv, E. (1976). *Neurosci. Lett.*, **3**, 157–62

38
Naloxone administration in chronic hallucinating schizophrenic patients

Philip A. Berger, Stanley J. Watson, Huda Akil and Jack D. Barchas
(Psychiatric Clinical Research Center and
Nancy Pritzker Laboratory of Behavioral Neurochemistry,
Department of Psychiatry and Behavioral Sciences,
Stanford University School of Medicine, Stanford, California 94305, U.S.A.)

The recent discovery of the endogenous opiate peptides has been followed by a massive research effort aimed at defining the role of these substances in both normal and abnormal physiology. A part of this research has focused on the possible role of the opiate peptides in psychiatric disorders. Controversial evidence has recently been presented suggesting a role for endogenous opiate systems in mood and psychoses. Terenius *et al.* (1976) reported that some opiate peptide fractions were elevated in unmedicated schizophrenic and manic patients. These concentrations decreased when the schizophrenic patients were medicated and when the manic patients became depressed (Terenius *et al.*, 1976). Gunne *et al.* (1977) then attempted to reverse the theorized opiate peptide contribution to schizophrenia by administering the opiate antagonist naloxone (0.4 mg, i.v.). They reported decreased auditory hallucinations in four of six schizophrenic patients tested. This study was single blind, did not use standard rating scales or explicit subject selection criteria (Gunne *et al.* 1977). Yet, the report of decrease or loss of auditory hallucinations was intriguing. Several groups then attempted to replicate this study without much success. Volavka *et al.* (1977) used the same dose of naloxone (0.4 mg) in carefully selected subjects, observed them for several hours and observed no effect on schizophrenic symptoms. Davis *et al.* (1977) gave between 0.4 and 10 mg of naloxone i.v. (usually, 0.4 mg) to patients from several diagnostic categories. These patients were studied for 1 hour and while they may have had improved cognition, no change in hallucinations was reported. Most recently Janowsky *et al.* (1977) have infused 1.2 mg of naloxone to a general population of schizophrenic subjects and observed no important changes over an hour.

We chose a different study design than the four investigations cited above. Our first concern was the dose of naloxone. The experience of many laboratories (including our own) in reversing the endogenous opiate peptides suggested that 10-60 times as much naloxone was required to reverse the endogenous opiate peptides than was required to reverse the effects of the plant opiate alkaloids (Martin *et al.*, 1976; Kosterlitz and Hughes, 1975). We therefore decided to use a much higher dose of naloxone for this study (10 mg, i.v.). The second major concern was duration of evaluation for drug effects. In the studies of Davis *et al.* (1977) and Janowsky *et al.* (1977) subjects were observed for only up to 1 hour. Pharmacological reversal of morphine by naloxone does occur very rapidly and passes quickly. Yet, physiological studies of the effects of naloxone showed effects on stress and electrical analgesia lasting for several hours (Akil *et al.*, 1976*a*; 1976*b*). Based on this time frame, we rated our subjects at intervals, up to 4 hours. The last major design feature of this study was the patient selection system. Subjects were chosen for chronicity of illness, stability of symptoms, and persistence of hallucinations.

Thus, we used higher doses of naloxone, observed longer, and chose to study a rarer subject pool, in the hope of testing the pharmacological effects of naloxone on schizophrenic symptoms under optimal conditions.

METHODS

All 11 subjects were males between the ages of 26 and 47, with a diagnosis of either chronic paranoid or chronic undifferentiated schizophrenia. These diagnoses were based on the Diagnostic and Statistical Manual of the American Psychiatric Association (DSM-H) and the diagnostic criteria suggested for use in psychiatric research by Feighner *et al.* (1972) and the diagnostic system of Taylor *et al.*, (1975). All patients volunteered and gave informed consent to participate in the study. Patients were chosen because of the presence of relatively stable psychotic symptoms, either on or off neuroleptic medications. Subjects were also selected only if they reported very frequent or nearly constant auditory hallucinations, that is, voices heard at least twice an hour, throughout the study period. All patients had psychotic symptoms that were active, obvious and easily rateable on two standard psychiatric rating scales. Each subject had easily rateable symptoms on at least one of the following subscales: anxiety, paranoia, anger, or general agitation, of the Brief Psychiatric Rating Scale (BPRS) (Overall, 1974) and NIMH psychiatric rating scales (Green *et al.*, 1977). Most subjects had rateable symptoms on several of these subscales. Subjects were also free of major physical disorders and did not have a history of extensive self-administration of psychoactive drugs of abuse. Thus, all subjects were given an extensive physical and psychiatric evaluation.

The strict requirements for participation in this study resulted in a fairly homogeneous pool of eleven patients, screened from approximately 1000 psychiatric patients. Six subjects had not received neuroleptic medications for at least 2 weeks before the study; the other five were maintained on their usual stable dose of neuroleptic medication throughout the study period.

The first two patients were studied on one day, using a single-blind design. The next nine subjects were studied using a double-blind, randomized cross-over paradigm, with naloxone and placebo infusions separated by at least 48 hours. Naloxone (10 mg) (Endo Labs, Inc.) or an equal volume of placebo, was administered i.v.

The patients were interviewed and rated by two raters who were trained in the use of the NIMH and BPRS Rating Scales. The raters did not know the sequence of administration. All interviews were videotaped. The ratings were recorded on the NIMH rating scale and the BPRS. Subjects also rated their current mood and hallucinatory state on a 100 mm visual analogue scale. One end of the 100 mm mood line read 'very sad', the other end 'very happy'. The hallucinatory state line read 'not at all' on one end, 'as bad as usual' in the center, and 'worse than usual' at the other end. The subject was asked to place a mark on each line to indicate his current state.

Patients were studied in a comfortable chair with an indwelling i.v. line for infusion. The baseline interview and ratings took place after the i.v. line was established and a saline injection was given. The two single-blind subjects were then given 10 mg of naloxone i.v. The double-blind patients were given either naloxone 10 mg or an equal volume of placebo after the baseline interview. The interview and ratings were repeated 30 min after the second infusion, and several times over the next few hours. Subjects did not know which infusions contained naloxone, and were not told the nature of the expected effect. During the nine randomized double-blind infusions, neither patients nor staff knew whether naloxone or placebo was given on a particular day.

RESULTS

The ratings recorded on the NIMH rating scale are the basis of the data and statistical analyses in this report. The BPRS and the subjective visual analogue scales were a part of the evaluation sessions and were in agreement with the NIMH scale, but are not analyzed in this preliminary report.

The two patients studied in a single-blind design both reported a loss of auditory hallucinations which lasted for several hours (table 38.1). One of these subjects (S2) became more irritable and had increased paranoid ideation after naloxone infusion. This irritability lasted about 45 min and then decreased. Except for this brief period of irritability in one subject both patients given naloxone in a single-blind design reported a feeling of well-being and relaxation that they described as unusual for them.

The nine subjects given naloxone in a placebo controlled, randomized double-blind, cross-over design (table 38.2) are the basis for statistical analysis. A one-way analysis of variance (ANOVA) on the difference scores between the response to drug and the response to placebo was carried out. A response score was defined as the difference between that day's baseline NIMH score and the score at 1.5 to 2.0 hours after infusion. This ANOVA revealed no significant effect of the sequence of administration of naloxone and placebo. There was, however, a statistically significant effect of naloxone on hallucinations ($F\ 1{,}7 = 5.62$, $P < 0.05$) (table 38.2).

Six of the nine patients reported a definite decrease or a complete loss of auditory hallucination. One patient (S6) reported an equivocal decrease. Two patients did not exhibit a response beyond that reported during placebo administration (table 38.2). Five of the six responding patients also reported an improvement in mood with decreased anxiety. Although the NIMH scale scores reflect this trend, the effect was not statistically significant (table 38.3). Several patients also reported subjectively better sleep the evening following the naloxone

Table 38.1 Subjective response to naloxone

Subject no.	Age and diagnosis	Study design	Neuroleptic medication	Drug sequence	Subject's and investigator's impressions of the response to naloxone*
S1	33, Pa	SB	No	P/N	++, 6 h, slightly less anxious, no hallucinations
S2	32, Un	SB	No	P/N	++, 96 h, transiently irritable, then calm, fewer voices
S3	28, Pa	DB	Yes	P/N	++, 48 h, less rapid thinking, less depressed and anxious, calm
S4	41, Pa	DB	Yes	P/N	++, 24 h, calmer, slept well, less tense
S5	26, Pa	DB	No	N/P	0 'hears his thoughts'. Both infusions 'helped'
S6	47, Pa	DB	Yes	P/N	± becoming more ill before study, naloxone suppressed 'voices'
S7	45, Pa	DB	No	N/P	0 very delusional, continued hallucinating
S8	26, Un	DB	Yes	N/P	+, 6 h, briefly irritable, then felt 'good'
S9	29, Un	DB	No	P/N	+, 3 h, transiently irritable, then less anxious and relaxed
S10	27, Pa	DB	Yes	N/P	+, 4 h, transiently irritable, then calm and even smiled
S11	22, Pa	DB	No	N/P	++, 3 h, slower thoughts, relaxed and felt 'good'

Diagnosis: Un, Chronic undifferentiated schizophrenia; Pa, chronic paranoid schizophrenia.
Study design: SB, Single-blind design; DB, double-blind design.
Sequence of testing: P/N, Placebo-naloxone; N/P, naloxone-placebo.
*The 0 to ++ ratings are the subjective impressions of the investigators: 0, no response; ±, equivocal improvement, +, detectable improvement with decrease in auditory hallucinations, ++, substantial loss of hallucinations. The time (for example, 6 h) is the patient's report of number of hours after infusion at which auditory hallucinations returned.

infusion (table 38.1). Three of these six subjects also described the biphasic mood change similar to that reported by S2. These three subjects generally felt and acted irritably or dysphorically for up to 45 min following the infusion and then described a calm and relaxed state.

Table 38.2 Effects of naloxone (10 mg i.v.) on hallucinations in schizophrenic patients

Subject no	Placebo day Hallucination ratings‡	Placebo day Difference	Naloxone day Hallucination ratings‡	Naloxone day Difference	Subjective impressions of the investigators†
S1	B– P–	–	B6 P0	6	++
S2	B– P–	–	B3 P0	3	++
S3	B– P2	1	B4 P0	4	++
S4	B2 P1	1	B4 P0	4	++
S5	B3 P3	0	B3 P4	–1	0
S6	B2 P2	0*	B6 P3	3	±
S7	B6 P6	0	B6 P6	0	0
S8	B5 P3	2	B5 P1	4	+
S9	B6 P6	0	B6 P3	3	+
S10	B5 P1	4	B6 P4	2	+
S11	B5 P5	0	B6 P0	6	++
	$\bar{X} = 0.88$ S 3–11: s.e.m. = 0.45 $F_{1,7}$ for order or sequence of presentation = 1.55; N.S.		$\bar{X} = 2.78$ S 3–11: s.e.m. = 0.72 $F_{1,7}$ for drug effect = 5.62, $P < 0.05$		

*Subject lost hallucinations later that day for several days, became more ill and was hospitalized.

†The 0 to ++ ratings were the subjective impressions of the investigators: 0, no response; ±, equivocal improvement; +, detectable improvement with decrease in auditory hallucinations; ++, substantial loss of hallucinations.

‡The larger the rating, the greater the pathology. B, Baseline rating that day, before infusion of drug; P, rating 75–120 min after drug infusion on the basis of the NIMH subscale. Difference, the difference between baseline rating and postinfusion rating. The larger the number, the greater the improvement, on the basis of the NIMH subscale.

Table 38.3 Effects of naloxone (10 mg i.v.) on anxiety in schizophrenic patients

Subject no	Placebo day: Anxiety ratings†	Placebo day: Difference	Naloxone day: Anxiety ratings†	Naloxone day: Difference
S1	B– P–	–	B1 P0	1
S2	B– P–	–	B3 P0	3
S3	B3 P3	0	B3 P0	3
S4	B2 P1	1	B3 P1	2
S5	B3 P3	0	B3 P3	0
S6	B6 P0	6*	B5 P4	1
S7	B3 P2	1	B4 P3	1
S8	B0 P0	0	B0 P0	0
S9	B5 P5	0	B5 P3	2
S10	B0 P1	−1	B7 P2	5
S11	B5 P4	1	B5 P0	5
	$\bar{X} = 0.88$ S 3–11, s.e.m. = 0.68 $F_{1,7}$ for order or sequence of presentation = 0.67, N.S.		$\bar{X} = 2.12$ S 3–11, s.e.m. = 0.63 $F_{1,7}$ for drug effect = 1.09, N.S.	

*Subject extremely anxious first day (placebo); calmed rapidly once study commenced
†The larger the number the greater the pathology. B, Baseline rating that day, before infusion of drug; P, rating 75–120 min after drug infusion on basis of NIMH subscale. Difference = the difference between baseline rating and postinfusion ratings. The larger the number, the greater the improvement, on the basis of the NIMH subscale.

The response of S6 was described as equivocal. This patient (S6) was difficult to evaluate because his clinical status worsened just before the study. The public health nurse who knew this patient reported that he was agitated and sleeping less a few days before the study. These symptoms often preceded hospitalization for this patient. This subject did not report changes in his hallucinations within the first few hours after saline injection, but 7 hours after saline he reported a decrease in hallucinations, and an increase in paranoid delusions over the next few days. On the day of the naloxone infusion he had elevated baseline ratings on both the global illness and hallucination subscales. Still, the naloxone infusion was associated with a decrease in hallucinations lasting several hours. This outpatient (S6) required hospitalization 2 days after the study.

One of the non-responders (S7) was grossly delusional and did not give reliable reports. There were no major changes in his ratings on any subscale. The second non-responder (S5) had a general improvement after both saline and naloxone. This subject (S5) had hallucinations that he characterized as hearing his own thoughts out loud. All other subjects described their voices as having an external source.

Thus, six of nine subjects given naloxone in double-blind design exhibited significant changes following naloxone infusion. At 1.5 to 2.0 hours after the infusion, naloxone produced a significant decrease in auditory hallucinations ($P < 0.05$) (table 38.2). There was also a non-significant tendency toward a decrease in anxiety. Several subjects had some decrease in anxiety and hallucination ratings following placebo infusion. None of the nine subjects demonstrated major changes in orientation, memory, or delusions during the study.

The changes associated with naloxone were of longer duration than might be expected from a knowledge of naloxone duration activity in reversing the effects of exogenous opiates like morphine. Of the six responders, the four shortest responses (S8, S9, S10, S11) lasted between 3 and 6 hours. Hallucinations then returned. Two other subjects reported a decrease, or loss, of hallucinations lasting 24–48 hours (S3 and S4). During that period these two subjects reported an improved mood state. These subjects also reported less trouble falling asleep and staying asleep. Two patients attributed changes in sleep patterns to the loss of 'voices', which usually disrupted their sleep.

As hallucinations returned, several patients described the hallucinations as 'very faint' or 'in the distance'. One subject said he could not hear the voices, but that the people who caused them were present, like a 'running (but) blank tape'. This patient seemed to feel the presence of his voices without actually hearing them before they returned completely. These statements are similar to the verbal report by one of the subjects described by Gunne *et al.* (1977).

The following case reports are of S3 and S9 (responders) and S7 (a non-responder).

S3: D. T. is a 28-year-old Caucasian male with several hospitalizations with the diagnosis of chronic undifferentiated schizophrenia. D. T. presented to the hospital with the complaint that he was losing his temper because 'I was hearing voices'. On examination, D. T. was anxious and often silent. He said his voices had been telling him 'to kill himself', or ordering him to dress in women's clothing. D. T. claimed he was silent because he couldn't distinguish real voices from auditory hallucinations, and he didn't want to strike out at the person he was talking to, thinking it was the 'voices'.

The first day he received a placebo infusion. That day's baseline was marked by these statements: 'voices yelling at me', 'I'm tired of listening to them'. He appeared very restless, angry, and very distracted. As the study continued that day, he was somewhat less tense with no 'voices' during the interviews, but heard them between sessions. The second study period (naloxone) was 2 days later. During that baseline interview he heard voices saying, 'Why don't you get rid of your wife?' They told him to be a female and then to be a male, with several voices arguing over it. He seemed to be the 'referee' between the voices. He was anxious, slightly angry and irritable. After naloxone (100 min) he showed less anxiety, guilt, hostility, and confusion. He appeared calmer and spoke of his ability to think more clearly because his thoughts were slower. He said, 'Today is very good'; he felt like Christmas Day (a good day for him as a child). He slept well that evening; reported no hallucinations until 48 hours later. This subject was judged to have a two plus response because of his decreased anxiety and absence of hallucinations.

S7: W. H. is a 41-year-old Caucasian male with a history of multiple hospitalizations with the diagnosis of chronic undifferentiated schizophrenia. On initial examination, W. H. was unkempt, had long, unclean hair and beard, long nails and obvious body lice. W. H. talked both to the examiner and to unseen persons in the room, with a narrative characterized by loose associations, circumstantiality, lack of clarity, irrelevance, over-abstraction heavily laced with religious, mystical and fairy tale-like delusions. W. H.'s affect was generally pleasant, but included periods of inappropriate laughter and giddiness, as well as periods of sadness without obvious provocation. He admitted to constant auditory hallucinations with 'gods', 'elves', 'demons', and other mythical creatures.

Both naloxone and placebo days were very similar. W. H. spoke in an agitated, pressured and highly delusional fashion about Norse gods, Odin, Thor and elves. He talked of his wife, the 'elf', his 'Olympian world', control of the clouds, being guilty over insulting Melina Mercouri and told us that 'on Mt Olympus, all they do is eat baklava and marzipan'. It was not possible to conduct extensive interviews, nor were we able to differentiate naloxone from placebo. This was judged to be an '0' response to naloxone.

S9: P. M. is a 29-year-old divorced Caucasian male who presented for his first psychiatric hospitalization with a 3-year history of a gradual withdrawal from his friends and school work. During the past 3 months he had briefly held several odd jobs. On examination P. M. was a neat, polite and cooperative young man, whose speech was overly abstract with pseudologic, neologisms, and loose associations. P. M. had a fluid delusional system, but stated that computers controlled by unknown people or groups were 'putting thoughts in my head', or 'taking over my body. . . changing my stomach muscles into women's muscles. . . trying to force me to use my mind to hurt people'. P. M. consistently heard voices that gave orders or commented on his behavior or his situation. His diagnosis is chronic undifferentiated schizophrenia with paranoid features.

In the baseline period of the first study day (naloxone), P. M. spoke of an extensive delusional system. He stated that he was blamed for 'all the deaths in California', that his stomach muscles actually belonged to a woman and that people read and controlled his mind. About 30 min after naloxone he said he felt 'slowed down', somewhat sadder, with some decrease in hallucinations. At 90 min after naloxone, he stated he felt 'relaxed', 'like I might be able to think without jeopardizing others'. He seemed to be less tense than at baseline or 30 min and reported decreased frequency of voices. By 4 hours, the voices had returned in full. This response was seen as a one plus response in that he was less anxious and exhibited a decrease in hallucinations. On the placebo day, he exhibited a similar delusional pattern during baseline. At the 30 and 90 min points, he spoke of his ability to broadcast his thoughts to one million people, of the voices telling him to kill, and of hearing buzzing sounds.

DISCUSSION

In this preliminary investigation of the effects of naloxone on some schizophrenic symptoms in chronic schizophrenic patients, we report significant decreases in auditory hallucinations and the suggestion of decreases in anxiety. Obviously, there are several limitations inherent in this study design. One problem is that by infusing on only 2 days, the effects of starting and stopping can be confused with drug effects. Further, even our most naive subject voiced some expectation for change on one of the two days. Each subject was rated several times during each test day; the potential for substantial effects of repeated interviews on psychotic symptoms must be considered. Auditory hallucinations are highly variable phenomena and may be subject to change induced by levels of activity, suggestion, social interactions, stress or anxiety. Finally naloxone is short acting, even if some effects can be seen hours after administration. It is very difficult, if not impossible, to study the consistency and reliability of its effects, especially on an intrinsically subjective and variable symptom such as auditory hallucinations. It is possible that the effects we have observed are primarily due to an effect of naloxone on the responsiveness to stress (Akil *et al.*, 1976*a*), and that they only apply to a small subgroup of schizophrenic patients.

After the completion of this study, we learned of the positive report by Emrich *et al.* (1977) in Germany. Their study design was similar, in that frequently hallucinating subjects were infused with a relatively high dose of naloxone (4 mg), and these subjects were evaluated for several hours.

Despite the limitations of the study design, the effects of naloxone on hallucinations in these investigations raises some important questions.

(1) Is naloxone likely to act on the endogenous opiate peptides? Naloxone has been an important pharmacological tool for investigating the opiate systems. Naloxone has demonstrated effects when the endogenous opiates are released by electrical stimulation (Akil *et al.*, 1976*b*; Oliveras *et al.*, 1977; Hosobuchi *et al.*, 1977; Jacob *et al.*, 1974). In addition, there are some limited but successful studies of the effect of opiate antagonists in regulating pain responsiveness (Jacob *et al.*, 1974; Grevert and Goldstein, 1977) and in stress-induced analgesia (Akil *et al.*, 1976*a*; Bodnar *et al.*, 1977). In the stress studies both biochemical changes in peptide levels and naloxone reversal were reported (Akil *et al.*, 1976*a*).

(2) Is it possible that the effects of naloxone on opiate peptides cause secondary effects on other neuronal systems? Despite the exponential growth of data on the endogenous opiate systems, the systems are still only poorly characterized. The anatomical localization of the opiate systems suggests they are well positioned for a role in regulation of mood and affect and for the possibility of extensive interactions with the catecholamines, particularly in limbic structures. The lateral septal nucleus, the nucleus accumbens, several amygdaloid nuclei, stria terminalis, and the hypothalamus have major opiate peptide contributions (Watson *et al.*, 1977*a*; Hökfelt *et al.*, 1977; Simantov *et al.*, 1977; Elde *et al.*, 1976; Watson *et al.*,

1977*b* and this volume). Thus while it is pure speculation, one could envisage both a direct effect of the opiate systems on mood or psychosis and an interaction with catecholamines leading to the production of abnormal mood or psychotic symptoms. In addition, animal pharmacological studies offer preliminary evidence that manipulation of the opiate systems can affect catecholaminergic systems and that pharmacological manipulation of the catecholaminergic system can affect the opiate system (Lal, 1975; Henderson and Hughes, 1976; Cicero *et al.*, 1974; Korf *et al.*, 1974; Nakamura *et al.*, 1973; Loh *et al.*, 1976; Holzman, 1974). Thus when the catecholamine hypothesis of affective disorders (Berger, 1977) or the dopamine hypothesis of schizophrenia (Berger *et al.*, 1978) is considered, the possible role of the endogenous opiates in these disorders should not be ignored. Clearly, extensive investigation at the basic science level is necessary to disentangle these important interactions.

(3) If the endogenous opiate system is involved in schizophrenia, why don't exogenous plant alkaloid opiates have much effect on schizophrenia or cause schizophrenic symptoms in normal subjects? It is certainly true that early studies which examined the effects of plant opiate alkaloids on schizophrenia have generally led to negative results. Wickler has summarized several European studies using morphine in schizophrenia and mania (Wickler, 1958). Although these patients were physically addicted, there were no major signs of improved or worsened psychotic symptoms.

However, it is clear that the endogenous opiate system is composed of two anatomically and biochemically discrete systems (Watson *et al.*, 1977*a, b* and this volume) and perhaps several pools of receptors (Lord *et al.*, 1976; Watson *et al.*, 1977*a, b* and this volume; Martin *et al.*, 1976). These investigators propose a theory involving three opiate receptors to account for differences in the physiological effects of several classes of plant alkaloid opiates. Morphine and similar agents are thought to act on the μ receptor, producing decreased pulse, respiration, and response to pain, while ketocyclazocine acts on the κ receptor producing no pulse or respiratory changes but decreasing response to pain. Finally, SKF 10 047 is postulated to act on the σ receptor producing increased pulse and respiration with decreased response to pain. These three types of opiate agonists (morphine, μ; ketocyclazocine, κ; and SKF 10 047, σ) exhibit differential patterns in the development of tolerance and dependence. They also exhibit different sensitivities to reversal by antagonists (Martin *et al.*, 1976). It is also interesting that both ketocyclazocine and SKF 10 047 produce intense dysphoria and very unpleasant hallucinations in normal human subjects.

SUMMARY

The administration of opiate antagonists to schizophrenic patients was based on a possible relationship between the endogenous opiate systems and schizophrenic systems. High doses of the opiate antagonist naloxone (10 mg) were given i.v. to chronic schizophrenic patients with nearly constant auditory hallucinations. In nine patients given naloxone in a placebo-controlled, randomized double-blind cross-over design, statistically significant decreases in auditory hallucinations were observed. This putative effect of naloxone may be due to its action on endogenous opiate systems or to the interaction of these opiate systems with other physiological systems, such as the central catecholaminergic system. However, naloxone may also have anxiolytic, mood or stress-altering abilities that may influence such schizophrenic symptoms as hallucinations, through other physiological or psychological mechanisms.

ACKNOWLEDGEMENTS

This research was supported in part by NIMH Mental Health Clinical Research Center Grant MH-30854 and NIMH Program-Project Grant MH-23861. We are grateful to Endo Laboratories Inc. for their gift of naloxone-HCl and matched i.v. vehicle placebo. We appreciate the dedicated efforts of the staff of the Stanford Psychiatric Clinical Research Center, especially Mrs Foradell Ogle and Mrs Meredith Stuckey. Huda Akil is a Sloan Foundation Fellow in the Neurosciences B.R. 1609. Stanley J. Watson is a recipient of a Bank of America, Giannini Post-Doctoral Fellowship in Medical Sciences and MH 11028.

REFERENCES

Akil, H., Madden, J., Patrick, R. and Barchas, J. D. (1976*a*). In *Opiates and Endogenous Opioid Peptides*, (ed. H. W. Kosterlitz). Elsevier/North Holland Press, Amsterdam, pp. 63–70

Akil, H., Mayer, D. J. and Liebeskind, J. C. (1976*b*). *Science,* **191**, 961–2

Berger, P. A. (1977). In *Neurotransmitter Function: Basic and Clinical Aspects*, (ed. W. Fields). Stratton Intercontinental, New York,

Berger, P. A., Elliott, G. R. and Barchas, J. D. (1978). In *Psychopharmacology: A Generation of Progress*, (eds. M. Lipton, A. DiMascio, and K. F. Killam). Raven Press, New York. pp. 1071–95

Bodnar, J. R., Kelley, D. D., Spiaggia, A. and Glusman, M. (1977). *Fedn Proc.*, **36**, 3896

Cicero, T. J., Meyer, E. R. and Smithloff, B. R. (1974). *J. Pharmac. exp. Ther.*, **189**, 72–82

Davis, G. C., Bunney, W. E., DeFraites, E. G., Kleinman, J. E., vanKammen, D. P., Post, R. M. and Wyatt, R. J. (1977). *Science,* **197**, 74–7

Elde, R., Hökfelt, T., Johansson, O. and Terenius, L. (1976). *Neuroscience,* **1**, 349–51

Emrich, H. M., Cording, C., Piree, S., Kolling, A., Uzerssen, D. and Herz, A. (1977). *Pharmakopsychiatrie,* **10**, 265–70

Feighner, J. P., Robins, E., Guze, S. B., Woodruff, R. A., Jr., Winokur, C. and Munoz, R. (1972). *Archs gen. Psychic.,* **26**, 57–63

Green, R., Bigelow, L. B., O'Brien, P. E., Stahl, E. and Wyatt, R. J. (1977). *Psychol. Rep.,* **40**, 543

Grevert, P. and Goldstein, A. (1977). *Proc. natn. Acad. Sci. U.S.A.,* **74**, 1291–4

Gunne, L. M., Lindstrom, L. and Terenius, L. (1977). *J. Neural Transmission,* **40**, 13–9

Henderson, G. and Hughes, J. (1976). *Br. J. Pharmac.*, **57**, 551–7

Hökfelt, T., Elde, R., Johansson, O., Terenius, L. and Stein, L. (1977). *Neurosci. Lett.*, **5**, 25–31

Holzman, S. G. (1974). *J. Pharmac. exp. Ther.*, **189**, 51–60

Hosobuchi, Y., Adams, J. E. and Linchitz, R. (1977). *Science,* **197**, 183–6

Jacob, J. J., Tremblay, E. C. and Colombel, M. C. (1974). *Psychopharmacologia,* **37**, 217–23

Janowsky, D. S., Segal, D. S., Bloom, F., Abrams, A. and Guillemin, R. (1977). *Am. J. Psychiat.*, **134**, 926–7

Korf, J., Bunney, B. S. and Aghajanian, G. K. (1974). *Eur. J. Pharmac.*, 165–9

Kosterlitz, H. W. and Hughes, J. (1975). In *Neurochemical Mechanisms in Analgesia and Dependence,* (ed. A. Goldstein). Pergamon Press, New York, pp. 245–50

Lal, H. (1975). *Life Sci.*, **17**, 483–96

Loh, H. H., Brase, D. A., Sampath-Khanna, S., Mar, J. B., Way, E. L. and Li, C. H. (1976). *Nature,* **264**, 567–8

Lord, J. A. H., Waterfield, A. A., Hughes, J. and Kosterlitz, H. W. (1976). In *Opiates and Endogenous Opioid Peptides,* (ed. H. W. Kosterlitz). Elsevier/North Holland Press, Amsterdam, pp. 275–8

Martin, W. R., Eades, G. G., Thompson, J. A., Huppler, R. E. and Gilbert, P. E. (1976). *J. Pharmac. exp. Ther.,* **197**, 518–32

Nakamura, K., Kuntzman, R., Maggio, A. C., Augulis, V. and Conney, A. H., (1973). *Psychopharmacology,* **31**, 177–89

Oliveras, J. L., Hosobuchi, Y., Redjemi, F., Guilbend, G. and Benson, J. (1977). *Brain Res.,* **120**, 221

Overall, J. E. (1974). *Modern Problems in Pharmacopsychiat.,* 7, 67–8

Simantov, R., Kuhar, M. J., Uhl, G. R. and Snyder, S. H. (1977). *Proc. natn. Acad. Sci. U.S.A.,* **74**, 2167–71

Taylor, M. A., Abrams, R. and Gaytanoga, P. (1975). *Comp. Psychiat.,* **16**, 91–6

Terenius, L., Wahlstrom, A., Lindstrom, L. and Widerlov, E. (1976). *Neurosci. Lett.,* **3**, 157–62

Volavka, J., Mallya, A., Baig, S. and Perez-Cruet, J. (1977). *Science,* **196**, 1227–8

Watson, S. J., Akil, H., Sullivan, S. O. and Barchas, J. D. (1977*a*). *Life Sci.,* **25**, 733–8

Watson, S. J., Barchas, J. D. and Li, C. H. (1977*b*). *Proc. natn. Acad. Sci. U.S.A.,* **74**, 5155–8

Wikler, A. (1958). *Public Health Monograph No. 52,* U.S. Printing Office, Washington, D.C.

39

Effects of naloxone in normal, manic, and schizophrenic patients: evidence for alleviation of manic symptoms

David S. Janowsky, Lewis L. Judd, Leighton Huey and David Segal
(Department of Psychiatry, School of Medicine,
University of California at San Diego,
La Jolla, California 92037, U.S.A.)

Considerable attention has focused recently on the possibility that endogenous peptides with opioid-like activity (endorphins) may have a role in the regulation of normal and abnormal human behavior. Animal studies support the possibility that endorphins may have behavioral effects, apart from their known analgesic properties. Bloom *et al.* (1976) and Segal *et al.* (1977) noted that centrally administered β-endorphin induces rigidity and immobility in rats, and Bloom *et al.* (1976) noted that i.v.t. β-endorphin induces a 'catatonic-like state, reminiscent of some aspects of schizophrenia, reversible with the relatively pure narcotic antagonist naloxone'. In addition, naloxone has been reported to inhibit apomorphine-induced stereotyped behavior in the rat (Cox *et al.*, 1976); to enhance chlorpromazine's effects on schedule-controlled behavior in pigeons (McMillan, 1971); to inhibit *d*-amphetamine-induced increases in locomotor activity (Holtzman, 1974; Segal *et al.*, this volume) and continuous avoidance responding in rats (Holtzman, 1974); and to reverse the effect of morphine and *d*-amphetamine on intracranial self-stimulation in rats (Holtzman, 1974).

Partly on the basis of the above experimental evidence, several investigators have attempted to explore the role of the endogenous opiate-like peptides in the regulation of human mood and psychotic phenomena. Stated most simply, the hypotheses which have been explored are that: (1) schizophrenic symptoms are activated by endorphins and antagonized by naloxone and (2) that euphoria and mania are activated by endorphins and antagonized by naloxone (Byck, 1976). With respect to schizophrenia, Terenius *et al.* (1976) observed elevated endorphins in the CSF of four chronic schizophrenics and Gunne *et al.* (1977) noted, in a single blind study, that 0.4 mg i.v. naloxone rapidly abolished hallucinations in four of six chronic schizophrenics. In contrast, Volavka *et al.* (1977) and Janowsky *et al.* (1977) found no rapidly-occurring antipsychotic effect from naloxone in schizophrenics; and Davis *et al.* (1977) noted a change in only one Brief Psychiatric Rating Scale (BPRS) item (unusual thought content) out of many in this study. In a more recent study, Emrich *et al.* (1977) noted that, although no significant antipsychotic effects occurred in the first hour after injection, a significant percentage of acute schizophrenics showed decreased psychotic symptoms during the period (2 to 7 hours) after injection of 4 mg naloxone.

With respect to the regulation of mood, Byck (1976) and Belluzzi and Stein (1977) proposed that an excess of endorphins may underlie euphoria, amphetamine-induced psychostimulation and mania. Byck (1976) postulated that the antimanic and anti-euphoric properties of lithium carbonate may be mediated through the endorphin system, as may the antimanic effects of haloperidol and pimozide. Certainly, endogenous opiates could parallel the euphoriant properties of such recreational opiates as heroin (Mirin *et al.*, 1976). Kline *et al.* (1977) have reported that β-endorphin alleviated depression in a limited number of subjects. Although they found no changes during a drug trial of naloxone, Terenius *et al.* (1977) noted that depression intensified in two of five depressed patients following withdrawal of a chronic naloxone regime. Furthermore, these authors noted increased CSF endorphin levels in their depressed patients.

The following work reports the results of several of our studies exploring the role of endorphins in the regulation of human behavior. We have studied normal subjects, schizophrenic patients, and affective disorder patients, using naloxone as a relatively specific endogenous opioid antagonist. We hypothesized that naloxone would exert significant behavioral effects in our subjects.

METHODS

Effects of naloxone on schizophrenic symptoms

The patient group consisted of eight male Caucasian schizophrenics (three paranoid, three schizo-affective, two chronic undifferentiated), ranging in age from 19–48 (average age 30). All were receiving neuroleptics (fluphenazine 10, 40, 80, or 100 mg/day; chlorpromazine 300 or 600 mg/day; haloperidol 50 mg/day; trifluoroperazine 30 mg/day). All were diagnosed as being schizophrenic, on the basis of classifications of the American Psychiatric Association Diagnostic and Statistical Manual of Mental Disorders (DMS-II, 1968). All were grossly psychotic at the time of testing and could be considered to be process schizophrenics. None was a chronically hospitalized inpatient.

The effect of naloxone on hallucinations and other schizophrenic symptoms was determined using a double-blind, cross-over design, with counterbalanced order of administration. Intravenous naloxone (Narcan) (1.2 mg) was rapidly given, followed or preceded by 24 hours by saline placebo. Each patient was interviewed by a psychiatrist beginning 15 min before and ending 60 min after receiving each i.v. infusion. Patients were rated on a 0–5 point scale at 15 min intervals using the items of the BPRS. They were also asked to describe any psychological or physical effects. The total BPRS score and individual item scores were obtained in each patient by averaging the scores obtained at baseline, 15, 30, 45 and 60 min after naloxone infusion. Statistical analysis was performed using analysis of variance (ANOVA) for repeated measures.

Effect of naloxone on affective symptoms in normal subjects and affective disorder patients

Subjects were male or non-pregnant female patients from the psychiatric wards of the San Diego Veterans Administration Hospital. All were diagnosed using information from the Schedule for Affect Disorder and Schizophrenia applying Research Diagnostic Criteria as well as using DSM-II diagnostic criteria. In addition, a sample of normal subjects was studied. Subjects were screened by a research psychiatrist to eliminate those with a history of drug or alcohol abuse. All subjects were required to have normal values on a battery of laboratory tests.

A total of 12 psychiatric patients (seven patients with manic depressive illness-manic or hypomanic phase, three depressed patients, one schizo-affective patient [with hypomanic symptoms] and one schizophrenic patient) and seven normal subjects met screening criteria. Normal subjects ranged in age from 22 to 31 years (mean = 27 years), and psychiatric patients ranged in age from 22 to 57 years (mean = 44 years). Of the 12 patients, 11 were male and 1 was female. Of the seven manic patients, two were receiving lithium alone and two others were receiving lithium and an antipsychotic drug at the time of the experiment. One other manic patient received an antipsychotic drug. No other patient received medication at the time of the experiment. Three manics had a history of alcoholism.

Subjects underwent two identical tests on consecutive days, each lasting approximately 3 to 4 hours. Each session consisted of a non-structured interview by a research psychiatrist, observed and rated by two research psychology technicians. Sessions took place in research space with videotaping and observation occurring through a two-way mirror. A two-factor design, using diagnosis as a between-groups factor and drug condition as a within-subjects factor was used. Subjects in each diagnostic group received both active and placebo naloxone in random order. Drug conditions were managed by the hospital pharmacy to keep the research staff 'blind' and order of administration was counterbalanced.

Subjects had an i.v. catheter inserted to allow repeated drug administrations and blood sampling. Observer behavioral ratings were made by the two research psychology technicians and the research psychiatrist using the following instruments

(1) Beigel–Murphy manic rating scale: 0–5 points, 19 items, 3 subscales (Beigel and Murphy, 1971);

(2) NIMH Behavior Rating Scale: 1–7 points, 24 items.

Also, the subjects self-completed the following tests and mood measurements described elsewhere (Judd *et al.*, 1977)

(1) Profile of Mood States (POMS): 0 to 4 points, 78 items, 5 subscales;

(2) Subjective High Assessment Scales (SHAS): a set of 82 items rated on a continuous 100 mm scale anchored at each end with opposite adjectives;

(3) 'High' lines—100 mm scales in both horizontal and vertical formats, designed to rate the extent of overall 'high' or euphoria experienced;

(4) Digit Symbol Test—A subtest of the WAIS, from which several equivalent forms have been developed. This test involves converting digits to abstract symbols.

As shown in figure 39.1, behavioral ratings were obtained (1) before and (2) just after injection of a 'pre-experimental' series of four 5 ml placebo injections, and (3) immediately following double-blind administration of experimental drug consisting of four 5 ml injections of placebo or four 5 ml (1 mg/ml) injections of

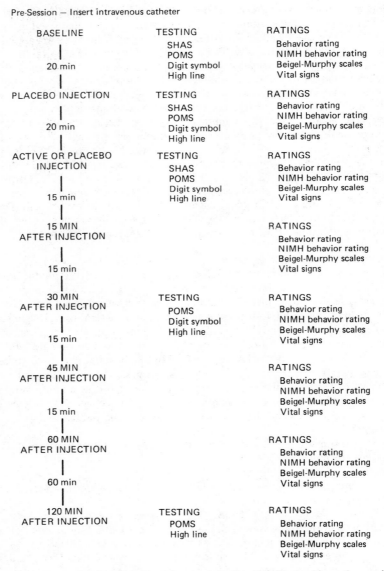

Pre-Session – Insert intravenous catheter

BASELINE	TESTING SHAS POMS Digit symbol High line	RATINGS Behavior rating NIMH behavior rating Beigel-Murphy scales Vital signs
20 min		
PLACEBO INJECTION	TESTING SHAS POMS Digit symbol High line	RATINGS Behavior rating NIMH behavior rating Beigel-Murphy scales Vital signs
20 min		
ACTIVE OR PLACEBO INJECTION	TESTING SHAS POMS Digit symbol High line	RATINGS Behavior rating NIMH behavior rating Beigel-Murphy scales Vital signs
15 min		
15 MIN AFTER INJECTION		RATINGS Behavior rating NIMH behavior rating Beigel-Murphy scales Vital signs
15 min		
30 MIN AFTER INJECTION	TESTING POMS Digit symbol High line	RATINGS Behavior rating NIMH behavior rating Beigel-Murphy scales Vital signs
15 min		
45 MIN AFTER INJECTION		RATINGS Behavior rating NIMH behavior rating Beigel-Murphy scales Vital signs
15 min		
60 MIN AFTER INJECTION		RATINGS Behavior rating NIMH behavior rating Beigel-Murphy scales Vital signs
60 min		
120 MIN AFTER INJECTION	TESTING POMS High line	RATINGS Behavior rating NIMH behavior rating Beigel-Murphy scales Vital signs

Figure 39.1 Sequence of procedures and tests evaluating the effects of i.v. naloxone in 19 subjects.

naloxone. Behavioral ratings were also obtained at 15, 30, 45, 60 and 120 min after experimental drug (naloxone or placebo) administration. Blood samples, pulse and blood pressure measurements were also obtained at 15 min intervals throughout the experiment.

The data obtained were statistically analyzed using ANOVA for repeated measures. Data were analyzed in two ways. First, all data points, including the baseline observations made prior to injection of 'pre-experimental' placebo were included. Second, since the baseline observations made before 'pre-experimental' placebo injection, were not based on the patients' experience in the experiment, followed immediately after venepuncture, and since much variance was noted in these observations, data were analyzed excluding these initial baseline observations.

In both experiments, witnessed signed informed consent was obtained from each subject after he/she had been fully informed, both verbally and in written form, of the purpose, procedures, and possible hazards of the experiment. All patients were made aware that their treatment was in no way contingent on their participation in the experiment and all were voluntary subjects.

RESULTS

Study of schizophrenics

For the group of eight schizophrenic patients studied, ANOVA of all individual BPRS items and total BPRS scores revealed no significant or near significiant differences between placebo and active naloxone trials. No drug-time or placebo-time or order effects were noted. Specifically, as shown in table 39.1, no significant changes occurred in the following BPRS items indicative of schizophrenia: hallucinations, conceptual disorganization, unusual thoughts, mannerisms, grandiosity, or blunted affect. None of the patients, initially reporting hallucinations, reported or were noted to have a decrease in auditory hallucinations. The effects of placebo and naloxone on these patients' hallucination and delusion scores are presented in table 39.2. Two patients said they felt less nervous after naloxone infusion, compared to one after placebo infusion; and two felt drowsy after naloxone infusion, compared to one after placebo. No other naloxone-related mood changes were noted.

Table 39.1 Effect of naloxone (1.2 mg, i.v.) on brief psychiatric rating scale scores in eight schizophrenic patients

BPRS item	Placebo	Naloxone	*F*	d.f.	*P* <
Conceptual disorganization	2.0 ± 0.2	2.5 ± 0.2	0.42	4/24	NS
Grandiosity	1.5 ± 0.2	1.5 ± 0.3	0.36	4/24	NS
Hallucinations	1.3 ± 0.2	1.4 ± 0.2	0.07	4/24	NS
Unusual thoughts	2.3 ± 0.2	2.1 ± 0.3	0.09	4/24	NS
Blunted affect	1.6 ± 0.3	1.6 ± 0.2	0.12	4/24	NS
Total BPRS	17.9 ± 1.2	19.5 ± 0.10	0.05	4/24	NS

Big placebo responses w/in subject over time; 5-pt. scale. Nothing dramatic here.

Table 39.2 Effects of naloxone (1.2 mg, i.v.) and placebo on BPRS hallucination and delusion scores in eight schizophrenic patients

Patient no.	Trial	Baseline H/D*	+ 15 min H/D	+ 30 min H/D	+ 45 min H/D	+ 60 min H/D
1	Placebo	0/4	1/3	2/3	2/3	0/0
	Naloxone	0/4	0/3	0/3	0/4	0/3
2	Placebo	0/4	0/4	0/2	0/1	0/3
	Naloxone	0/3	0/4	0/4	2/2	0/1
3	Placebo	0/0	0/3	0/2	0/2	0/2
	Naloxone	0/0	0/0	0/0	0/0	0/0
4	Placebo	1/4	1/3	1/3	1/3	2/3
	Naloxone	0/3	3/4	3/4	1/4	2/4
5	Placebo	0/0	0/0	0/4	2/4	0/3
	Naloxone	0/2	0/2	0/3	0/2	0/2
6	Placebo	3/3	0/0	3/4	3/4	3/3
	Naloxone	3/3	3/3	3/4	3/3	3/4
7	Placebo	1/3	3/3	2/3	2/3	3/3
	Naloxone	3/3	3/3	3/4	3/3	3/3
8	Placebo	3/4	3/4	3/4	3/4	3/4
	Naloxone	3/4	3/3	3/3	3/4	3/4

*D, Delusions; H, hallucinations rated on a 0–5 point scale.

Table 39.3 Significant ($P < 0.05$) effects of naloxone (20 mg, i.v.) in seven normal subjects

Item	Change
POMS items (out of 72 items)	
'kindly'	Increase†
'good-natured'	Increase†
Behavior rating (out of 24 items)	
'communicative'	Decrease†
SHAS items (out of 82 items)	
'joyful'	Increase*
'nothing is right with the world'	Decrease*
'things were never worse'	Decrease*
'wish experience was over'	Increase*
'less irritable'	Increase†
'steadier thoughts'	Decrease†

*When pre-experimental baseline values are dropped these items are not significant.
†When pre-experimental baseline values are dropped these items become significant.
POMS, Profile of Mood States; SHAS, Subjective High Assessment Scales.

Study of affective disorder patients and normal subjects

In the normal volunteer subject subgroup, as shown in table 39.3, the effects of naloxone, compared with placebo, suggest an increase in several items indicating increased feelings of well being. However, the number of items which were statistically significant is small and could have occurred by chance alone. When the observations made before the 'pre-experimental' placebo injections occurred are eliminated from the data analysis, several new items become significant and several items lose significance.

As shown in table 39.4, for the overall group of 12 psychiatric patients, naloxone significantly affected a number of items and scales. Generally, these items reflect decreased activation, decreased manic symptoms, and increased dysphoria. However, when the observations made before the pre-experimental placebo injections are eliminated from the data analysis, most items and scales lose their statistical significance.

Table 39.4 Significant ($P < 0.05$) effects of naloxone (20 mg) in 12 psychiatric patients

Item	Change
POMS items (out of 72 items)	
'nervous'	Increase
'resentful'	Increase†
'anxious'	Increase†
Behavior ratings (out of 24 items)	
'lethargic'	Increase*
'drowsy'	Increase*
'cheerful'	Decrease*
NIMH rating (out of 24 items)	
'elated mood'	Decrease†
Beigel–Murphy rating (out of 19 items)	
'happy and cheerful'	Decrease*
Elation–Grandiosity Scale (4 items)	Decrease*
Total Beigel–Murphy (15 items)	Decrease*
SHAS items (out of 82 items)	
'ability to communicate'	Increase
'not helped by this experience'	Increase

*When pre-experimental baseline values are dropped these items are not significant

†When pre-experimental baseline values are dropped these items become significant

As shown in table 39.5, when the seven patients diagnosed as having hypomanic or manic symptoms are considered separately, a number of significant naloxone effects are evident, indicating an antimanic effect. However, as with the normal control subjects and the overall patient group, elimination of those observations made before 'pre-experimental' placebo injection caused most significant items

Table 39.5 Significant ($P < 0.05$) effects of naloxone (20 mg, i.v.) in seven manic patients

Item	Change
POMS items (out of 72 items)	
'active'	Increase†
'resentful'	Increase†
'bitter'	Increase†
Behavior rating (out of 24 items)	
'charming'	Decrease*
NIMH rating (out of 24 items)	
'disorganized speech'	Decrease*
'elated mood'	Decrease*
'motor hyperactivitv'	Decrease*
Beigel–Murphy rating (out of 19 items)	
'talking'	Decrease*
'jumps from one subject to another'	Decrease*
'happy and cheerful'	Decrease
'verbalizes feeling of well-being'	Decrease*
Elation–Grandiosity Scale (4 items)	Decrease*
Total Beigel–Murphy (15 items)	Decrease*
SHAS items (out of 82 items)	
'nothing bothers me'	Decrease
'rapid changing emotions'	Decrease*
'worried about self'	Decrease*
'highest I've ever been'	Decrease

*When pre-experimental baseline values are dropped these items are not significant
†When pre-experimental baseline values are dropped these items become significant

and scales to become only near significant. Furthermore, analysis of individual patient results revealed that only two of the patients (both bipolar manic-depressive patients, manic phase) had shown dramatic changes on naloxone, as compared to placebo. The other patients had shown relatively small, or no such changes. Thus, a small proportion of the patients accounted for most of the variance.

The antimanic effects of naloxone were demonstrated in a 22-year old actively manic, manic-depressive male patient. Before, during, and after administration of the 'pre-experimental' placebo infusion, the patient exhibited extreme pressure of speech, flight of ideas, clang associations, garrulousness, and verbal intrusiveness. He exhibited mild elevation of mood. Within 15 min of receiving 20 mg i.v. naloxone, he had shown mild, fleeting depressive symptoms, expressed a feeling of being very tired, and had exhibited periods of putting down his head in his arms and remaining silent. When he did speak, he demonstrated occasional mild pressure of speech, but spoke coherently, logically, and with insight into his emotional state. He said that he felt good, and relaxed, and he showed little, if any, flight of ideas, and no clang associations. Between 30 and 45 min after naloxone

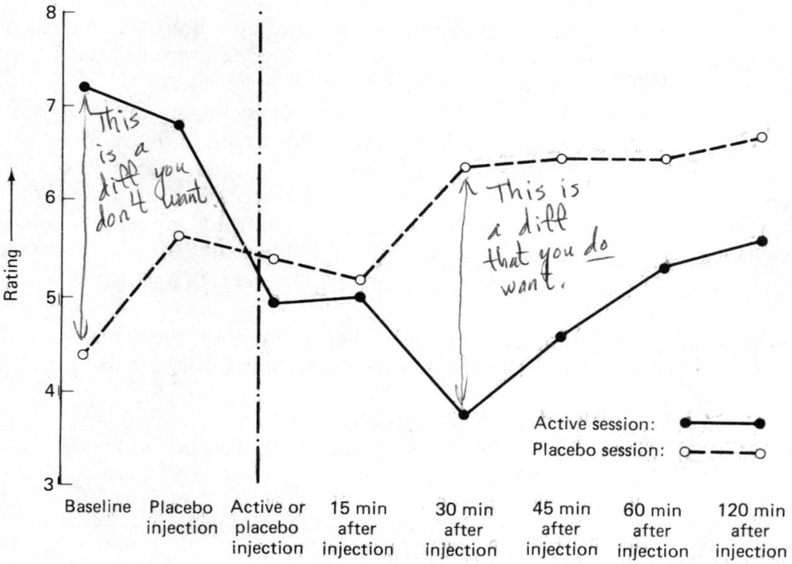

Figure 39.2 The effect of naloxone (20 mg) on the Elation–Grandiosity Subscale of the Beigel–Murphy manic rating scale in seven hypomanic patients.

Table 39.6 Effects, in seven patients with hypomanic symptoms, of intravenous naloxone (20 mg) on the Elation–Grandiosity subscale of the Beigel–Murphy mania rating scale

	Elation–Grandiosity Subscale scores*					
	Placebo			Active drug		
Patient	Post-placebo baseline	30 min post-placebo	Change score†	Post-placebo baseline	30 min post-naloxone	Change score
1	3	5	+2	8	2.5	−5.5
2	10	15	+5	10	5	−5
3	1	4	+3	6	4	−2
4	7.5	5	−2.5	8	8.5	+0.5
5	7.5	6	−1.5	5	3	−2
6	5	4.5	−0.5	4	3	−1
7	5	6	+1	7.5	0	−7.5
			Total = +6.5			Total = −22.5

*$P < 0.05$ for differences in changes from baseline following placebo and naloxone using a Student's t test for paired results

†Change score= post 'pre-experimental' placebo baseline score subtracted from 30 min post-experimental placebo or naloxone score

infusion, the patient's manic symptoms returned and by 1 hour after naloxone infusion, he had returned to his baseline state. During the preceding day's placebo infusion, he had shown a mild intensification of his manic state.

The effect of naloxone on the Beigel-Murphy Elation-Grandiosity Subscale scores of the seven hypomanic-manic patients is illustrated in figure 39.2. This mania subscale appeared most sensitive to naloxone's effects. Table 39.6 demonstrates the changes from baseline in Elation-Grandiosity Subscale scores in the seven subjects diagnosed manic or hypomanic 30 min following placebo and active naloxone infusion, respectively. Table 39.7 illustrates the paucity of items which are significant when the results from all 19 subjects (12 patients, 7 normals) are combined.

As shown in figure 39.3, with regard to changes in pulse, the overall patient group ($N = 12$) showed a significant relative decrease in pulse rate following active

Table 39.7 Significant ($P < 0.05$) effects of naloxone (20 mg, i.v.) in all 19 subjects (pre-placebo baseline omitted)

Item	Change
POMS items (out of 72 items)	
'resentful'	Increase
'anxious'	Increase
Pulse rate	Decrease

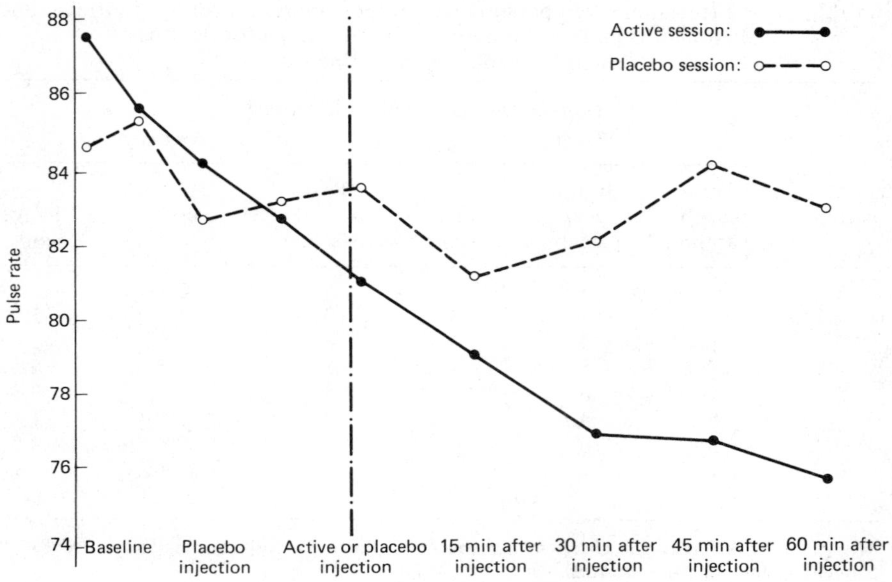

Figure 39.3 The effect of naloxone (20 mg) on pulse in 12 psychiatric patients.

naloxone infusion. This change was also noted in the overall subject group ($N = 19$), but was not evident in the normals or the manic subgroup. Blood pressure was not significantly affected by naloxone in the patients or normal subjects.

DISCUSSION

With respect to our observations of schizophrenics, we have not been able to confirm the reports of some (Gunne *et al.*, 1976; Emrich *et al.*, 1977) that i.v. naloxone has antipsychotic properties. We did not modify schizophrenic symptoms using a 1.2 mg dose of i.v. naloxone, followed by 1 hour of observation, and thus our results are consistent with those of some, but not others. Significantly, our patients, like those of Gunne *et al.* (1977), were receiving neuroleptics and were severely and chronically ill. Thus, in our patients, naloxone does not appear to have immediate anti-hallucinatory and/or antipsychotic effects when administered in i.v. doses three times as high as those given by Gunne *et al.* (1977).

However, our results do not preclude the possibility (1) that, since all suggestive animal experiments utilized doses of naloxone much higher than those given in the current experiment, higher and/or more chronic doses of naloxone might have antipsychotic effects; (2) that naloxone may ameliorate symptoms in a subgroup of other psychotic patients; (3) that, since the antipsychotic agents used might have exerted the maximum possible therapeutic influence, naloxone given alone might relieve psychotic symptoms in schizophrenics not receiving antipsychotic drugs; and (4) that as suggested by Emrich *et al.* (1977), naloxone may exert anti-psychotic effects relatively late after its injection. Thus, our results, although not supporting naloxone's exerting an antipsychotic effect, do not rule out the possibility that such an effect may occur under some circumstances.

The following points concerning the effects of naloxone in affective disorder patients are noteworthy. In these experiments we used a relatively large dose of naloxone (20 mg) which, in similar doses, has been found to antagonize β-endorphin effects in rats (Segal, unpublished work). Also, our naloxone was tested in morphine-treated rats and found to be behaviorally active. Our methodology utilized a double-blind cross-over, counterbalanced order design, with all subjects being 'desensitized' before experimental drug administration by 'pre-experimental' baseline placebo injections. Subjects were self-rated, as well as observer-rated. Thus, we feel our experimental design is quite comprehensive. Our results, using normal controls ($N = 7$) are probably negative, as are our results in the entire subject group ($N = 19$). Our cardiovascular results are significant and of interest. Naloxone appears to decrease pulse rate, a phenomenon of unknown cause.

Our results suggest that naloxone exerts general anti-activating, mildly depressing, antimanic effects in patients with an affective component to their illness, and more specifically in patients who are hypomanic or manic. The finding that naloxone may exert effects on affective symptoms contrasts with the observations of Davis *et al.* (1976), and Terenius *et al.* (1977), who found no such effects in affective disorder patients. However, it should be noted that our dose of naloxone considerably exceeded that used by the latter investigators.

Although, when all data points are used in the analysis, including observations made before injection of 'pre-experimental' placebo, naloxone appears to exert a mild, significant antimanic, anergic, dysphoric effect, this statistically significant observation is rather tenuous. When only the observations made after injection of 'pre-experimental' placebo are used in the data analysis, most of the significant changes become only near-significant. This loss of significance may be due to the decrease in degrees of freedom, and may thus be methodologic, or may be due to 'pre-placebo' baseline values falsely altering the behavioral curve. Furthermore, analysis of the effects of naloxone in individual patients demonstrates that naloxone apparently caused dramatic 'antimanic' effects in only two manic patients and only mild or no effects in the rest of the 12-patient group. Thus, we feel that the statistical significance of our results must, for the present, remain an open question.

However, we do believe that it is likely that a subgroup of manic patients, as illustrated by two of our subjects, responded to naloxone with alleviation of their mania. A design utilizing alternate injections of naloxone and placebo over a period of days would seem indicated to determine whether apparent naloxone responders indeed exist. Furthermore, although the dose of naloxone utilized in our study was relatively high (20 mg), it is possible that still higher doses of naloxone (such as 1 mg/kg) are needed to occupy opiate receptors (Hollt and Herz, 1978), or that a longer observation or drug administration period is indicated to detect more consistent changes.

Thus, we feel our results are of probable theoretical and practical interest, and worth confirming or rejecting by expanding the number of subjects.

ACKNOWLEDGEMENTS

With research support from San Diego Veterans Administration Hospital MRIS No. 4576 and NIMH Grant No. 1 P50 MH 30914-01.

REFERENCES

Beigel, A. and Murphy, D. (1971). *Am. J. Psychiat.*, **128**, 688–94

Belluzzi, J. D. and Stein, L. (1977). *Nature*, **266**, 556–8

Bloom, F., Segal, D., Ling, N. and Guillemin, R. (1976). *Science*, **194**, 630–2

Byck, R. (1976). *Lancet*, **ii**, 72–3

Cox, B., Ary, M. and Lomax, P. (1976). *J. Pharmac. exp. Ther.*, **196**, 637–41

Davis, G. C., Bunney, W. E. Jr, de Fraites, E. G., Kleinman, J. E., van Kammen, D. P., Post, R. M. and Wyatt, R. J. (1977). *Science*, **197**, 74–7

Emrich, H. M., Cording, C., Piree, S., Kolling, A., Zerssen, D. and Herz, A. (1977). *Pharmacopsychiatrie*, **10**, 265–70

Gunne, L. M., Lindstrom, L. and Terenius, L. (1977). *J. Neural Transmission*, **40**, 13–9

Hollt, V. and Herz, A. (1978). *Fedn. Proc.*, in press

Holtzman, S. G. (1974). *J. Pharmac. exp. Ther.*, **189**, 51–60

Janowsky, D. S., Segal, D. S., Abrams, A., Bloom, R. and Guillemin, R. (1977). *Psychopharmacology*, **53**, 295–7

Judd, L. L., Hubbard, B., Janowsky, D. S., Huey, L. Y. and Attewell, P. A. (1977). *Archs gen. Psychiat.*, **34**, 346–51

Kline, N. S., Li, C. H., Lehmann, H. E., Lajtha, A., Laski, E. and Cooper, T. (1977). *Archs gen. Psychiat.*, **34**, 1111–3

McMillan, D. E. (1971). *Psychopharmacologia (Berl.)*, **19**, 128–33

Mirin, S. M., Meyer, R. E. and McNanuee, B. (1976). *Archs gen. Psychiat.*, **33**, 1503–8

Segal, D. S., Browne, R. G., Bloom, F., Guillemin, R. and Ling, N. (1977). *Science*, **198**, 411–4
Terenius, L. A., Wahlström, A., Lindstrom, L. and Widerlov, E. (1976). *Neurosci. Lett.*, **3**, 157–62
Terenius, L., Wahlström, A. and Agron, H. (1977). *Psychopharmacology*, **54**, 31–3
Volavka, J. A., Mallya, A., Baig, S. and Perez-Cruet, J. (1977). *Science*, **196**, 1227–8

40

Behavioral effects of opioid peptides: implications for future clinical research

Lewis L. Judd, David S. Segal, and David S. Janowsky
(Department of Psychiatry, School of Medicine,
University of California, San Diego,
La Jolla, California, 92093, U.S.A.)

In the previous chapter, the findings from the clinical studies conducted by our group at the University of California, San Diego, are described and commented upon. Davis *et al.* (1977) reported a decline in unusual thought content and Berger *et al.* (1977) noted a reduction in auditory hallucinations in schizophrenics following naloxone infusion. This short chapter will highlight the way in which animal work generated the human investigations and describe the overall conceptual framework which has guided our research in this area.

The aim in both animals and humans has been to define the function of endogenous opioids in the regulation of normal and abnormal behavior. Within this framework, the exogenous agonist and antagonist agents are viewed as pharmacological tools to manipulate the opioid peptides in order to delineate their role in behavior. This pharmacological manipulation of an endogenous system provides the opportunity for the identification of the full spectrum of opioid peptide effects in both animals and man.

Recently Bloom *et al.* (1977) and Segal *et al.* (1977) reported profound behavioral effects in rats after i.v.t. administration of the opioid peptide, β-endorphin. The most striking feature of this response profile was a marked catatonic-like state, which was reversed by the administration of naloxone, an opiate antagonist. These findings suggested that endogenous opioids might be involved in the regulation of a broad spectrum of behaviors, and that defects in the mechanisms regulating these peptides might play a part in the pathophysiology of psychiatric disorders. It was further proposed that those disorders which result from an excess activation of opiate receptors might be therapeutically responsive to opiate antagonists.

A series of clinical studies assessing i.v. naloxone in schizophrenics has been reported (Davis *et al.*, 1977; Gunne *et al.*, 1977; Janowsky *et al.*, 1977; Terenius *et al.*, 1976; and Volavka *et al.*, 1977) and no obvious consistent naloxone effects have been identified. Thus it could be concluded from the naloxone studies that the endogenous opiate-like peptides may not be involved in the etiology or the pathophysiology of schizophrenia. However, it is possible that higher doses of naloxone more closely approximating those given in animals may be necessary to exert an 'antipsychotic' effect. Further, until now, studies have generally used acute rather than chronic administration of naloxone and it may be unrealistic to expect that acute administration of naloxone could induce observable persistent changes in a severely disordered patient population.

It should also be noted that there are intriguing data from several studies indicating that while naloxone does not exert a dramatic effect on schizophrenia, there is, nevertheless, evidence that certain specific behaviors characteristic of schizophrenia are altered. Bunney *et al.* (1977) reported a decline in unusual thought content; Berger *et al.* (this volume) noted a reduction in auditory hallucinations, and Davis *et al.* (1977) also noted attenuation of unusual thought content in schizophrenics following naloxone infusions. Therefore, it is possible that only specific aspects of schizophrenic behavior are responsive to naloxone.

Finally, it should be emphasized that although β-endorphin produced a broad spectrum of behavioral effects in rats, the most prominent feature of the behavior profile was a naloxone-reversible catatonic-like state. Therefore schizophrenics with catatonia may be uniquely responsive to naloxone treatment. In a non-blind trial we administered 1.4 mg of naloxone i.v. to a severely motor-retarded catatonic schizophrenic with no noticeable effect. In contrast, both i.v. sodium amytal and diazepam were markedly effective in this patient. Thus, despite the lack of response in one patient, a controlled study of naloxone in catatonic schizophrenia remains a potentially promising investigation.

As was reported in the previous chapter our most recent clinical studies have concentrated upon patients with affect disorder. This research was stimulated by the findings of Segal *et al.* (1977) which indicated that at lower doses opioid peptides and opiates induce a naloxone-reversible behavioral activation in rats. In addition, it has been found that naloxone antagonizes stimulant-induced activation (Holtzman, 1974; Segal *et al.*, 1977). These findings in the animal, together with our experience and that of others which indicated that stimulants exacerbate mania, suggested that endogenous opioid peptides might be involved in affect disorder, with an excess in opiate receptor activity being responsible for mania and a deficiency for depression.

The effects of 20 mg i.v. naloxone on seven manic or hypomanic patients with bipolar depression can be viewed as a continuum. Specifically, one patient manifested a slight increase in manic behavior, two did not change, two manifested a mild to moderate attenuation of their manic behavior, and two patients evidenced dramatic and marked attenuation of manic behavior. In the case of these latter two patients, both were bipolar depression, Type I (out of a total of four such patients). Furthermore, the time course of the naloxone responders was strikingly similar in that the response was rapid and was fully manifested 15 to 30 min after infusion, with a return to baseline levels within 1 to 2 hours. Since normal subjects, under the same experimental conditions basically did not change following naloxone infusion, this finding in this particular group of patients appears even more intriguing.

Our results may be interpreted as indicating that a subpopulation of bipolar patients are uniquely responsive to naloxone; however, it is also possible that with higher doses and a chronic treatment regimen, a larger percentage of the manic population might be affected by naloxone.

One indication of another clinical use for naloxone stems from the finding that naloxone altered the response pattern of rats to novel stimuli (Segal *et al.*, 1977). In the animal model rats were observed to attend to novel stimuli for a longer time following the administration of naloxone. Thus, an investigation into the effects of naloxone on various parameters of attention and cognition in humans appears to be warranted. Indeed, if naloxone, by its effect on the endogenous opioid system induces focused attentional behavior, it may be that compounds of this pharmacological class will be beneficial to patient populations such as hyperkinetic children, in which distractibility and problems of attention are present. Clinical trials of a specific narcotic antagonist in this specific clinical sample would be of obvious interest.

The use of endogenous opioids as research tools, especially in man, has been problematic because of their scarcity and cost. Thus there may be an advantage in substituting exogenous opiates for the endogenous compounds, given the fact that certain opiates seem indistinguishable in many of their behavioral effects from those of the opioid peptides. For example, Segal *et al.* (1977) recently reported that in all the behavioral measures which were observed, the effects of β-endorphin and methadone HCl in rats were identical. This seems to be true for the other opiates as well, with the exception of morphine, which may be somewhat more atypical in its behavioral effects (Herz *et al.*, this volume). Therefore, this should be taken into consideration when evaluating past anecdotal clinical studies and in the design of new ones, since the other opiates and not morphine may be more comparable in their behavioral effects to those of the endogenous peptides. Nevertheless, the methodological issue to be emphasized is that there may be some advantages in using exogenous opiates to elucidate the behaviors subserved by the endogenous opioids.

It is obvious that many of the hypotheses we are testing in the clinical studies have been significantly influenced by, or actually derived from, the animal model. It is our intention to continue this tightly integrated interaction since it has beem particularly fruitful. We hope that, as the clinical observations emerge they will feed back and enrich the animal studies, to the mutual advantage of the animal and human studies.

ACKNOWLEDGEMENTS

Aspects of the research cited here were supported by Medical Research Service, Veterans Administration and Grant No. 1 P50 MH 30914-01, National Institute of Mental Health. D.S.S. is the recipient of NIMH Research Scientist Award MH 70183.

REFERENCES

Bloom, F., Segal, D., Ling, N. and Guillemin, R. (1976). *Science,* **194**, 630–2

Davis, G. C., Bunney, W. E. Jr, de Fraites, E. G., Kleinman, J. E., Van Kammen, D. P., Post, R. M. and Wyatt, R. J. (1977). *Science,* **197**, 74–7

Gunne, L. M., Lindstrom, L. and Terenius, L. (1977). *J. Neural Transmission*, **40**, 13–8
Holtzman, A. G. (1974). *J. Pharmac. exp. Ther.*, **189**, 51–60
Janowsky, D. S., Segal, D. S., Abrams, A., Bloom, F. and Guillemin, R. (1977). *Psychopharmacology*, **53**, 295–7
Segal, D. S., Browne, R. G., Bloom, F., Guillemin, R. and Ling, N. (1977). *Science*, **198**, 411–4
Terenius, L. A., Wahlström, A., Lindstrom, L. and Widerlov, E. (1976). *Neurosci. Lett.*, **3**, 157–62
Volavka, J. A., Mallya, A., Baig, S. and Perez-Cruet, J. (1977). *Science*, **196**, 1227–8

41

Actions of naloxone in different types of psychoses

H. M. Emrich, C. Cording, S. Pirée, A. Kölling, H.-J. Möller,
D. von Zerssen and A. Herz
(Max-Planck-Institut für Psychiatrie, Munich, F.R.G.)

The possibility of a therapeutic action of the specific morphine antagonist naloxone in psychotic patients was raised by the work of Terenius *et al.* (1976) who found increased levels of endorphins in CSF of patients with chronic schizophrenia. Consequently, Gunne *et al.* (1977) studied a possible antipsychotic effect of naloxone and observed, in a single-blind study, an immediate reversal of auditory hallucinations in four schizophrenic patients after i.v. injection of 0.4 mg of this drug. However, Volavka *et al.* (1977) could not reproduce these results in seven schizophrenic patients under similar conditions, using a double-blind design. Furthermore, a study of Davis *et al.* (1977) on the action of naloxone (0.4–10.0 mg) in fourteen schizophrenic patients and five patients with affective psychoses failed to demonstrate a clear naloxone-induced improvement of hallucinations, mannerisms and posturing, conceptual disorganization and psychosis, whereas the item 'unusual thought content' did show a statistically significant improvement ($P < 0.04$). The affectively ill patients were not influenced by the drug. In eight schizophrenic patients Janowsky *et al.* (1977) observed no improvement in seven psychosis-specific items after 1.2 mg naloxone. It should be mentioned that the psychopathological ratings did not extend for more than 1 hour after injection in the studies of Davis *et al.* (1977) and of Janowsky *et al.* (1977). On the other hand, Akil *et al.* (1978) using 10.0 mg naloxone, found a statistically significant reduction of hallucinations and of psychotic anxiety in six patients with schizophrenia. The maximal effect in this study occurred about 2 hours after injection.

Previously, Emrich *et al.* (1977) investigated the effect of 4.0 mg naloxone (in 3 cases, 1.2 mg) in 20 psychotic patients with frequent hallucinations and/or actual delusional experience. Thirteen of these 20 patients suffered from an acute episode of schizophrenia or schizoaffective psychosis, 4 from chronic schizophrenia. Furthermore, 2 patients with an alcoholic hallucinosis (DD: schizophrenia) and 1 patient with a paranoid involutional psychosis were included in the study.

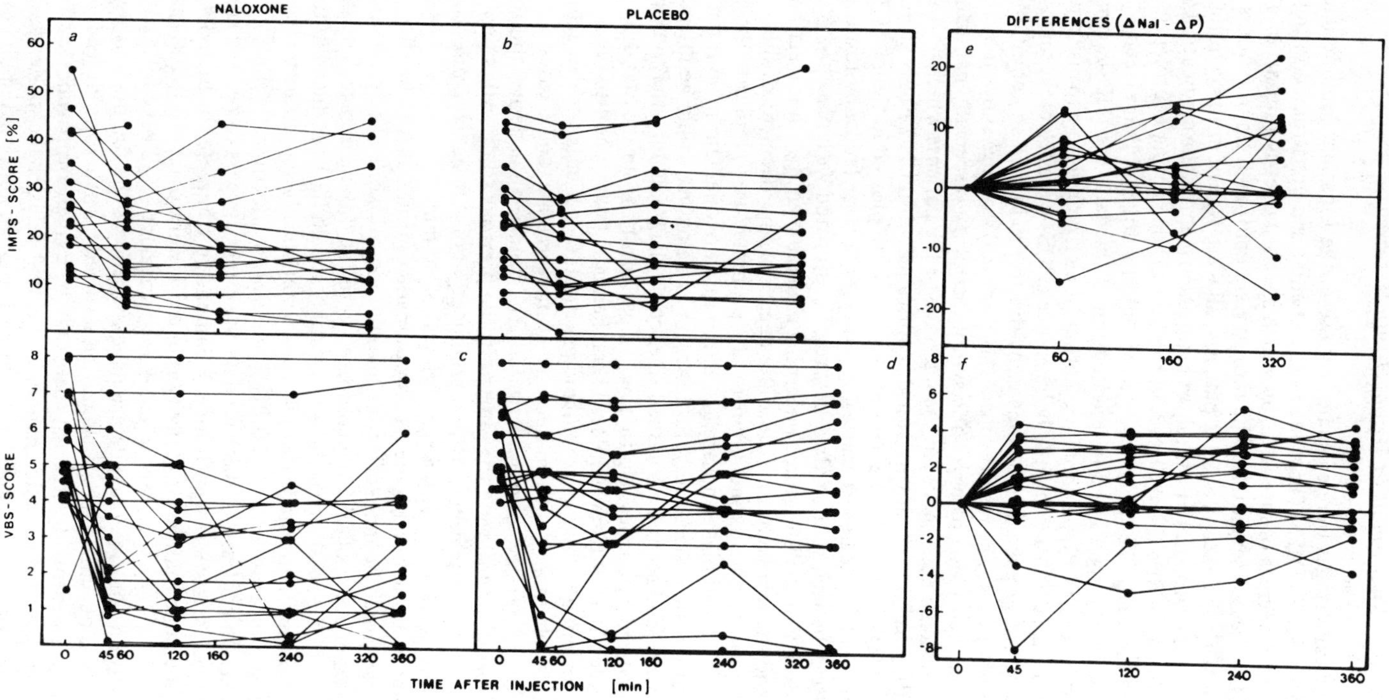

Figure 41.1*a*, *b*, Mean IMPS-score (factors PCP+PAR+GRN+EXC+HOS) as a function of time in 20 psychotic patients. At 0 min, injections of 4.0 mg naloxone (in three cases 1.2 mg) (or placebo) were given. *c*, *d*, Mean VBS (*V*erlaufs-*B*eurteilungs-*S*kala = course-assessment-scale) score (assessment of hallucinations and of actual delusional experience) as a function of time. *e*, *f*, Difference between naloxone effect and placebo effect.

Psychopathological changes were evaluated by use of the Inpatient Multidimensional Psychiatric Scale (IMPS) (Lorr *et al.*, 1962) and a self-constructed rating-scale (VBS) with 8 degrees of intensity, by which special target-symptoms of a patient could be assessed separately. The ratings were continued up to 6 hours after injection. With the exception of 2 patients, all were free of antipsychotic drugs; in the case of pretreatment with short acting neuroleptics the medication was discontinued 7 days before the trial and, in the case of long acting neuroleptics 4 weeks before the trial. The trials were performed in a double-blind placebo-controlled cross-over design. For a first evaluation of the data, the IMPS-factors perceptual distortion (PCP), paranoid projection (PAR), grandiose expansiveness (GRN), excitement (EXC) and hostile belligerence (HOS) were selected, since these subscales were suspected to be most sensitive to productive and emotional symptoms of psychoses. The results of the IMPS and VBS-ratings showed a naloxone-induced reduction of psychotic symptomatology (especially hallucinations/actual delusional experience) in the majority of the patients which—compared with placebo—reached statistical significance within 2–7 hours after injection ($P = 0.007 - 0.036$). The data of this study are plotted in figure 41.1. The results show a high degree of scattering; however, a clear tendency towards improvement can be seen in the naloxone-data, as compared with placebo.

The controversy in the literature concerning a possible antipsychotic action of naloxone and the relatively small absolute degree of improvement of the psychotic symptoms on naloxone in our results prompted us to replicate the same investigation with a still higher dosage (24.8 mg) of naloxone. Our main intention was to find out whether the antipsychotic action of naloxone would be intensified at a higher dosage, and second we wished to exclude the possibility that our initial results had occurred by chance. Up to now, 12 patients (3 from the Max-Planck-Institut für Psychiatrie; 9 from the Bezirkskrankenhaus Haar) who had been diagnosed as suffering from a schizophrenic psychosis (6 patients with an acute episode of schizophrenia, 1 of them in a post-stuporous state, and 6 cases of chronic schizophrenia) have been investigated. The double-blind design and the psychopathological ratings were the same as in the previous study. All patients were free of antipsychotic drugs. After a pre-injection of 0.8 mg naloxone, two doses of 12.0 mg were given with a time-interval of 30 min.

A preliminary evaluation (figure 41.2) was made to find out whether the 24.8 mg dosage would be more effective than 4.0 mg naloxone. The present data show no higher efficacy of 24.8 mg compared with the 4.0 mg dosage. The slight antipsychotic effect, observed in the 4.0 mg study, could be reproduced in the IMPS data, showing—compared with placebo—a statistically significant reduction of psychotic symptomatology ($P < 0.01$, 5 hours after injection; $P < 0.05$, 7 hours after injection). In contrast, in the VBS data the effect appears to be even smaller and did not reach statistical significance. We intend to complete the high-dosage series up to the same number of patients as in our lower dosage study (20 cases). The main result of our experience in naloxone-treatment of 32 psychotic patients with hallucinations and/or actual delusional experience is the finding that psychotic symptoms of schizophrenia cannot be reversed by naloxone, at least not by a short-acting treatment, although there may be a small antipsychotic effect, particularly with respect to hallucinations and actual delusional experience. This result is a strong argument against the hypothesis that an abnormal opioid or an

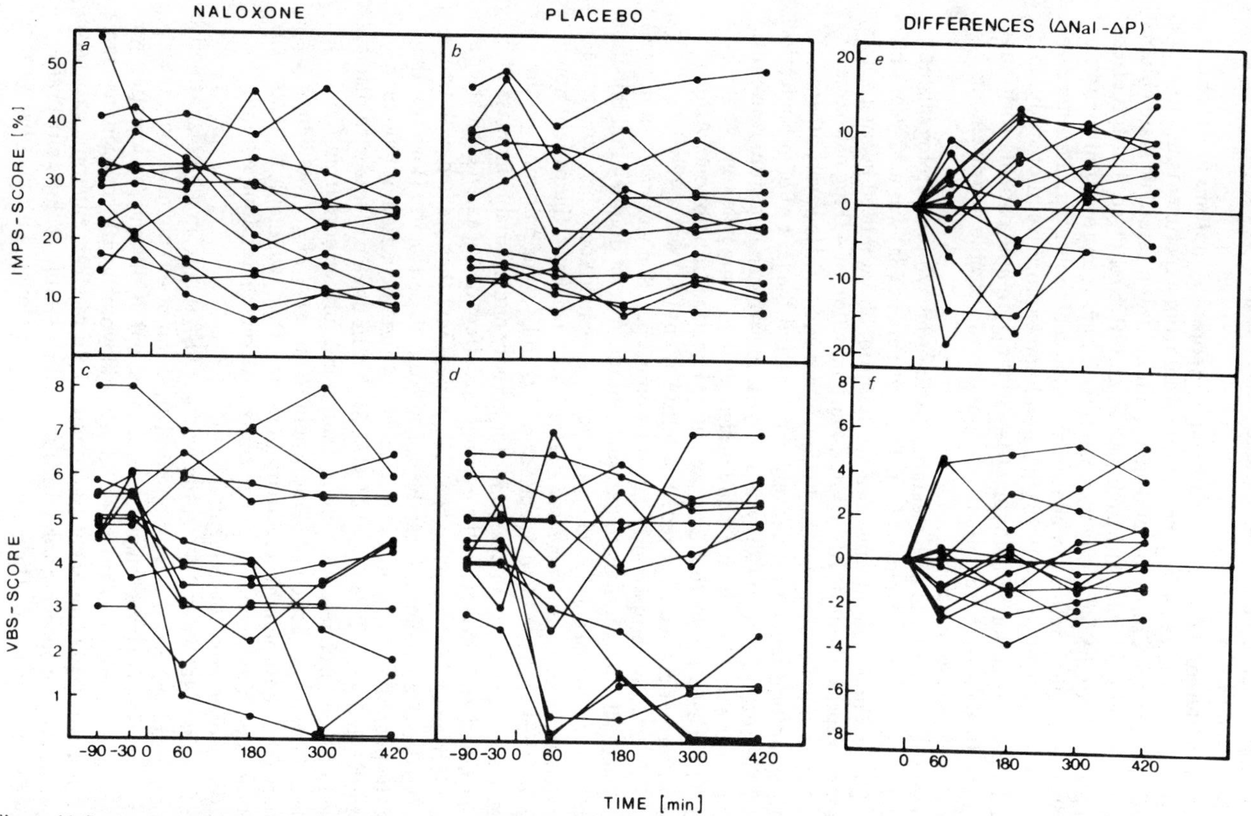

Figure 41.2*a*, *b*, Mean IMPS-score (factors PCP+PAR+GRN+EXC+HOS) as a function of time in 12 patients with schizophrenia. At 0 min, injections of 12.8 mg naloxone were given followed by second injections of 12.0 mg 30 min later (or placebo). *c*, *d*, Mean VBS score (assessment of hallucinations and of actual delusional experience) as a function of time. *e*, *f*, Difference between naloxone effect and placebo effect.

endorphin-hyperactivity may have a causative role in the pathogenesis of schizophrenia. However, endorphins may modulate biochemical processes underlying the psychotic symptoms.

A possible action of naloxone on catatonic/stuporous symptoms in patients with catatonic schizophrenia may be hypothesized from experiments in rats, according to which i.v.t. injection of β-endorphin induces a catatonic state (Bloom *et al.*, 1976) in these animals. Although Herz *et al.* (1978) showed that this effect is induced in exactly the same way by opiates with high receptor affinity and that it parallels the analgesic action, an abnormal opioid metabolism in catatonic cannot be excluded. Schenk *et al.* (1978) in a non-blind explorative pilot study, investigated a possible action of naloxone (0.4–30.0 mg) in nine patients with catatonic stupor. In eight of these patients, they observed a sizable improvement, according to clinical impressions.

We treated three patients with a catatonic-stuporous symptomatology using 0.4–10.0 mg naloxone i.v. (figure 41.3). The first patient (3a) was a 32-year-old woman. She was uncommunicative and nearly mute. She admitted hearing voices, but refused to speak about it. After a non-blind injection of 4.0 mg naloxone, speech-production increased and she became more excited. However, other psychotic symptoms remained relatively constant and the lack of communication persisted. The second patient (3b) was a 47-year-old woman in a stuporous-mute state. She was treated in a double-blind design with 24.8 mg naloxone versus placebo. The speech-production increased after injection of naloxone. After placebo no further change occurred. The third patient (3c) was a 42-year-old woman with catatonic stupor and frequent stereotypes. She was nearly mute and showed practically no reactions to external stimuli. After a double-blind injection of placebo no change occurred, whereas after 0.4 mg naloxone the stereotypies disappeared and speech-rate increased dramatically. However, the patient now developed delusions. Non-blind injections of 2.0 and 4.0 mg naloxone on the next day were followed by increased motor activity and a variable increase of speech-production. However, in the evening this effect disappeared even after a further injection of 10.0 mg naloxone. The patient was then treated with neuroleptics. No decisive conclusions can be drawn from these results. However, they suggest the possibility of an anti-stuporous/anti-catatonic action of naloxone.

From the finding of Terenius *et al.* (1976) that in three patients with mania, increased CSF endorphin levels were measured and furthermore from the possible antidepressive action of β-endorphin (Kline *et al.*, 1977), one may hypothesize an endorphin hyperactivity in mania. Thus two manic patients were treated by us with naloxone, one in an open trial, one under double-blind, placebo-controlled conditions (figure 41.4).

The first case (4a) was a 29-year-old woman, suffering from a bipolar affective psychosis (manic phase). After a non-blind injection of 4.0 mg naloxone, the manic symptomatology was enhanced and she asked, if this was 'an injection for laughter'. The second case (4b) was a 33-year-old woman with endogenous mania. Her psychopathology (prominent symptoms: flight of ideas, euphoria, expansiveness, overactivity of speech-production) showed no sizable changes either after naloxone or after placebo. These findings are in agreement with the observations of Davis *et al.* (1977) in two patients with hypomania.

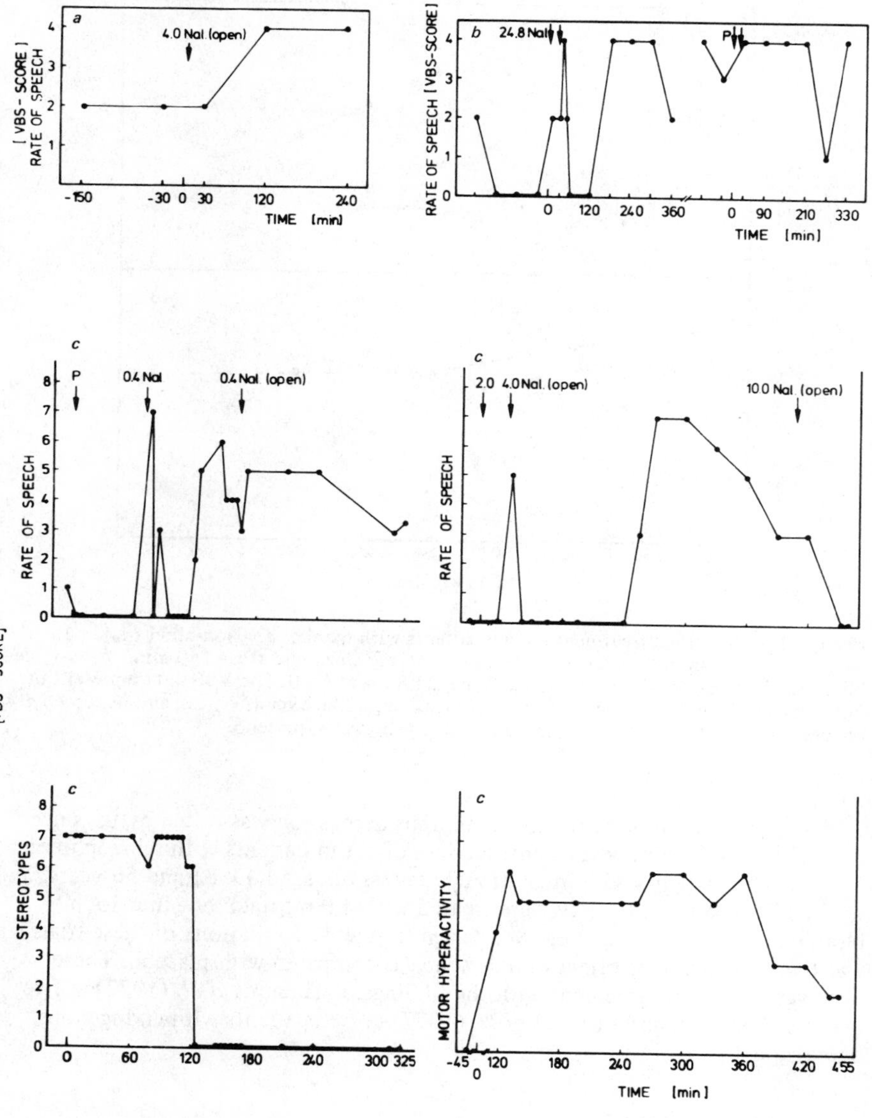

Figure 41.3 Naloxone treatment of three patients with catatonia. *a*, Non-blind trial in a 32-year-old woman; *b*, double-blind trial in a 47-year-old woman; *c*, trial, initially double-blind, later non-blind in a 42-year-old woman. Ratings of speech rate, stereotypes and motor hyperactivity by use of the VBS scale.

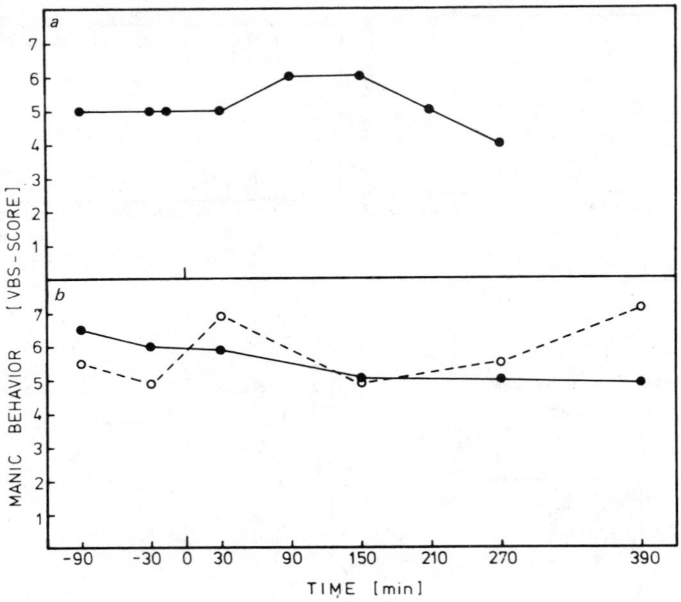

Figure 41.4 Naloxone treatment of two patients with mania. *a*, Non-blind trial in a 29-year-old woman, naloxone 4.0 mg at t = 0; 50 mg clozapine at t = 150 min. *b*, double-blind trial in a 33-year-old woman, naloxone, 24.8 mg at t = 0. The VBS data represent the mean values of the VBS ratings of flight of ideas, euphoria, expansiveness, and hyperactivity of speech-production. Filled circles, naloxone; open circles, placebo.

A possible action of naloxone on anxious depression was tested by us, since Akil *et al.* (1977) observed an anti-anxiety effect in patients with schizophrenia. Three female patients with involutional depression, aged 49, 51 and 56 years, with a high degree of anxiety were treated with 4.0 mg naloxone in a double-blind placebo-controlled cross-over design (figure 41.5). In none of these trials was there a convincing effect of naloxone—as compared with placebo. These observations are in agreement with the findings of Terenius *et al.* (1977) in five depressed patients and of Davis *et al.* (1977) in two patients with endogenous depression.

ACKNOWLEDGEMENT

Thankful appreciation is extended to director Dr Ch. Schulz, Dr L. Achner, Dr I. Meisel-Kosik, Dr J. Staudinger, Dr R. Oechsner, Dr H. Dwinger, Bezirkskrankenhaus Haar, and their coworkers for their generous support of this study. We thank Dr M. J. Ferster, Endo Laboratories Inc., Brussels, for kindly supplying naloxone. This work was supported by a grant from the Fritz Thyssen Stiftung, Cologne.

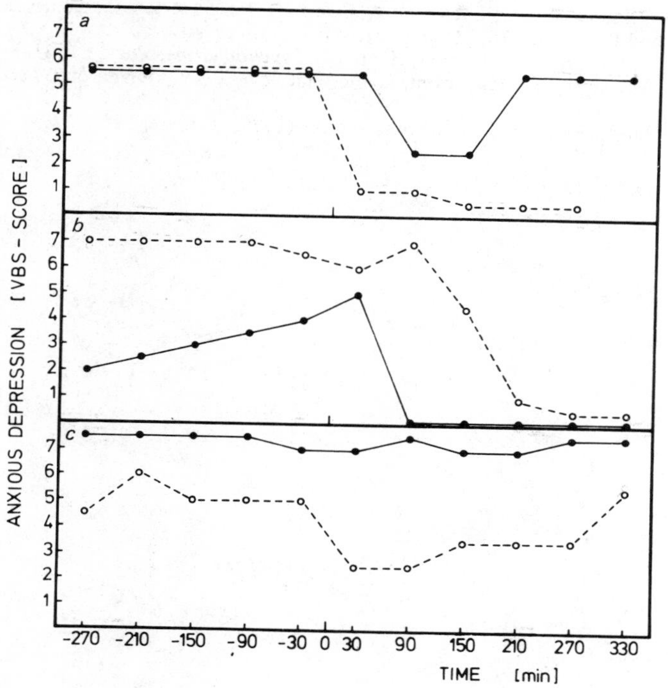

Figure 41.5 Naloxone treatment of three patients with involutional depression with a high degree of anxiety. The VBS data represent the mean values of VBS ratings of anxiety and of anergy. The trials were done in a double-blind cross-over placebo-controlled design. Naloxone: 4.0 mg at $t = 0$. Filled circles, naloxone; open circles, placebo.

REFERENCES

Akil, H., Watson, S. J., Berger, P. A. and Barchas, J. D. (1978). In *Advances in Biochemical Psychopharmacology 18.* (eds. E. Costa and M. Trabucchi). Raven Press, New York, pp. 141–7

Bloom, F., Segal, D., Ling, N. and Guillemin, R. (1976). *Science,* **194**, 630–2

Davis, G. C., Bunney, W. E. Jr, de Fraites, E. G., Kleinman, J. E., van Kammen, D. P., Post, R. M. and Wyatt, R. J. (1977). *Science,* **197**, 74–7

Emrich, H. M., Cording, C., Pirée, S., Kölling, A., v. Zerssen, D. and Herz, A. (1977). *Pharmakopsychiatrie,* **10**, 265–70

Gunne, L.-M., Lindström, L. and Terenius, L. (1977). *J. Neural Transmission,* **40**, 13–9

Herz, A., Bläsig, J., Emrich, H. M., Cording, C., Pirée, S., Kölling, A. and v. Zerssen, D. (1978). In *Advances in Biochemical Psychopharmacology 18.* (eds. E. Costa and M. Trabucchi). Raven Press, New York, pp. 333–9

Janowsky, D. S., Segal, D., Bloom, F., Abrams, A. and Guillemin, R. (1977). *Am. J. Psychiat.,* **134**, 926–7

Kline, N. S., Li, C. H., Lehmann, H. E., Lajtha, A., Laski, E. and Cooper, T. (1977). *Archs gen. Psychiat.,* **34**, 1111–3

Lorr, M., Klett, C. J., McNair, D. M., Lasky, J. J. (1962). *Inpatient Multidimensional Psychiatric Scale (IMPS).* Consulting Psychologists Press (Palo Alto, California)

Schenk, G. K., Enders, P., Engelmeier, M.-P., Ewert, T., Herdemerten, S., Köhler, K.-H., Matz, D. and Pach, J. (1978). *Arzneimittel-Forsch.* (in press)
Terenius, L., Wahlström, A. and Ågren, H. (1977). *Psychopharmacology*, **54**, 31–3
Terenius, L., Wahlström, A., Lindstrom, L. and Widerlov, E. (1976). *Neurosci. Lett.*, **3**, 157–62
Volavka, J., Mallya, A., Baig, S. and Perez-Cruet, J. (1977). *Science*, **196**, 1227–8

42
Effects of naloxone on schedule-controlled behavior in monkeys

R. T. Kelleher and S. R. Goldberg
(Laboratory of Psychobiology, Department of Psychiatry, Harvard Medical School, Boston and New England Regional Primate Research Center, Southborough, Massachusetts, U.S.A.)

The many unanswered questions about the influence of the endorphins on behavior have enhanced interest in the behavioral pharmacology of the narcotic antagonists. Because narcotic antagonists can effectively block opiate receptors, which mediate the actions of the endorphins, the behavioral effects of appropriate doses of narcotic antagonists might reveal functional characteristics of the endorphin system. Studies in several species have indicated that naloxone, an effective narcotic antagonist, has no remarkable effects on behavior at doses that are known to block opiate receptors (Byrd, 1976; Downs and Woods, 1976; El-Sobky *et al.*, 1976; Goldberg *et al.*, 1976; Goldstein *et al.*, 1976). These results have led some investigators to suggest that the endorphin system, like some other neurohumoral or hormonal systems, is dormant until activated by certain types of events. Because the opiates are known to be effective analgesics, it has been assumed that naloxone would be most likely to affect behavior controlled by painful or noxious stimuli.

Some investigators, using procedures in which behavior is controlled by noxious stimuli, have found that responding is enhanced in rats given naloxone (for example, Frederickson *et al.*, 1976, 1977; Jacob *et al.*, 1973), whereas other investigators, using similar procedures, have found that responding is unaffected by naloxone (for example, Goldstein and Lowry, 1975; Goldstein *et al.*, 1976). Although these seemingly discrepant results may be reconciled by attention to variables not previously considered, such as diurnal rhythms (Frederickson *et al.*, 1977), the effects of naloxone have been small relative to the effects of other drugs used clinically to modify behavior. It may be inappropriate to concentrate on behavior controlled by noxious stimuli since many studies have indicated that the opiates can have marked effects on behavior controlled by other types of stimuli (for example, Downs and Woods, 1976; Holtzman, 1974; Goldberg *et al.*, 1976). It seems that opiate receptors can modulate a variety of behavioral activities.

The purpose of this chapter is to consider the behavioral pharmacology of naloxone in two species of monkeys. We will present data on: (1) the potency and efficacy of naloxone as an antagonist of the behavioral effects of morphine; (2) the behavioral effects of a full range of doses of naloxone; (3) the influence of morphine pretreatments on the behavioral effects of naloxone; and (4) the effects of repeated daily administrations of naloxone on behavior. The results indicate that repeated administration of naloxone as well as pretreatment with morphine, can markedly enhance the behavioral effects of naloxone so that relatively low doses are effective.

NALOXONE AS AN ANTAGONIST

The behavioral effects of naloxone are most appropriately considered in the context of its potency and efficacy as an opiate antagonist. Although it is well established that naloxone can effectively antagonize many of the behavioral effects of morphine, there are few quantitative data on the potency of naloxone in shifting morphine dose–effect curves. Many problems arise in doing behavioral experiments of this type because of the long periods required to determine several dose–effect curves for morphine when each dose can be given only after several intervening control sessions in which no drug is given. We have developed a technique for establishing reliable cumulative dose–effect curves for behavioral effects of i.v. morphine in single experimental sessions. This technique was used to study shifts of morphine dose–effect curves after various doses of naloxone.

Rhesus monkeys deprived of food were trained under a multiple fixed-interval (FI), fixed-ratio (FR) schedule of food presentation (three 250 mg food pellets). The monkeys were studied individually while restrained in a primate chair inside a sound-attenuating experimental chamber. A response key was mounted on a wall in front of the monkey, and stimulus lights were mounted overhead. During the 5 min FI schedule component, food was presented at the first key-pressing response that occurred after at least 5 min had elapsed in the presence of a red stimulus light. During the 30-response FR schedule component, food was presented at the 30th key-pressing response in the presence of a green stimulus light. During the 2 min time-out component, the experimental chamber was dark, and responding had no specified consequences. If the monkey did not respond, FR components terminated after 2 min and FI components after 12 min, and the sequence of components advanced automatically. Each cycle of components began with the time-out component, followed by two consecutive FR components and then the FI component. An experimental session comprised 21 cycles. Rates of key pressing (responses per second) under each schedule component were averaged over every three cycles.

For i.v. drug injections an indwelling catheter was implanted by way of the right or left internal jugular vein into the superior vena cava. The distal end of the catheter was passed through the skin in the middle of the monkey's back. The monkeys wore leather jackets at all times to protect the catheters. During experimental sessions, the catheter was connected to polyvinyl chloride tubing which was led outside the experimental chamber where it could be attached to a Harvard Apparatus constant infusion syringe pump. A solution of saline or drug was injected into the dead space of the tubing and then rapidly infused into the

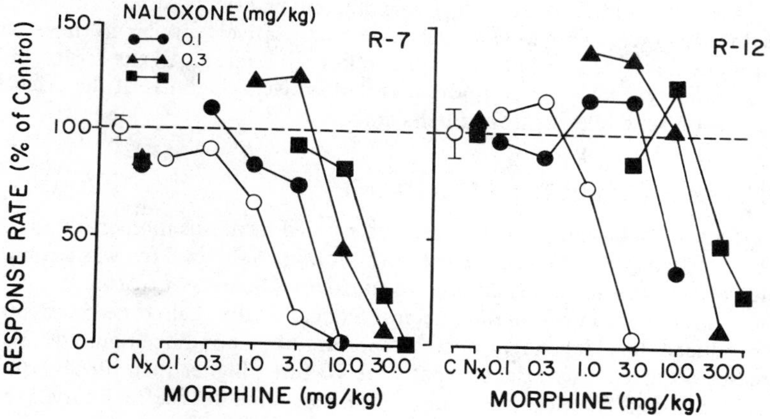

Figure 42.1 Effects of morphine i.v. after saline (○) or after naloxone (●, ▲, ■) i.v. on average response rate under a 30-response FR schedule in rhesus monkeys R-7 and R-12. The horizontal dashed line represents average control response rate. The control rate of responding was 1.64 (s.e. ± 0.12; N = 10) responses per second for R-7 and 1.65 (s.e. ± 0.21, N = 7) responses per second for R-12. Naloxone hydrochloride was injected i.v. at the start of cycle 4. Increasing doses of morphine sulfate were injected intravenously at the start of every third subsequent cycle; the abscissa indicates the cumulative dose of morphine. The open symbols represent means of two observations; the closed symbols represent single observations.

monkey by saline from the syringe pump. Intravenous injections were completed during the 2 min time-out component that began a cycle. The standard procedure was to inject saline or naloxone hydrochloride before cycle 4 and then to inject increasing doses of morphine sulfate before cycles 7, 10, 13 and 19. When responding ceased, no further doses were injected.

Characteristic rates and patterns of responding were maintained under each schedule component. Since the drugs had similar effects on FI and FR schedules, the effects on only FR performances will be presented here. Intravenous injections of increasing doses of morphine decreased responding in a dose-dependent fashion (figure 42.1). The doses of naloxone that were studied had no effect on responding. The morphine dose–effect curves of each monkey were shifted to the right about 0.5 log unit after 0.1 mg/kg of naloxone and about 1 log unit after 1 mg/kg of naloxone. After some doses of naloxone, certain doses of morphine produced small increases in responding; for example, 1 or 3 mg/kg of morphine after 0.3 mg/kg of naloxone.

The present results are consistent with those of previous studies of antagonism of the behavioral effects of morphine by naloxone. In a study of rhesus monkeys responding under a multiple FI FR schedule of food presentation, Downs and Woods (1976) found that naloxone (0.3 mg/kg, i.m.) could restore FR responding that had been completely suppressed by morphine (5.6. or 10 mg/kg, i.m.). The present results are also consistent with previous studies in the squirrel monkey of the antagonism by naloxone of the effects of morphine on responding maintained under schedules of electric-shock presentation (Byrd, 1976), of electric-shock postponement (Holtzman, 1976) and of food presentation (Goldberg *et al.*, 1976).

The present technique for studying the antagonistic effects of naloxone appears to yield results which are qualitatively and quantitatively similar to those obtained when single doses of morphine are studied in each session. All the results indicate that in monkeys, naloxone is a potent and effective antagonist of the effects of morphine on schedule-controlled behavior.

BEHAVIORAL EFFECTS OF NALOXONE

The effects of naloxone on behavior were studied in rhesus monkeys under the same conditions described in the previous section. Naloxone i.v. was administered in increasing doses until responding was decreased below control values. Although increases in responding occurred occasionally, naloxone characteristically produced dose-dependent decreases in rate of responding (figure 42.2). These decreases occurred only at doses that were 10 times higher than those required to produce a shift of about one log unit in the morphine dose–effect curve (see figure 42.1). After the cumulative dose of 10 mg/kg of naloxone, the monkeys still ate food pellets readily. They occasionally showed muscle tremors, but generally they seemed normal. The present behavioral results are similar to those obtained by Downs and Woods (1976) after single i.m. injections of naloxone to rhesus monkeys responding under a similar multiple schedule of food presentation. In two of their monkeys, which had experience under various schedules of food or drug presentation but which had never been given narcotics or narcotic antagonists, naloxone induced tremors and salivation.

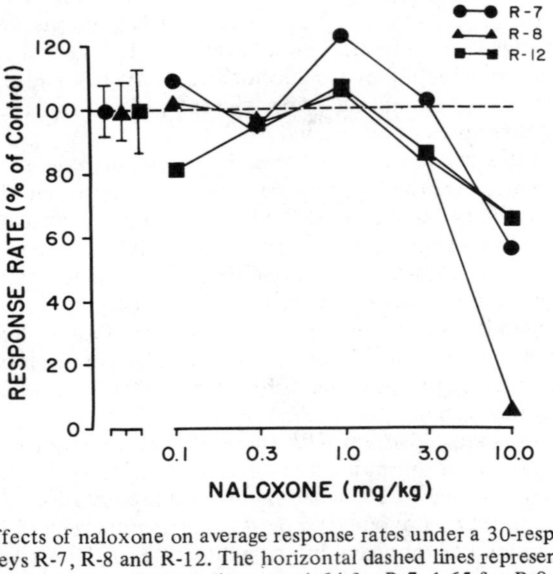

Figure 42.2 Effects of naloxone on average response rates under a 30-response FR schedule in rhesus monkeys R-7, R-8 and R-12. The horizontal dashed lines represent average control response rate. Control rates of responding were 1.64 for R-7, 1.65 for R-8 and 3.11 for R-12. Vertical bars at the left indicate s.e. Saline was injected i.v. at the start of cycle 4 and naloxone was injected i.v. in increasing doses at the start of every third subsequent cycle; the abscissa indicates the cumulative dose of naloxone. Each point is based on the mean of two observations.

Several studies of the effects of naloxone on various types of schedule-controlled behavior have been conducted in the squirrel monkey. Under multiple F1, FR schedules of food presentation, responding was decreased only at a dose of naloxone (10 mg/kg, i.m.) that produced salivation and vomiting (Goldberg *et al.*, 1976). Naloxone (0.01 to 1.0 mg/kg, i.m.) had no effect on responding maintained under a schedule of electric-shock postponement (Holtzman, 1976) nor under an FI schedule of electric-shock presentation (Byrd, 1976). Smith and McKearney (1977) studied the effects of naloxone (0.3 to 17 mg/kg, i.m.) on squirrel monkeys under titration schedules in which responding altered the intensity of continuously presented electric shock. Under the escape titration schedule, in which responses decreased the intensity of electric shock that otherwise increased at a fixed rate, naloxone increased rates of responding in three of four monkeys at doses of 1.0 or 3.0 mg/kg, but did not decrease responding even at 17 mg/kg. Under the punishment titration schedule, in which responding under a schedule of food presentation increased the intensity of an electric shock that otherwise decreased at a fixed rate, responding was markedly decreased by 10 mg/kg of naloxone. The effects of naloxone were qualitatively similar to those of morphine under both titration schedules.

The most consistent effect of naloxone on schedule-controlled behavior in monkeys is to decrease responding at doses that are much higher than those required to antagonize the effects of morphine. Lower doses of naloxone have been found to affect behavior in some monkeys under some experimental conditions, but it is difficult to characterize these effects yet. The notion that blocking the opiate receptors with naloxone might have consistent effects on behavior and that these effects might be opposite to those of morphine has not been supported.

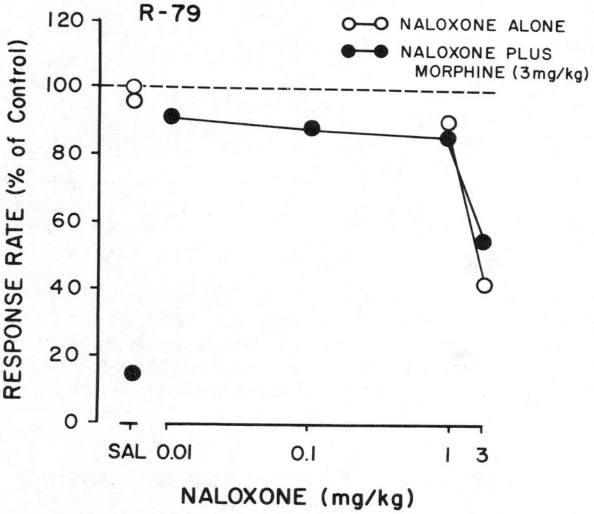

Figure 42.3 Effects of naloxone i.m. alone or naloxone plus a high dose of morphine i.m. on responding under a FR schedule of food presentation in rhesus monkey R-79. The control rate of responding was 2.32 responses per second (± s.d. 0.33; $N = 5$). Note that the effects of 3 mg/kg of naloxone were about the same whether or not morphine was present.

The effects of high doses of naloxone in decreasing responding are generally considered to be nonspecific; however, there have been few attempts to analyze these effects as yet. Some relevant information is provided by a study in which high doses of naloxone and morphine were combined. A rhesus monkey responded under a 30-response FR schedule of food presentation with a 1 min time-out period after each food presentation. Each session, in which drug or saline was injected i.m., was preceded by several sessions in which no injections were given. Naloxone (3 mg/kg, i.m.) decreased responding, whereas a lower dose of naloxone or injection of saline had no effect on responding (figure 42.3). When 3 mg/kg of naloxone was given in combination with a dose of morphine (3 mg/kg, i.m.) that decreased responding, the effects of morphine were not as well antagonized as by lower doses of naloxone. Moreover, the effects of this relatively large dose of naloxone were not altered by the presence of morphine. Goldberg *et al.* (1976) reported similar findings with combinations of relatively large doses of naloxone (10 mg/kg, i.m.) and morphine (1 mg/kg, i.m.) in squirrel monkeys responding under a multiple 10 min FI, 30-response FR schedule of food presentation (figure 42.4). The results consistently indicate that high doses of naloxone continue to decrease responding in monkeys even in the presence of morphine.

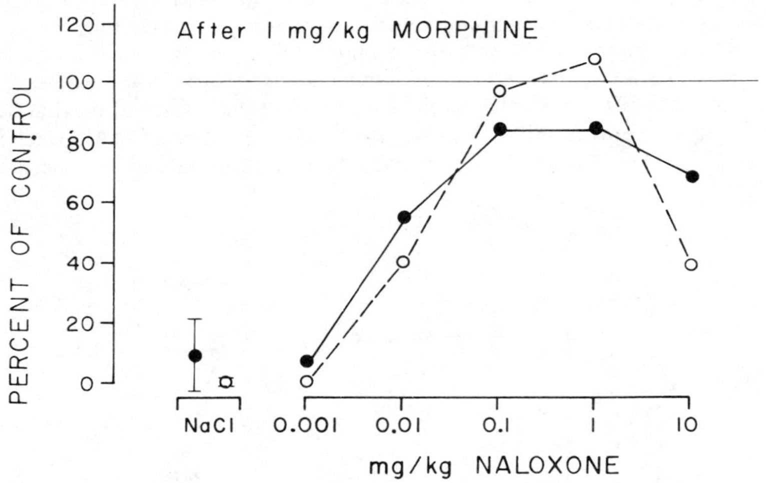

Figure 42.4 Effects of a fixed dose of morphine (1 mg/kg, i.m.) on responding under a multiple FI (•), FR (○) schedule of food presentation. Each NaCl point is based on the mean of two observations in each of three squirrel monkeys; brackets represent s.e. The solid line at 100 per cent indicates control levels of FI and FR responding. Naloxone alone at 10 mg/kg decreased response rates to about 50 per cent of control levels. (From Goldberg *et al.*, 1976, with permission).

BEHAVIORAL EFFECTS OF NALOXONE AFTER MORPHINE

The relation between dose of naloxone and its behavioral effects can be altered in animals that have been given repeated injections of morphine (for example, Villarreal and Karbowski, 1973) or even a single injection of morphine (for example, Jacob *et al.*, 1973). We studied the effects of naloxone on the behavior of rhesus monkeys that had been pretreated with morphine. The monkeys had been trained under the multiple 30-response FR, 5 min FI schedule of food presentation described earlier. A solution of saline or morphine was continuously infused intravenously for 20 hours before an experimental session. During the experimental session, saline i.v. was injected at the beginning of cycle 4 and then increasing doses of naloxone were injected at the beginning of every third subsequent cycle.

The effects of naloxone after the first infusion of saline were similar to those described previously. Rates of responding under the FR schedule were decreased by a cumulative dose of 10 mg/kg of naloxone (figure 42.5). Intravenous infusions of total doses of 1 or 3 mg/kg of morphine, which had no consistent effect on performance in the cycles after saline injection, shifted the naloxone dose–effect curve about 2 log units to the left. No clear signs of physiological disturbance were observed while behavior was disrupted by naloxone. After a subsequent infusion of saline, the redetermined naloxone dose–effect curve was about 0.5 to 1 log unit to the left of the first naloxone dose–effect curve, indicating that some sort of sensitization to the effect of naloxone had occurred.

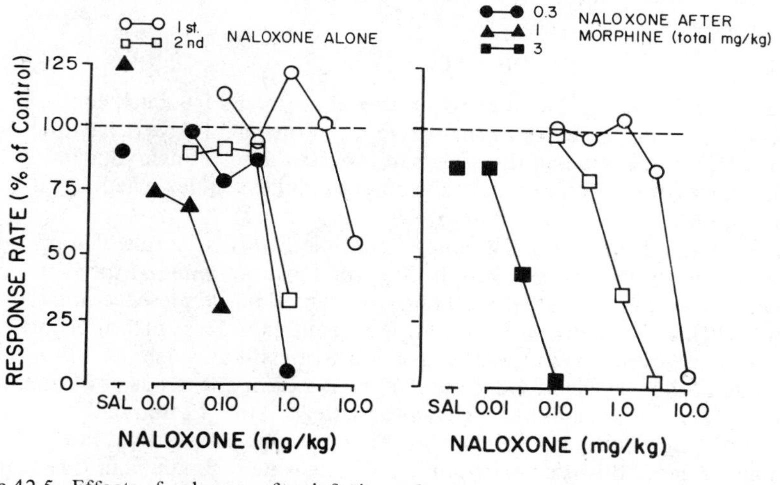

Figure 42.5 Effects of naloxone after infusions of saline (○, □) or morphine (●, ▲, ■) on responding under a 30-response FR schedule of food presentation in rhesus monkeys R-7 (left panel) and R-8 (right panel). Note that pretreatment with morphine shifted the naloxone dose–effect curves to the left.

It has been well-established that naloxone can severely disrupt the behavior of animals that have been chronically treated with morphine. Using morphine-dependent (3 mg/kg, s.c. daily every 6 hours) rhesus monkeys, Villarreal and Karbowski (1973) found that low doses of naloxone (0.1 mg/kg, s.c.) produced 'gross behavioral and physiological disturbances closely resembling the disturbances occurring after withdrawal of morphine'. Several studies have shown that relatively low doses of naloxone can produce signs of morphine withdrawal or disruptions of behavior in mice or rats that have received only a single dose of morphine (for example Jacob *et al.*, 1973; Sparber *et al.*, 1978). In a study of the behavior of rats under a 15-response FR schedule of food presentation, Sparber *et al.* (1978) found that a previously ineffective dose of naloxone (2.5 mg/kg, i.p.) markedly decreased responding three hours after the animals had been injected with morphine (15 or 30 mg/kg, i.p.).

The present results with rhesus monkeys are consistent with those of previous studies with other species in indicating that low doses of naloxone can induce clear behavioral effects in animals that have had a relatively brief exposure to morphine. It is unclear whether this type of finding should be interpreted in terms of naloxone's producing a morphine withdrawal syndrome by revealing a rapidly developing state of dependence on morphine or in terms of pretreatment with morphine enhancing behavioral effects of naloxone. At an empirical level, the present results can be most simply described as a shift to the left of the naloxone dose–effect curve after pretreatment with morphine.

The reason for the change in the dose–effect curve for naloxone after saline infusions is unclear. We have occasionally observed that monkeys became sensitive to low doses of naloxone at times when they were receiving naloxone frequently. The present findings and our earlier observations suggested that it might be fruitful to study the effects of repeated injections of naloxone.

REPEATED INJECTIONS OF NALOXONE

If the endorphin system involves some type of hormonal feedback control, repeated or prolonged block of the opiate receptors might have behavioral consequences. We have studied the effects of repeated doses of naloxone on the performances of squirrel monkeys and rhesus monkeys under schedules of food presentation.

Squirrel monkeys responded under a multiple FI, FR schedule of food presentation. Under a 10 min FI schedule, food was presented at the first response occurring after at least 10 min had elapsed in the presence of a red stimulus light. Under the 30-response FR schedule, food was presented at the 30th response occurring in the presence of a green stimulus light. A 1 min time-out period followed each food presentation. If a component was not terminated by a response, the time-out occurred automatically after 12 min in the FI component or 2 min in the FR component. Characteristic patterns and rates of responding under this type of multiple schedule were maintained in three squirrel monkeys. Naloxone (10 mg/kg, i.m.) was given daily for 16 days, either 5 min before the session or at about the same time of day on weekends and holidays.

Naloxone initially decreased responding in each schedule component (figure 42.6). Although response rates occasionally increased toward control levels in subsequent sessions, responding was about as suppressed on days 14 to 16 as on days 1 to 3. The monkeys salivated profusely and often vomited after the daily injections. Responding remained suppressed during the first session after naloxone injections were stopped, but then recovered.

The monkeys did not develop tolerance to the suppression of schedule-controlled responding or the physiological disturbances induced by this high dose of naloxone. The behavioral effects of naloxone persisted for at least 24 hours after the last dose of naloxone. During the 6 months after this study, these squirrel monkeys received various combinations of naloxone and nalorphine or

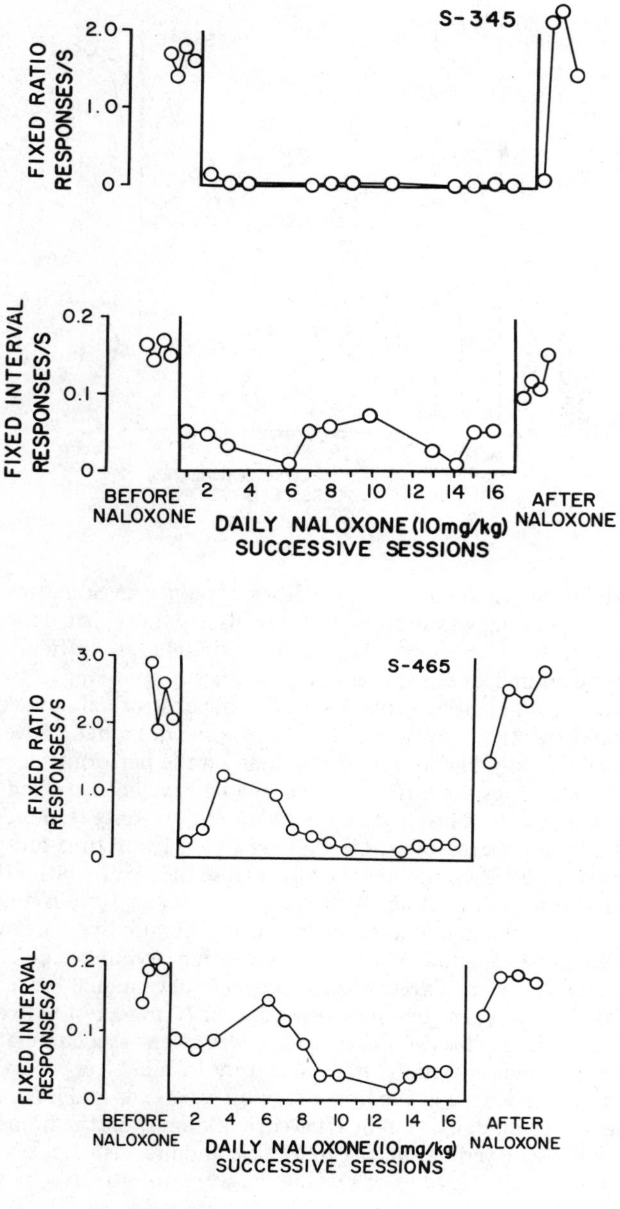

Figure 42.6 Suppression of responding under a multiple FI, FR schedule of food presentation by naloxone i.m. (squirrel monkeys S-345, S-465 and S-540). Note the lack of tolerance to repeated doses of naloxone and the continued suppression of responding in the first sessions after naloxone injections were stopped.

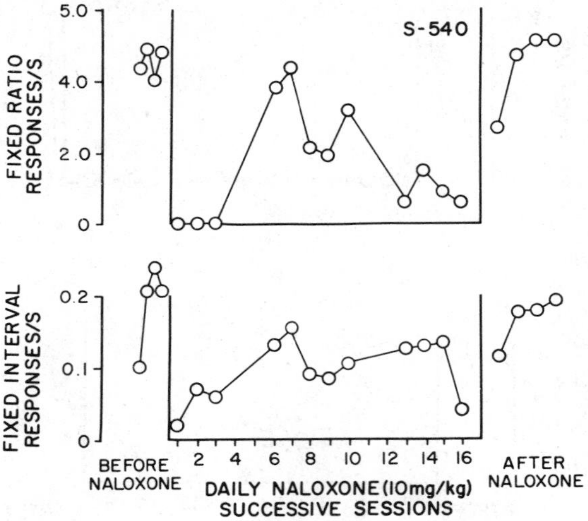

Fig. 6. (cont.)

naloxone and *d*-amphetamine or single doses of naloxone or naltrexone. During this period, responding was suppressed by relatively low single doses of naloxone or naltrexone in these monkeys. Although the findings are difficult to interpret because of the complicated experimental histories, responding in two of the three monkeys could still be suppressed by a low dose of naloxone (1 mg/kg, i.m.) about 4 years after the daily injections of naloxone described above.

The effects of daily high doses of naloxone on the performance of a rhesus monkey under a 20-response fixed-ratio schedule have been studied. In the presence of a green stimulus light, every twentieth response resulted in the delivery of a food pellet (Noyes, 1 g) followed by a 1 min time-out period. A cycle comprised 10 FR components or the elapse of 20 min without the completion of 10 components. After each cycle, there was a 10 min time-out period. The experimental session ended after five cycles. Cumulative dose–effect curves were established by injecting naloxone or saline i.m. 5 min before each cycle. Initially, the effects of naloxone after saline were determined twice in sessions separated by 4 days. Then the monkey was given 10 mg/kg of naloxone i.m. each day for 22 days. This dose of naloxone was given: as a cumulative dose during the experimental session; as a single dose 15 min after the experimental session; or as a single dose in the home cage on weekends and holidays. After 22 days, saline was given daily 15 min after each session or in the home cage.

When saline was given before the first cycle and increasing doses of naloxone before subsequent cycles, rates of responding were not affected by total doses of 0.1 to 3.0 mg/kg, but were increased by 10 mg/kg (figure 42.7). With further daily doses of naloxone, the dose–effect curves were altered. Both increases and decreases in responding were produced by lower and lower doses of naloxone. By the tenth day of repeated daily injections, 1.0 mg/kg of naloxone almost completely suppressed responding. Further changes in the dose–effect curve

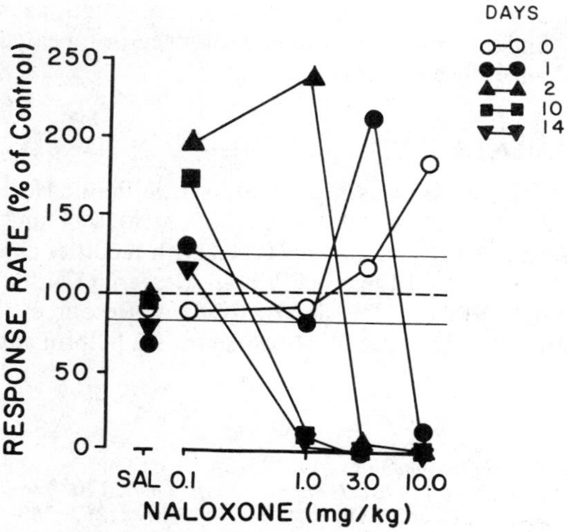

Figure 42.7 Effects of naloxone on responding under a FR schedule of food presentation after repeated injections of naloxone (rhesus monkey R-346). The dashed horizontal line represents mean control rate; continuous horizontal lines represent the range of rates during control sessions in which saline was administered before each cycle. Mean control rate was 1.27 responses per second. Saline was injected 5 min before cycle 1 (points at left of graph) and increasing doses of naloxone were injected 5 min before subsequent cycles; the abscissa indicates the cumulative dose of naloxone. Note the increasing sensitivity to the behavioral effects of naloxone.

could not be reliably established because response rates became extremely low even when naloxone was not given during the session. By the last session in which naloxone had been injected on the previous day, the average rate of responding was only 0.06 response per second. When saline injections were given daily 15 min after the session, responding slowly recovered toward control levels over about 10 days. On the sixth day after saline injections were begun, 1 mg/kg, i.m. of naloxone still completely suppressed responding.

CONCLUSIONS

Under diverse experimental conditions, including those in which behavior is controlled by noxious stimuli, naloxone suppresses schedule-controlled responding in monkeys only at doses which are much higher than those which antagonize the effects of morphine. The effects of these high doses of naloxone are not altered by the concurrent administration of morphine.

After short or long-term treatment with morphine, the dose-effect curves for the behavioral effects of naloxone are shifted markedly to the left.

Monkeys show little or no tolerance to the behavioral effects or physiological disturbances produced by naloxone. Indeed, repeated daily injections of high doses of naloxone shift the dose–effect curve for the behavioral effects of naloxone to the left. This sensitization to the effects of naloxone may be long lasting.

The endorphin system seems to have either limited functional significance or low tonic activity under normal conditions. Prolonged or repeated block of opiate receptors may enhance the activity of the system.

ACKNOWLEDGEMENTS

Preparation of this manuscript was supported by U.S. Public Health Service Research Grants MH07658, DA00499, DA01505, MH02094 and Research Career Program Award 1-K05-MH22589 (RTK) with facilities and services furnished by the New England Regional Primate Research Center (U.S. Public Health Service Grant RR00168, Division of Research Resources, National Institutes of Health). We thank Dr W. H. Morse for his helpful advice.

REFERENCES

Byrd, L. D. (1976). *Psychopharmacology,* **49**, 225–34

Downs, D. A. and Woods, J. H. (1976). *J. Pharmac. exp. Ther.,* **196**, 298–306

El-Sobky, A., Dostrovsky, J. O. and Wall, P. D. (1976). *Nature,* **263**, 783–4

Frederickson, R. C. A., Burgis, V. and Edwards, J. D. (1977). *Science,* **198**, 756–8

Frederickson, R. C. A., Nickander, R., Smithwick, E. L., Shuman, R. and Norris, F. H. (1976). In *Opiates and Endogenous Opioid Peptides*, (ed. H. W. Kosterlitz). Elsevier, Amsterdam, pp. 239–46

Goldberg, S. R., Morse, W. H. and Goldberg, D. M. (1976). *J. Pharmac. exp. Ther.,* **196**, 625–36

Goldstein, A. (1976). *Science,* **193**, 1081–6

Goldstein, A. and Lowry, P. J. (1975). *Life Sci.,* **17**, 927–31

Goldstein, A., Pryor, G. T., Otis, L. S. and Larsen, F. (1976). *Life Sci.,* **18**, 599–604

Holtzman, S. G. (1974). *J. Pharmac. exp. Ther.,* **189**, 51–60

Holtzman, S. G. (1976). *J. Pharmac. exp. Ther.,* **196**, 145–55

Jacob, J. J. C., Barthelemy, C. D., Tremblay, E. C. and Colombel, M. C. (1973). In *Narcotic Antagonists: Advances in Biochemical Psychopharmacology,* Vol. 8, (eds. M. C. Braude, L. S. Harris, E. L. May, J. P. Smith and J. E. Villarreal). Raven Press, New York. pp. 299–318

Smith, J. B. and McKearney, J. W. (1977). *J. Pharmac. exp. Ther.,* **200**, 508–15

Sparber, S. B., Gellert, V. F., Lichtblau, L. and Eisenberg, R. (1978). In *Factors Affecting the Action of Narcotics*, (eds. M. W. Adler, L. Manara and R. Samanin). Raven Press, New York, in press

Villarreal, J. E. and Karbowski, M. G. (1973). In *Narcotic Antagonists: Advances in Biochemical Psychopharmacology,* Vol. 8, (eds. M. C. Braude, L. S. Harris, E. L. May, J. P. Smith and J. E. Villarreal). Raven Press, New York, pp. 273–289

43

Possible role of β-endorphin in heat adaptation

John W. Holaday*, Horace H. Loh†, Eddie Wei‡, and Choh Hao Li∮
(*Department of Medical Neurosciences, Division of Neuropsychiatry, Walter Reed Army Institute of Research, Washington, D.C. 20012; †Department of Pharmacology and ∮Hormone Research Laboratory, University of California, San Francisco, California 94143; and ‡School of Public Health, University of California, Berkeley, California, 94720, U.S.A.)

We have recently demonstrated that hypophysectomy enhances the potency of β-endorphin or morphine. This effect was not solely a result of adrenal dysfunction following extirpation of the pituitary (Holaday *et al.*, 1977*a*). While conducting those studies, we observed unique behavioral effects of i.v.t. injections of β-endorphin that were never observed with equi-antinociceptive doses of morphine. Wet-dog shakes were seen within the first 5 min of drug injection, a phenomenon previously described by Bloom *et al.* (1976). When these wet-dog shakes ceased, we occasionally observed a clonic, seizure-like state accompanied by copious salivation. This effect was never observed in hypophysectomized rats (Holaday *et al.*, 1977*b*; Holaday *et al.*, 1978*a*). Both wet-dog shakes and these 'sialogic-seizures' were potentiated by heat exposure.

A predominant feature of these collective observations was their association with altered thermoregulatory states. Consequently, we wished to test the hypothesis that the potent thermoregulatory changes observed after pharmacological β-endorphin administration may indicate that endorphins are involved in adaptation to altered environmental temperatures (Holaday *et al.*, 1978*b*).

In previous work, Goldstein and Lowry (1975) had demonstrated a lack of colonic temperature change in chronically cold-exposed rats injected with the specific opiate-antagonist, naloxone (2 °C for 16 hours; 10 mg/kg naloxone). From these studies, it was inferred that endorphins do not play a predominant part in cold adaptation. Since hypothermia is the ultimate consequence of increasing dosages of opiates, we evaluated the effects of naloxone in both acutely and chronically heat-exposed rats. Moreover, the effects of hypophysectomy on these behaviors were also studied. The results of these experiments demonstrating a possible role for endorphins in adaptation to heat have been reported, in part, elsewhere (Holaday *et al.*, 1978*b*).

MATERIALS AND METHODS

In studies designed to assess the unique behavioral effects of β-endorphin, male Long-Evans rats (Charles River Laboratories), weighing 190 ± 10 (s.d.) g, were hypophysectomized by the parapharyngeal approach. Sham-operated control rats were treated identically, except that pituitary glands were not removed. Simultaneously with the above surgery, intracranial guides were affixed to the cranium for subsequent i.v.t. opiate injections. In order to ensure survival in the absence of the pituitary, hypophysectomized and control rats were housed two to a cage in a temperature-controlled environment (26.5 ± 0.5°C) with water and food *ad libitum*.

Animals were tested with β-endorphin, synthesized as previously reported, morphine sulfate (Mallinckrodt (Chemical Works, Inc.), and/or naloxone HCl (Endo Laboratories). Two weeks following surgery, drugs were injected i.v.t. in the right-lateral ventricle in 20 μl normal saline following light anesthetization in a bell jar with halothane vapor (Holaday *et al.*, 1977*a*). Doses of either peptide or morphine sulfate were injected i.v.t. without regard to body weight since brain weights were the same regardless of surgery. Naloxone HCl (4 mg/kg) was injected i.p. (0.1 ml per 100 g body weight).

Salivation was scored 0 for dry mouth, 1 for moist surfaces within the mouth, 2 for wet mouth, 3 for drooling, and 4 for drooling accompanied by a seizure-like state. These measures were made at discrete intervals and were continued until pharmacological effects ceased (see figure legends). Other details of the above surgical and pharmacological procedures appear in previous reports (Holaday *et al.*, 1977*a*; 1977*b*; 1978*a*).

To evaluate the effects of naloxone on heat-exposed animals in the first acute study, male Sprague-Dawley rats weighing 260–300 g were chosen because of previous use of such rats in evaluating opiate withdrawal effects at various ambient temperatures (Wei *et al.*, 1974). Initial colonic temperatures were measured in the room where animals were housed (22.0 ± 0.5°C) by means of a thermistor probe rectally inserted to a depth of 6 cm. Rats were then placed in glass jars approximately 12 inches high and 8 inches in diameter within a hot room (37.0 ± 0.5°C, 20–30 per cent humidity) for 1 hour (Holaday *et al.*, 1978*b*). Physiological saline or naloxone in saline (10 mg/kg) was injected i.p. (0.1 ml per 100 g body weight) in a blinded fashion. The number of escape attempts from the jars were counted in 5 min intervals for a total of 15 min after injections. Colonic temperatures were again measured 45 min after injections.

To assess the possible role of the pituitary gland in modifying thermoregulatory behavior in response to naloxone, male Long-Evans rats (180–220 g) were hypophysectomized or sham operated and maintained for at least one week after surgery as described above. For the short-term study, rats were placed within glass jars in the hot room (37.0 ± 0.5°C, 20–30 per cent humidity) for 1 hour. Since pilot studies demonstrated that sham-operated control rats would not survive

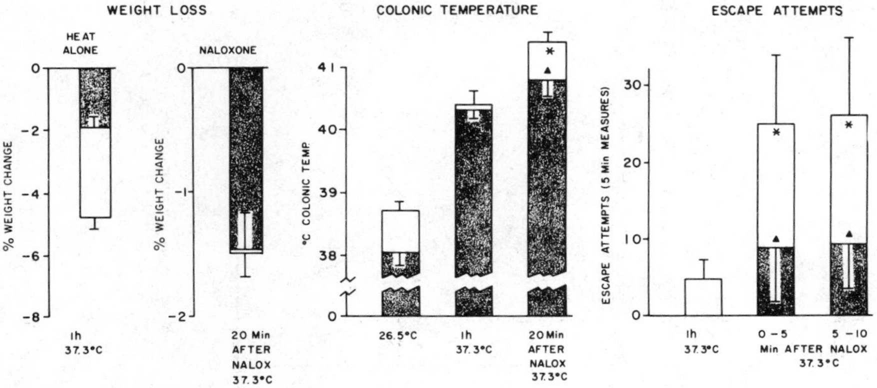

Figure 43.1 Effects of naloxone in acutely heat-exposed rats (1 h at 37.3 °C). Vertical bars are s.e.m.; clear histograms represent sham-operated controls, shaded histograms are hypophysectomized rats. Statistical comparisons are made only within the same surgical group (n = 6 per group). All effects occurred 20 min post-naloxone. *$P < 0.05$; ▲, no difference

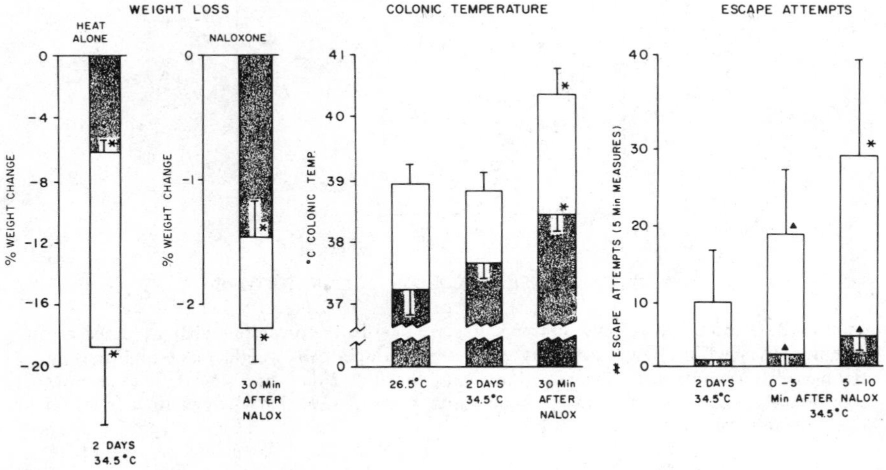

Figure 43.2 Effects of naloxone in chronically heat-exposed rats (2 days at 34.5 °C). Hypophysectomized rats (shaded histograms, n = 6) were compared with sham-operated control rats (clear histograms, n = 5) as in figure 43.3. *$P < 0.05$, ▲, no significant difference. Effects were measured 30 min post-naloxone.

long-term exposure to temperatures above 35°C, chronic heat-exposed rats were kept at 34.5 ± 0.5°C (20–30 per cent humidity) for 2 days.

Body weight and colonic temperature measures were made before sham injections. After evaluating pre-naloxone escape attempts for 5 min, naloxone (10 mg/kg) was injected i.p. and escape attempts were re-evaluated during the

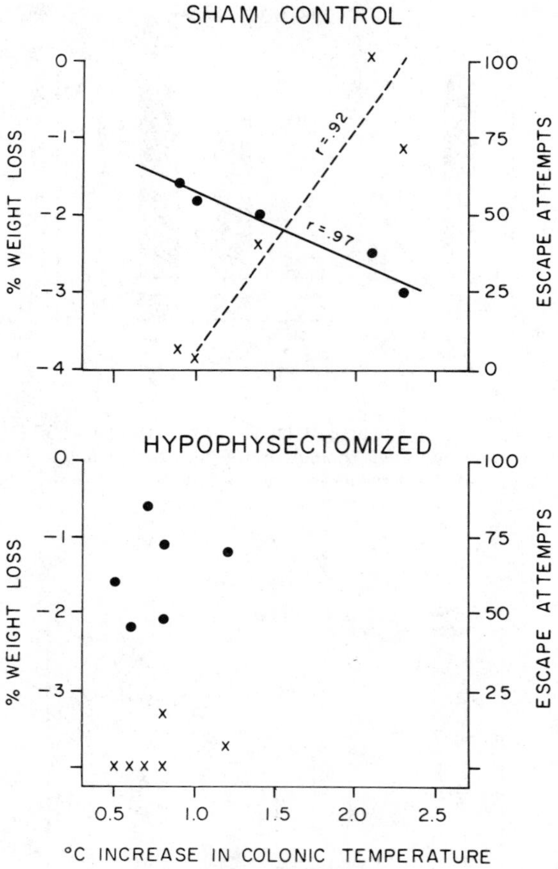

Figure 43.3 Increased colonic temperatures are positively correlated with increased escape attempts (dashed line) and negatively correlated with per cent weight loss (solid line) in sham-operated control rats after chronic heat exposure (2 days at 34.5°C). These events are significantly correlated in sham-operated control rats ($P < 0.02$), whereas no correlation was found in hypophysectomized animals.

following two consecutive 5 min intervals. Twenty to 30 min after naloxone, body weights and colonic temperatures were again measured.

Statistical significance for percentage weight loss, as well as for change in colonic temperature, was analyzed by means of the Student's *t* test. Escape attempts in the first study of naloxone effects after acute-heat exposure were statistically evaluated by the Mann-Whitney U test (Siegel, 1956); anticipation of positive results allowed for one-tailed statistical analysis (figure 43.1). To compare pre and post-naloxone effects in hypophysectomized and sham control rats, the Wilcoxon's matched-pair, signed-ranks test was used (Siegel, 1956) (figures 43.2 and 43.3). Statistical significance was ascribed if $P < 0.05$ unless otherwise noted.

Table 43.1 Effects of hypophysectomy and ambient temperature on β-endorphin-induced sialogogic activity

Surgery	No. of rats	Dose β-endorphin (μg)	Room temperature (°C)	15 min sialogogic score (0–4) $\bar{x} \pm$ s.e.m.	% seizure	Change in colonic temperature 1st 15 min (°C) $\bar{x} \pm$ s.e.m.	Colonic temperature at end of 15 min (°C) $\bar{x} \pm$ s.e.m.
Sham	16	5–10	23.0	0.3 ± 0.2	20	−0.6 ± 0.2	38.7 ± 0.2
Sham	6	7.5	26.5	2.0 ± 0.9	50	0 ± 0.2	38.8 ± 0.2
Sham	5	7.5	34.5	3.6 ± 0.4	80	+1.0 ± 0.2	41.9 ± 0.4
Hypophysectomized	8	7.5	26.5	0	0	−0.4 ± 0.1	37.0 ± 0.1
Hypophysectomized	6	7.5	34.5	0	0	+0.4 ± 0.2	39.4 ± 0.2

Potentiation of β-endorphin-induced sialogogic seizures by increased ambient temperatures. Ambient temperatures were increased 4°C, then an additonal 8°C to stimulate a progressive 'dose' effect. In sham-control rats, sialogogic scores, percentage of rats undergoing seizures (and changes in colonic temperature all increase in response to increasing ambient temperature. Hypophysectomized rats were not observed to salivate or have seizures after similar treatment.

RESULTS

β-endorphin induction of sialogogic-seizure effects

After cessation of wet-dog shaking behavior, occasionally rats would spontaneously initiate a clonic, seizure-like behavior (Holaday *et al.*, 1977*b*; Holaday *et al.*, 1978*a*). In this state, copious salivation was accompanied by a rhythmic movement of the forepaws toward the mouth in synchrony with biting movements. While in this 'eating' posture, these spasms were observed to occur once or twice per second and persisted for 2-3 min after initiation. Eyes were partially closed during the seizure-like state. The onset of this behavior occurred 10–15 min after β-endorphin injection and continued at irregular intervals for as long as 60 min following administration of as little as 7.5 μg of this peptide. This pre-cataleptic state was further characterized by hyperexcitability, Episodes were often triggered by handling the animals; whereupon they sat upright on their hindpaws for the duration of the clonic-seizure state. If presented with a food pellet during these episodes, the animals would bite the food and intersperse chewing motions between the rhythmic bites.

If doses of β-endorphin were excessive (> 15-20 μg) and righting reflexes were lost, the animals would pass through the threshold for this seizure-like behavior to a state of complete catalepsy, although excess salivation continued. Nonetheless, a dose-response relationship for increasing sialogogic scores was observed to result from successively larger doses of β-endorphin (Holaday *et al.*, 1977*b*; Holaday *et al.*, 1978*a*). Morphine sulfate i.v.t. injected in doses which produced equi-antinociception with β-endorphin, was not observed to produce this behavior. In addition, hypophysectomized rats were not observed to have these sialogogic-seizure responses after β-endorphin (table 43.1).

The opiate specificity of this sialogogic behavior was confirmed by the naloxone reversal of ongoing sialogogic activity after 30 μg β-endorphin i.v.t in sham-operated control rats. The sialogogic-response area, integrated over 320 min for naloxone-injected rats (4 mg/kg i.p.; 30 min after β-endorphin), was significantly lower

Table 43.2 Effects of naloxone on thermoregulatory responses after acute exposure to heat (1 hour, 36.6 °C)

		Average no. of escape attempts (post-drug) ($\bar{x}$ ± s.e.m.)			Colonic temperature		
Drug (i.p.)	No. of rats	0–5 min	5–10 min	10–15 min	Pre-drug	45 min Post-drug	Change
Saline	8	1.1 ± 1.1	1.0 ± 0.7	1.4 ± 1.4	40.5 ± 0.1	40.1 ± 0.1	–0.4 ± 0.1*
Naloxone (10 mg/kg)	8	4.0 ± 2.9	5.0 ± 2.3	9.4 ± 4.0†	40.4 ± 0.1	40.5 ± 0.1	+0.1 ± 0.2

Naloxone-induced behavior in acutely-heated rats. Either saline or naloxone (10 mg/kg) were injected after 1 h exposure to 36.6°C. Raters were blinded as to which drug was injected. Colonic temperatures in saline-injected control rats declined over 45 min post-injection (* = $P < 0.05$, whereas naloxone-injected rats maintained the same colonic temperature. Naloxone-injected rats also had a progressively increasing escape frequently over time († = $P < 0.05$). See text for details.

than the sialogogic response area in saline-injected animals (38 ± 20 s.e.m., naloxone; 184 ± 20 s.e.m., saline; $P < 0.01$; $n = 4$ per group).

In table 43.1, it can be seen that as the environmental temperature is increased progressively, sialogogic scores, percentage of animals undergoing seizures, and changes in colonic temperatures also increase in response to a relatively low dose of β-endorphin (i.v.t.) in sham-operated control rats. Thus, the potentiation of all three of these measures by increasing ambient temperatures strongly suggests their involvement with thermoregulatory mechanisms. By contrast, similarly-treated hypophysectomized rats did not exhibit sialogogic behavior or the associated-clonic, seizure-like state; albeit their elevated colonic temperatures were well within the range of temperatures observed in heat-exposed, sham-operated control rats (table 43.1, right side).

In these studies, it was also shown that exposure to elevated temperatures alone (1 hour, 40°C) can elicit salivation in rats (Holaday *et al.*, 1978*b*). This is in agreement with the findings of Hainsworth and Epstein (1966) who reported that salivation and saliva-spreading are the predominant cooling mechanisms in rats.

Naloxone effects in acutely heated rats

Acute exposure to heated environments has been shown to result in attempts to escape from a confining enclosure (Wei *et al.*, 1974; Hainsworth, 1967). In table 43.2, this response is demonstrated to be potentiated by 10 mg/kg naloxone when compared with saline-injected rats exposed to 36.6°C for 1 hour (see Holaday *et al.* (1978*b*) for details). As the effects of the naloxone injections become progressively greater over time, there is a concomitant increase in number of escape attempts. However, not until the 10–15 min post-drug interval does the number of escape attempts in naloxone-injected rats significantly exceed escape attempts in saline-treated rats. There was no increase in escape behavior over time in saline-injected controls (table 43.2).

The average increase in colonic temperature as a consequence of 1 hour heat exposure alone was 1.73°C. Over the ensuing 45 min after saline injections, a significant decline in colonic temperature was observed (table 43.2). By contrast, this adaptation of colonic temperatures over 45 min was blocked by naloxone injections. A slight increase in colonic temperatures occurred in this group of animals (table 43.2).

Effects of hypophysectomy on acutely-heated, naloxone-treated rats

Hypophysectomized rats were approximately 1.3°C colder than sham-operated control rats at the maintenance temperature of 26.5°C (figure 43.1). After 1 hour acute-heat exposure alone, both groups attained the same elevated colonic temperature (41.3°C) accompanied by a significant decline in body weight.

Subsequent naloxone injections in sham-operated control rats further potentiated body weight loss ($P < 0.001$), and, in addition, resulted in an increased number of escape attempts ($P < 0.025$) and an increase in colonic temperature ($P < 0.01$). By contrast, naloxone injection in hypophysectomized rats did not significantly increase escape attempts or colonic temperature even though the same elevated colonic temperatures before drug injection were observed in both groups (figure 43.1). Weight loss after naloxone in hypophysectomized rats was significant, however ($P < 0.001$).

Effects of hypophysectomy on chronically-heated, naloxone-treated rats

In order to determine whether or not the naloxone-induced changes after subjecting rats to acute heat were a consequence of the sudden stress of heat exposure, we repeated the same procedure in rats exposed to elevated temperatures for 2 days. Unlike actuely-heated rats, colonic temperatures in chronically-heated rats were no different than pre-exposure control temperatures, possibly indicating adaptation to this raised temperature. Otherwise, the differences in naloxone effects after acute and chronic heat exposure were minimal (figure 43.2). The same general patterns of responses were seen in sham-operated control rats (compare figures 43.1 and 43.2). As before, hypophysectomized rats had greatly attenuated responses to naloxone.

In addition to the three signs of naloxone effects demonstrated above, naloxone-injected control rats, in both acute and chronic studies, exhibited enhanced saliva-spreading behavior as well as increased diarrhea and abnormal posturing. As with other measures, these signs of hyperthermia were more infrequent in hypophysectomized rats.

Figure 43.3 demonstrates the association between increases in escape attempts and elevations in colonic temperature in sham-operated control rats injected with naloxone (10 mg/kg). Moreover, the naloxone-induced decreases in body weight are also correlated with increased colonic temperature. In hypophysectomized rats, significant decreases in body weight and increases in colonic temperature were again observed as in figure 43.2, however no correlated relationships among these three measures were observed in these animals (figure 43.3, bottom).

DISCUSSION

The occurrence of mild hyperthermia with low doses of opiates has been reported by us and others (Holaday *et al.*, 1977*a*; Cox *et al.*, 1976; Tseng *et al.*, 1977). We have also demonstrated that the wet-dog shakes that occur after i.v.t. injections of relatively low doses of β-endorphin in rats are positively correlated with increased colonic temperatures (Holaday *et al.*, 1978*a*). Furthermore, upon cessation of wet-dog shaking behavior, a clonic, seizure-like state accompanied by profuse salivation was occasionally seen (Holaday *et al.*, 1977*b*; Holaday *et al.*, 1978*a*). Hainsworth and Epstein (1966) reported that salivation and saliva-spreading are the predominant cooling behaviors exhibited by rats in response to heat exposure. We therefore subjected rats to progressively elevated ambient temperatures and subsequently administered a relatively low-dose of β-endorphin i.v.t. to determine if we could potentiate these effects. The parallel increases in sialogogic scores, percentage of animals having seizure episodes, and colonic temperatures which appear to result from exposure to increases in ambient temperature (table 43.1) suggest that these measures are complementary indicators of a β-endorphin-induced alteration in thermoregulation. Is it possible that these pharmacological effects of β-endorphin indicate a role for endorphins in adaptation to changes in environmental temperature?

Goldstein and Lowry, noting that low doses of opiates are hyperthermic, subjected rats to cold exposure and subsequently injected naloxone to test the hypothesis that endorphins subserve a role as endogenous hyperthermic agents (Goldstein and Lowry, 1975). They were unable to find any significant effects of this specific-opiate antagonist in altering body temperature under conditions of cold exposure. Since higher opiate doses ultimately result in a fall in body temperature, we tested the hypothesis that endorphins may function in heat adaptation (Holaday *et al.*, 1978*b*).

The data in table 43.2 demonstrate a significant increase in escape attempts in heat-exposed, naloxone-injected rats. Escape attempts have been shown to be behavioral indicators of real or 'sensed' hyperthermia (Holaday *et al.*, 1978*b*; Wei *et al.*, 1974, Hainsworth, 1967), an observation which was confirmed by the positive relationship between escape attempts and colonic temperature in figure 43.3 (top). Therefore, the potentiation of these effects by naloxone infers that endorphins may specifically function in adaptation to heat stress. This observation is further substantiated by the colonic temperature results depicted in table 43.2. Colonic temperatures in saline-injected rats significantly decline over time during heat exposure, whereas naloxone-injected rats fail to demonstrate this adaptation of colonic temperatures.

These effects of naloxone on acutely-heated rats were verified in additional studies (figure 43.1). Once again, naloxone was observed to rapidly produce a significant increase in escape attempts in control rats. Also shown to accompany the naloxone-induced increases in escape frequency were elevations in colonic temperature and decreases in body weight. In addition, these rats salivated copiously and spread the saliva on exposed skin surfaces, had increased diarrhea, and exhibited an abnormal, spread posture. The actual increases in body temperature were therefore complemented by the expected signs believed to be associated with activation of heat-loss behaviors (such as escape attempts, salivation and abnormal posture).

It has been reported that in rats rendered physically dependent on morphine, naloxone produces a variety of abstinence signs which share a common association as behavioral indicators of altered thermoregulation (Wei *et al.*, 1974). Thus, in heat-exposed rats, naloxone likewise potentiates adaptive thermoregulatory signs. However, in rats rendered physically dependent to morphine, both heat loss and heat gaining effects were seen after naloxone (Wei *et al.*, 1974). Since only heat-loss behaviors were observed in these studies of naloxone effects on heat-exposed rats, the parallelism between abstinence signs and heat-stress signs is not absolute. This difference is probably due to the effects of chronic morphine on altering body temperature baselines (Gunne, 1960), whereas the studies reviewed here were performed on opiate-naive rats.

Since the pituitary gland is known to be a rich source of endorphins (Li and Chung, 1976; Goldstein, 1976), we were interested in evaluating the effects of pituitary removal on these naloxone-induced behaviors. As seen in figure 43.1, hypophysectomized rats failed to show the significant increases in colonic temperature and escape attempts that were observed in sham control rats. Moreover, other signs such as salivation, diarrhea, and the abnormal posturing were also observed far less frequently in these rats. The resulting conclusion that pituitary endorphins may have a functional role in thermoregulatory behaviors is further strengthened by the lack of correlated changes in body weight loss, escape attempts, and colonic temperatures in rats surgically deprived of normal pituitary function (figure 43.3).

In a previous report (Holaday *et al.*, 1978*b*), we discussed the possibility that circulating pituitary β-endorphin may gain access to opiate receptors in the brain through areas where a functional blood-brain barrier is missing, for example, the area postrema or sub-fornical regions. This would allow for diffusion of functional concentrations of circulating β-endorphin to nearby areas known to mediate opiate effects. Alternatively, recent anatomical evidence for the direct secretion of pituitary peptides into the brain has been obtained by Bergland and Page (1978) in nine different mammalian species. These speculations and findings must be reconciled, however, with repeated observations that hypophysectomy does not alter the static levels of pituitary peptides in the brain (Chung and Goldstein, 1976; Fuxe *et al.*, 1977; Kreiger *et al.*, 1977). It is possible that turnover studies will clarify these discrepancies.

To ensure that the effects of naloxone in acutely heat-exposed rats were not a consequence of the sudden stress of exposure to a heated environment, a similar study was performed after chronic heat exposure. The same pattern of effects was observed in both studies (compare figures 43.1 and 43.2), thus supporting the hypothesis that these phenomena are more generally heat specific as opposed to stress non-specific.

The main conclusion of our naloxone studies is that endorphins have a role in adaptations to heat stress, possibly as endogenous hypothermic modulators. If the converse were assumed, for example, that endorphins are endogenous hyperthermic agents, one would have expected to see an effect of naloxone in cold-exposed rats. In the thorough studies of Goldstein and Lowry, no such effect was obtained in naloxone-injected, cold-exposed rats. Moreover, an expected concomitant of this postulated role of endorphins as important physiological hypothermic modulators would be that rats made tolerant to morphine would likewise be tolerant to the endogenous hypothermic effects of endorphins. Indeed, tolerant rats have a significantly higher resting temperature than non-tolerant rats (Gunne, 1960) and are less able to survive heat exposure (Wei, 1973).

It has been assumed that the primary physiological function of endorphins is to decrease the perceived intensity of painful stimuli. The data reviewed here suggest that the common neuroanatomical pathways for the perception and integration of pain and temperature may be more than coincidental since thermoregulation not only depends on these peripheral inputs but also seems to be modulated by endorphins.

REFERENCES

Bergland, R. M. and Page, R. B. (1978). *Endocrinology* (in press)
Bloom, F., Segal, D., Ling, N. and Guillemin, R. (1976). *Science*, **194**, 630–2
Chung, A. L. and Goldstein, A. (1976). *Life Sci.*, **19**, 1005–8
Cox, B., Ary, M., Chesarek, W. and Lomax, P. (1976). *Eur. J. Pharmac.*, **36**, 33–9
Fuxe, K., Hökfelt, T., Eneroth, P., Gustafson, J.-A. and Skett, P. (1977). *Science*, **196**, 899–900

Goldstein, A. (1976). *Science*, **193**, 1081–6

Goldstein, A. and Lowry, P. J. (1975). *Life Sci.*, **17**, 927–32

Gunne, L. M. (1960). *Archs int. Pharmacodyn.*, **129**, 416–28

Hainsworth, F. R. (1967). *Am. J. Physiol.*, **212**, 1288–93

Hainsworth, F. R. and Epstein, A. N. (1966). *Science*, **153**, 1255–7

Holaday, J. W., Law, P.-Y., Tseng, L.-F., Loh, H. H. and Li, C. H. (1977*a*). *Proc. natn. Acad. Sci. U.S.A.*, **74**, 4628–32

Holaday, J. W., Li, C. H. and Loh, H. H. (1977*b*). *Soc. Neurosci. Abstr.*, **3**, 347

Holaday, J. W., Loh, H. H. and Li, C. H. (1978*a*). *Life Sci.*, **22**, 1525–36

Holaday, J. W., Wei, E., Loh, H. H. and Li, C. H. (1978b). *Proc. natn. Acad. Sci. U.S.A.*, **75**, 2923–7

Kreiger, D. T., Liotta, A. and Brownstein, M. J. (1977). *Proc. natn. Acad. Sci. U.S.A.*, **74**, 648–52

Li, C. H. and Chung, D. (1976). *Proc. natn. Acad. Sci. U.S.A.*, **73**, 1145–8

Li, C. H., Lemaire, S., Yamashiro, D. and Doneen, B. A. (1976). *Biochem. biophys. Res. Commun.*, **71**, 19–25

Siegel, S. (1956). *Nonparametric Statistics for the Behavioral Sciences*, New York, McGraw-Hill

Tseng, L.-F., Loh, H. H. and Li, C. H. (1977). *Biochem. biophys. Res. Commun.*, **74**, 390–6

Wei, E. (1973). *Psychopharmacologia (Berl.)*, **28**, 35–41

Wei, E., Tseng, L.-F., Loh, H. H. and Way, E. L. (1974). *Nature*, **247**, 398–400

44
Naloxone-induced mood and physiologic changes in normal volunteers

Reese T. Jones, and Ronald I. Herning
(Department of Psychiatry, University of California San Francisco,
San Francisco, California 94143, U.S.A.)

Given the possibility that endorphins may have a role in the regulation of mood and perception, perhaps as neurotransmitters or neuromodulators (Goldstein, 1976; Hughes and Kosterlitz, 1977), we thought it useful to investigate the effects of naloxone administered to normal volunteer subjects. The relatively few studies of naloxone in normal volunteers focus on very specialized areas such as pain relief (Goldstein and Hilgard, 1976; Grevert and Goldstein, 1977), sexual behavior (Goldstein, 1977), respiratory function (Sadove, 1963), or have given small, intramuscular doses (Wang *et al.*, 1974). Most of the older data on naloxone effects on mood and subjective symptoms come from populations of formerly opiate dependent individuals, surgical patients and so on (Jasinski *et al.*, 1965; Fink *et al.*, 1968). In the few instances where naloxone was noted to have subjective or physiological effects, it was assumed to be a consequence of protracted opiate abstinence.

When we began this work it was already obvious that any naloxone effects in humans might well be only evident by rather subtle changes in mood or physiology (Goldstein, 1976). The use of volunteers who are not mentally ill or drug dependent offers certain advantages when attempting to measure minimal subjective changes. If one is concerned that naloxone has more of an effect on subjective state or perception than it does on behavior, man's ability to provide verbal reports offers obvious advantages over experimental animals.

Since naloxone appears to have similar antagonist properties on both opiate peptides and exogenous opiates, we thought that an attempt to measure the signs and symptoms expected during precipitated opiate withdrawal would be useful. This preliminary report describes the effects of naloxone as measured by a battery of subjective and physiological tests very similar to those used to characterize opiate abstinence (Kolb and Himmelsbach, 1938; Wang *et al.*, 1974; Haertzen *et al.*, 1970).

METHODS

We have tested 18 young adult subjects (ages 18 to 31 years). They were selected on the basis of their being in good physical and mental health and having no history of illicit or prolonged medical administration of opiate or opiate-like drugs. If there was any question of possible opiate drug use, the subject was not included in the study. An occasional subject may have had opiates on one or two occasions 10 to 15 years before the experiment; for example, before or following tonsillectomy. Other than these occasional exposures many years earlier, we are reasonably confident that none of the subjects tested was an opiate user.

An attempt was made to test subjects in a quiescent, basal state. During the 3 to 4 hour experimental session they reclined in bed in a quiet, temperature and humidity-controlled room. An indwelling i.v. catheter of the type used for central venous pressure measurements was threaded through a forearm vein such that the tip lay in the area of the subclavian vein, thus allowing injections producing only minimal pressure and temperature cues. The naloxone was injected into a 5 per cent dextrose in water solution that was maintained throughout the experimental period. The injections were made without the subject or observeis being aware of the exact timing or the content of the injection. Care was taken so that the subjects were at rest and in a relatively stable physiological state around the time of any injection.

The naloxone was injected in 3 to 20 mg doses in the form of rapid bolus injections. The 10 mg per ml concentration allowed for rapid injection. Eight subjects were given 20 mg doses, five given 10 mg and five given 3 mg. Some were tested on a second occasion, but only first test session data are reported here. Injections of similar volumes of both physiological saline and injections of the vehicle in which the naloxone was prepared were given in a balanced order before or after naloxone injections.

An array of physiological and psychological measures thought to be sensitive to opiate abstinence phenomena are listed in table 44.1. The physiological measures were collected throughout the experimental period, for the most part continuously, using an on-line computer data reduction system. Every 20 to 30 min the subject was asked to place the dominant hand in a hand rest so that finger tremor measures could be obtained. The injections were timed around this procedure. This allowed for a 5 min period when the subject was quite still, not talking, and focusing attention on a visual fixation spot. Subjective symptom and mood ratings were made immediately before this period and following it; that is, about 10 min after the injection. Subjective symptoms commonly experienced during opiate withdrawal were recorded on a Himmelsbach-like scale with each symptom scored 0 to 4 as to intensity (Jasinski *et al.*, 1965; Wang *et al.*, 1974; Haertzen *et al.*, 1970). Mood was assessed with the Profile of Mood Scale administered by the observer. Subjects were asked to report any experiences, no matter how trivial, to the observer who sat quietly in the experimental chamber.

Data analysis compared pre and post-injection changes after placebo, after vehicle and after naloxone. Physiological measures were taken as the 5 min average pre-injection and at 1 min, 2 min, 10 min, 15 min and, in some cases, 30 min post-injection. Values were analyzed with a repeated measures analysis of variance. Subjective symptom and Profile of Mood Scale data was also analyzed with a stepwise discriminant analysis (Dixon, 1975).

Table 44.1 Physiological and subjective report measures obtained before and after naloxone or placebo injections

Physiological measures	
	Body temperature (tympanic membrane thermocouple)
	Skin temperature (finger thermistor)
	Heart rate (EKG)
	Respiratory rate
	Blood pressure
	Skin conductance
	Pupil size (Photograph)
	Salivary flow (Total unstimulated, 2 min)
	EEG-C_3 F_3 0_1 0_2 (Spectral analysis)
	Tremor (finger accelerometer–frequency spectra)
Subjective reports	
	Opiate withdrawal symptoms
	Profile of mood scale
	Ongoing verbal reports

RESULTS

Naloxone effects were mostly evident as changes in subjective symptom reports. Analysis of variance of the physiological data comparing pre and post-placebo, vehicle and naloxone administration revealed only a statistically significant difference between placebo and naloxone on the heart rate measure. Heart rate increased three beats per minute 4 min after the naloxone injection ($P < 0.05$). This small change was gone 10 min following injection. Body temperature (0.1 °C decrease 10 min after injection) and skin temperature (0.6 °C increase, 15 min after injection) changes did not reach the 0.05 level of statistical significance. No drug-time or placebo-time or order effects were noted. Dose effects over the range from 3 to 20 mg of naloxone were not evident. A variety of analyses, both looking at dose effect correlation and grouping of subjects into various dose levels were examined without any evidence of a dose effect.

Subjective symptom mean scores reported 5 min following placebo injection and naloxone injection are listed in table 44.2. It is evident that both low intensity symptoms were experienced and that individual variability was large. A stepwise discriminant analysis (Dixon, 1975) was used to determine whether differences in responses after naloxone and placebo injection could be used to construct an objective weighting of items that discriminated treatments. Then, by applying the weights to the item discriminating placebo and naloxone, a single number along a continuum could be given. In a sense, this procedure is not very different from calculating a single 'Himmelsbach' score (Jasinski *et al.*, 1965). However, determining symptoms and weights is a little more objective with the discriminant analysis technique. In addition, the analysis picks only items which are important in discriminating the two populations of response (placebo or

Table 44.2 Effect of intravenous naloxone or placebo on subjective symptoms reported 5 min after injection, item means and standard errors

Symptoms	Placebo		Naloxone	
Yawning	0.53	0.13	0.83	0.23
Tears	0.09	0.05	0.39	0.23
Rhinorrhea	0.06	0.06	0.17	0.12
Sweating	0.09	0.05	0.22	0.10
Gooseflesh	0.16	0.07	0.17	0.09
Restlessness	0.75	0.11	1.06	0.22
Nausea	0.00	0.00	0.05	0.05
Tense	0.25	0.08	0.33	0.14
Tremor	0.06	0.04	0.06	0.05
Irritability	0.12	0.06	0.28	0.14
Muscle discomfort	0.09	0.05	0.00	0.00
Bone or joint aches	0.06	0.04	0.22	0.10
Feeling hot	0.03	0.03	0.22	0.13
Feeling cold	0.53	0.12	0.28	0.13
Abdominal discomfort	0.03	0.03	0.00	0.00
Decreased appetite	0.00	0.00	0.17	0.00
Number of cases	32		18	

naloxone) along a continuum. A multivariate F test of mean differences between the two groups of item scores was calculated. This test is similar to a univariate test made between placebo and naloxone item scores except only one test is made of all the differences between item scores at once. Of course, if the test is non-significant, no meaningful weighting scheme can be constructed or a continuum built.

The 7 of the 15 symptoms useful in distinguishing placebo condition from naloxone are shown in table 44.3 along with the weights assigned. The two

Table 44.3 Symptoms useful in discriminating between placebo and naloxone-induced states

Symptoms	Weights
Loss of appetite	−3.27321
Feeling cold	1.21211
Tears	−0.82606
Yawning	−0.29821
Muscle discomfort	2.02858
Restlessness	−0.45132
Sweating	−0.95760

Symptoms selected by stepwise discriminant analysis and raw score weights (multivariate F, −3.60, d.f. 7, 47). Symptoms with negative weights occur with naloxone. Symptoms with positive weights do not occur with naloxone.

items with positive weights, feeling cold and muscle discomfort, represent symptoms that tended to be absent following naloxone. All the others are symptoms that best discriminated the naloxone and placebo condition. The symptoms all represent those commonly seen during mild opiate withdrawal (Haertzen *et al.*, 1970). The multivariate *F* test from the stepwise discriminant analysis was significant beyond the 0.005 level ($F = 3.60$, d.f. 7, 42). Using the weights from these seven symptoms, a value was assigned to the symptom following each injection. That is something akin to a Himmelsbach abstinence score. When this is done, only four placebo injections are misclassified along with the naloxone scores and four naloxone injections misclassified with the placebo treatments. Thus, there appears to be a subset or constellation of subjectively reported symptoms useful in distinguishing the effects of a placebo injection from the effect of naloxone given to healthy human subjects with no history of opiate dependence or use.

On a similar discriminant analysis of the Profile of Mood State data, the multivariate *F* test of the selected mood states between placebo and naloxone injections was only significant at the 0.05 level. Only one of the six mood states was selected, confusion. In this instance, the test is similar to a univariate *t* test. However, with this one variable the classification of individual injections into the two injection groups was not as clear as with the opiate withdrawal symptoms. Fifteen of the placebo group and 16 of the naloxone group were misclassified. Thus, in terms of mood states, confusion appears to be most important but the variability and low intensity of symptoms as recorded by the Profile of Mood Scale did not allow us to build a powerful set of weights for developing a classification.

The comments that subjects made to the observer sitting in the experimental chamber indicated naloxone effects consistent with those reported on the symptom checklist, but in many ways providing data with less constraints than a structured symptom list quite often imposes. Observers did much better than chance in guessing which injection was naloxone. Reports of a generalized warm feeling throughout the body, particularly the trunk, feelings of fatigue, decreased vigor and irritability were commonly reported following naloxone and only very rarely described after the vehicle or placebo injections. Whereas vehicle not infrequently produced warm or cold feelings in the arm in the location of the catheter tip, the vehicle never produced such symptoms in the trunk.

Three subjects reported intense changes in mood and affect following naloxone. Approximately 45 s following the injection of 4 mg of naloxone, one subject reported what he termed overwhelming waves of depression. He began crying profusely and wailing and described feelings of hopelessness, worthlessness. At the same time he stated he was aware that it was 'crazy' to have such feelings in this situation, but they were there nevertheless. The depressed state lasted approximately 20 min, gradually lessening. An injection of placebo following it elicited no symptoms. An injection of 4 mg of naloxone 4 days later was followed by a similar, though less intense, period of depression. Injections of vehicle and placebo on that occasion were followed by no mood changes. Another subject, following a 4 mg injection of naloxone, experienced what he termed very vivid visual images and called them hallucinations. On detailed inquiry, they seemed to represent more illusions than true hallucinations. At the same time he experienced a variety of old memories and slight paranoid feelings regarding the experimenters. These also occurred within 1 min of the injection and lasted about 30 min. This subject compared the experience to one that he had previously had after LSD ingestion. Placebo or vehicle in this instance produced no symptoms whatsoever. Many subjects stated they felt mildly irritable in the 15 min period following naloxone injections. However, one subject became so irritable and annoyed with the experimenters following the naloxone that he requested to be allowed to terminate the experiment. Following the placebo and vehicle injections, he had experienced no such mood changes. He was asked if he would at least sit quietly for 20 or 30 min to allow us to collect the rest of the data. After about 30 min he said that he felt rather foolish about the way he had previously acted. He wished to continue the experiment and was given an injection of placebo with no particular change following. These three subjects stood out because of the intensity of their changes following naloxone injection. Although the group data was not as impressive, a similar pattern existed. For example, on the Profile of Mood Scales, although not statistically significant, subjects experienced increases in tension and depression and anger following naloxone injections, decreases in vigor, increases in fatigue and increased confusion. In many instances the narrative report appeared to capture changes in mood better than did the Profile of Mood rating instrument.

DISCUSSION

Naloxone given to subjects in a relatively unstimulated and relaxed state produces effects most evident as subtle changes in mood and subtle, but reasonably consistent, bodily sensations. The physiological changes in an occasional subject were marked, but in the grouped data did not reach statistically significant levels other than for a small heart rate increase. Thus, there was not a complete lack of effect as has been often claimed, but the magnitude of change and the individual variability were such that further work is needed to fully describe the naloxone related changes.

Given the absence of a change following naloxone administration, there are an enormous number of other explanations (Hughes and Kosterlitz, 1977). Our data does establish that it is safe and practical to administer at least up to 20 mg rapidly injected doses of naloxone to healthy individuals. No serious adverse acute effects occurred. It may well be that higher doses of naloxone are necessary to occupy a larger fraction of the opiate receptors in the body and would produce more evidence of some effect (Emrich *et al.*, 1977). Many psychoactive drugs produce mainly subjective effects at low doses.

Besides an inadequate dose, it may well be that the enkephalinergic system is not tonically active, and naloxone effects would only be evident under certain conditions such as stress or pain (Goldstein, 1976). The few subjects who showed dramatic mood changes after naloxone were individuals who appeared (in retrospect) unusually stressed by the experimental situation or were people undergoing personal or environmental stresses in the life outside the laboratory.

A great redundancy may exist in the 'normal' enkephalinergic or endorphinergic systems with arrays of multiple opiate receptors with differing sensitivity to naloxone. So it may be unreasonable to expect dramatic effects. Some might even question the importance of effects mainly manifested by subjective reports. There is reason to think that subjective reports of perceptual and mood changes, when collected under properly controlled conditions with placebos; appropriate blinding of observers, and so on, are more sensitive and at least as reliable as physiological or biochemical measures.

One problem with the physiological measures was a great deal of variability during the pre-injection 'baseline' period, despite a vigorous attempt to allow subjects to reach a truly basal level of activity. Even after 1 hour or more of rest in the quiet bed, the simple act of clicking a camera to obtain a measure of pupil size caused a variety of perturbations in a previously stable battery of physiological measures. Variability in such responsivity between subjects could obscure subtle naloxone effects. We are attempting some other types of analysis of the vast amount of physiological data collected and may yet demonstrate a physiological correlate of the subjective effects. Also, because of our uncertainty as to the expected time course of the naloxone effects (should they occur), it may well be that our recording periods following injection were too brief. Some effects might be evident at longer intervals following injection than the 30 min that we usually had available (Emrich *et al.*, 1977).

The application of discriminate analyses might be criticized by some. We thought it worth reporting as an attempt to sort through an array of weak opiate withdrawal symptoms so as to come up with at least a tentative weighting scheme with some advantages over the more traditional Himmelsbach type checklist. The symptoms selected by the analyses make some intuitive sense if one expects naloxone interactions with endogenous opiate-like substances to be similar to those occurring with exogenous opiates. Loss of appetite, tears, yawning, restlessness, and sweating are among the earliest symptoms of naturally occurring or precipitated opiate abstinence. The selection of symptoms and rankings, of course, need replication in another study, since the pitfalls of discriminant analysis are well known. We offer them mainly as a suggestion to other investigators who might not otherwise enquire of schizophrenics and others concerning such events. Similarly, though not statistically significant, the trends on the Profile of Mood Scale clusters are consistent with the observed naloxone effects in animal studies where the drug resembles an aversive substance (Downs and Woods, 1975). The increased levels of tension, depression, anger, decreased vigor, increased fatigue and increased confusion, represent a trend that may well turn out to be statistically significant at higher dose levels or with selected subjects. Such reports were common in the comments made spontaneously by the subjects.

In summary, it appears the most readily observed effects of naloxone when given to volunteer subjects not previously exposed to opiates are on such phenomena as mood and bodily sensations. The individual differences in experienced intensity of such effects may well represent individual differences in the enkephalinergic system. Individual differences in response should make the whole subject all the more interesting for one interested in human behavior.

ACKNOWLEDGEMENT

This work was supported by Research Grant No. DA4RG012 and Research Scientist Award No. DA00053 from the National Institute on Drug Abuse.

REFERENCES

Dixon, W. J. (Ed.) (1975). *Biomedical Computer Programs, Los Angeles,* University of California, pp. 411–51

Downs, D. A. and Woods, J. H. (1975). *Pharmac. Rev.,* **27**, 397–406

Emrich, H. M., Cording, C., Piree, S., Kolling, A., Zerssen, D. V. and Herz, A. (1977). *Pharmakopsychiatrie,* **10**, 265–70

Fink, M., Zaks, A., Sharoff, R., Mora, A., Bruner, A., Levit, S. and Freedman, A. M. (1968). *Clin. Pharmac. Ther.,* **9**, 568–77

Goldstein, A. (1976). *Science,* **193**, 1081–6

Goldstein, A. (1977). *Archs gen. psychiat.,* **34**, 1179–80

Goldstein, A. and Hilgard, E. R. (1975). *Proc. natn. Acad. Sci. U.S.A.,* **72**, 2041–3

Grevert, P. and Goldstein, A. (1977). *Proc. natn. Acad. Sci. U.S.A.,* **74**, 1291–4

Haertzen, C. A., Meketon, M. J. and Hooks, N. T. Jr. (1970). *Br. J. Addiction,* **65**, 245–55

Hughes, J. and Kosterlitz, H. W. (1977). *Br. med. Bull.,* **33**, 157–9

Jasinski, D. R., Martin, W. R. and Haertzen, C. A. (1965). *J. Pharm. exp. Ther.,* **157**, 420–6

Kolb, L. and Himmelsbach, C. K. (1938). *Am. J. Psychiat.,* **94**, 759–79

Sadove, M. S., Balagot, R. C., Hatano, S. and Jobgen, E. A. (1963). *J. Am. Med. Assoc.,* **183**, 666–8

Wang, R. I. H., Wiesen, R. L., Lamid, S. and Rob, B. L. (1974). *Clin. Pharmac. Ther.,* **16**, 653–8

Section Three
Clinical Studies

(A) Therapeutic Use of Endorphins

45

FDA requirements for the study of endorphins

Edward C. Tocus
(Division of Neuropharmacological Drug Products, Bureau of Drugs, U.S. Food and Drug Administration, U.S.A.)

This chapter will discuss the conditions which the U.S. Food and Drug Administration (FDA) will require for the study of the endorphins in man.

The first question concerns the FDA's involvement in the first place. In the best of all possible worlds, there would be no FDA and there would be no regulations. Since this real world is far from being the best possible, the FDA does exist and Congress has required that certain conditions be met for studies in humans. The principles which have led to the FDA requirements are based on those broad principles which developed from the Nuremberg code following the Second World War. The Helsinki agreement in Finland in 1964 and, more recently, the second Helsinki agreement, which was reached in Tokyo in 1975, addressed the question of clinical research. Generally, the FDA is concerned with the pharmaceutical industry and regulating the development of drugs which will be offered to the American public for treatment of various diseases on a commercial basis. FDA is also responsible for monitoring the investigation of substances of academic interest in medicine which have not been approved for interstate commerce to ensure the scientific and ethical merits of the studies. One might argue that the endorphins are natural substances and therefore not subject to interstate commerce or to FDA regulations. This is a reasonable point of view with one major fallacy; and that is, when a reasonable point of view does not coincide with a legal requirement, the legal requirement will prevail. In this case, exogenous endorphins are proposed for administration to man and, therefore, subject to the Food and Drug Regulations. This means that an Investigational New Drug Application (IND) must be submitted and found not to present any safety problems before clinical studies can proceed.

Many investigators are familiar with the IND requirements and have submitted investigational drug applications to the FDA. Those who have submitted applications are aware of the reasons for the requirements that are imposed on the investigator on these investigations. Most investigators would agree that our requirements are in the realm of good scientific procedure and would perform similar studies without the requirements. Therefore, no additional work has been imposed other than that of filling out application forms, submitting the protocols, and preparing annual reports. With that introduction then, let us look at the real requirements.

In the area of drug research, the program may be considered in three distinct stages. The first stage is entirely devoted to chemistry. The second stage is devoted to non-human pharmacology and toxicology. The third stage is devoted to human pharmacology and toxicology. A certain amount of information must be developed in one stage before work can proceed in the next. Therefore, one must initially look at the chemistry of the material which is to be involved. The FDA requires that the material to be investigated is characterized in its chemical structure, formulation and preparation such that a reproducible material may be obtained consistently with each new procedure of preparation. Ideally, the material would be pure within the limits of existing methodology for characterizing the substance. It would be prepared in a reasonably simple pharmaceutical preparation for administration with a minimum of excipients. The complete synthesis would be known and the purity and properties of all of the materials involved in the synthesis also would be known. With this information the investigator is assured that any effects seen in biological systems are due to the active ingredient of the preparation, and not due to an impurity or some variation of the active ingredient. Perhaps most important is that the product which is prepared each time is reproducible and contains the same materials with each new batch of preparation. Unless this is so, the data generated from the material prepared may be of no value because the results could depend on an unknown substance.

The second stage is the non-human pharmacology and toxicology. It could be said that at one time pharmacology in animals was used to assay the purity of a chemical material by way of the results obtained from the drug in an animal model. Over the past 4 years, with the endorphins, we have heard much of the effects of various preparations on the mouse vas deferens and the guinea pig ileum. These model systems and the interpretation of responses in the biological system to morphine-like substances had been a classical example of developing knowledge in pharmacology. This pre-clinical pharmacology continues and will continue as new information leads to new questions and new protocols for study. When pre-clinical pharmacology studies indicate that the material under investigation has some application in understanding or in treating a human disease condition, protocols are developed for investigating the material in the human for its pharmacological effects. It is at this point that the FDA becomes involved, and the Investigational New Drug Application is necessary. Because pharmacological activity of drugs and other substances may have both beneficial and detrimental effects on the human, both aspects of the drug's activity must be determined before it is given to the human. One of the basic principles agreed upon in the Helsinki Declaration, revised in 1975, was 'Every biomedical research project involving human subjects should be preceded by careful assessment of predictable risks in comparison with forseeable benefits to the subject, or to others. Concern for the interest of the subject must always prevail over the interests of science and society'.

It is a determination of the predictable risks that the animal toxicity studies are designed to fulfill. The endorphins are in extremely short supply and are extremely expensive materials and, therefore, the toxicity data which must be generated in animals needs to be met with a minimum of expenditure of this valuable resource material.

The amount of pre-clinical or animal data necessary to support the safety of a proposed clinical protocol is primarily determined by the length of time the drug will be administered to humans. For the vast majority of Phase I clinical studies, administration of the experimental substance is restricted to a single dose. The animal data necessary to support such a protocol would consist of both acute toxicity studies and some subacute toxicity studies. The acute toxicity of the compound should be determined in three or four species, one of which should be a non-rodent, by the route to be used clinically. It is most desirable to determine acute toxicity by more than one route of administration, however, since the amount of useful information generated by this procedure is significantly increased. The subacute toxicity studies should consist of administration of the compound for 2 weeks at three dosage levels by the route to be used clinically. Two species of animals should be used, one of which is a non-rodent. At least ten rodents per sex per group should be included and at least two non-rodents per sex per dosage group. The purpose of the subacute toxicity studies is to establish a maximum tolerated dose, the toxicity profile of the compound and an estimate of the 'no-effect' dosage. During these studies the following parameters should be observed: body weights, food consumption, behavior, hematology (both pre-testing and final), clinical chemistry (pre-test and final) including urine analysis. At the conclusion of the study major organs should be examined both grossly and histopathologically. Special studies are sometimes required, depending on the nature of the individual compound. For example, for parenteral products, suitable intramuscular and/or perivascular tolerance studies and blood compatibility studies are required. Clinical testing beyond Phase I single-dose studies requires more extensive animal studies, such as reproductive and teratological studies before administration to females of childbearing age.

An FDA publication outlining the type of animal studies required to support clinical testing is available from the FDA for the asking. In addition, FDA pharmacologists are available for any investigator to consult as to the type and design of pre-clinical studies.

To some it may seem unnecessary or meaningless to perform such animal studies for compounds such as enkephalins and endorphins, since they occur endogenously. However, it must be kept in mind that other endogenous compounds have been developed as therapeutic agents and have revealed toxic effects, usually because such agents are being administered in pharmacological rather than physiological amounts. It must also be remembered that normally-occurring compounds administered by new routes may behave differently from the endogenous substance and that tissues or organs not normally exposed to these substances under physiological conditions may be exposed under clinical testing.

With the successful completion of these animal studies, the target organs most likely to be affected by excess quantities of the test material will have been determined. If excessive doses have been given to experimental animals without target organ toxicity, one may reasonably assume that the toxic profile of the drug is not sufficiently severe to prevent the early clinical studies of the drug.

It must be reiterated, however, that the animal studies precede the human studies, so that work in humans always begins from a data base which has been established in animals. Now we are ready to proceed to the human studies. In the United States human studies have been divided into three phases. Phase I includes the initial administration and clinical pharmacology studies of the drug in man; this is generally in normal, healthy, human volunteers to determine levels of tolerance and pharmacokinetics of the drug. The upper limitations of the Phase I study are evidence of undesirable side effects or effects predicted by the animal studies, such that there is assurance that no irreversible harm will be done to the human volunteers during the course of the investigations. Alternatively, with some new drugs the initial introduction into man may, ethically or scientifically, more properly be done in selected patients, thereby combining tolerance and early efficacy studies. When normal volunteers are the initial recipients of a drug, the very early trials in patients which follow are also considered part of Phase I.

The number of subjects and patients in Phase I will, of course, vary with the drug but may generally be stated to be in the range of 20-80 on drug. Drug dynamic and metabolic studies, in whichever stage of investigation they are performed, are considered to be Phase I clinical pharmacological studies. While some, such as absorption studies, are performed in the early stages, others, such as efforts to identify metabolites, may not be performed until later.

Phase II is sometimes referred to as the clinical investigating phase. During this phase the drug is given for the condition for which it is intended. An intensive study is made of the effects of the drug in the disease and on the various physiological and psychological functions of the individual with the condition. It is also during this stage that the drug may be compared either with a placebo or with an active control drug depending upon the condition being investigated. Phase II studies are generally best carried out by clinical pharmacologists or by those physicians with particular expertise in the condition which is being treated. During Phase II it is determined whether the material actually produces the desired clinical effects. During Phase II, variations of the preparation may be tested and compared in developing the final dosage form. Phase II studies are used to plan the final investigation of the drug to determine the limitations of its usefulness in treatment. This final stage is Phase III, where the drug dosage form and preparation have been completed. Generally, all animal toxicology and the effects on animal reproduction have been completed. Phase III studies are clinical trials designed to gather additional information in establishing efficacy and further evidence of safety, tolerance, and definition of the adverse effects. The drug will be used in Phase III in a manner similar to that which is proposed following marketing of the drug.

The endorphins are in the earliest phase of clinical study. With respect to the chemistry, the process of determining the proper route, the proper dosage form and the limits of the human dose has only begun. Currently there is no clear-cut therapeutic indication for the endorphins. The clinical studies are based on the assumption that endogenous material with a pharmacological profile, such as the endorphins, must serve some function in maintaining the homeostatic balance of the organism. Because endorphins exist in all species of vertebrates, it is assumed that they have a basic role in neurochemistry. It is this definitive role which the animal and human studies will determine in the next several years. It is FDA's intention to work with the investigators in this exciting new field and hope that the results generated will be beneficial to preserving the health of mankind.

46
β-Endorphin therapy in psychiatric patients

Nathan S. Kline and Heinz E. Lehmann
(Rockland Research Institute, Orangeburg, New York, U.S.A.
McGill University, Montreal, Canada)

Several years ago our interest was aroused when the effects of several polypeptides were described. In view of the fact that opiates have a long history in the folk as well as modern medical treatment of depression, the availability of opiate peptides was intriguing. Preliminary agreement was therefore reached with C. H. Li two years ago that when synthesized and purified in adequate quantities, we would have the opportunity of evaluating the therapeutic action of the opiate peptides. In June of this year we administered small doses of β-endorphin to the first five patients. Patients were selected on the following criteria

(1) Severity of illness;
(2) Failure of extensive previous treatment.

We also sought

(3) Typicality;
(4) Variety of diagnosis (as far as possible);
(5) Patients well known to the investigators.

We were presented with an unusual problem of experimental design since the supply of material was so limited; we had less than 250 mg. Since we started with very small doses in view of the fact that this was the first administration to psychiatric patients, we were able to give a total of 42 injections. Clinical responses appeared in a few patients at the initial 1.5 mg dose and, later in a few patients, we noticed no great difference between the 6 mg and 9 mg dose. Therefore we settled somewhat arbitrarily on 10 mg as the upper limit for our clinical trials (table 46.1). It would be of great interest to learn the action of higher doses. If the cataleptic animal responses obtained by Bloom *et al.* (1976) are indicative of the toxicity level, there is an enormous margin of safety since the dose in human equivalent by body weight would have been well over 1,000 mg.

Table 46.1

Diagnosis	No. of patients	Doses of endorphin	Dose range (mg)
Schizophrenics	4	15	1.5–9
Depression	2	4	1.8–9
Anxiety disorder (agoraphobia)	2	7	0.5–5
Obsessive-compulsive	1	4	6–9
Personality disorder (affective)	3	7	1–9
Mental deficiency	1	1	2
Autism	1	2	5–10
Control	1	2	9
	15	42	

Decisions as to whether treatment was indicated on a particular day and, if so, at what dose level were made on the basis of the patient's clinical report and appearance, in a typically clinical fashion since the patient's therapeutic welfare was the primary basis of decision. The stereotyped 'pre-packaged' experimental design would have been totally unsuitable. As will be discussed subsequently, had we not reverted to the earlier traditional methods of clinical investigation, we would probably have missed the unexpected sequence of responses. Our emphasis on prolonged careful observation, aided by review of videotape recordings, allowed us to avoid the restrictions and preconceptions which are ordinarily built into such a design.

In hypothesis-forming investigations, when the trial substance is limited and its effects unknown, the single-blind placebo control, in our opinion, is the most appropriate. Most patients were first given placebo. A questionable placebo-response was reported in only one patient and, interestingly, he was one of the few who showed no therapeutic response. In the case of the control subject (Dr Laski), we assumed that he might deduce that we would give placebo and follow this with active substance. We gave a placebo, followed by another placebo, followed by the active material.

We have started double-blind studies which will not be discussed here.

As control substances, in addition to placebo, we administered i.v. sodium amytal to two of the three patients who showed no response and obtained typical barbiturate effects. The control subject was given i.v. morphine; one patient who was experienced in the effects of cannabis was able to draw a comparison. In preparation for possible adverse effects, we had prepared an emergency syringe already loaded with naloxone and ready for use with each patient on each treatment occasion. Ironically, it would appear that the naloxone would have been useless since on the half dozen occasions when we deliberately tried to terminate the response which followed β-endorphin administration, naloxone was without effect except in one case where its action was questionable and of minor significance, possibly reducing sleepinesss; possibly the 0.4-mg dose was too low.

One anticipated factor which was confirmed early on was the relevance of concomitant administration of major antipsychotic drugs. In general, the schizophrenics responded much more favorably to β-endorphin when the major tranquilizers were discontinued. Surprisingly this has held true even when the antipsychotic drugs were stopped after the β-endorphin had been given. We would obviously recommend stricter control of this variable in future studies. since at times patients show temporary improvement following withdrawal of medication.

In view of the limited supply of material available for human use both at present and probably in the near future, we feel it is important that all of us working with patients share our experiences as rapidly as possible.

GENERAL EFFECTS OF i.v. β-ENDORPHIN IN HUMAN SUBJECTS

Although we cannot yet describe the general characteristics of β-endorphin administration to human subjects with all desirable and reproducible precision, we have observed the following features up till now

(1) *Immediate effects* that manifest themselves as symptoms of the autonomic nervous system (for example, dry mouth or flushing) or as paresthesias (for example, tingling sensations). They appear within a few seconds and last for 1 or 2 min.

(2) *Delayed effects* which may be differentiated into three phases

Phase I may be described as *antidysphoric* in nature. It produces activated and disinhibited behavior and is associated with anxiolytic, antidepressant and mildly analgesic effects. It occurs within 5-10 min and lasts from 1-6 hours.

Phase II is *inhibitory* in nature. It is characterized by sedation, drowsiness, perplexity and impaired concentration. It may occur after 1–4 hours and last from 2 to 3 hours.

Table 46.2 Effects of intravenous administration of β-endorphin

Immediate	Autonomic affects and paresthesias
Onset	2–30 s
Duration	30–120 s
Delayed	
Phase I	Antidysphoric (activating; disinhibiting; anxiolytic; antidepressant)
Onset	5–10 min
Duration	1–6 h
Phase II	Inhibitory (sedation; drowsiness; perplexity; impairment of cognitive processes)
Onset	2–4 h
Duration	2–3 h
Phase III	Therapeutic (disappearance or attenuation of symptoms: for example, hallucinations, delusions, depression, anxiety, compulsive rituals; return of lost personality features; gaining of insight)
Onset	1–5 d
Duration	1–10 d or longer

Phase III is characterized by *therapeutic* action. A psychiatric patient may experience loss or attenuation of psychotic as well as neurotic symptoms (for example, hallucinations, delusions, anxiety, depression or compulsive rituals), and may show return of insight and of long-lost features of his old, healthy personality. This phase may be observed within 1-5 days following the injection and may last from 1 to 10 days or longer (table 46.2).

CASE HISTORIES

The following are brief descriptions of 14 psychiatric patients who have received β-endorphin treatment. One volunteer subject, a graduate pharmacologist and psychiatrist, has also been given β-endorphin injections on two occasions.

Case 1

This 59-year-old man had unipolar depression. He had had three depressive episodes since 1955, for which he was treated with psychotherapy, electroconvulsive therapy (ECT), and pharmacotherapy, before entering treatment with one of us in 1968. He had been working as a businessman, but at the age of 42 he decided to go into medicine and graduated at a foreign university in 1966. Later, against our advice, he entered a psychiatric residency in the United States, which he completed in 1971. However, the final evaluation of the training center's director stated that 'it seems impossible for him to function in any type of situation which would require decision under pressure'. He was marginally responsive to various antidepressant medications until 1 year ago. Since that time, he has been continuously depressed and unable to work, complaining of severe insomnia and spending many hours in bed during the day.

Case 2

This man, aged 34, had chronic paranoid schizophrenia. His mental disorder began at age 16 when he was hospitalized for symptoms of acute agitation, manneristic and uncooperative behavior, rambling, incoherent speech, severe thought disorder, and lack of insight. He was repeatedly hospitalized and treated with insulin coma and several courses of ECT until the age of 26 when he began treatment with us. He has received various antipsychotic drugs and he can now manage in the community where he lives with his mother. Pleasant and cooperative, with fair insight, he exhibits moderate thinking disorder, occasional bouts of anxiety, and continual auditory hallucinations. He is unable to work.

Case 3

This man, aged 35, had chronic schizophrenia (undifferentiated). His first breakdown occurred at age 22, and he was hospitalized on several occasions for as long as 1 year at a time. He was treated extensively with psychotherapy and antipsychotic drugs for ideas of reference, preoccupation with homosexuality, attacks of severe anxiety and panic, inability to concentrate, and frequent auditory hallucinations. In treatment with us since 1967–and under continuous antipsychotic pharmacotherapy–he is able to live with his parents (but not alone) and functions as a part-time gardener for a local church.

Case 4

This 41-year-old man was diagnosed as having chronic paranoid schizophrenia. There was good personality functioning until age 16 when he became careless, indifferent and inefficient. At age 18, he was admitted to a psychiatric hospital for a period of 10 months and thereafter was hospitalized for years in at least seven different psychiatric facilities, receiving the full range of psychiatric treatments, for example, psychotherapy, insulin coma, ECT, and antipsychotic pharmacotherapy. His course has been stormy and his behavior on occasion violent. Since 1966, he has been treated by us and now receives a recent antipsychotic drug (clozapine). For the past 3 years he has lived with his mother, holding a steady, responsible job. His social life is defective, his emotional response inadequate, and he still has almost continuous auditory hallucinations, which he considers 'a nuisance'.

Case 5

This 63-year-old man has recurrent unipolar depression. His first depressive episode, for which he was not treated, occurred at age 33 and lasted a year. In 1975, he again became depressed and attempted suicide (overdose); he was treated with ECT and subsequently improved for 6 months. In 1976, he relapsed and has since been continuously depressed with symptoms of severe dejection, psychomotor retardation, indecisiveness, insomnia, hopelessness, and suicidal ideation. He has been unresponsive to recent treatment with antidepressant drugs. Under treatment by us for only a few days, the patient is now hospitalized.

Case 6

This man, aged 65, was diagnosed as having bipolar affective disorder (depressed). His illness began at age 49 after a divorce from his first wife by whom he had two sons. He remarried 2 years later. Since then, he has had at least yearly attacks of depression or mania. During free intervals, he functions as a successful lawyer, publishes his work in law journals, and has a satisfactory social life. He has been treated by us since 1964 and has received lithium carbonate treatment since 1966. His current depression began 2 months ago. He is receiving antidepressant drug treatment to which he has not yet responded. At present, he is unable to work, has no initiative, has depressive ruminations, suicidal thoughts, and attacks of panic.

Case 7

This 24-year-old, single man has been diagnosed as suffering from schizophrenia, catatonic type. Two years ago, while attending college, he was in a car accident where the driver was killed. Since then, the patient has complained that a computer is controlling him. He has had auditory hallucinations and thought insertion. Always a loner, he is now completely withdrawn. His only activity consists of watching television. Most of the time, he is mute and unresponsive and sits motionlessly, one hand held over his mouth. His face is blank. Previous treatment includes various neuroleptic and antiparkinsonism drugs.

Case 8

This 36-year-old married man, with two children, has been diagnosed as suffering from an anxiety disorder, mainly agoraphobia. He works as an accountant. Ten years ago, while in a parade, he suddenly felt 'lousy' and has never felt well since then. He has 'passed out' twice and was once hospitalized for this. All physical tests were negative. He complains of anxiety, nervousness, difficulty with concentration, inability to be as sociable as he used to be, constant worries about job and money. Appetite and sex life are not impaired but he sleeps poorly. His chief complaints are his panicky feelings in crowds and in all public places. For instance, he is unable to go to train stations or to go shopping in large stores because he becomes panicky and is afraid of passing out. Previous treatment includes megavitamin and thyroid treatment, tryptophan and pharmacotherapy with anxiolytic as well as tricyclic antidepressant drugs and stimulants, for example Ritalin.

Case 9

This 45-year-old woman has been diagnosed as suffering from anxiety neurosis and agoraphobia. She has been twice married and has an adopted daughter. For some 15 years she has had severe anxiety, can never be at home or go out alone, is unable to make decisions, is often depressed and sometimes thinks of suicide. She has no energy and often is unable to perform her household duties. After a brief remission she relapsed again 2 years ago and since then has had only minimal relief from medication. Previous treatments include intensive psychotherapy and pharmacotherapy with anxiolytic, neuroleptic and antidepressant drugs, including MAO inhibitors and Dexamyl.

Case 10

This 32-year-old, single man has been diagnosed as suffering from an obsessive-compulsive neurosis. He is college-educated and for some time worked as an auditor in a bank, then as a driver on an airport-shuttle service and finally had to give up all work. Compulsive even as a child, his symptoms began to seriously interfere with his life at age 18. He felt 'caught in a web' from which he could not free himself. At times, he is almost helpless. Some ordinary 5 min routines might take him hours or days to complete. Some days, he cannot even open a letter. Recently, it took him 16 hours, spent over 4 days, to arrange for payment of a monthly electricity bill. Often, he cannot take a bath because of the need for cleaning the tub. Sometimes he sleeps on the floor, afraid to disarrange the pillows on the bed. He lives alone but depends on his parents for continuous help with ordinary life activities. Occasionally, he becomes extremely tense and irritable. Once, in an outburst of rage, he pushed his father, causing him to break his arm. His mother is a compulsive person who has suffered from depression. The patient has previously been treated by three other psychiatrists with psychotherapy and with the following drugs: Dilantin, Valium, Mellaril, Taractan, Artane, Cogentin, Benadryl, Triavil, Marplan, Nardil and lithium. He has been twice hospitalized for this condition.

Case 11

This 15-year-old, severely retarded girl was diagnosed at $3\frac{1}{2}$ years of age as an autistic child. She was toilet-trained at age 3, dressed at age 6 and learned to speak single words at age 5. She still does not speak in sentences. Until the age of 12 she attended a special school for the emotionally disabled. During the last year she regressed and now requires constant reminding for feeding, toileting and so on. She is not unfriendly, cooperative, but has little eye contact and displays many mannerisms, such as rocking, slapping her thigh and face, biting her hand. She can carry out simple instructions and write her name, but is unable to hold a conversation. Her speech consists of single words with much echolalia and perseveration. Previous treatment includes special psychosocial remedial measures and pharmacotherapy with neuroleptics and antiparkinsonism drugs.

Case 12

Normal volunteer.

Case 13

This 30-year-old married woman, with one child, has been diagnosed as suffering from a neurotic depressive personality disorder. Her father was an alcoholic. The patient has been depressed and angry for the last 6 years, frequently thinking of suicide. '. . . indifferent toward life and not being myself, even when I am not severely depressed', she complains of irritability, disgust and lack of interest even in her daughter. Off and on, she has had colitis. Her husband is supportive. She has been in intensive psychotherapy for 2 years. She was hospitalized in 1972 for this condition. Her pharmacotherapy which has been unsuccessful until now, includes Valium and other antianxiety agents, for example, Seconal, several tricyclic and antidepressant drugs, an MAO-inhibitor and lithium.

Case 14

This 24-year-old, single man, is a college student. He has been diagnosed as suffering from a depressive personality disorder. His depression developed at age 14 when he was experimenting with a variety of street drugs, including hard drugs and hallucinogens. There is a family history of depression in the maternal grandfather and an aunt. The patient complains of lack of ambition, anhedonia, difficulty in concentration and decision making. He is tired all the time, has difficulty falling asleep or sleeps all the time. With effort, he can socialize, but he says that all his feelings are numbed. He has not much interest in sex. Previous treatment includes several years of individual and group psychotherapy as well as pharmacotherapy with four different tricyclic and three MAO inhibitor antidepressants, alone and in combination; also tryptophan and Ritalin.

Case 15

This is an unmarried young man, 18 years of age. In early childhood he was diagnosed as suffering from autism. Motor development was fairly normal, speech development delayed. He never went to regular school, but has attended a special school for the last 6 years. He is tall, cooperative, but one has difficulty in obtaining and holding his attention. His speech displays a surprisingly good vocabulary but is uttered in a loud, abrupt and very manneristic way. He also displays various motor mannerisms. He can draw at the level of an 8-year-old, tends to perseverate and likes to fill in empty spaces with solid shading. He relies almost completely on his parents' guidance and instructions and, being very distractible, he tends frequently to become inappropriate in his behavior. There is no family history of psychiatric disorder.

INDIVIDUAL EFFECTS OF INTRAVENOUSLY ADMINISTERED β-ENDORPHIN IN 15 HUMAN SUBJECTS

Our limited sample of psychiatric patients, belonging to seven different diagnostic categories, does not enable us to make a statistical evaluation of our observations. However, there were differences in β-endorphin effects in different patients and in the control subject. These can probably best be described in the following individual tabulation of observations for each patient, arranged according to his or her diagnostic category (table 46.3).

RADIOIMMUNOASSAY (RIA) RESULTS

Blood samples were collected by means of a butterfly valve in a vein in the antecubital fossa. The samples were collected pre-injection and 15, 30, 45, 60, 90 and 120 min post-injection. These samples were immediately placed in ice water and kept in the cold until centrifuged (refrigerated centrifuge) and the plasma frozen.

The antisera and pure β-endorphin were kindly supplied by Dr C. H. Li. Pure β-endorphin was iodinated using an enzymatic (lactoperoxidase) procedure as described by Aubert *et al.* (1974). Iodinated β-endorphin was separated by column chromatography on a 60 × 0.6 cm column containing Sephadex G-25 in 0.1 M acetic acid containing 0.25% bovine serum albumen. The RIA procedure used was essentially that of Li *et al.* (1977). In our hands the antisera at a final dilution of 1/5000 gave a curve with half maximal displacement at 2–300 pg and a usable range of 100 pg to 5 ng.

We have six subject experiments in which single bolus injections of 3 to 9 mg β-endorphin were given. These data were readily fitted with a single exponent and the half-life of elimination calculated from these data had a mean of 19.6 min (range 12–35 min).

Table 46.3 Effects of β-endorphin

Diagnosis	Patient no.	Dose and date	Autonomic effects	Changes in mood, cognition, perception, behavior Phase I	Phase II	Phase III
Schizophrenia (undifferentiated)	2	1.5 mg (6/29/77)	Feeling of heat in mouth	More talkative; thought disorder increased	–	–
		3 mg (7/12/77)	Dry mouth; feeling of heat in mouth	More talkative; thought disorder increased; hallucinations diminished (?)	–	Hallucinations diminished; behavior more appropriate
		6 mg (7/21/77)	Feeling of heat in mouth; dry mouth; numbness in mouth	More talkative; hallucinations diminished (?)	Reports feeling more tired; improved after Naloxone (?)	Hallucinations diminished; behavior more appropriate; brighter, improved appearance. Markedly improved. Had 'two heavenly days without voices'.
		6 mg (11/17/77)	'Acidity' in stomach	Grandiose, talkative, smiling, marked thought disorder	–	–

Schizophrenia (paranoid)	4	1.5 mg (6/29/77)	–	More irritable; thought disorder increased	–	–
		3 mg (7/12/77)	–	More irritable; thought disorder increased; hallucinations diminished (?)	–	–
		6 mg (7/21/77)	–	More friendly; hallucinations diminished	–	More active; less withdrawn
Schizophrenia (catatonic)	7	9 mg (8/11/77)	–	–	–	–
		9 mg (9/21/77)	–	–	–	–
Schizophrenia (schizoaffective)	3	1.5 mg (6/29/77)	–	Slightly elated	–	Fewer anxiety attacks
		3 mg (7/12/77)	Dry mouth	More energetic; talks faster; feels 'like after amphetamine'.	Tiredness; terminated by naloxone	Paranoid delusions gone; gaining better insight
		6 mg (7/21/77)	Dry mouth	Mildly elated; talkative	Tired	Schizophrenic symptoms replaced by depression (of insight?); stopped working
		9 mg (8/11/77)	Dry mouth	More talkative; less depressed	Tired	Less depressed; long suppressed personality features return; for example, sense of humor; resumed working

Table 46.3 (Continued)

Diagnosis	Patient no.	Dose and date	Autonomic effects	Changes in mood, cognition, perception, behavior Phase I	Phase II	Phase III
		6 mg (10/17/77)	Dry mouth	More talkative Still increased pressure of speech		Working through his problems, but indulges in 'too much day-dreaming'. Has come to terms with his problems. No paranoid symptoms, panic or depression. Works regularly. Makes plans for future. More sensitive; seeking personal contact
		3 mg (11/3/77)	Dry mouth	More talkative; elated	–	
Depression (Unipolar)	5	1.8 mg (6/29/77)	Dry mouth	Marked activation; less depressed	Drowsy	–
		9 mg (7/21/77)	Dry mouth	Marked activation; less depressed; able to smile; increased spontaneity	Drowsy	–
Depression (bipolar)	6	9 mg (7/12/77)	Dry mouth; warmth in neck	Increased spontaneity; panic gone; guilt and suicidal urges diminished	–	–

		9 mg (7/21/77)	Dry mouth; warmth in neck	Increased spontaneity; no panic; guilt and suicidal urges diminished	–	–
Anxiety disorder (agoraphobia)	8	1 mg (9/9/77)	–	–	–	'Pressure in head relieved'; sexually more active
		6 mg (10/6/77)	'Burning' in back of neck; facial flush	More talkative; joking	–	'Felt great'. Concentrates better. 'Loosening up'. No agoraphobia. Sociable
		3 mg (10/13/77)	'Burning' in neck	More talkative mildly elated	–	Wife states: '...for 10 days he was just like 10 years ago–then the bottom fell out'.
		5 mg (11/3/77)	'Burning' in neck	Mildly elated	–	'About 5 days after each injection I felt much better for about a week; but I have difficulty sleeping'
		6 mg (11/17/77)	'Burning' in neck, facial flush, tongue tingling	Mild elation	–	–

Table 46.3 (Continued)

Diagnosis	Patient no.	Dose and date	Autonomic effects	Changes in mood, cognition, perception, behavior Phase I	Phase II	Phase III
Anxiety disorder (Agorophobia)	9	1 mg (9/27/77)	–	Feeling 'high; like an amphetamine high'; able to cross street alone	–	All week much calmer; more courage; could make decisions she could not before
		0.5 mg (10/6/77)	–	Continues to feel 'high'	–	Continues to feel much better than in the past in spite of unusual stress in her environment; is more assertive
Obsessive-compulsive	10	9 mg (9/15/77)	Numb feeling in cheek; facial flush	Looks brighter, smiles	–	During next 2 weeks had three unusually good days, but also some that were worse than before
		6 mg (10/6/77)	Numb feeling and facial flush	Talkative	–	Had 'best day in years'; did routine easily he could not do before
		6 mg (10/13/77)	Numb mouth; facial flush	Smiling; but more tense	–	More active and 'more himself', but also more anxious and much more irritable

		6 mg (11/3/77)	Numbness in face	More talkative; tense	–	'One of the best weeks in the last 2 years, felt peaceful and cheerful; irritability and tension gone; daily routines take half the time; less stubborn; dreams much more; spends much time reminiscing; plans future
Personality disorder (affective)	1	1.5 mg (6/29/77)	–	Slight, questionable activation	–	–
		3 mg (7/12/77)	–	–	–	–
Personality disorder (affective)	14	6 mg (10/13/77)	Tingling sensation of heat in neck	Feeling better, 'eased up'; depression 'muted', like novocain on the brain	–	Slightly improved for a week
		9 mg (11/3/77)	Tingling, numbness, warm sensation all over	Feels much better but only 'as though the depression is just covered up'.	–	Not feeling better than when on drugs not as 'feverish' but relative wellbeing. Symptoms 'muted', lasts a few days

Table 46.3 (Continued)

Diagnosis	Patient no.	Dose and date	Autonomic effects	Changes in mood, cognition, perception, behavior Phase I	Phase II	Phase III
		9 mg (11/17/77)	Tingling and numbness	Short 'rush' which gradually decreased. Feeling relaxed, less distressed, smiling but 'not much hope for future'.	—	Relative wellbeing. Slight improvement which lasted a few days. 'Like smoking pot but without anxiety which I usually feel'
Personality disorder	13	1 mg (9/29/77)	—	No subjective change, but appeared more relaxed, and lively	—	—
		6 mg (10/6/77)	—	No subjective change, but appeared more relaxed and lively	—	—

Mental deficiency	11	2 mg (9/15/77)	–	–	–	–
Autism	15	5 mg (11/29/77)	Marked facial flushes	Quieter speech and behavior, less manneristic	Drowsiness	Quieter, more controlled
		10 mg (12/8/77)	Marked facial flushes	Friendlier, more talkative, better organized	–	–
Control	12	9 mg (7/21/77)	Dry mouth	–	Drowsy, slowed, perplexed, impaired concentration. Naloxone: no effect	–
		9 mg (8/11/77)	Dry mouth	–	Drowsy, slowed, impaired concentration. Naloxone: immediate unpleasant effects, that is, nausea, tingling–lasting 2–3 min; no effect on drowsiness	

Preliminary attempts to measure endogenous levels of β-endorphin in the above patients have not proved successful, indicating that in man endogenous levels, if present, are in the pg/ml range.

DISCUSSION

At this point our study is still in an early exploratory stage, and it is difficult to construct a comprehensive theoretical model for the observed action of β-endorphin in its various phases, nor are there enough observational data patterns to formulate distinct hypotheses to be tested.

In a first approximation to a summary of our observations, one may state that in the 42 injections, the various reactions to β-endorphin were observed in the following order of frequency

Phase I (antidysphoric)–35 times
Phase III (therapeutic)–27 times
Autonomic reactions–27 times
Phase II (inhibitory)–9 times

In the control subject the only observed reaction was the inhibitory phase II on the two occasions when he received β-endorphin. The most pronounced and sustained therapeutic effects (phase III) were seen in the schizo-affective and the undifferentiated schizophrenics, in the two agoraphobic and in the (one) obsessive-compulsive patients. Transient improvement (phase I) only was observed in the two depressed patients. No or insignificant improvement occurred in the catatonic and the paranoid schizophrenic, in the autistic, the mentally retarded and in two of the three personality disorder patients.

The outline of a pattern seems to manifest itself in that the best therapeutic results were observed in patients complaining of distinct neurotic or psychotic anxiety, while patients whose main symptoms were anger and hostility or who had settled into a rigid, unprotesting behavior pattern failed to respond.

It is interesting that the mute and negativistic catatonic patient who showed no reaction to β-endorphin responded, nevertheless, in the typical, dramatic fashion to the disinhibiting action of i.v. amobarbital, thus demonstrating that the mechanism—and probably also the site—of action is different for β-endorphin and amobarbital. One patient described the phase I effect of β-endorphin as similar to his experience with cannabis, but without the anxiety that he personally always feels when he smokes marijuana. Finally, the control subject was given morphine i.v. on two occasions and found these experiences to be different from those after β-endorphin.

Thus, β-endorphin causes behavioral and experimental reactions that may differ distinctly from those produced by i.v. amobarbital, inhaled cannabis and i.v. morphine. Only future investigations can reveal whether different fragments of β-endorphin are responsible for the spectrum of its effects and for the time lag between them. If the intriguing therapeutic phase III can be confirmed in future studies, indirect and complex action mechanisms—possibly involving negative feedback processes—must be considered for its explanation.

REFERENCES

Aubert, M. L., Grumbach, M. M. and Kaplan, S. L. (1974). *Acta Endocr.*, 77, 460–76
Bloom, F., Segal, D., Ling, N. and Guillemin, R. (1976). *Science,* **194**, 630–2
Li, C. H., Jagannadha Rao, A., Doneen, B. A. and Yamashiro D. (1977). *Biochem. biophys. Res. Commun.*, 71, 576–80

47

Preliminary results of treatment with β-endorphin in depression

J. Angst, V. Autenrieth, F. Brem, M. Koukkou, H. Meyer,
H. H. Stassen and U. Storck
(Research Department, Psychiatric University Clinic, Zurich,
PO Box 68, CH-8029 Zurich, Switzerland)

In the summer of 1977, N. S. Kline and H. E. Lehmann reported their first results with synthetic β-endorphin in psychiatric patients (Kline *et al.*, 1977). They put at our disposal trial material for six injections and, on the basis of their own findings, advised us to look at possible antidepressive effects during the first hours after the injection. We decided to treat six hospitalized depressive female patients, and we took special care to choose patients whose symptoms had been stable for at least 8 days, so that a sudden change would be noticed immediately. The question was whether a change of the depressive state would occur during the 5 hours after i.v. injection and whether a mania or hypomania could be induced. In addition, we wanted to examine possible changes in body temperature, blood pressure, pulse rate and EEG.

METHODOLOGY

Sample

Six female patients each received 10 mg of synthetic β-endorphin in a single dose, which was slowly injected i.v. during 5 min; four patients (1–4) were bipolar, two were unipolar depressives (cases 5 + 6). Their average age was 45.5 ± 8.3 years (range 34 to 56).

Interruption of previous medication

In all cases, antidepressive medication was stopped at least 3 days before the trial injection. In four cases the last sleep medication was given 48 hours before β-endorphin; in two cases, 12 hours before the injection. In these circumstances, an interaction with psychotropic drugs cannot be excluded, since it is well known that they remain in the body for a long time. For ethical reasons we could not interrupt medication for longer.

Schedule of investigation

All data were collected in the morning within 5 hours and 15 min, at seven examinations: before the injection, and 30, 60, 120, 180, 240 and 300 min after the injection. Thus, the patients were closely observed for more than 5 hours. In each examination, the following variables were measured: body temperature, systolic and diastolic blood pressure in sitting position, pulse rate, and from both hemispheres, temporo-parietal and parieto-occipital EEG. The EEG was analysed for 2 min with eyes closed, then 1 min with eyes open, and then again 2 min with eyes closed. In addition, the examiner rated the depressive state using a global rating scale (1 to 6). The patient also rated his subjective condition on seven different analogue scales (0–100) at each examination. The items were: body feeling; inner unrest; anxiety; feeling of illness; general feeling; energy; mood. Furthermore the patient filled out a questionnaire with 15 items, which were taken partly from the scale of ZUNG with graduations from 0–3 (no, questionable, yes, pronounced).

The clinical examination was completed with a neurological examination which included reflexes, pyramidal signs, muscle tone, gait, posture, tremor, diadochokinesis, ocular motor control, pupillary reactions, corneal reflexes, and senory functions (touch, position, temperature, pain). All measurements were made once before β-endorphin injection and six times after the application, as described above.

Setting

All examinations were conducted in an air-conditioned EEG recording chamber. The patients reclined during the injection, then they were permitted to move. They sat down at a table to fill out the questionnaires and they lay down for the EEG recordings. Between examinations they would walk freely to their rooms to lunch, and to do some needlework.

Analysis of the data

The EEG data from both channels of both hemispheres were screened as paper records, and were analysed into power spectra during the 1 min before and the 1 min after eye opening, using a Fourier transformation. For technical details see table 47.1. The spectra were averaged over subjects for each channel and each examination. In this preliminary evaluation, we shall consider some results in the alpha band and slow beta band. For both bands we computed the power(s), and the power distribution and symmetry of band.

The other data were transferred to punch cards and analysed using the university computing system. The small sample ($N = 6$) permits only a tentative evaluation, and possibly hypotheses. In spite of the small sample and in order to survey the data, we computed a one-way analysis of variances for repeated measurements.

Table 47.1 Technical characteristics of the EEG analysis

Patients	6	
Time series	640 × 32 s	
Digitizing	256 Hz	
α-band	7.5 – 12.5 Hz	
β_1-band	12.5 – 22.5 Hz	
Channels	4 (temp/par, par/occ left and right)	
Accuracy	0.25 Hz	
Parameters	$P = \int_{\alpha_1}^{\alpha_2} p(\omega)d\omega$	power/s
	$-1 \leqslant S \leqslant +1$	power-distribution and symmetry of band

RESULTS

Psychopathology

Changes in subjective state, such as inner unrest, anxiety, feeling of illness, energy, emotion, were measured with the aid of the analogue self-rating scales and then assembled to a total score. Since the average score of the six cases provided little

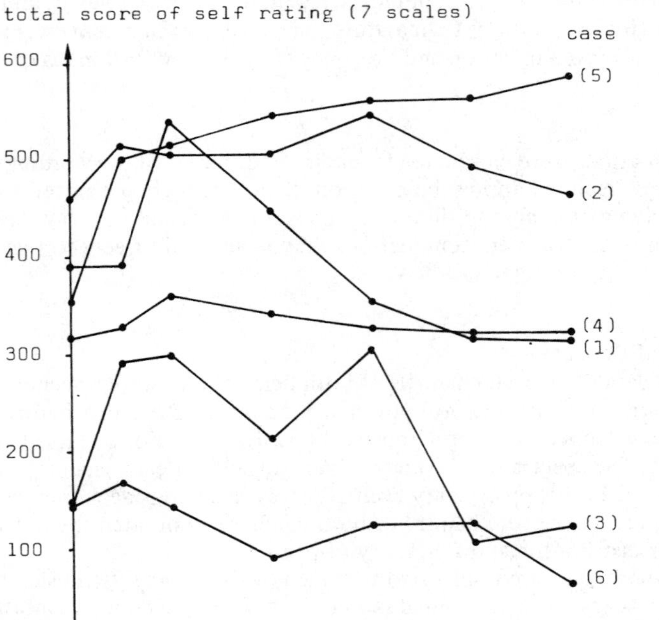

Figure 47.1 Individual self-rating scores of six patients.

effective information, we show individual curves with each patients' total score (figure 47.1). The individual curves demonstrate that during the first hour all six patients showed increased scores: in general, the score decreased during the following hour. Improvement persisted only in one case (case 5). The other five cases showed a smaller or equal score at the end of the observation period than before the injection.

The seven subjective items measured by analogue scales from 0 to 100 were also analysed separately. Item 1 (body feeling) and item 4 (feeling of illness) did not show a substantial change during the trial. The other five items showed a trend to an improvement (that is, inner unrest, anxiety, general feeling, energy, mood'). As an example, figure 47.2 shows the individual scores of each patient for the item 'energy'. It is evident that within the first 30 min there was a marked increase of energy in most cases followed by a marked decrease at the end of the trial in four cases; two patients remained at an increased score. A similar change was found in the other items mentioned above. The other self-rating scale (a modified version of the ZUNG-scale including some additional items) did not show a substantial change (table 47.2). On the other hand the doctor's global rating showed some improvement after 2, 3 and 4 hours of the trial and a relapse at the end (table 47.2).

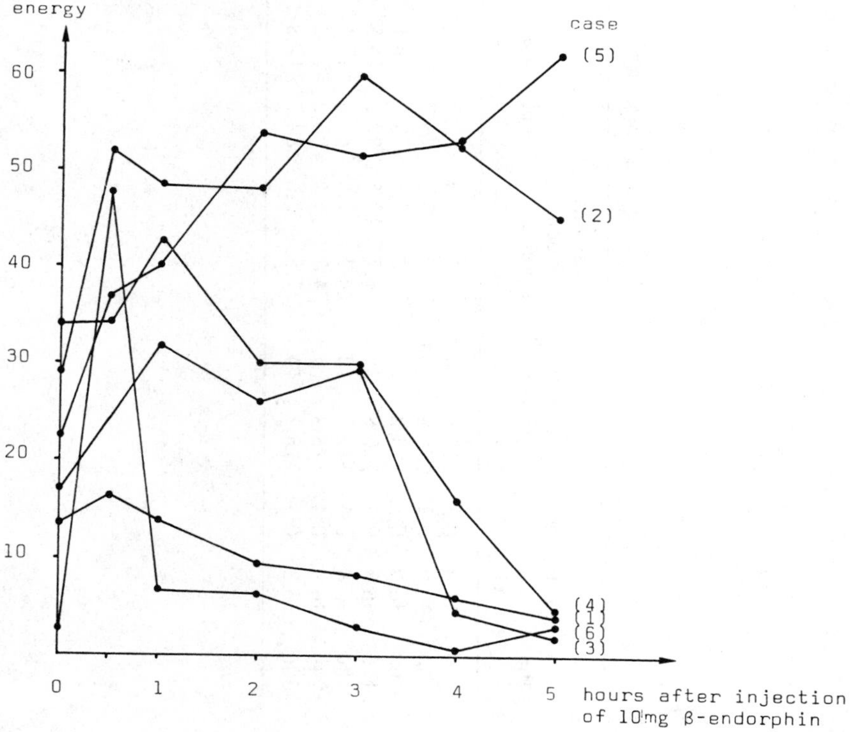

Figure 47.2 Self-rating of energy of six patients.

Table 47.2 Measurements

Min	Temperature		Systolic blood pressure		Diastolic blood pressure		Pulse rate		Total self-rating score		'ZUNG-modification'		Physician's rating	
	$\bar{x}$	s	$\bar{x}$	s	$\bar{x}$	s	$\bar{x}$	s	$\bar{x}$	s	$\bar{x}$	s	$\bar{x}$	s
0	36.9	0.3	117.5	24.4	78.3	12.9	87.0	18.8	301.8	131.1	22.3	4.4	4.2	1.0
30	36.9	0.3	125.8	24.0	76.7	13.3	76.7	7.9	365.3	131.5	20.5	5.2	4.2	1.0
60	36.9	0.1	114.2	22.2	75.8	12.8	79.7	18.1	393.7	156.3	19.2	6.7	4.0	1.1
120	36.8	0.5	120.8	25.2	76.7	12.5	82.0	14.5	356.4	177.8	20.5	6.5	3.8	1.3
180	36.8	0.4	112.5	12.5	74.2	11.6	84.0	9.1	371.5	157.0	20.3	5.0	3.8	1.3
240	36.9	0.4	115.8	9.1	74.2	11.1	84.0	16.2	323.3	181.2	22.0	6.7	3.8	1.7
300	36.8	0.5	118.3	14.7	77.5	7.6	84.7	17.8	308.7	198.6	21.7	5.0	4.2	1.3

Switch into hypomania

In three of the six cases a switch into hypomania or mania was observed during or after the trial. In one case (case 3), the change seemed to be induced by the sleep deprivation (provoked by the withdrawal of a hypnotic) before the trial. This patient remained for a few days in a dysphoric hypomanic state and relapsed after that into a depression again. In a second case (case 5), a unipolar depressed patient, there was a clear hypomanic state, developing in the afternoon and evening after the injection and followed by a relapse into depression the next day. This patient was euphoric, talkative and overactive. A third patient (case 4) suffering from a bipolar disorder, switched the day after the trial definitively into a manic episode that required haloperidol treatment for a few weeks. The fact that in three of the six cases a switch into hypomania or mania was observed is of some interest but should not be overinterpreted. Despite the effect of the injection of β-endorphin, other factors may also be involved such as poor sleep during the night before the experiment, withdrawal of previous medication, and stress induced by the whole experiment.

Somatic findings

The neurological examinations showed no major changes. Body temperature and systolic and diastolic blood pressure remained constant during the whole observation period of 5 hours (table 47.2). The pulse rate decreased in the first 30 min from 87 to 77 pulses per s on the average, and then increased again to the previous rate.

Side effects

Despite the lowering of the pulse rate within the first 30 min described above, there were no clear side effects. The decrease of the pulse rate could also be explained by the relaxation of the patients after the injection. Neurological side effects were not observed. Two patients have to be mentioned individually. One patient (case 4) has suffered for years from stenocardiac attacks. Ten minutes after the injection such an attack reappeared and was improved by one capsule of nitroglycerine. Monitoring of the ECG did not show any new changes. Since the patient had not slept the night before (because we had omitted a sleep medication) this factor could also have contributed to the development of a new attack. In a second case (case 6) the patient experienced pains during the injection, first in the stomach, then at the left side of the neck. The ECG was normal. Pains were changing and also reproducible by an injection of physiological solution of NaCl. In this case the pains were psychosomatic because they had been observed the days before and after the trial.

EEG data

Conventional visual analysis of the EEG showed no systematic changes of the background activity during the repeated examinations. There were no epileptic discharges, and no asymmetries. The spectral analysis showed basically similar changes over time in both frequency bands, and all four channels (figures 47.3

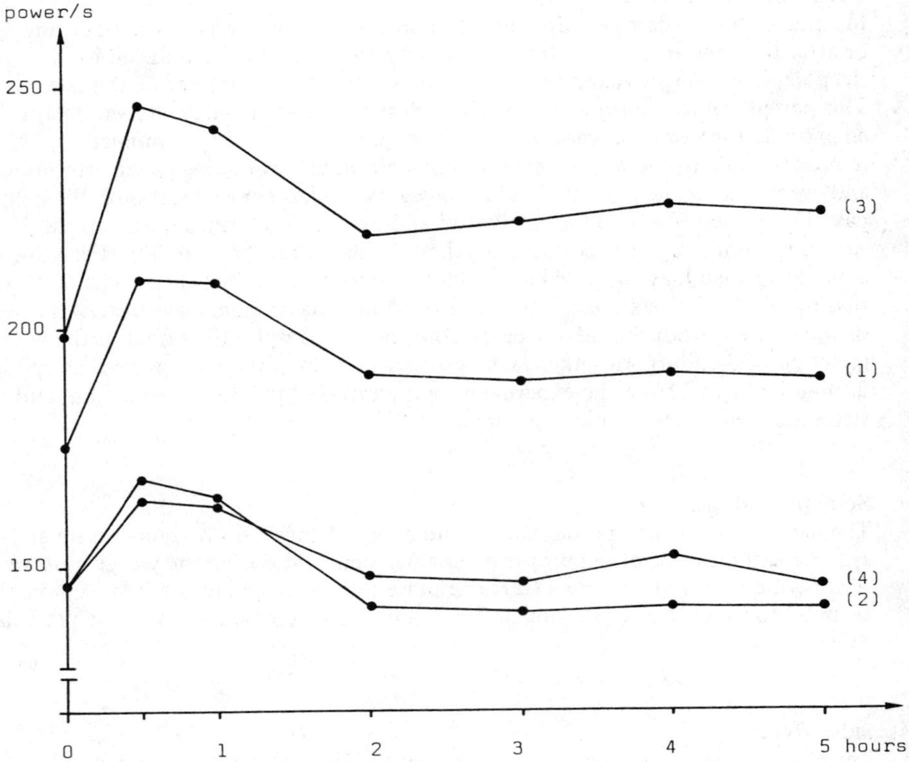

Figure 47.3 Mean values of α-band power, four channels. (1) Temporo-parietal left; (2) Temporo-parietal right; (3) parieto-occipital left; (4) parieto-occipital right.

and 47.4). An increase in alpha and beta power was found after injection; thereafter a decrease was seen which, however, did not reach predrug levels in the temporo-parietal leads. The power distribution and symmetry of bands did not change substantially over time.

SUBJECTS

Case 1

45-year-old, bipolar female patient, unchanged depressive for years, permanently hospitalized, resistant to various psychopharmaca and electroshock therapy. State of moderately retarded depression. After the injection this patient had only a light feeling of warmth in the upper part of the body, but no effects or side effects afterwards. The day after the trial, the depression was unchanged.

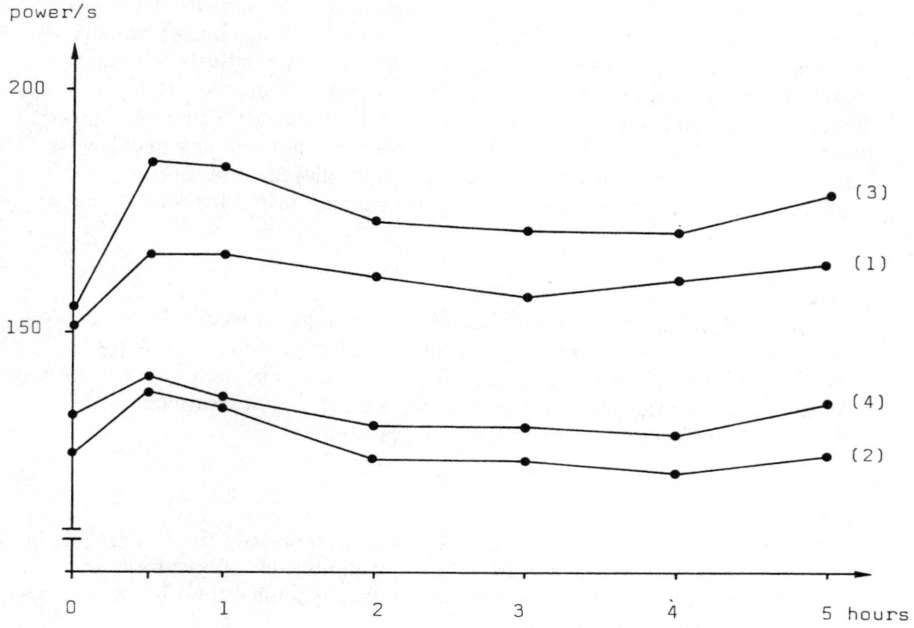

Figure 47.4 Mean values of β-band power, four channels. (1) Temporo-parietal left; (2) temporo-parietal right; (3) parieto-occipital left; (4) parieto-occipital right.

Case 2

34-year-old, bipolar female patient with periodic depression and slightly hypomanic periods in the interval. Depressive for $2\frac{1}{2}$ months, resistant to antidepressants. Somewhat fluctuating condition. A date for the trial was fixed with this patient, but on this day, the depression had practically disappeared, so that 5 ml saline were injected. The remission lasted 14 days. Then the patient became depressive again and we gave her an injection of β-endorphin. This injection was followed 1 hour later by an evident but transient subjective and objective improvement.

Case 3

56-year-old, bipolar female patient with chronic depression, and short manic episodes of a few consecutive days every few months. At the time of the injection, the patient was deeply depressive. A subjective and objective improvement occurred 1 hour after the injection; in this context, the reduction of the anxiety of expectation also had some effect. Four hours after the injection, the condition had deteriorated again, and the trial was a disappointment for the patient. The improvement had manifested itself 30 min after the injection and affected mood, feeling of illness, anxiety and inner unrest and relaxation. One hour later the patient was relaxed, lively, no longer had any anxious expectations, began to speak and to knit and subjectively felt somewhat irritated. The appetite had increased. Two hours later, the patient felt dysphoric again and felt nausea. After lunch and 3 hours after the injection the patient was depressive again, she was no longer able to do any needlework. The day after the trial, the patient was somehow relieved of tension, less depressive, still somewhat irritated. The improvement lasted for several days.

Case 4

52-year-old, female patient with bipolar depression, for weeks deeply depressive. One hour after the injection a pronounced improvement took place, which gradually disappeared in the following hours. The next day, the patient became hypomanic and finally extremely manic, so that treatment with haloperidol of up to 12 mg a day was necessary.

Case 5

38-year-old, female patient, a retarded unipolar depressive for 1 year. One hour after the injection, the depressive symptoms diminished subjectively and objectively. In the evening, she was manic, agitated and euphoric; the following day, she was depressive again.

Case 6

38-year-old, unipolar female patient, deeply retarded-illusory, depressive with delusions. Anxiety, hopelessness, helplessness. A piercing epigastric ache began during the injection, therefore the injection was stopped after one half of the dose was given. ECG control showed no pathological signs.

DISCUSSION

Several factors have to be considered in discussing the observed changes. Previous medication, for example tricyclic antidepressants and hypnotics, was stopped. It is well known that such stoppage of medication can induce a change of psychopathology or even a marked improvement. Furthermore some of the patients showed a partial or total sleep deficit before the experiment because they were left without medication; it is also known that sleep deprivation may induce some change. Finally the experiment was carried out in a special setting, in an EEG chamber. The patients were aware of the whole technical situation. They were exposed to a rather intensive physical and psychological examination and had prolonged and close contacts with physicians and other staff who were taking care of them. Finally the expectation of the patients for improvement with the i.v. injection was in some cases extraordinarily high.

In these circumstances one would expect that some of the patients should show some changes of their condition independent of the i.v. injection of β-endorphin. In one case of a sleep deprivation the patient was clearly improved before the experiment and did not change during the experiment. All patients showed some improvements in the first hour after the injection, and in some of these cases placebo reactions have to be considered and cannot be excluded because there was no placebo control.

Despite these considerations we think that in two patients there was an unexpected marked and persistent improvement induced by the injection. One of these patients developed hypomania for half a day. In a third patient the experiment induced a switch from depression to mania that persisted for weeks. On the basis of these observations the hypothesis is justified that β-endorphin may have antidepressive properties and may have potential for switching depression to hypomania and mania.

The interpretation of the EEG findings is not easy: we found an increase of power/s in the alpha and beta band. The increase of the alpha band power could be interpreted as the result of relaxation. However, the subsequent trend towards reduction of the alpha power suggests an additional transient drug effect. In addition the increase of beta power is usually not associated with relaxation, and may also be an effect of β-endorphin. The observed increase of both the alpha and beta power is not a common drug effect but has been described by Itil *et al.* (1972) as an initial transient effect of anticholinergic antidepressants. The hypothesis of a morphine-like EEG effect of β-endorphin is not confirmed. An alpha power increase would be consistent with morphine-like effects, but morphine reduces beta power activity (Saletu, 1976).

SUMMARY

Four bipolar and two unipolar severely depressed hospitalized patients were each treated in a non-blind drug trial with a single injection of 10 mg β-endorphin i.v. Measurements were taken before and for the 5 hours after the injection. The injections were well tolerated except in one case where an attack of pre-existent angina pectoris was precipitated. Body temperature and blood pressure did not change. Pulse rate decreased within the first 60 min, returning after that to the pre-drug level. EEG power in the alpha and beta band increased after the injection of β-endorphin similarly to the initial effect of anticholinergic antidepressants on EEG.

A change of depressive psychopathology measured by self-ratings was observed in all six patients within the first 20 to 30 min. There was an initial increase of energy and mood and a decrease of anxiety, depression and restlessness. These changes persisted in general for 2 hours; thereafter, four patients relapsed and were very disappointed. In two cases the improvement remained stable and was confirmed by doctors' ratings. Two patients showed a switch from depression to hypomania and one patient to mania; however, the necessary withholding of sleep medication the night before the experiment may confound this observation. Nevertheless, our data suggest that the following hypotheses deserve further investigation.

(1) β-endorphin may have some antidepressive properties;

(2) β-endorphin may have the potential to switch depression to hypomania and mania.

ACKNOWLEDGEMENT

We are greatly indebted to Choh Hao Li and Nathan S. Kline who placed a supply of β-endorphin at our disposal.

REFERENCES

Itil, T. M., Polvan, N. and Hsu, W. (1972). *Curr. ther. Res.*, **14**, 395–413

Kline, N. S., Li, C. H., Lehmann, H. E., Lajtha, A., Laski, E. and Cooper T. (1977). *Archs gen. Psychiat.*, **34**, 1111–3

Saletu, B. (1976). *Psychopharmaka, Gehirntätigkeit und Schlaf.* S. Karger, Basel, New York

48
Demonstration of the analgesic activity of human β-endorphin in six patients

Y. Hosobuchi* and C. H. Li†
(*Department of Neurological Surgery
and †The Hormone Research Laboratory
School of Medicine, University of California,
San Francisco, California 94143, U.S.A.)

It has been demonstrated that the untriakontapeptide β-endorphin produces more potent analgesia in animals than morphine, on a molar basis (Loh *et al.*, 1976; Tseng *et al.*, 1976*a*; Meglio *et al.*, 1977; Feldberg and Smyth, 1976). The present study was undertaken in an attempt to show a similar mode of action of β-endorphin in humans.

MATERIALS AND METHODS

β-endorphin was isolated from human pituitary glands as previously described (Li *et al.*, 1976). Sterile solutions of the peptide at various concentrations were prepared in normal saline and sterilized by micropore filtration.

Six patients on the Neurological Surgery Service of the H.C. Moffitt Hospital of the University of California Medical Center, San Francisco, were selected for i.v.t. and/or i.v. administration of β-endorphin. (The research protocol has been approved by the Committee on Human Research of the University of California, San Francisco, according to guidelines established by the Department of Health, Education and Welfare. Informed consent was obtained from patients who participated in these experiments). All patients were suffering from intractable pain that had been managed with opiate analgesics. Although the dose level necessary to alleviate their pain had been increased over time, none of the patients had developed a tolerance to opiates.

For patients 1, 2 and 3, electrical stimulation of the central grey matter was chosen as the neurosurgical method of treatment (Hosobuchi *et al.*, 1977*a*); a unilateral thoracic cordotomy was chosen for the treatment of patients 4 and 5, and a sacral neurectomy for patient 6.

As part of the stereotactic procedure for implantation of electrodes, under local anasthesia, the first three patients had bilateral burr holes placed in the frontal area 2.5 cm from the midline and 1 cm anterior to the coronal suture. Through one of the burr holes, a lateral ventricle was tapped with a catheter, which was then advanced through the foramen of Monroe to the third ventricle. Target points for electrode implantation were selected on the basis of a ventriculogram performed through the catheter with air and contrast material. The catheter was then connected to an Ommaya reservoir (Wood *et al.*, 1977), which was implanted under the scalp at the site of surgery.

A few days after surgery, patients were taken off opiate analgesics at least 6 to 8 hours before the administration of the peptide; it is not possible to go beyond this point because of severe pain. In a double blind manner, β-endorphin (100, 200, and 400 μg doses in 1-2 ml of normal saline) was administered by percutaneous puncture into the Ommaya reservoir. Only one dose was administered in a 48 hour period to avoid the possible rapid development of tolerance seen in animals (Hosobuchi *et al.*, 1977*b*). Opiate analgesics, rather than brain stimulation, were used for pain control during the testing period.

The analgesic effect of β-endorphin was evaluated for each case with regard to its effect on the patients' original pain, by the patients' subjective 'pain estimate' on the basis of a 0 to 10 scale, and the patients' response to acute pain tested by the Hardy-Wolf-Goddell graded thermal dolorimeter (Hosobuchi *et al.*, 1977*a*). Vital signs and electrocardiograms were monitored closely. In addition to the patients' subjective reaction to analgesia, neurological function and possible alteration in behavior were monitored for 6 to 8 hours. After the analgesic effect of β-endorphin was established in the three patients, 0.4 to 1.0 mg of naloxone was injected i.v. to delineate the opiate-like analgesic action of β-endorphin.

Because of the extremely limited supply of the compound, it was administered i.v. (5 to 15 mg in 2 ml of normal saline) in four patients only (patient 3 and, before their surgery, patients 4, 5 and 6). The pharmacological effect of the compound was evaluated as above.

RESULTS

A clear analgesic effect was observed in three patients after i.v.t. administration of 200 μg of β-endorphin (figure 48.1B). Clear clinical relief of pain in each patient preceded by 10 to 20 min a significant alteration of the threshold of acute pain determined by thermal dolorimeter. In fact, pain relief lasted much longer than the elevation of the acute pain threshold; patients were relatively free of pain for 4 to 6 hours. Similarly, a 400 μg dose of the compound produced clinical pain relief that preceded the elevation of the dolorimetric threshold (figure 48.1C). The analgesic effect at 400 μg was profound and prolonged: the patient was free of clinical pain for about 8 hours. At any dose level, there were no alterations in vital signs, neurological function, or behavior of the patients, except that they appeared to be more relaxed, cheerful and generally more talkative, which we felt was due primarily to relief from their pain. There was no evidence of euphoria or hallucination.

Immediately after rapid i.v.t. administration of 200 μg of β-endorphin in 2 ml of normal saline or, in another experiment, after rapid administration of 2 ml of

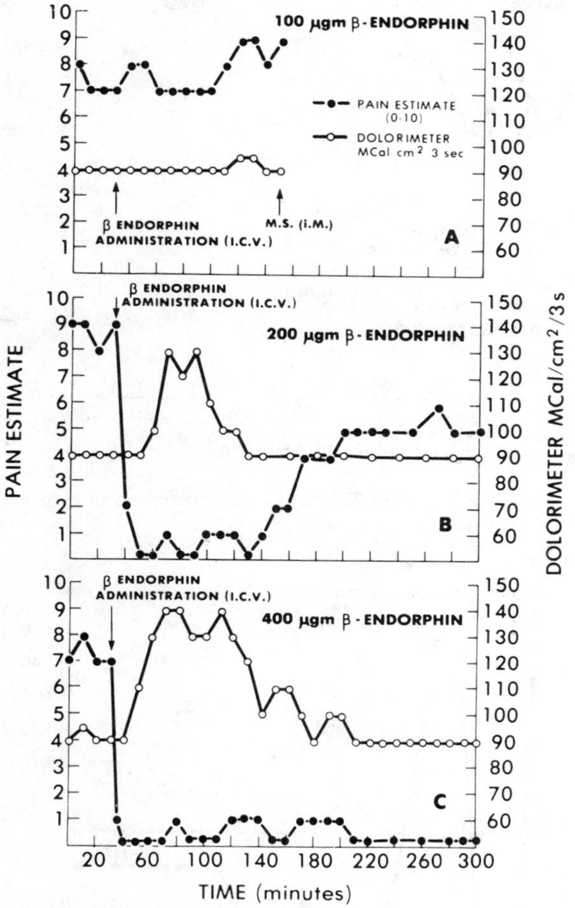

Figure 48.1 The response of patient 1 to i.v.t. administration of human β-endorphin. A, 100 μg; B, 200 μg; C, 400 μg respectively. In (A), the patient received 15 mg of morphine (M.S.) i.m. due to his increasing pain; the observation was terminated at this point. The left hand ordinates are the patient's subjective 'Pain Estimate' scale. The right hand ordinates are the dolorimetric scale in millicalories per cm^2 per 3 s.

normal saline placebo, patient 1 complained of transient 'dizziness' lasting 10 to 15 s. This reaction appeared to be related to the speed of administration rather than to β-endorphin, since the effect was absent after a much more slowly-administered 400 μg dose of the compound in normal saline.

At the 100 μg dose level, the observation period had to be reduced in all patients due to the common, time-related increase in pain intensity between administrations of analgesic agents (figure 48.1A). Increased pain intensity reflected only the absence of any analgesic effect of β-endorphin at this dose level.

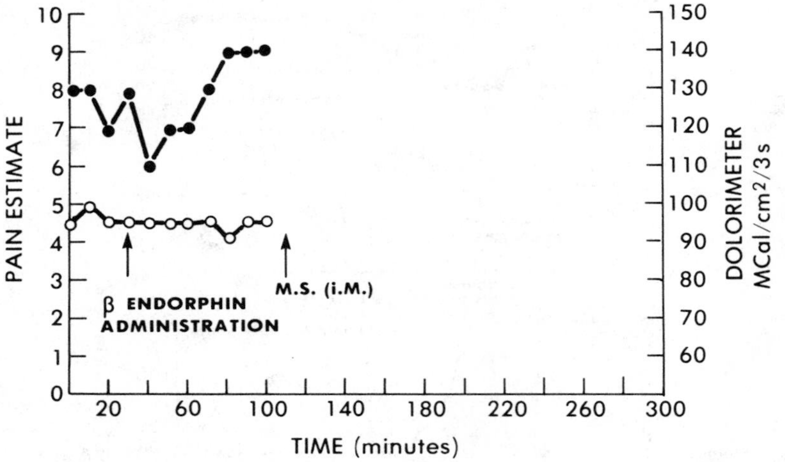

Figure 48.2 The response of patient 3 to the i.v. administration of β-endorphin. The scales are the same as in figure 48.1.

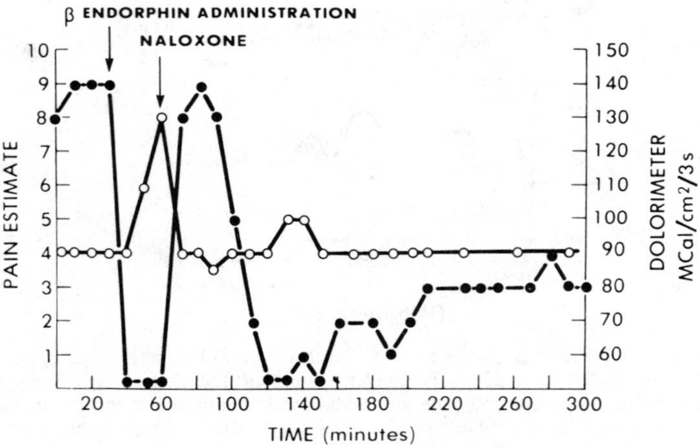

Figure 48.3 The response of patient 3 to the i.v.t. administration of 400 μg of β-endorphin, followed by the i.v. administration of 0.8 mg of naloxone. The scales are the same as in figure 48.1.

A possible transient analgesic effect of i.v. administered β-endorphin was seen only in patients 3 and 6 at a 15 mg dose level (figure 48.2), without significant alteration of dolorimetric threshold. In patients 4 and 5 there was no significant effect at 15 mg. However, at this dose level all patients complained of varying degrees of a 'hot sensation' all over their bodies, and nausea or unpleasant sensations in the epigastrium accompanied by mild tachycardia, without changes in either EKG or blood pressure. Patients 3 and 4 appeared to be somewhat anxious, although no other behavioral alteration or psychological effect was noted. The reaction appeared a few minutes after intravenous injection and lasted for 10 to 15 min. Because of this unpleasant side effect, further administrations of high doses of the compound were not performed.

DISCUSSION

Intraventricular administration of human β-endorphin to patients produced significant analgesic effects accompanied by long periods of relief from clinical pain. There was no observable behavioral or psychological alteration, as seen in animals, over the dose range tested. The analgesic effect of β-endorphin was totally reversed by i.v. administered naloxone, a specific opiate antagonist (figure 48.3).

Intravenous administration of β-endorphin at a 15 mg dose level, however, showed questionable analgesic properties, accompanied by moderately unpleasant hot sensations and epigastric discomfort similar to the effect of ventral periaqueductal grey stimulation in humans reported by Nashold *et al.* (1969) and Hosobuchi *et al.* (1977*a*). Because of this side effect, we did not attempt comparison of β-endorphin analgesic efficacy with i.v. administered morphine. Similarly, because i.v.t. administration of the compound was separated by 48 hours to avoid the possible development of the acute tolerance observed in animals (Hosobuchi *et al.*, 1977*b*; Tseng *et al.*, 1976*b*; Wei and Loh, 1976), no evidence of tolerance development to β-endorphin in humans was observed in this study.

Despite the fact that three patients received prolonged partial to total relief of their intractable pain by i.v.t. administration of β-endorphin, they reported relatively short periods of alteration of acute pain threshold as graded by the thermal energy scale. We do not yet understand how the afferent mechanism involved in chronic pain differs from that operating in cases of acute pain. It is quite possible that the actual afferent input signal of persistent pain is far less intense than that of acute pain, and that persistence in duration causes suffering. For such low amplitude input, the success of β-endorphin-produced pain relief does not require any prolonged alteration in the acute pain level.

The current study in a very small group of patients indicates a powerful analgesic action, without undesirable side effects, of i.v.t. administered β-endorphin. However, this is certainly not the most readily applicable mode of administration for routine clinical use. The possible tolerance development observed in animals has to be evaluated in humans before the true clinical value of β-endorphin as an analgesic agent can be evaluated.

This work was supported in part by NIMH Grant MH-30245.

REFERENCES

Feldberg, W. S. and Smyth, D. G. (1976). *J. Physiol., Lond.*, **260**, 30–1

Hosobuchi, Y., Adams, J. E. and Linchitz, R. (1977*a*). *Science*, **197**, 183–6

Hosobuchi, Y., Meglio, M., Adams, J. E. and Li, C. H. (1977*b*). *Proc. natn. Acad. Sci. U.S.A.*, **74**, 4017–9

Li, C. H., Lemaire, S., Yamashiro, D. and Doneen, B. A. (1976). *Biochem. biophys. Res. Commun.*, **71**, 19–25

Loh, H. H., Tseng, L. F., Nei, E. and Li, C. H. (1976). *Proc. natn. Acad. Sci. U.S.A.*, **73**, 2895–8
Meglio, M., Hosobuchi, Y., Loh, H. H., Adams, J. E. and Li, C. H. (1977). *Proc. natn. Acad. Sci. U.S.A.*, **74**, 774–6
Nashold, B. S., Wilson, W. P. and Slaughter, D. G. (1969). *J. Neurosurg.*, **30**, 14–24
Tseng, L. F., Loh, H. H. and Li, C. H. (1976*a*). *Nature,* **263**, 239–40
Tseng, L. F., Loh, H. H. and Li, C. H. (1976*b*). *Proc. natn. Acad. Sci. U.S.A.*, **73**, 4187–9
Wei, E. and Loh, H. H. (1976). *Science,* **193**, 1262–3
Wood, J. H., Poplack, D. G., Lleyer, W. A. and Ommaya, A. K. (1977). *Science,* **195**, 499–501

49

β-Endorphin: initial clinical studies

Don H. Catlin*†, Ka Kit Hui†, Horace H. Loh‡ and Choh Hao Li§
(Departments of Pharmacology* and Medicine† University of California
Los Angeles, California 90024
Department of Pharmacology‡ and The Hormone Research Laboratory§
University of California, San Francisco, California 94143, U.S.A.)

β-endorphin is an endogenous opiate-like peptide isolated from human pituitary glands in 1976 by Li and associates (Li *et al.*, 1976). Subsequently, human β-endorphin has been synthesized (Li *et al.*, 1977), and its pharmacological effects extensively studied (see Loh and Li, 1977). In animal studies, one of the most consistent observations is that β-endorphin has antinociceptive properties (Li *et al.*, 1976, 1977; Loh *et al.*, 1976; Meglio *et al.*, 1977; Cox *et al.*, 1976; Feldberg and Smyth, 1977). Tolerance to, and physical dependence on β-endorphin have been demonstrated (Wei and Loh, 1976; Tseng *et al.*, 1976*c*; van Ree *et al.*, 1976; Hosobuchi *et al.*, 1977), and it will inhibit the jumping response associated with abrupt withdrawal of morphine in mice (Tseng *et al.*, 1976*a*). On the basis of the studies cited above, it is reasonable to anticipate that β-endorphin may possess analgesic activity in man, and that it may suppress the narcotic abstinence syndrome. In this chapter we discuss our experience (Catlin *et al.*, 1977; 1978) with the intravenous (i.v.) administration of synthetic human β-endorphin to human subjects with pain and to narcotic addicts undergoing abrupt withdrawal of methadone.

The studies were designed to determine if β-endorphin is pharmacologically active by the i.v. route of administration; our data are consistent with the view that it is. Intravenous β-endorphin produces analgesia in the cat (Feldberg and Smyth, 1977) and mouse (Tseng *et al.*, 1976*b*) and Kline *et al.* (1977) have reported that 3–9 mg doses of β-endorphin may have an effect on schizophrenia and affective disorders. Additional objectives of our work are to determine the dose, duration of action, and toxicity of β-endorphin. At doses as high as 30 mg we have not observed any toxicity and the duration of action appears to be brief.

MATERIALS AND METHODS

Drugs

Human β-endorphin was synthesized as previously described (Li *et al.*, 1977). Morphine sulfate was obtained from Eli Lilly and Company (Indianapolis, Indiana). Intravenously infused drugs were added to a reservoir (Volutrol) manufactured by Travenol Laboratories, Inc. (Deerfield, Illinois). The infusate was either 5 per cent dextrose or saline. Pulse doses of drugs were injected directly into the i.v. tubing and rapidly flushed into a peripheral vein.

Subjects

The subjects, ranging between 27 and 62 years of age, were studied at the UCLA Clinical Research Center or hospital ward. Before acceptance for the study, a complete medical history was taken, a physical examination was performed, and the informed consent was explained and signed. Laboratory studies included urinalysis, hemogram, electrolytes, creatinine, blood urea nitrogen, serum glutamic oxaloacetic transaminase, serum glutamate pyruvate transaminase, alkaline phosphatase, chest X-ray and EKG. Some of these tests were repeated at 2-7 day intervals following completion of the protocol.

Analgesia protocol

The detailed protocol has been described (Catlin *et al.*, 1977). In brief, three subjects (A, B, C) with chronic pain due to cancer received single doses of β-endorphin or saline as a substitute for a regularly scheduled dose of narcotic. Clinical signs and self-reports were monitored at frequent intervals for several hours. The experimental design varied slightly with each subject, the constant elements being an evaluation of analgesia by a blind observer, and one or more injections of saline before endorphin.

On experimental day 1, the subject is told that saline will be substituted for one dose of narcotic, but is not informed which dose will be substituted. If the subject reports analgesia following placebo, the narcotic is withheld until pain returns to a maximum level. If there is no response to placebo within 0.5-1.0 hour, the narcotic is administered. On experimental day 2, an i.v. infusion is initiated, and the patient is informed that β-endorphin or placebo will be administered. The subject is aware that drug is administered while the investigator is in the room, but cannot tell exactly when the drug is administered.

Suppression of abstinence protocol

Subject 1 was a 27-year-old female who had a 7 year history of heroin abuse, and who had been maintained on 50-80 mg of methadone per day for 6 years. Subject 2, a 35-year-old male, had been a regular user of heroin for several years before enrolling in a methadone program 7 years prior to this study. Immediately before this study, subjects 1 and 2 were, respectively, receiving 20 and 50 mg of methadone per day.

The last dose was administered on the day the subject was admitted to the Clinical Research Center. Signs and symptoms of methadone abstinence usually begin 36-72 hours after drug discontinuation (Martin *et al.*, 1973); accordingly, the initial 24 hours were utilized to obtain the baseline physical and laboratory examinations.

Measurements

The intensity of the abstinence syndrome was assessed by a modification of the method described by Himmelsbach (1939), in which points are assigned for the presence of various signs or symptoms typical of narcotic abstinence. One point was assigned for each of the following measurable signs: each 2.0 mmHg increase in systolic blood pressure over baseline (limit 10 points); each 1 respiration/minute increase in respiratory rate over baseline (limit 10 points); and each 0.1 °C increase in temperature over baseline (limit 10 points). The presence of the following signs during a 3 min observation period were assigned one point each: lacrimation, piloerection, perspiration, rhinorrhea, yawning, rhythmic tremor of a muscle group, and restlessness. If the subject could not be readily engaged in conversation or answered questions with one or two words, an additional point was added to the total. In addition to the above, the subjects were asked to rate their current subjective state. An ordinal feeling scale with the following items was used: very good, good, average, slightly bad, bad, and very bad, which were assigned values of −2, −1, 0, 1, 2, and 3. The intensity of the abstinence syndrome was quantitated by summing the points to arrive at an abstinence intensity score (AIS). The AIS was determined at 0.5-1.0 hour intervals during infusions, and at frequent intervals throughout the remainder of the day. In addition, the heart and respiratory rates were constantly monitored by a telemetry system (Catlin *et al.*, 1977).

Experimental design

The protocol lasted 8 days. Intravenous infusions of 2-5 hour's duration were initiated on those days when the AIS equalled or exceeded 20 points. About 1 hour after beginning infusion a successive series of 3-7 periods of 30 min each was initiated. At the onset of each period, either an experimental drug or saline was added to the infusion reservoir. The infusion equipment was positioned behind a curtain such that the subject was unaware of the time at which drugs or saline were administered. An observer, who was aware of the nature of the study, but was not informed of the drug administration schedule, evaluated the subjective drug effects at 0.5 to 1.0 hour intervals. A more detailed description of the individual protocols is available (Catlin *et al.*, 1977; 1978).

RESULTS

Analgesia protocol

Subject A was a 46-year-old female with an infiltrating ductal carcinoma of the breast. Before β-endorphin administration she had received irradiation and extensive chemotherapy. She had complained of deep back and chest pain for several months and was receiving daily methadone (20 mg) and dihydromorphone

(10 mg) at the time of study. Objective and subjective drug effects were assessed following morphine sulfate and saline controls on experimental day 1. β-Endorphin (0.5 mg; 6.25 μg/kg) was administered i.v. on day 2. One of the investigators was aware of the drug administered, other observers were not aware (strict double-blind conditions did not prevail). At the time of placebo administration (day 1) the subject was informed that either placebo or morphine would be administered. Since analgesia was reported following placebo, the morphine was not administered until 5 hours later. Similarly at the time of β-endorphin administration, the subject was told that either placebo or active drug would be administered. The subject reported excellent analgesia following placebo and β-endorphin. The duration of analgesia was longer (15 hours) after β-endorphin compared to placebo (4 hours).

Subject B was a 42-year-old male with adenocarcinoma of the right superior sulcus and metastases to bone. Immediately before study he was receiving 15 mg of morphine sulfate i.m. every 3 hours. His pain was judged to be as severe as occurs in clinical medicine. Thirty min after placebo he reported a reduction in pain, but at 45 min and 1 hour he had no relief and indicated that he must have received 'the blank'. Five minutes after two 0.25 mg test doses of β-endorphin, 4.5 mg was infused over 5 min (total: 100 μg/kg). Between 15 and 45 min later the subject reported a slight reduction in pain. A blinded observer felt that he had good relief at 30 min, on the basis of the observation of increased freedom of movement and a relaxed expression compared to the subject's usual tense and rigid posture. At 70 min the subject complained of great pain and morphine was administered. There was no objective evidence that β-endorphin produced any acute effects and minimal evidence of subjective effects.

Subject C was a 63-year-old male with carcinoma involving the body and tail of the pancreas. The principal findings were marked weight loss and an abdomen distended and tense with ascitic fluid. Before β-endorphin administration, he was receiving 70–100 mg of morphine sulfate per day in divided doses. The primary pain was deep in the abdomen and back. It was partially relieved 30 min after morphine and maximally, but not completely, relieved at 1–2 hours. His pain was difficult to accurately quantitate with the rating scale (self-report); nevertheless, it could be assessed by other observations, such as sleeping time, speech content, and facial expression.

Saline was given i.m. and 1 hour later it was apparent that he had no relief and was vigorously demanding morphine. On protocol day 2, the saline was given i.v. at the time of a scheduled morphine injection; 30 min later he had some relief, but at 60 min he complained a great deal. At 105 min he was angry and hostile, and morphine was administered with good effect. On protocol day 3, subject C received 9 mg (180 μg/kg) of β-endorphin over 11 min. Five min later he reported pain relief and indicated a desire to sleep. At 22 min his eyes were closed and he appeared to be asleep. Twenty-four minutes after endorphin, the ward physicians, who had been evaluating the subject daily for 14 days, paid their routine visit. They were not aware that endorphin had been administered and remarked that he seemed quite different: more outgoing, less tense; relaxed; he actually smiled; he seemed comfortable. At 2 hours he complained of considerable pain, but did not demand morphine and went back to sleep. At 3 hours morphine was administered. The nurses' notes for the day read '. . .appears to be in better spirits today'.

The acute administration of β-endorphin to subjects A, B and C did not result in any significant changes in vital signs and no other acute clinical changes were identified. In particular, none of the subjects reported euphoria, dysphoria, or other changes in mental status. Pupillary constriction and respiratory depression were not observed. Follow-up for a period of 5 patient months has not revealed any late clinical or laboratory sequelae that can be attributable to β-endorphin.

Abstinence suppression protocol

Abstinence intensity

Subject 1. During the 8 day protocol, subject 1 received two doses of β-endorphin, one of morphine sulfate, and three of saline, as summarized in figure 49.1. By the third day of abstinence, the AIS exceeded 20 points. On day 4, an AIS of 23 was recorded at 1200 h, and a pulse dose of saline was administered. During the next hour the AIS decreased and then returned to a value of 22 by the end of the third hour. At that point, a pulse dose of β-endorphin (6.0 mg) was administered and 6–10 min later, additional 2.0 mg pulse doses were given (total: 222 μg/kg). At 30 min the AIS had decreased to 15, it remained unchanged for 2 hours and then decreased again to less than 10. Three pulse doses of morphine sulfate totalling 10 mg were administered over 10 min on the fifth day; the AIS steadily decreased from 23 to less than 10 over the next 2.5 hours, increased at 5 hours, and then decreased again.

On the sixth day, the AIS remained less than 20 until the late afternoon. At 1800 h, when the AIS was 33, a pulse dose of saline was administered; 1 hour later, there was a slight decrease in the AIS; at 3 hours, the score was 25, and by 5 hours, the score was 16. On the seventh and eighth days, infusions of β-endorphin and saline were carried out. By the end of the 30 min infusion of 20 mg (444 μg/kg) of β-endorphin, the AIS had decreased from 26 to 15, and one hour after concluding the infusion, the score was 10; over the next 5 hours, the AIS increased and then sharply decreased again. In contrast, 30 min after initiating a 30 min infusion of saline, the AIS had slightly increased, and at 1 and 2 hours, there was a modest fall to 16 before rising again.

A more detailed comparison between the saline and β-endorphin responses are provided in figure 49.2. In this figure the abstinence intensity scores following each of the 3 saline and 2 β-endorphin doses are plotted on the same coordinates with time zero representing the time of drug administration. In contrast to saline curves D and E, the two β-endorphin curves (A and B) have steep slopes for the initial 0.5 (B) or 1.5 (A) hours. One of the saline curves (C) also has a steep initial slope, but the magnitude of the change in AIS was small. The initial 2 hours of the morphine curve (not shown) is virtually identical to endorphin curve A. The lowest AIS (7.5) occurred following the 444 μg/kg dose of β-endorphin; following the lower dose (222 μg/kg) values of less than 10 were also found, however, not until the fourth to sixth hour. The lowest values recorded following saline were 15–16, and in the case of curve E, this was not achieved until the sixth hour.

Subject 2. The summary graph of abstinence scores for subject 2 has been published (Catlin *et al.*, 1978). The 10 mg dose of morphine sulfate was admin-

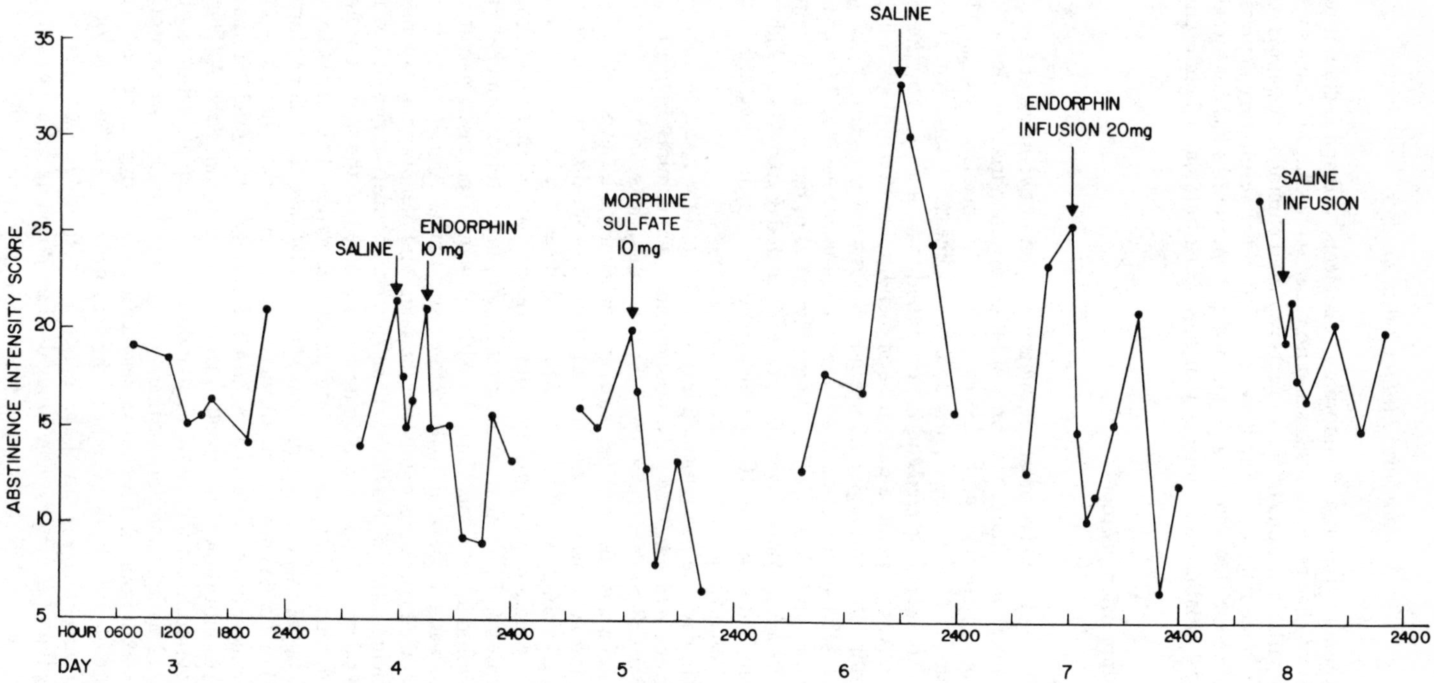

Figure 49.1 Abstinence intensity scores for subject 1 at various hours of the day for days 3–8 of methadone abstinence. The vertical arrows on days 4–8 represent the time at which doses of saline, β-endorphin or morphine sulfate were administered. The details of the drug administration schedule are described in the materials and methods.

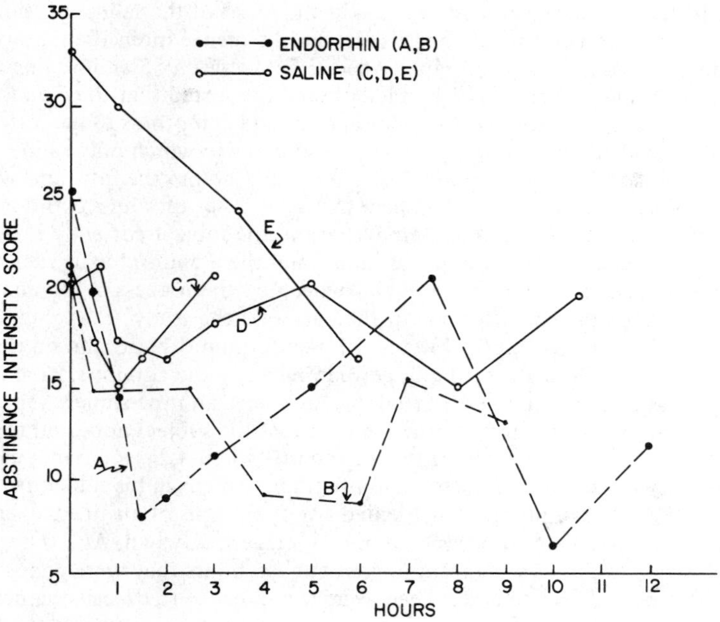

Figure 49.2 Abstinence intensity scores for subject 1 determined at frequent intervals for up to 12 hours following single doses (curves B, C, and E) or infusions (curves A and D) of saline (C, D, and E) or β-endorphin (A and B) on protocol days 4 (B, C), 6 (E), 7 (A), and 8 (D). The dose was administered or the infusion initiated at time zero.

istered when the AIS was 30, thereafter, the score steadily decreased for 3 hours reaching a minimum of 8 points. During two different 3 hour infusions of saline (day 5 and 8) the AIS did not significantly change; on both saline days the AIS scores fluctuated between 18 and 22 points. Thirty milligrams (375 μg/kg) of β-endorphin were infused during one 30 min period of a 4 hour infusion of saline on the sixth experimental day. At the beginning of the endorphin period, the AIS was 18, at the midpoint it was 10, and 30 min after the infusion was completed, the score was 6, and remained at this level for an additional 3 hours.

Self-reports, observer reports and behavioral observations

A detailed chronology of the self-reports of subject 1 have been presented (Catlin *et al.*, 1977). In summary, 8 min after the infusion of β-endorphin (444 μg/kg) was initiated, subject 1 spontaneously reported a decrease in the intensity of abstinence, and by 25 min, reported feeling completely normal. It should be noted that the severity of the abstinence syndrome was particularly marked before the infusion; in contrast, 30 min later, the subject was alert, lucid and hungry. The subject specifically denied any subjective effects other than a return to the normal state, and could not identify any effects that were similar to a narcotic. Compared to the β-endorphin infusion, the intensity of the abstinence syndrome, both subjectively and objectively, was less at the onset of the saline infusion. During the early part of the saline infusion, the abstinence intensified; however, the intensity spontaneously and rapidly decreased between 55 and 60 min after initiating the saline infusion. The blinded observer reported that the β-endorphin infusion produced definite improvement in signs and symptoms of narcotic abstinence. He also reported improvement on the day in which only saline was infused. After completing the pulse dose studies and before the infusions were initiated, subject 1 was asked to compare the pulse doses of saline, β-endorphin, and morphine sulfate. Without any equivocation, the subject correctly identified the saline as a 'blank', the morphine as 'dope' and the β-endorphin as such. Correct identification of the last could have been by the process of elimination since the subject had been informed of the nature of the study.

Subject 2 received 375 μg/kg (30 mg) of β-endorphin over 30 min on the sixth day of abstinence. During the 30 min period preceding the administration of β-endorphin, there was no self-reported improvement, and the subject reported moderately severe abstinence. During the infusion, the subject appeared to be asleep; when aroused at the end of the infusion (0.5 hour), he spontaneously reported a dry mouth and indicated definite improvement in his subjective symptoms. Fifteen minutes later he denied any symptoms of abstinence, and the only objective signs were an occasional myoclonic jerk or yawn. At 1.0 hour he indicated that symptoms were returning, but at 1.5 hours they were gone, and at 4 hours he reported feeling better than average and began to do calisthenics. Between 2 and 10 hours after β-endorphin, yawning and myoclonic jerks were occasionally observed, however, he appeared relaxed and was quite friendly and garrulous. The blinded observer reported that the drug administered suppressed abstinence and commented specifically that the subject appeared less agitated. About 15 hours after β-endorphin the nurse observed that he was anxious and restless, and 7.5 mg of morphine sulfate was administered.

Subject 2 also reported subjective improvement during the saline infusion. During the first hour he appeared to be asleep, except for occasional myoclonic jerks. At the end of 1 hour he reported definite improvement that lasted for about 15 min. This report corresponded to a time at which his respiratory rate was increasing. For the next 2 hours his self-report indicated mild symptoms, representing an improvement in his subjective state compared with that before infusion, and signs of mild abstinence were present. The blinded observer reported a reduction in abstinence during the infusion of saline. Compared with the β-endorphin, the observer reported that the magnitude of the saline effect was similar, but the duration of the saline response was much shorter.

DISCUSSION

We have administered β-endorphin to five subjects; consequently, our data constitute a preliminary report and definitive conclusions cannot be reached. The first question to be posed is whether or not we have observed a pharmacological effect of β-endorphin. We do not have enough data to answer this question, however, our data are consistent with pharmacological activity. In the abstinence suppression subjects, we have observed responses that are of sufficient magnitude to represent a primary effect. The comparison of abstinence intensity scores after infusion of saline and β-endorphin to abstinence subject 1 (figure 49.2) indicates a difference in the temporal sequence of events and magnitude of the response. In both cases, the decrease in AIS following β-endorphin was faster and greater as compared with the saline responses. Subject 2 showed little change in AIS following two doses of saline, and a decrease following β-endorphin or saline. The decreases in respiratory rate appear to be temporally related to infusion of β-endorphin; however, it is clear that marked spontaneous changes may also occur during saline infusions. Aside from the objective measurements, the self-reports and observer reports are consistent with pharmacological activity of β-endorphin. It is clear from this report and many others that both analgesia and opiate abstinence are conditions that respond to placebo administration, therefore, the unequivocal demonstration of pharmacological activity will require a greater number of subjects, a higher dose, or further evidence that endorphin and placebo responses differ with respect to temporal sequence and magnitude.

The general question of whether or not β-endorphin is active by the i.v. route of administration has been addressed by other investigators. (Kline *et al.*, 1977; Guillemin *et al.*, 1977; Tseng *et al.*, 1976*b*; Rivier *et al.*, 1977; Feldberg and Smyth, 1977). We have observed (unpublished) excitement and emesis in two cats at the same dose. Other endorphins (generic) produce analgesia following both i.v. and oral administration (Roemer *et al.*, 1977; Dutta *et al.*, 1977).

Our second objective was to establish a dose and dosage regimen. Pain subject A, who received 6.25 μg/kg, most certainly did not receive a sufficient dose to produce analgesia, and the report of improvement was probably a placebo response. The failure of pain subject B to experience analgesia could be due to insufficient dosage (100 μg/kg) or, since he was receiving high doses of morphine sulfate, cross tolerance between morphine sulfate and β-endorphin may have obscured an effect. Pain subject C, who received 180 μg/kg, showed the most impressive response, although he too was receiving modest doses of morphine sulfate. In contrast, in our abstinence suppression studies we used much higher doses (up to 444 μg/kg) and still cannot be certain if these doses represent the lower or upper level of the dose-response curves. The fact that a 444 μg/kg dose appeared to give a greater response compared to the 222 μg/kg dose in subject 1 suggests the former possibility. It must also be considered, however, that the responses we monitored are characterized by a low degree of sensitivity to i.v. β-endorphin, and that doses of 400 μg/kg represent the upper level of the dose-response curves. Conditions other than narcotic abstinence and responses other than the ones we monitored may have an entirely different dose-response curve. We anticipated that the narcotic abstinence subjects would be very sensitive to opiates and this was shown by the positive response to 10 mg of morphine sulfate. If we assume that the responses we observed following the high doses of β-endorphin were equivalent to the responses after 10 mg of morphine sulfate, then on a molar basis β-endorphin would be 4–5 times more potent than morphine. A similar potency was found by Tseng *et al.* (1976*b*).

It should be noted that none of our subjects has experienced or demonstrated any of the typical opiate effects. For example we have not observed pupillary constriction, low respiratory rates, dysphoria or euphoria. Some subjects have reported a return toward normal, but not true euphoria. Two of our subjects spontaneously reported a dry mouth. Neither have we observed any clinical or laboratory evidence of toxicity to β-endorphin. We have followed most of our subjects for several weeks with laboratory and physical examinations and have not identified any problems that can be attributed to β-endorphin.

In summary we have presented preliminary evidence that β-endorphin may be safely administered to man in doses up to 400 μg/kg and that it may have analgesic and narcotic abstinence suppressing properties.

ACKNOWLEDGEMENTS

This work was supported in part by MH30245 (C.H.L.) and the Aetna Foundation (D.H.C.). The Clinical Research Center is supported by USPHS RR-865. We thank Patricia Sanders for assistance with the clinical studies and for typing the manuscript.

REFERENCES

Catlin, D. H., Hui, K. K., Loh, H. H. and Li, C. H. (1977). *Commun. Psychopharmacol.*, **1**, 493–500

Catlin, D. H., Hui, K. K., Loh, H. H. and Li, C. H. (1978). In *Advances in Biochemical Psychopharmacology*, (eds. E. Costa and M. Trabucchi). Raven Press, New York

Cox, B. M., Goldstein, A. and Li, C. H. (1976). *Proc. natn. Acad. Sci. U.S.A.*, **73**, 1821–3

Dutta, A. S., Gormley, J. J., Hayward, C. F., Morley, J. S., Shaw, J. S., Stacey, G. J. and Turnbull, M. T. (1977). *Life Sci.*, **21**, 559–62

Feldberg, W. and Smyth, D. G. (1977). *Br. J. Pharmac.*, **60**, 445–53

Guillemin, R., Vargo, T., Rossier, J., Minick, S., Ling, N., Rivier, C., Vale, W. and Bloom, F. (1977). *Science*, **197**, 1367–9

Himmelsbach, C. K. (1939). *J. pharmac. exp. Ther.*, **66**, 239–49

Hosobuchi, Y., Meglio, M., Adams, J. E. and Li, C. H. (1977). *Proc. natn. Acad. Sci. U.S.A.*, **74**, 4017–9

Kline, N. S., Li, C. H., Lehman, H. E., Lajtha, A., Laski, E. and Cooper, T. (1977). *Archs gen. Psychiat.*, **34**, 1111–3

Li, C. H., Chung, D. and Doneen, B. A. (1976). *Biochem. biophys. Res. Commun.*, **72**, 1542–7

Li, C. H., Yamashiro, D., Tseng, L.-F. and Loh, H. H. (1977). *J. med. Chem.*, **20**, 325–8

Loh, H. H., Tseng, L.-F., Wei, E. and Li, C. H. (1976). *Proc. natn. Acad. Sci. U.S.A.*, **73**, 2895–8

Martin, W. R., Jasinski, D. R., Haertzen, C. A., Kay, D. C., Jones, B. C., Mansky, P. A. and Carpenter, R. W. (1973). *Archs gen. Psychiat.*, **28**, 286–95

Meglio, M., Hosobuchi, Y., Loh, H. H., Adams, J. E. and Li, C. H. (1977). *Proc. natn. Acad. Sci. U.S.A.*, **74**, 774–6

Rivier, C., Vale, W., Ling, N., Brown, M. and Guillemin, R. (1977). *Endocrinology*, **100**, 238–41

Roemer, D., Buescher, H. H., Hill, R. C., Pless, J., Bauer, W., Cardinaux, F., Closse, A., Hauser, D. and Huguenin, R. (1977). *Nature*, **268**, 547–9

Tseng, L.-F., Loh, H. H. and Li, C. H. (1976*a*). *Proc. natn. Acad. Sci. U.S.A.*, **73**, 4187–9

Tseng, L.-F., Loh, H. H. and Li, C. H. (1976*b*). *Nature*, **263**, 239–40

Tseng, L.-F., Loh, H. H. and Li, C. H. (1976*c*). *Biochem. biophys. Res. Commun.*, **74**, 390–6

van Ree, J. M., de Wied, D., Bradbury, A. F., Hulme, E. C., Smyth, D. G. and Snell, C. R. (1976). *Nature*, **264**, 792–4

Wei, E. and Loh, H. H. (1976). *Science*, **193**, 1262–3

Section Three
Clinical Studies

(B) Endorphins in Body Tissues

See Lindström et al (1978) Acta Psychiat. scand.

50
Possible role of endorphins in schizophrenia and other psychiatric disorders

Lars-M. Gunne, Leif Lindström and Erik Widerlöv
(Psychiatric Research Center, S-750 17 Uppsala, Sweden)

The impressive mood-manipulating effects of opiates, as well as the psychotomimetic properties of some opiate antagonists have long been familiar to pharmacologists. When the brain endorphins were discovered (Terenius and Wahlström, 1975*a*; Pasternak *et al.*, 1975; Hughes, 1975; Cox *et al.*, 1975) it soon became evident that the activity state of the newly postulated peptidergic neuronal system (Elde *et al.*, 1976) might help to elucidate some psychiatric diseases, which had hitherto only been clinically defined. After Terenius and Wahlström (1975*b*) had developed a technique for the semiquantitative measurement of two major endorphin fractions (I and II) in cerebrospinal fluid (CSF), this method was applied in various psychiatric disorders (Terenius *et al.*, 1976; Lindström *et al.*, 1977). Preliminary reports have shown that before treatment some cases of schizophrenia had supranormal CSF levels of fraction I and the same was true of certain phases of manic-depressive psychosis. Another approach to these problems consisted in trials of an opiate antagonist in schizophrenia. In a pilot study schizophrenic hallucinations were found to be temporarily reversed by administration of naloxone (Gunne *et al.*, 1977). The present chapter reports an extension of these studies.

MATERIAL AND METHODS

CSF levels of endorphins

Table 50.1 gives some background data on the subjects of the present study. The healthy volunteers were asked concerning drug use, earlier psychiatric problems, hospital stays and heredity of psychiatric disease. All gave an unremarkable case history.

Lumbar punctures were undertaken between 8-9 a.m. with the subjects in a supine position. Twelve millilitres of CSF were withdrawn, centrifuged and stored

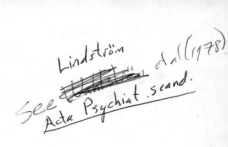

Table 50. 1 Categories of individuals subjected to lumbar puncture

Diagnostic group	No. of subjects	Age in years (median and range)	Age at first onset (median and range)	Number of CSF samples per subject
Healthy volunteers				
Male	10	24.5 (21–38)		2
Female	9	24.0 (20–35)		2
Manic-depressive				
Male	3	49.0 (44–60)	33 (20–33)	2–7
Female	1	30	17	2
Puerperal psychosis	4	28.5 (21–30)		2
Schizophrenic				
Male	19	27.5 (21–47)	21 (16–36)	1–2
Female	5	31.0 (18–49)	18 (14–23)	1–2

at −80 °C until assay within a month. The lumbar punctures were repeated after an interval of 1–3 months. In the psychotic patients this generally occurred when the clinical condition had improved or, in the case of the manic-depressives, when there had been a major change of mood. All psychotic cases received neuroleptic treatment and the four manic-depressives were given lithium. On the day of CSF sampling, ratings of the psychic state were performed according to the Comprehensive Psychopathological Rating Scale (CPRS) (Åsberg *et al.*, 1978).

The CSF levels of endorphins were assayed according to Terenius and Wahlström (1975*b*). The method is based on a Sephadex G10 column separation of endorphins followed by an *in vitro* radioreceptor assay. For details, see Wahlström and Terenius (this volume).

Trials of narcotic antagonists

Ten schizophrenic patients (median age: 33.5, range: 18–52 years; median duration of illness: 9.0, range: 1–20 years) were selected due to their repeated complaints concerning auditory hallucinations. They were studied for 10 days during consecutive weeks. Inclusion criteria were complaints about 'voices' on at least three out of five mornings during the first week of observation. During the second week for 5 days, placebo (saline) or naloxone (0.8 mg) was injected i.v. at 9 a.m. under double blind conditions in a randomized order. Naloxone was given on two or three mornings during that week and the patients self-rated the intensity and frequency of their hallucinatory experiences, retrospectively, after 4 hours.

In a double-blind cross-over study of naltrexone, 50 mg tablets (or placebo) were administered twice daily at 0800 h and 2000 h. Observers' ratings of the clinical state were performed twice weekly by 3 independent raters according to the Nurse's Observation Scale for Inpatient Evaluation (NOSIE) (30) and the CPRS scales (Honigfeld *et al.*, 1966; Åsberg *et al.*, 1978). Altogether 10 schizophrenic patients participated (seven males, three females; median age: 25.0, range: 21–57 years; median duration of illness: 5.5, range: 1–34 years). Half of the group received placebo and the other half naltrexone for 2 weeks, followed by a cross-over for another 2 weeks. During both drug trials neuroleptic administration (haloperidol, chlorpromazine, perphenazine, flupenthixol, clozapine) was maintained at a constant dose level, each patient receiving one or two of the above neuroleptic drugs. This medication reduced, but did not eliminate, the schizophrenic symptomatology.

RESULTS

CSF levels of endorphins

Figure 50.1 shows the levels of fraction I in healthy volunteers (controls), manic-depressive psychosis (MD), puerperal psychosis and schizophrenia both before (○) and during treatment with neuroleptics (●). Figure 50.2 shows the corresponding levels of fraction II. Both the MD group and the untreated schizophrenic group

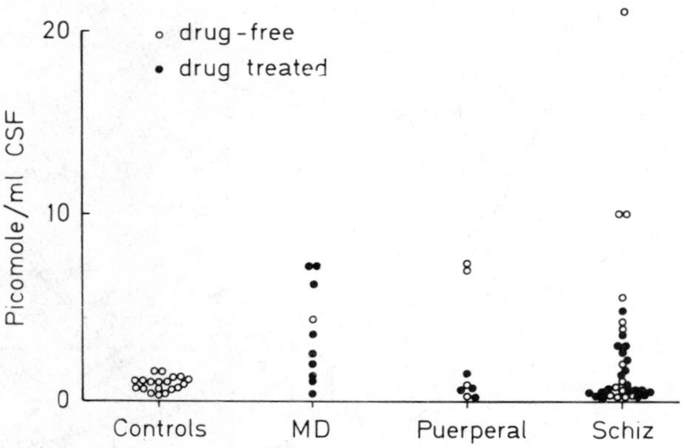

Figure 50.1 CSF endorphins belonging to fraction I (Terenius and Wahlström, 1975*b*) in healthy volunteers (controls), manic-depression (MD), puerperal and schizophrenic psychosis.

had significantly elevated mean levels of fractions I and II ($P < 0.05$). Figure 50.3 shows the tendency in schizophrenic cases and puerperal psychosis of a reduction of the initially elevated fraction I towards the control range during treatment with antipsychotic medicines (chlorpromazine, thioridazine, haloperidol or clozapine). At the same time some cases had a rise in fraction II.

Trials of narcotic antagonists

The i.v. injection of 0.8 mg naloxone eliminated the hallucinations in only one case (on three separate days) whereas saline was ineffective (on two days). In another case all injections caused a cessation of hallucinosis (placebo-reactor)

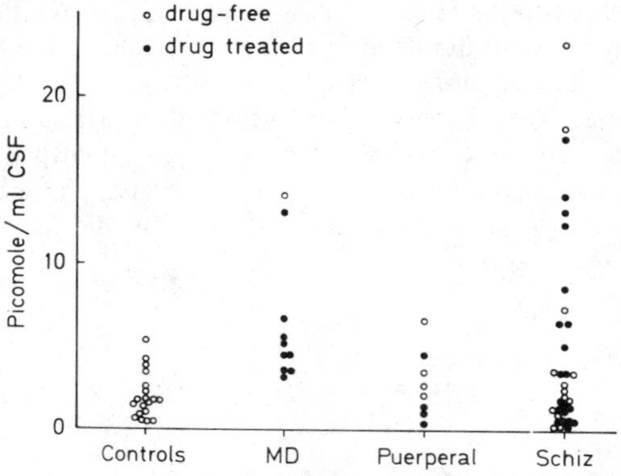

Figure 50.2 CSF endorphins belonging to fraction II (for explanation see figure 50.1)

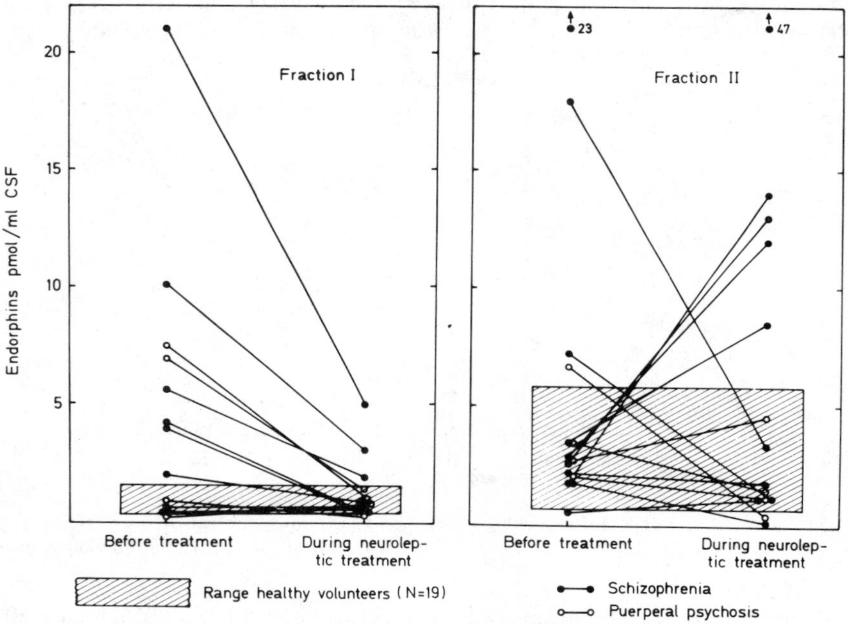

Figure 50.3 CSF endorphin levels before and during treatment in schizophrenia (•) and puerperal psychosis (○); left: fraction I, right: fraction II.

and in the other eight patients the reaction pattern was ambiguous. There was no response to one or more naloxone injections (continued hallucinations) and occasional placebo effects (reduced intensity of hallucinations).

The mean response to naltrexone 100 mg/day was negative. The subjects showed no clinical improvement when observers ratings were treated statistically. However, also in this study one patient responded favourably, whereas in the rest placebo was slightly superior to the active compound (figure 50.4).

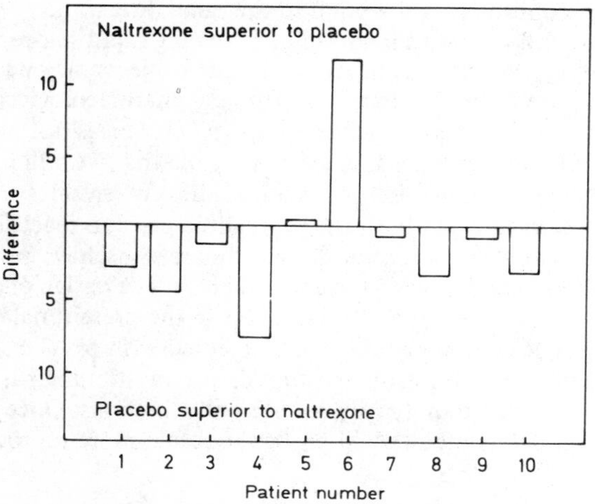

Figure 50.4 Mean individual differences in total CPRS scores between naltrexone and placebo treatment in 10 chronic schizophrenic subjects.

DISCUSSION

Our earlier study of CSF endorphins in endogenous psychosis has been enlarged and the new data still confirm the observed high fraction I endorphin levels in about half the cases of untreated schizophrenic or puerperal psychosis. We are not yet aware of any clinical differences between cases who initially had high and cases with normal or low CSF endorphins, but more detailed studies in the future might elucidate that question. Our MD cases have shown some elevation of fraction I at all stages of their disease. The level during mania tended to be somewhat higher than during depression, the mean during symptom-free intervals falling between these two. In schizophrenic and puerperal psychoses there was a reduction of the elevated fraction I to normal or slightly supranormal levels during treatment. In fraction II on the other hand, some cases showed an increase during treatment. It is speculated that fraction II, which may be a pituitary endorphin, might have been increased due to some compensatory mechanism, when fraction I was reduced. In support of this it was noticed that the rise in fraction II occurred only in cases where fraction I was reduced during treatment. Our observations of high endorphin levels in initial, disturbed phases of schizophrenia and a decline during treatment, seems to link CSF endorphins to observable manifestations of psychotic behavior.

The two trials with naloxone and naltrexone were negative from a statistical point of view, although in both studies 1 out of 10 seemed to be a responder. Although some authors (Volavka *et al.*, 1977; Davis *et al.*, 1977; Janowsky *et al.*, 1977) have failed to replicate our initial results with naloxone (Gunne *et al.*, 1977) this matter may still not be altogether settled. Emrich *et al.* (1977) using higher doses, found a reducing effect with naloxone on schizophrenic hallucinations and other unpublished results point in the same direction.

The methodological problems involved in recording rapid self-reported changes of experienced psychotic material in schizophrenic subjects may need more attention when we are beginning to work with new pharmacological tools, the opiate antagonists or β-endorphin (Kline *et al.*, 1977). This is not merely a matter of creating double-blind conditions. It seems possible that we will have to define which patient categories can be useful in such studies. When selecting experimental subjects we must learn to avoid both the suggestible placebo reactors and those patients who, due to disease manifestations or other reasons, have great difficulty in communicating their experiences to the experimenter. The design of such experiments should probably not be a retrospective rating (as in the present naloxone study), due to the disturbance of time sense often connected with psychotic states. On the other hand it should be remembered that direct questioning has an arousing effect, which may in itself temporarily reverse hallucinations. Once the technical problems have been overcome, we will probably obtain more reproducible results in this new field.

ACKNOWLEDGEMENT

This study was supported by a Swedish Medical Research Council grant no B79-21x-5095. The authors wish to thank Endo Laboratories Inc. for naloxone and naltrexone.

REFERENCES

Åsberg, M., Montgomery, S. A., Perris, C., Schalling, D. and Sedvall, G. (1978). *Acta. psychiat. scand.*, Suppl. 271

Cox, B. M., Opheim, K. E., Teschemacher, H. and Goldstein, A. (1975). *Life Sci.*, **16**, 1777-82

Davis, G. C., Bunney, W. E. Jr. and De Fraites, E. G. (1977). *Science*, **197**, 74–7

Elde, R., Hökfelt, T., Johansson, O. and Terenius, L. (1976). *Neuroscience*, **1**, 349–51

Emrich, H. M., Cording, C., Pirée, S., Kölling, A., Zerssen, D. v. and Herz, A. (1977). *Pharmakopsychiatrie*, **10**, 265–70

Gunne, L.-M., Lindström, L. and Terenius, L. (1977). *J. Neural Transmission*, **40**, 13–9

Honigfeld, T., Gillis, R. D. and Klett, C. J. (1966). *Psychol. Rep.*, **19**, 180–2

Hughes, J. (1975). *Brain Res.*, **88**, 295–308

Janowsky, D. S., Segal, D. S., Bloom, F., Abrams, A. and Guillemin, R. (1977). *Am. J. Psychiat.*, **134**, 926–7

Kline, N. S., Li, C. H., Lehmann, H. E., Lajtha, A., Laski, E. and Cooper, T. (1977). *Archs gen. Psychiat.*, **34**, 1111–3

Lindström, L., Gunne, L.-M. and Terenius, L. (1977). *VI World Congress of Psychiatry, Honolulu 1977* (in press)

Pasternak, G. W., Goodman, R. and Snyder, S. H. (1975). *Life Sci.*, **16**, 1765–9

Terenius, L. and Wahlström, A. (1975*a*). *Acta physiol. scand.*, **94**, 74–81

Terenius, L. and Wahlström, A. (1975*b*). *Life Sci.*, **16**, 1759–64

Terenius, L., Wahlström, A., Lindström, L. and Widerlöv, E. (1976). *Neurosci. Lett.*, **3**, 157–62

Volavka, J., Mallya, A., Baig, S. and Perez-Cruet, J. (1977). *Science*, **196**, 1227–8

51

Endorphins in human cerebrospinal fluid and their measurement

Lars Terenius, Agneta Wahlström and Lars Johansson
(Department of Pharmacology, University of Uppsala,
Box 573, S-751 23 Uppsala, Sweden)

The identification of the endorphins in 1975 (Goldstein, 1976) raises several questions regarding their possible significance. The apparent inactivity of narcotic antagonists such as naloxone in morphine-naive individuals is hard to explain if these substances have a profound role. However, if it is presumed that endorphins share such actions of morphine as changes in the state of mind, these actions are difficult to define. This problem is no less in humans. During the past 2 years our aim has been to approach the possible role of endorphins in human physiology and pathology. How can one measure CNS endorphin activity in humans? Obviously there are no direct ways. The best approximation might be the measurement of endorphins in the lumbar cerebrospinal fluid (CSF), an approach proven to have some validity for monoamine systems (Post and Goodwin, 1978).

A pilot study was initiated. We developed a simple chromatographic fractionation procedure which was followed by the testing of endorphin activity in a radioreceptor assay. This is a biological assay and the activity read will be a function of both the quantity and the receptor affinity of the tested substance. As has been reported for brain extracts (Goldstein, 1976), the CSF contains not just a single but a family of endorphins (figure 51.1). The two major fractions, I and II, were measured in a series of CSF samples from patients suffering from severe somatic pain and neurological diseases with symptoms other than pain, respectively. The results were surprisingly consistent, the cases with pain showed lower Fraction I endorphin levels than the other cases (Terenius and Wahlström, 1975). A similar study in chronic psychosis showed grossly elevated levels of Fraction I, Fraction II or of both fractions (Terenius *et al.*, 1976). Apparently, the endorphin systems, as reflected in the CSF analysis, are far from constantly engaged in different individuals, and furthermore, there was an indication of a relationship between human pathology and endorphin levels. The observation of high levels in psychosis led to clinical trials with narcotic antagonists (Gunne *et al.*, 1977; Terenius *et al.*, 1977).

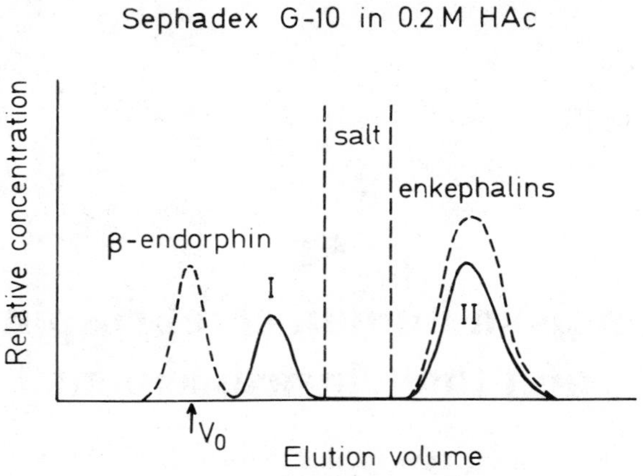

Figure 51.1 Chromatographic elution characteristics of β-endorphin, the enkephalins and Fractions I and II from human cerebrospinal fluid.

CHEMICAL ASPECTS

The publication of the chemical structures of the enkephalins (Hughes *et al.*, 1975), and the endorphins (Guillemin *et al.*, 1976; Bradbury *et al.*, 1976) stimulated us to compare the chemical properties of the active component in the CSF fractions with the properties of the known compounds. In chromatographic analysis on Sephadex gels, β-endorphin was found to elute before Fraction I, indicating their non-identity, while the enkephalins and Fraction II co-eluted. The amounts of Fraction I endorphin(s) are very small and we have, for obvious reasons, not been able to obtain large quantities of lumbar CSF. Ventricular CSF from hydrocephalic patients is more readily available and has provided us with enough Fraction I endorphins to allow subfractionation. Samples were run in a high-pressure liquid chromatography (h.p.l.c.) system on a reversed phase silica gel column (figure 51.2). The main active component from Fraction I does not co-elute with the enkephalins or with longer endorphins. Furthermore, it shows no reactivity in radioimmunoassays (RIA) with antibodies directed against met-enkephalin or β-endorphin. Still it seems to be a peptide, since proteolytic enzymes like Pronase reduce its activity. Trypsin, on the other hand, reduces its activity almost completely in contrast to the enkephalins. In conclusion, the active component in Fraction I appears to be distinct from and maybe even unrelated to, the previously characterized endorphins. Its peptide nature also distinguishes it from the non-peptides with opioid receptor activity described by Schulz *et al.* (1977) and Gintzler *et al.* (1976).

Fraction II endorphins occur in larger quantities and their chemical properties could be studied on samples of lumbar CSF from patients, most of them suffering from chronic pain (of non-cerebral origin). Also this fraction was subjected to h.p.l.c. on reversed phase silica gel columns. The major component was distinctly different from the enkephalins (which would appear in Fraction II if present). The major Fraction II component was not recognized by the met-enkephalin or

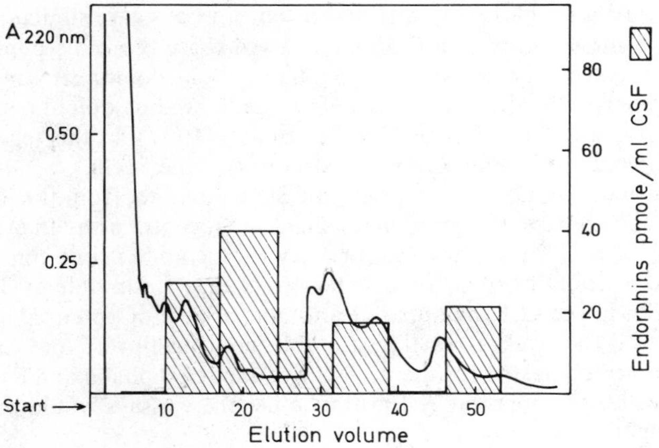

Figure 51.2 Distribution of opiate receptor activity ('endorphins') from Fraction I on high pressure liquid chromatography on reversed phase silica gel (solvent 50 per cent methanol in 2 mM phosphate buffer, pH 6.8). In this and the following figures the endorphin activity is expressed as if due to the presence of met-enkephalin in pmol/ml CSF.

Table 51.1 Opioid receptor selectivities of endorphins, narcotic analgesics and CSF fractions

Substance		K_D [^{3}H] Leu-enkephalin (D-Ala^2) / K_D Dihydromorphine
α-Endorphin		2.0
β-Endorphin		4.7
γ-Endorphin		1.9
Met-enkephalin		0.8
Leu-enkephalin		0.6
Morphine		31
Dihydromorphine		63
l-Methadone		30
Fraction II	Rapid	4.5
	Slow	2.3
Fraction I	Rapid	2.0
	Slow	3.0

Dissociation constants (K_D) were determined with [^{3}H] leu-enkephalin [D-Ala^2] and [^{3}H] dihydromorphine as radioindicators.

β-endorphin antibodies. Also this fraction was partially degradable by Pronase and almost completely degraded by trypsin. In a few samples, enkephalins were in fact detected. They had the expected retention behavior on Sephadex gels and on h.p.l.c. columns. Furthermore, they cross-reacted with the respective antibodies, and on a quantitative basis antibody and receptor assays gave similar results.

The active components in both Fraction I and II are typically 'peptide-like' in their receptor selectivity. In other words, the fractions do not discriminate between classical opiate agonist sites and sites preferentially binding opioid peptides (Lord *et al.*, 1977; Simantov and Snyder, 1976; Terenius, 1977). In this regard they behave as the opioid peptides of known structure (table 51.1).

In conclusion, the major endorphins in CSF are distinct from the known endorphins and we have therefore maintained the receptor assay in attempts to make clinical correlations. The receptor assay is much more time-consuming than the RIA and it would be of great advantage to change methodology. The presence of enkephalins in the CSF may provide another variable of potential diagnostic value. However, the levels, if at all measurable, are usually very low. Samples are now being routinely tested for the presence of met-enkephalin and β-endorphin by RIA. It will therefore soon be learnt whether these assays would provide useful information.

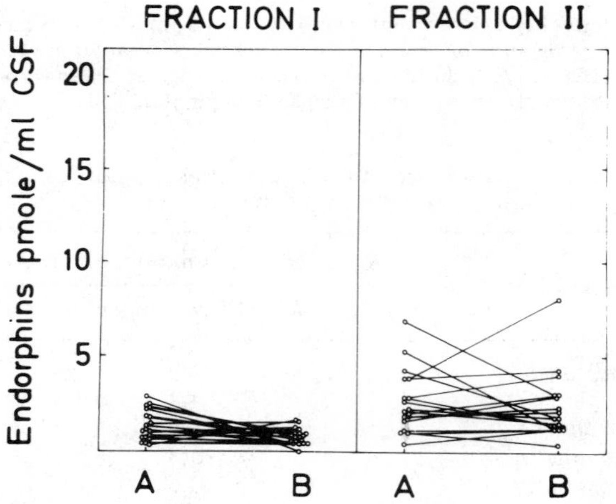

Figure 51.3 Endorphin levels in cerebrospinal fluid of healthy volunteers sampled twice at 3–4 week intervals.

CHARACTERISTICS OF THE TESTING PROCEDURE

All steps of the radioreceptor assay have been standardized very carefully. The procedure is checked at intervals with standard samples. At each occasion an assay is run, known concentrations of met-enkephalin are tested, a calibration curve is constructed, and the activity of the test samples are read from the calibration curve (Terenius *et al.*, 1976). The reproducibility of the assay is adequate. Eight aliquots of a sample of lumbar CSF were run and tested by two operators. The level of Fraction I in these samples was read as 1.2 ± 0.15 and of Fraction II as 9.0 ± 0.3 pmol met-enkephalin per ml CSF, respectively (Lindström *et al.*,

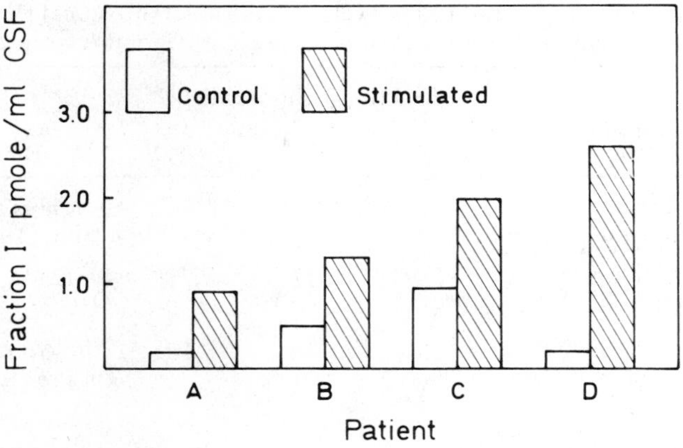

Figure 51.4 Increase in lumbar endorphin Fraction I levels on electroacupuncture. The stimulation involved the lumbar region. From Sjölund *et al.* (1977)

1978). One prerequisite for some utility of these assays would be a reasonably narrow concentration range in healthy individuals and its relative constancy over time. In a series of 19 healthy volunteers, these conditions seem to be fulfilled (figure 51.3). In Fraction II, a sex difference is possible and has to be taken into account in correlative studies. The relative constancy in healthy volunteers is in great contrast to differences observed in psychosis (Lindström *et al.*, 1978; see also Gunne *et al.*, this volume).

PROBLEMS OF INTERPRETATION

Our aim is to study the activity of endorphin systems in the CNS. Is the CSF assay able to provide a valid mirror image of what is going on in the brain? One problem is that the lumbar CSF is a sort of backwater which is geographically distant from the higher brain centers of interest in psychotic patients. In patients with chronic pain, this problem may be less acute, since enkephalins may modulate pain sensitivity to a significant extent via processes in the spinal cord and the lower brain stem (Basbaum *et al.*, 1976; Hökfelt *et al.*, 1977). We have made some observations regarding possible compartmentalization of CSF endorphins in the CSF-containing spaces. Levels of endorphins at the cervical level are comparable to those at the lumbar level. Secondly, CSF obtained from continuous lumbar drainage of patients which chronic pain or increased intracranial pressure shows rather constant levels of endorphins. Thirdly, ventricular CSF samples seem to give levels which are similar to those of lumbar samples. These observations do not, however, answer the basic question about the relation between CNS endorphin activity and CSF endorphin levels. Similar interpretative problems are present in the measurements of CSF metabolites of the monoamine neurotransmitters (Curzon *et al.*, 1976; Garelis *et al.*, 1974; Sjöström *et al.*, 1975). In the case of endorphins one observation may point to a direct relationship. If patients with severe, chronic pain of somatic origin are stimulated electrically and at low

Table 51.2 Fraction I endorphin levels in lumbar cerebrospinal fluid of patients with chronic pain and in healthy volunteers

Series	Patient category	Fraction I endorphin <0.6	0.6–1.2	>1.2*	Reference
I	Trigeminal neuralgia	7	1		Terenius and Wahlström (1975)
II	Chronic pain (neurogenic)	8	1		Sjölund *et al.* (1977)
III	Chronic pain (organic)	13	3	4	Almay *et al.* (in preparation)
	Chronic pain (psychogenic)	1	8	8	
IV	Healthy volunteers	3	12	4	Lindström *et al.* (1978)

*Expressed as if due to met-enkephalin

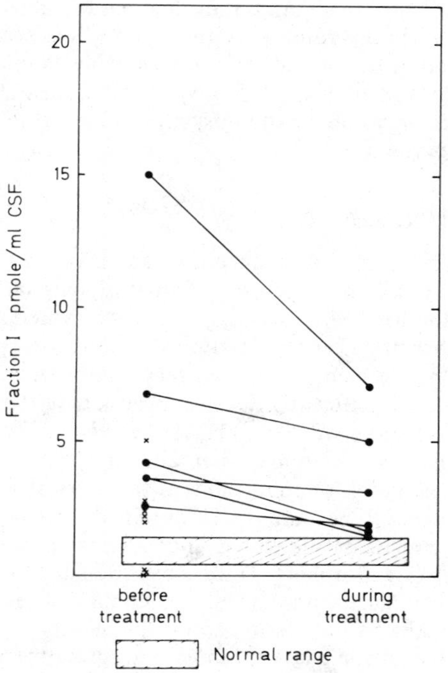

Figure 51.5 Endorphin Fraction I levels of cerebrospinal fluid in patients with affective depression. •, Patients who were sampled twice; before and after 2–3 week's treatment with naloxone injections. From Terenius *et al.* (1977).

frequency (given so-called electro-acupuncture), pain is relieved and there is a concomitant increase in CSF endorphins (figure 51.4). Incidentally, this treatment gives naloxone-reversible pain relief (Sjölund and Eriksson, 1976).

APPLICATIONS TO CLINICAL PROBLEMS

In addition to studies in psychosis (see Gunne *et al.*, this volume) the CSF endorphin assay has been applied to patients which chronic pain, extending our previous series, and to patients with depression. There are many reasons for studying these categories of patients. Chronic pain syndromes are hard to evaluate and to treat. In every patient the syndrome has its somatogenic and psychogenic components. The contribution of each to the reaction to pain may be very different. In some patients there may be no clear somatic component at all, and a pain syndrom in this situation may be related to a depressive syndrome. A common pathogenesis of pain and depressive syndromes has in fact been proposed (Sternbach, 1974). In our extended studies of patients which chronic pain syndromes, we seem to confirm our earlier findings of low Fraction I endorphin in patients with somatogenic pain, particularly in neurogenic pain (table 51.2). The difference from healthy volunteers is statistically significant. In pain with mainly psychogenic dimensions the Fraction I levels seem to be higher. With an increase in depressive symptomatology there is a proportional and statistically significant increase in Fraction I levels (Almay *et al.*, in preparation). In line with this observation is the finding of very high Fraction I levels in patients with affective depression (usually not suffering from pain). As illustrated in figure 51.5, a patient in severe depression may have a 10-fold increase over the 'normal' range (Terenius *et al.*, 1977). A pilot trial of naloxone over a period of 2 to 3 weeks in five of these patients resulted in some reduction of the CSF endorphins. The trial was clinically unsuccessful for reasons not fully understood.

CONCLUSIONS

The relatively simple method of analysing CSF endorphins in a receptor test has been proved to be a useful empirical tool for correlative studies in some human diseases. The results indicate that the endorphin systems are highly dynamic and may respond to drug treatment. A diagnostic potential of the test is already apparent and it could be used to evaluate drug responses. The full implications of the observations made here will have to await the chemical identification of the active components.

ACKNOWLEDGEMENTS

We are greatly indebted to clinical colleagues for stimulating cooperation, to Dr B. Sjölund for ventricular cerebrospinal fluid, to Ms Åsa Häggström for technical assistance and to the Swedish Medical Research Council for financial help.

REFERENCES

Basbaum, A. I., Clanton, C. H. and Fields, H. L. (1976). *Proc. natn. Acad. Sci. U.S.A.*, **73**, 4685–8
Bradbury, A. F., Smyth, D. G. and Snell, C. R. (1976). *Biochem. biophys. Res. Commun.*, **69**, 950–6
Curzon, G., Kantamaneni, B. D., Bartlett, J. R. and Bridges, P. K. (1976). *J. Neurochem.*, **26**, 613–5
Garelis, E., Young, S. N., Lal, S. and Sourkes, T. L. (1974). *Brain Res.*, **79**, 1–8
Gintzler, A. R., Levy, A. and Spector, S. (1976). *Proc. natn. Acad. Sci. U.S.A.*, 73, 2132–6
Goldstein, A. (1976). *Science*, **193**, 1081–6
Guillemin, R., Ling, N. and Burgus, R. (1976). *C.r. hebd. Séanc. Acad. Sci. Paris*, **282**, 783–5
Gunne, L.-M., Lindström, L. and Terenius, L. (1977). *J. Neural Transmission*, **40**, 13–9
Hughes, J., Smith, T., Kosterlitz, H. W., Fothergill, L. A., Morgan, B. and Morris, H. R. (1975). *Nature*, **258**, 577–9
Hökfelt, T., Ljungdal, Å., Elde, R., Nilsson, G. and Terenius, L. (1977). *Proc. natn. Acad. Sci. U.S.A.*, **74**, 3081–5
Lindström, L., Widerlöv, E., Gunne, L.-M., Wahlström, A. and Terenius, L. (1978). *Acta psychiat. scand.*, **57**, 153–64
Lord, J. A. H., Waterfield, A. A., Hughes, J. and Kosterlitz, H. W. (1977). *Nature*, **267**, 495–9
Post, R. M. and Goodwin, F. K. (1975). In *Handbook of Psychopharmacology* (eds L. L. Iversen, S. D. Iversen and S. H. Snyder), vol. 13, Plenum Press, New York, pp 147–86
Schulz, R., Wüster, M. and Herz, A. (1977). *Life Sci.*, **21**, 105–6
Simantov, R. and Snyder, S. H. (1976). *Molec. Pharmac.*, **12**, 987–8
Sjölund, B. and Eriksson, M. (1976). *Lancet*, **ii**, 1085
Sjölund, B., Terenius, L. and Eriksson, M. (1977). *Acta physiol. scand.*, **100**, 382–4
Sjöström, R., Ekstedt, J. and Änggård, E. (1975). *J. Neurol. Neurosurg. Psychiat.*, **38**, 66–8
Sternbach, R. A. (1974). *Pain Patients. Traits and Treatment*, Academic Press, New York
Terenius, L. (1977). *Psychoneuroendocrinology*, **2**, 53–8
Terenius, L. and Wahlström, A. (1975). *Life Sci.*, **16**, 1759–64
Terenius, L., Wahlström, A., Lindström, L. and Widerlöv, E. (1976). *Neurosci. Lett.*, **3**, 157–62
Terenius, L., Wahlström, A. and Ågren, H. (1977). *Psychopharmacology*, **54**, 31–3

52
Plasma β-lipotropin in the human

Dorothy T. Krieger, Anthony Liotta and Toshihiro Suda
(Department of Medicine, Mt Sinai Medical Center,
New York, New York 10029, U.S.A.)

To date there has been no specific immunoassay for human lipotropin (LPH). The importance of such an assay is evident with the realization that β-LPH, not β-MSH, is present in human pituitary and plasma. There is no evidence for the presence of a human β-MSH. This has been shown to be a breakdown product derived by cleavage from β-LPH during *in vitro* extraction procedures. Previous reports of the measurement of human LPH have relied on indirect evidence obtained from data derived by RIA for 'β_h-MSH'. These assays have utilized antibodies, raised either against ACTH or β-MSH. In some of these reports, but not all, it has been demonstrated that such antibodies partially or completely cross-react with β-LPH or γ-LPH and react with a material in plasma which has an elution pattern on gel filtration identical or closely related to that of the lipotropins. The studies to be reported are based on the development of a homologous RIA for human LPH which has no cross-reactivity with β-MSH. Data will be presented on the measurement of basal and stimulated plasma LPH concentrations in normal subjects, and in patients with abnormalities in ACTH and cortisol secretion, and correlation of these concentrations with those of plasma ACTH.

MATERIALS AND METHODS

An antibody to β_h-LPH was obtained by immunizing rabbits with β_h-LPH in complete Freund's adjuvant. β_h-LPH was iodinated with ^{125}I, by means of the chloramine T method, achieving a specific activity of 120–160 μCi/μg. Plasma at a concentration of 10 per cent or more of the incubation volume was demonstrated to interfere with the assay. 8 Anilino-1-naphthalene sulfonic acid (ANS) was added to all plasma samples and these were extracted with silicic acid. Such extraction procedures give average recovery of β-LPH added to LPH-free human plasma of 87 per cent. Antibody was used at a final dilution of 1/50 000. (This antiserum was purified by affinity chromatography to remove a binding site that recognizes β-endorphin.)

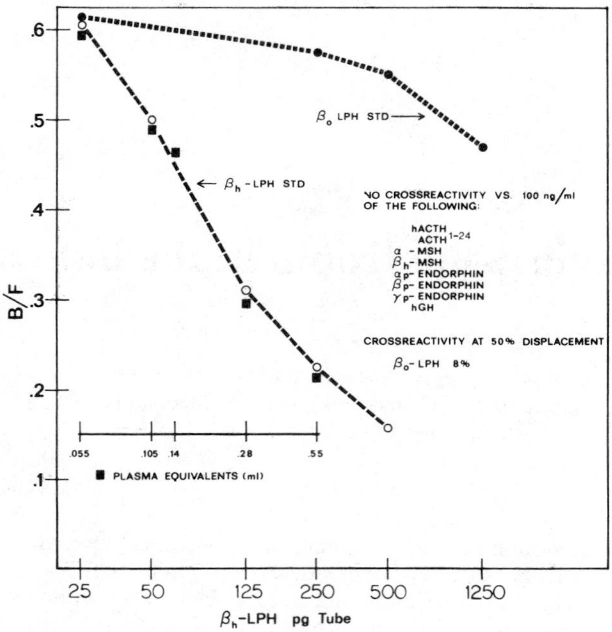

Figure 52.1 Standard curve for β_h-LPH. The ratio of bound to free labelled hormone is plotted on the ordinate. The abscissa depicts the dose of peptide on a logarithmic scale (pg/tube). Cross-reactivity studies with indicated peptides are also depicted. ■, Dilution curve of a plasma extract exhibiting parallel inhibition with that of the standard.

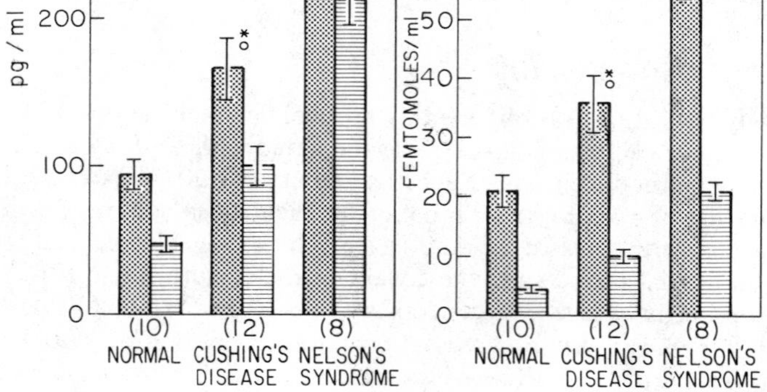

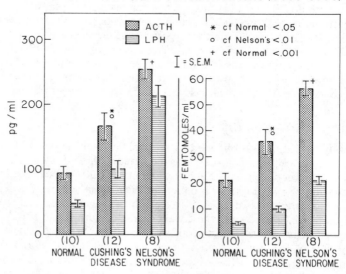

Figure 52.2 Molar concentrations of ACTH and LPH in plasma from normal subjects and patients with Cushing's disease and Nelson's syndrome.

Samples were assayed in duplicate, at up to four dilutions to establish parallelism. Incubation was carried out 4°C for 3 days. Separation of bound from free hormone was accomplished with charcoal dextran. The sensitivity of this asay is 75 pg/ml, using equilibrium incubation conditions and 20–25 pg/ml when non-equilibrium conditions are used; with an intraassay coefficient of variation of 8.3 per cent and an interassay coefficient of variation of 11.7 per cent. The antiserum used exhibits no cross-reactivity with ACTH, β-MSH or porcine α, β, or γ-endorphin (see figure 52.1), indicating that the antigenic determinant resides in the extreme N-terminus of the LPH molecule, corresponding to the species variant sequence. There is less than 10 per cent cross-reactivity (at 50 per cent displacement) with LPH of ovine, porcine and rodent origin. The present antibody recognizes β and γ-LPH with nearly equal affinity (Krieger *et al.,* 1977). Assays for plasma ACTH and plasma cortisol were performed by methods current in our laboratory (Liotta and Krieger, 1975; Murphy, 1977).

The normal subjects studied ranged from 24–30 years of age. Patient material consisted of subjects with untreated Cushing's disease, Nelson's syndrome, ectopic ACTH secretion, and Addison's disease. Blood samples were collected into previously heparinized plastic syringes, placed into pre-cooled plastic tubes, and centrifuged in a refrigerated centrifuge within 15 min. *N*-ethyl maleimide was added at a final concentration of 1 mM, and plasma stored at –20 °C until assayed. All specimens, including those for determination of basal concentrations, were obtained via an indwelling i.v. catheter that had been inserted at least 1 hour previously. Insulin tolerance tests and vasopressin tests were performed as previously described (Krieger and Glick, 1972).

RESULTS

Basal plasma LPH and ACTH concentrations

Plasma LPH concentrations (figure 52.2) (0800–0900 h) in normal subjects are in agreement with those reported for plasma 'β-MSH' by Tanaka *et al.* (1977) and are approximately twofold higher than those reported in two other studies (Bachelot *et al.*, 1977; Gilkes *et al.*, 1975) using antibodies not specific for LPH. Plasma LPH concentrations in patients with Cushing's disease, Nelson's syndrome and the ectopic ACTH syndrome fall within the range reported in other studies measuring 'β-MSH' in these disease states. On a molar basis, plasma ACTH concentrations were greater than those of LPH in all instances.

A highly significant correlation ($r > 0.9000$) was present between plasma ACTH and LPH concentrations in all of the above patient groups. A correlation of 0.5595 was seen in normal subjects.

Basal plasma ACTH/LPH ratios in normal subjects are similar to those noted by Gilkes *et al.* (1975). In the present study, ratios in patients with Cushing's disease were not significantly different from those seen in normal subjects, whereas those in patients with Nelson's syndrome and ectopic ACTH production were significantly lower than those in either the normal subjects or the patients with Cushing's disease (figure 52.3). In no instances were such concentrations equimolar. Gilkes *et al.* (1975) and Abe *et al.* (1967) have also noted lower ratios in patients with Nelson's syndrome. (Studies in additional patients have revealed a significantly lower ratio in patients with Cushing's disease.)

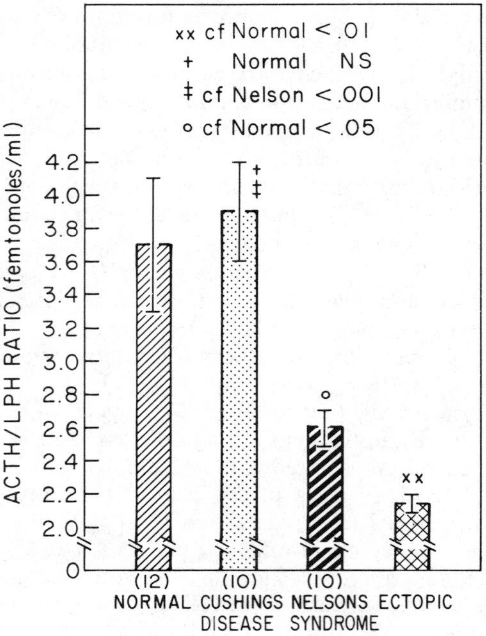

Figure 52.3 Molar ratios of ACTH and LPH in plasma from normal subjects and patients with Cushing's disease and Nelson's syndrome.

Response of plasma LPH and ACTH to insulin induced hypoglycemia
Plasma LPH and ACTH concentrations rose in parallel (figure 52.4) in response to effective hypoglycemia, both reaching peak concentrations at the same time following insulin administration. The mean percentage increases in plasma ACTH and LPH concentrations were 375 and 473 per cent, respectively. Peak ACTH/LPH molar ratios were 3.8 which were not significantly different from ratios of 4.4 seen in basal specimens. Molar ratios at 90 and 120 min were 1.8 and 1.3, respectively, both of which were significantly different from ratios observed in basal and peak samples (figure 52.5). It remains to be seen whether such altered ratios reflect differential rates of disappearance of ACTH and LPH, different distribution volumes, or different release mechanisms for each hormone. In recent studies we have demonstrated a greater metabolic clearance rate for β-lipotropin than for ACTH.

Response of Plasma ACTH and LPH to vasopressin administration
Studies have been performed in normal subjects and patients with Cushing's disease and Nelson's syndrome. In normal subjects and patients with Cushing's disease and Nelson's syndrome, plasma LPH and ACTH concentrations rose in parallel, both reaching peak concentrations at essentially the same time following vasopressin administration (figure 52.6). Similar percentage increases in plasma ACTH and LPH concentrations were seen in normal subjects and patients with

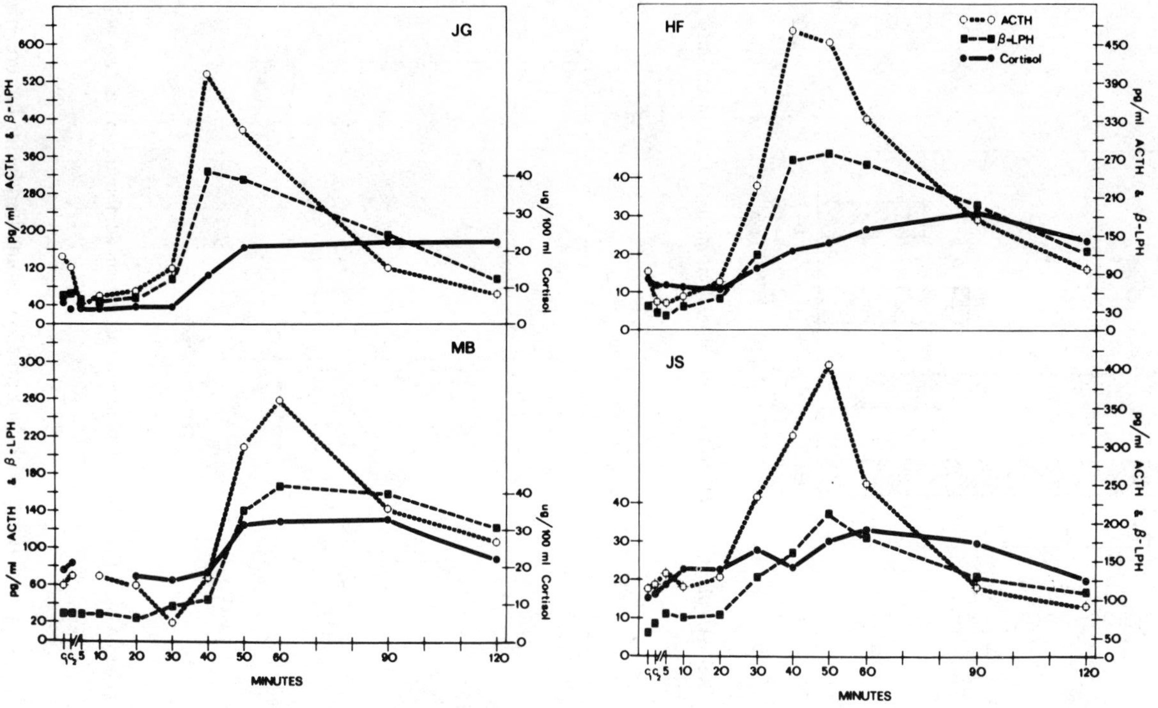

Figure 52.4 Plasma ACTH and LPH response to insulin induced hypoglycemia in four normal adult subjects.

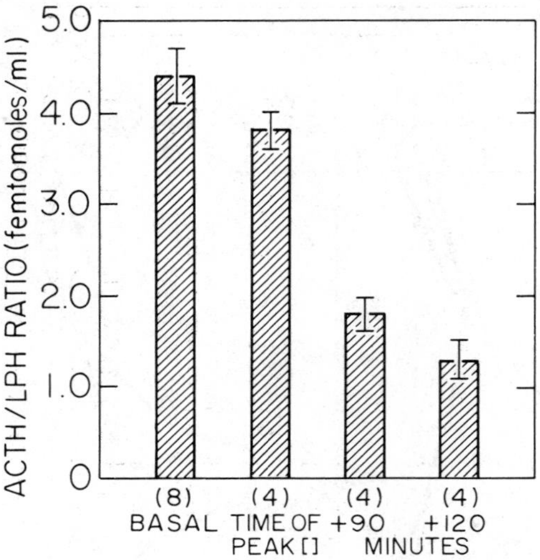

Figure 52.5 Ratio of plasma ACTH to LPH concentrations during course of insulin tolerance testing.

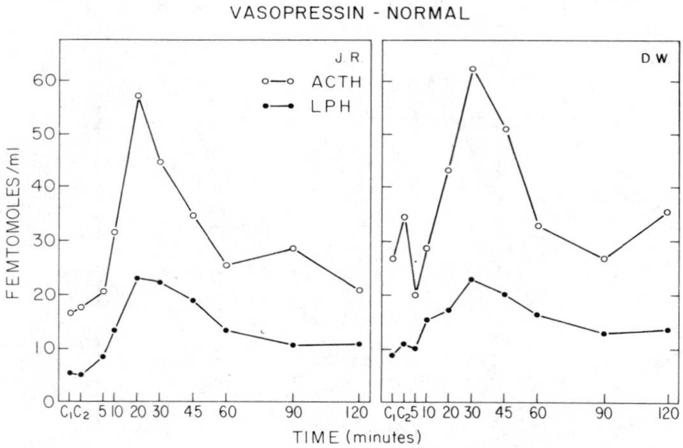

Figure 52.6 Plasma ACTH and LPH response to vasopressin administration in two normal subjects.

Cushing's disease, the patients with Nelson's syndrome had lesser increments. Unlike the findings noted in the insulin tolerance test, molar ACTH/LPH ratios did not vary significantly over time.

DISCUSSION

The present data are the first in which human plasma LPH-like activity and its response to two different stimuli in normal subjects, as well as in patients with pituitary-adrenal disease, has been measured using a specific antibody which demonstrates no cross-reactivity with either α, β-MSH, ACTH or synthetic ACTH fragments. As already noted, plasma LPH concentrations both in normal subjects and in patients with pituitary-adrenal disease, and ACTH/LPH ratios are similar to those reported in other studies using a less specific antibody. In the normal subject, as well as in patients with Cushing's disease, Nelson's syndrome, or the ectopic ACTH syndrome, there is a highly significant correlation of plasma ACTH and LPH concentration. Such a high correlation would support the observation that ACTH and LPH are first synthesized in the pituitary or in the ectopic tumor as part of a common prohormone (Mains *et al.*, 1977) which is subsequently degraded into its component moieties. Such correlation would not, however, mitigate against the possibility that LPH is further processed into smaller components before secretion or at peripheral sites. This might explain the different molar ratios of these substances found in plasma in various conditions. Pulse chase *in vitro* as well as determination *in vivo* of both peripheral LPH and endorphin concentrations, especially under the conditions of pituitary stimulation might help to clarify this problem.

In addition to the concordance of plasma ACTH and LPH concentrations, the other significant finding in these studies is that of the parallelism of reponse of these concentrations following either insulin-induced hypoglycemia or vasopressin administration. In the case of insulin-induced hypoglycemia, there was a decrease in plasma ACTH/LPH ratios following attainment of peak levels; no significant change in such ratios was seen following vasopressin administration. Whether this represents a different pituitary response to endogenous 'CRF' stimulation (as induced by hypoglycemia) than to vasopressin will have to be further assessed by *in vitro* studies in which ACTH and LPH responsiveness to median eminence extract and to vasopressin can be measured.

Gilkes *et al.* (1975) and Hirata *et al.* (1975) reported similar findings during the course of insulin tolerance testing; Hirata *et al.* (1975) reported an increase of ACTH but not of β-MSH, following vasopressin administration. (In the latter study lysine-vasopressin rather than Pitressin was used, and there is no information as to cross-reactivity of the antibody employed with β-LPH).

The decrease in molar plasma ACTH/LPH ratios following attainment of peak levels after insulin hypoglycemia might be explained by the longer half life of endogenous lipotropin compared to that of ACTH (Tanaka *et al.*, 1977; Gilkes *et al.*, 1977). As noted above, other possibilities, such as different distribution volume of these two peptides, or secretion or generation of molecular forms other than those of authentic LPH having different immunoreactivity may also explain these findings. There is evidence of secretion of smaller amounts of γ-LPH than of β-LPH during the course of insulin induced hypoglycemia (Donald and Toth, 1973), although basal levels of both forms of LPH seemed to be similar. These findings might suggest that β-LPH is preferentially secreted under acute stimulation, while under basal conditions there is pituitary or plasma conversion of β-LPH to γ-LPH. Thus far there have been no studies in normal subjects in which Sephadex chromatography has been utilized to determine the nature of plasma elution patterns in normal subjects under basal and stimulated conditions using both forms of LPH as markers.

The present data therefore indicate that LPH is secreted simultaneously with ACTH under basal and stimulated conditions. They also suggest that in patients with pituitary tumors and ectopic ACTH secretion there may be less intrapituitary conversion of LPH to smaller peptides or that the form of LPH present has a longer half life than normal LPH. It is obvious that measurement of plasma endorphin concentrations, and perhaps of other opiate-like substances derived from LPH will be necessary to fully assess the significance of this observation. We have recently reported (Suda *et al.*, 1978) the presence of significant basal plasma β-endorphin concentrations in patients with Nelson's syndrome, ectopic ACTH syndrome and Addison's disease. β-Endorphin is not detectable in plasma from normal subjects under basal conditions.

Simultaneous determination of these peptides and their ratios may give some clue as to the pathological process present in cases of ACTH hypersecretion. Should future studies demonstrate different ACTH/endorphin than ACTH/LPH ratios this may raise further questions as to the dynamics of the pituitary secret-tion and metabolism of these peptides, as well as leading to exploration of the possible effects in patients of the elevated endorphin levels present.

ACKNOWLEDGMENTS

This work is supported in part by the Lita Annenberg Hazen Charitable Trust. The technical assistance of Mr H. Hauser is gratefully acknowledged.

REFERENCES

Abe, K., Nicholson, W. E., Liddle, G. W., Island, D. P. and Orth, D. N. (1967). *J. clin. invest.*, **46**, 1609–16

Bachelot, I., Wolfsen, A. R. and Odell, W. D. (1977). *J. clin. Endocr. Metab.*, **44**, 939–46

Donald, R. A. and Toth, A. (1973). *J. clin. Endocr. Metab.*, **36**, 925–30

Gilkes, J. H., Bloomfield, G. A., Scott, A. P., Lowry, P. J. Ratcliffe, J. G., Landon, J. and Rees, L. H. (1975). *J. clin. Endocr. Metab.*, **40**, 450–7

Gilkes, J. J. H., Rees, L. H. and Besser, G. M. (1977). *Br. med. J.*, **1**, 996–8

Hirata, Y., Sakamoto, N., Matsukura, S. and Imura, H. (1975). *J. clin. Endocr. Metab.*, **41**, 1092–7

Krieger, D. T. and Glick, S. (1972). *Am. J. Med.*, **52**, 25

Krieger, D. T., Liotta, A. and Li, C. H. (1977). *Life Sci.*, **21**, 1771–8

Liotta, A. and Krieger, D. T. (1975). *J. clin. Endocr. Metab.*, **40**, 268–77

Mains, R. E., Eipper, B. A. and Ling, N. (1977). *Proc. natn. Acad. Sci. U.S.A.*, **74**, 3014–8

Murphy, B. E. P. (1967). *J. clin. Endocr. Metab.*, **27**, 983–90

Suda, T., Liotta, A. and Krieger, D. T. (1978). *Science* (in press)

Tanaka, K., Nicholson, W. E. and Orth, D. N. (1977). *Abstr. No. 73, 59th Annual Meeting Endocrinol. Soc.*, 93

53
Presence of a non-peptide morphine-like compound in human CSF and urine

S. Spector, J. Shorr, J. Finberg and K. Foley*
(Roche Institute of Molecular Biology, Nutley, New Jersey 07110 and
*Memorial Sloan-Kettering Cancer Center, New York,
New York, 10021, U.S.A.)

In our laboratory, we have been developing the formation of antibodies to drugs for a number of reasons but one that has been foremost in our thinking is whether these very specific proteins that have been generated for particular drug molecules can act as surrogate receptors. The antibody possesses many of the qualities of the receptor, and so it should be reasonable to assume that if there are endogenous substances in the body which impinge upon the opiate receptor, and if the receptor recognizes morphine, the antibody developed to bind morphine should also bind an endogenous opiate.

Because of the low molecular weight of drugs, they are usually incapable of stimulating the formation of antibodies. As a consequence, they have to be conjugated to a carrier protein in order to impart to them the critical molecular size. It is also known that one can generate antibodies that will be able to recognize various portions of the drug molecule dependent on the site on which the drug or hapten is conjugated to the larger molecular weight carrier.

We have used antibodies generated by a conjugated morphine-bovine serum albumin (BSA) immunogen in which the morphine molecule was coupled to the protein at two different sites to look for endogenous substances in tissues and biological fluids. The test system we initially used was the RIA technique (Berson and Yalow, 1959).

The conjugation of morphine to protein at C_3 position was done by first converting morphine to 3-O-carboxymethylmorphine and the carboxymethylmorphine was coupled to BSA in the presence of a water-soluble carbodiimide as described by Spector and Parker (1970). The *in vitro* binding of the antibody formed by this immunogen with various opiate alkaloids is shown in table 53.1. The congeners of morphine, codeine, normorphine and heroin all bind to the antibody to the same extent. Synthetic surrogates of morphine are bound by the

Table 53.1 Competition with ^3H-dihydromorphine for binding sites

Comp'd	Structure	Conc'n which inhibits labeled Ag–Ab complex 50%
	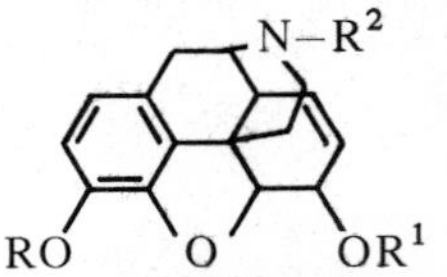 	
1) Morphine	R = H R^1 = H R^2 = CH_3	500 picograms
2) Codeine	R = CH_3 R^1 = H R^2 = CH_3	500 picograms
3) Normorphine	R = H R^1 = H R^2 = H	500 picograms
4) Morphine-3-monoglucuronide	R = 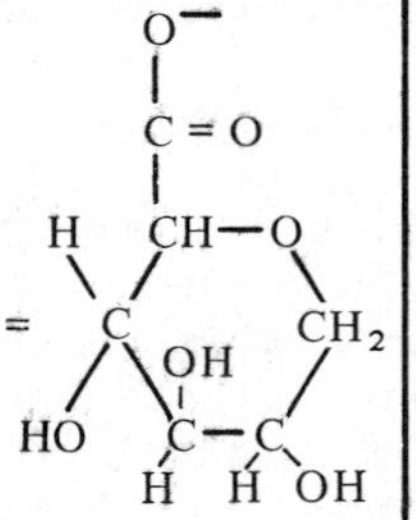 R^1 = H R^2 = CH_3	200 nanograms
5) Heroin	R = CH_3—C(=O) R^1 = CH_3—C(=O) R^2 = CH_3	500 picograms

antibody poorly if at all. Nalorphine and methadone require a concentration of at least 500 times that of morphine to produce 50 per cent inhibition of binding to labeled hapten–protein complex. The synthetic morphinans, dextrorphan and levorphan, were not recognized at all by the antibody combining sites at a concentration 500 times that of morphine.

We then prepared a morphine immunogen in which the carrier protein was conjugated to the nitrogen atom of the opiate alkaloid by initially forming N-methyl carboxymorphine and again in the presence of a water soluble carbo-

Table 53.2 Competition with ^{3}H-dihydromorphine for binding sites

Compound	Structure 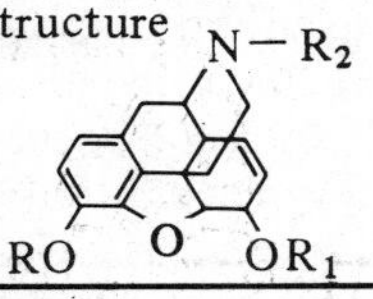	Conc'n which inhibits labeled Ag–Ab complex 50%
Morphine	R = H R_1 = H R_2 = CH_3	30 pg
Codeine	R = CH_3 R_1 = H R_2 = CH_3	> 50,000 pg
Normorphine	R = H R_1 = H R_2 = H	30 pg
Morphine glucuronide	R = 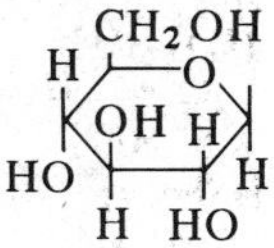 R_1 = H R_2 = CH_3	10,000 pg
Nalorphine	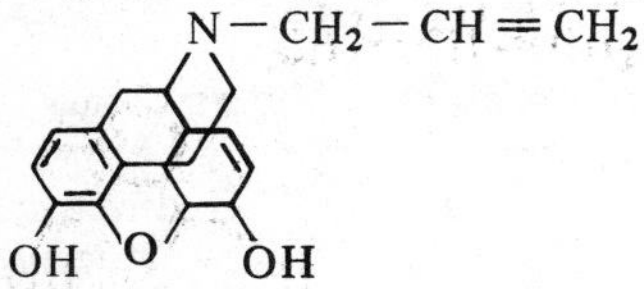	40 pg
Levallorphan	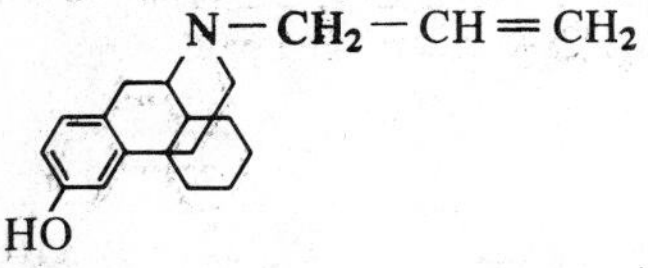	200 pg
Methadone	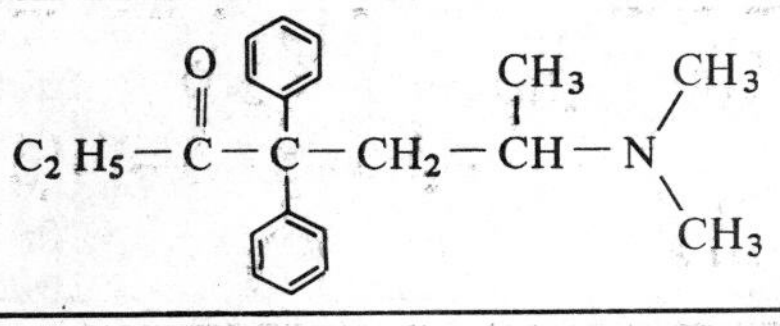	> 50,000 pg

diimide coupling it to BSA (Gintzler *et al.*, 1976). The specificity of the antibodies developed by this immunogen is shown in table 53.2. The congeners of morphine, normorphine, and nalorphine all bind to these antibodies at approximately the same concentration. However, these antibodies could now differentiate codeine from morphine. Modification of the furan ring of morphine also abolishes a determinant group which the antibody can recognize. Thus, we have now developed two antibodies which recognized different parts of the morphine molecule. Peptides with opiate-like properties have been isolated and characterized (Hughes *et al.*, 1975; Pasternak *et al.*, 1975; Terenius and Wahlström, 1975; Li *et al.*, 1976). These various peptides were tested to determine whether the antibodies developed against morphine would bind any of these peptides and table 53.3 shows that the antibodies are morphine specific as they failed to bind any of the peptides.

To detect the presence of an endogenous morphine-like material, brain extracts from beef, cat, rabbit, rat and guinea pig were incubated with labeled hapten and antibody; it was found that these brain extracts contained material which could compete with the labeled morphine for binding to the antibodies. This material being extracted from brain tissue was recognized equally well by both of our antibodies. Because these antibodies had such a high degree of binding specificity, we are tentatively calling the extracted substance, morphine-like compound (MLC). MLC was quantitated as morphine immunoequivalents and this was assessed by comparing the degree of inhibition of binding to the antibody of labeled hapten produced by non-radioactive morphine with the degree of inhibition of binding produced by MLC. Assuming that the specific morphine antibody binds MLC with an affinity equal to its affinity for morphine and that MLC has a molecular weight close to morphine one can also express MLC as molar equivalents of morphine. Ultrafiltration studies using UM2 membranes indicate that MLC has a molecular weight less than 1000. This molecular weight cut off is also obtained using the Biogel-P_2 resin.

Table 53.3 Antimorphine rabbit antibody specificity

Compound	Inhibition of [^{125}I] morphine binding to antibody by 50%
Morphine	0.1 ng
Naloxone	>5
Dextrorphan	100
Levorphan	1
L-Methadone	>1000
Met-Enkephalin	>1000
Leu-Enkephalin	>1000
β-Endorphin	>1000
Tyrosine	>1000
Tyr-Gly	>1000
Tyr-Gly-Gly	>1000
Gly-Gly-Phe-Met	>1000
Substance-P	>1000

Studies were done to eliminate the possibility that the presence of MLC was a consequence of the diet of some of our experimental animals. We, therefore put some of our laboratory animals, specifically the rats, rabbits, and guinea pigs on a synthetic diet for 2 weeks and found that it did not influence the brain MLC concentrations in these animals. Also, with all the emphasis being placed on opiate-like peptides we subjected MLC to various peptidases including Pronase, trypsin, carboxypeptidase A and aminopeptidase and to boiling in 6 N HCl and none of these treatments altered MLC activity as measured by RIA.

We have also reported (Blume *et al.*, 1977) that MLC isolated from central nervous tissue is not only recognized by a morphine specific antibody but can also be recognized and bind to opiate receptors. These receptors have been shown by Klee and Nirenberg (1974) to be present in intact cells or membrane fractions from mouse neuroblastoma × rat glioma hybrid cell line NG108-15. Using brain neuronal membrane preparation, which also has opiate receptors, gives similar results as the NG108-15 hybrid cell line. The affinity these opiate receptors have for MLC is 2–3 times greater than that of leu-enkephalin and 20 to 100 times stronger than that of naloxone or morphine.

Since MLC could be detected in brain tissue, we then investigated biological fluids, such as cerebrospinal fluid (CSF) and urine. There have been reports to indicate that some of the opiate-like acting peptides are present in CSF and we would like to report that MLC is present in the CSF. Samples were obtained from patients who were at the Memorial Sloan-Kettering Cancer Center in New York City. Table 53.4 shows that there were six females and two males in this study, that their ages ranged from 18 to 55 years, and that they were hospitalized because of meningeal carcinoma or had neurological syndrome associated with intracranial hypertension. The CSF was obtained under sterile conditions from an Ommaya reservoir. None of the patients received narcotic medication. These subjects had CSF values of MLC up to 1 ng morphine equivalent per ml. It is also interesting that Rubinstein (personal communication) analyzed some of these CSF samples using the column monitoring of peptides and amino acid analyses and was unable to detect any of the opiate peptides. The only activity that can be found using receptor binding assay is a small molecular weight substance. When we did an analysis of the small molecular weight substance, we found it to be MLC. The CSF was assayed for MLC using the RIA procedure for morphine determination. With three samples we also did a binding assay using intact cells from the mouse neuroblastoma and rat glioma hybrid clone NG108-15 in which the radioactive ligand was [^{3}H] leu-enkephalin (45.6 Ci/mmol). The receptor binding assay is not that specific, as it will recognize both MLC and opiate-like peptides. However, the antibodies only bind morphine and not the peptides so that the RIA is more specific for identifying the presence of MLC. Since the antibody used in the RIA was developed against morphine, rather than MLC, we find that the receptor assay gives us values of MLC which are 20 to 100 times more than the RIA. This is quite understandable since the receptor should bind an endogenous ligand far better than an antibody which has been produced for morphine.

The other biological fluid that we looked at for MLC was the urine. We obtained 24-hour samples from 19 human volunteers from our laboratory who were not on any medication. The concentrations of MLC in urine varied from a level of 1 ng/mg creatinine to about 2 ng/mg creatinine (table 53.5). We have no idea, at this point,

Table 53.4 Morphine-like compound in human CSF

Patient	Age	Sex	Diagnosis	Site	Drug treatment Non-narcotic	Narcotic	MLC ng equivalents/ml CSF
J.H.	38	F	B I H*	Lumbar	None	None	Below assay sensitivity
C.N.	18	F	B I H*	Lumbar	None	None	Below assay sensitivity
J.W.	38	F	B I H*	Vent.	None	None	0.12
G.O.	45	F	B I H*	Vent.	Aldomet	None	0.3
J.W.	55	M	Hodgkins meningeal ca.	Vent.	Prednisone	None	1
C.D.	51	F	Ca. breast Meningeal ca.	Vent.	None	None	0.3
B.S.	35	F	Malignant melanoma	Lumbar	Decadron	None	0.03
Pooled†	CSF	M	Normal	Lumbar	None	None	0.05

*Benign Intracranial Hypertension
†Obtained by the courtesy of Dr L. Terenius, University of Uppsala, Uppsala, Sweden.

Table 53.5 Presence of morphine-like compound (MLC) in human urine

(ng MLC equivalents/mg creatinine/ml urine) Male*	Female*
(n = 13)	(n = 6)
2.39 ± 0.25†	1.96 ± 0.4†

*Subjects were all normal volunteers from our laboratory.
†Mean ± s.e.m.

whether there is a diurnal rhythm regarding MLC, hormonal effects on the elaboration of MLC or the effects of drugs.

Finally, I should like to include some information regarding the behavioral effects of MLC. We are currently in the process of purifying enough of the MLC in order to characterize it chemically. We have gone through various chromatographic methods, including an affinity column on which morphine antibodies have been immobilized, and we have a few hundred nanograms morphine equivalents of MLC. Rats were injected with 10 ng morphine equivalents of MLC into the third ventricle. Four of the six rats initially became very agitated, running around the cage but not in a coordinated running behavior, rather it was as though they were jumping. This lasted for about 5 min and then they exhibited a catatonic behavior pattern. The other two rats immediately became catatonic. The catatonia persisted from 30 min to 2 hours.

In summary, we would like to point out that just as there may be more than one opiate receptor, this also applies to the presence of endogenous ligands and that peptides are not the sole endogenous substrate for the opiate receptors. We have included evidence that there is an endogenous non-peptide opiate which binds to opiate receptors,which is present in biological tissues and fluids in all mammals studied including man,which elicits behavioral effects, and is recognized by specific morphine antibodies. It must have structural characteristics much like morphine and yet it is not morphine, as it is not blocked by the narcotic antagonist naloxone. At the moment, there are too many things we don't know about MLC but time and effort will modify that.

REFERENCES

Berson, S. A. and Yalow, R. S. (1959). *Nature,* **184**, 1648–9

Spector, S. and Parker, C. W. (1970). *Science,* **168**, 1347–8

Gintzler, A. R., Mohaci, E. and Spector, S. (1976). *Eur. J. Pharmac.,* **38**, 149–56

Hughes, J., Smith, T. W., Kosterlitz, H. W., Fothergill, L. A., Morgan, B. A. and Morris, H. R. (1975). *Nature,* **258**, 577–9

Pasternak, G. W., Goodman, R. and Snyder, S. H. (1975). *Life Sci.,* **16**, 1765–9

Terenius, L. and Wahlström, A. (1975). *Life Sci.,* **16**, 1759–64

Li, C. H. and Chung, D. (1976). *Proc. natn. Acad. Sci. U.S.A.,* **73**, 1145–8

Blume, A. J., Shorr, J., Finberg, J. P. M. and Spector, S. (1977). *Proc. natn. Acad. Sci. U.S.A.,* **74**, 4927–31

Klee, W. A. and Nirenberg, M. (1974). *Proc. natn. Acad. Sci. U.S.A.,* **71**, 3474–7

54

Pronase P resistant endogenous opiate-like acting materials

Michael Wüster, Rüdiger Schulz, Petra Loth,
Herbert Schneider*, and Albert Herz
(Department of Neuropharmacology, Max-Planck-Institut für Psychiatrie,
Kraepelinstrasse 2, 8000 München 40, and
*Department of Neuropsychopharmacology,
Schering AG, 1000 Berlin, F.R.G.)

Endogenous opiate-like substances, possessing significantly different properties from the known opioid peptides, have been detected in blood (Schulz *et al.*, 1977*a*), urine (Goldstein and Cox, 1977; Schulz and Wüster, 1977), amniotic fluid (Schulz, unpublished), brain (Wüster *et al.*, 1978; Höllt, unpublished), liver (Simon, personal communication; Wüster, unpublished), and small intestine (Schulz *et al.*, 1977*a,b*). Interestingly, Pronase P or other peptidases fail to destroy their biological activity. This property, when considered together with analytical data previously reported, does not support the notion that these substances comprise opioid peptides. In the present communication data are given to further characterize these opiate-like acting compounds of unknown structure from brain and urine.

METHODS

In view of the lipophilic character of the substances, they were extracted by a solvent mixture consisting of heptane and chloroform (1:1, v/v). The freshly dissected brains of five rats were homogenized in 100 ml Tris buffer (0.1 M, pH 8.6). The homogenate was stirred at room temperature for 30 min with 200 ml heptane/chloroform. After separation of the phases, the organic layer was removed and evaporated to dryness. The residue was run on t.l.c. (silica gel, solvent 2-propanol/water, 7:3, v/v), and opiate-like activity was detected between R_f values of 0.8 and 0.9. For extraction of freshly obtained urine, 100 ml samples were stirred for 30 min with 200 ml heptane/chloroform. The organic phase was separated, evaporated to dryness, and the residue was placed onto a Sephadex LH 20 column (2 × 3 cm), equilibrated with heptane/chloroform (1:1, v/v).

Opioid activity was eluted with 50 ml heptane/chloroform (1:1). Tests for opiate-like activity were conducted with strips of the guinea pig ileum (GPI) (Schulz and Goldstein, 1972; ED_{50} for morphine 100 nM). Opiate-like effects on this preparation refer to naloxone-reversible inhibitions of electrically induced twitches.

RESULTS

The pharmacological activity of opioid materials from brain and urine on the twitch tension of electrically stimulated strips is illustrated in figure 54.1. The onset of action of the brain extract was slow with a 50 per cent depression of the electrically evoked response occurring after about 20 min. This inhibitory effect was completely reversed by naloxone (100 nM). The antagonistic effect of naloxone decreased as the antagonist was washed out, so that a persistent opiate-like action became apparent. Naloxone-reversible inhibition was observed even 3 hours after exposure of the preparation to the brain extract although washes were conducted in 10 min intervals (panel A). Material purified by paper electrophoresis did not exhibit the long acting depressive effect. So far, this characteristic pattern of slow onset and offset of opiate-like action resembles the kinetics observed with crude opioid material obtained from blood and small intestine (Schulz *et al.*, 1977*a*). Opiate-like material extracted from urine in comparison to that present in the brain extract showed a more rapid onset and offset of action. The maximal inhibition occurred within 15 min and the activity was washed off easily (panel B).

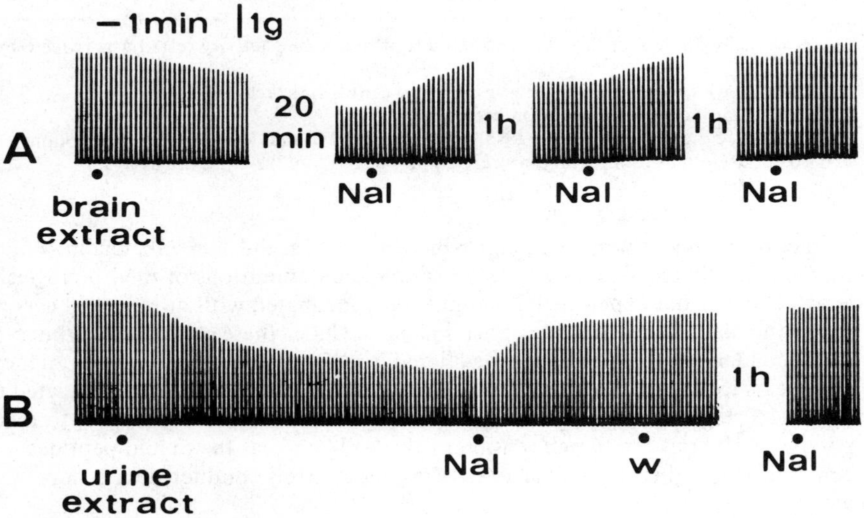

Figure 54.1 Naloxone-reversible opiate-like activity of extracts from brain (panel A) and urine (panel B) on the electrically stimulated (0.1 Hz, 60 V, 0.5 ms) longitudinal muscle-myenteric plexus preparation of the GPI. The opiate-like activity extracted from brain persisted for several hours despite washing (w) of the preparation at 10 min intervals, whereas the material from urine was easily removed by washing. Nal = 100 μM.

Tests of the brain extract on the isolated mouse vas deferens (Henderson *et al.*, 1972; ED_{50} for met-enkephalin 10 nM, for normorphine 400 nM) revealed a 30-fold decreased sensitivity to the opiate-like activity compared to that found on the GPI. Again, this finding is in accordance with the reported effects of opiate-like acting material from blood and small intestine on both bioassay systems.

In an effort to further elucidate the properties of these heptane/chloroform extracts from brain and urine, they were tested with the agent cyanogen bromide (CNBr) (Gross, 1967). Compounds like met-enkephalin having a S-methyl group on methionine, which is critical for the opiate receptor interaction, will show a substantial loss of biological activity after such treatment while others (such as leu-enkephalin) will not. Table 54.1 indicates that the heptane/chloroform

Table 54.1 Percentage loss of biological activity of opiate-like acting materials*

	Brain (chloroform/heptane extract)	Urine (chloroform/heptane extract)	Leu-enkephalin	Met-enkephalin	β-endorphin
Effect of cyanogen bromide†	No loss	No loss	5; 10	90; 95	70; 80
Effect of nitrous acid‡	No loss	No loss	100; 100	100; 100	100; 100

*Tests were conducted on the GPI. The amount of opiate-like activity tested was twice the ED_{50}.
†Samples were exposed to 25 mg CNBr in 70 per cent formic acid for 24 h at 4 °C. CNBr was removed by lyophilization before assay.
‡Samples were incubated with 1 mg $NaNO_2$ and 10 μl 250 mM formic acid (final volume 120 μl) for 90 min at room temperature. Samples were lyophilized before assay.

extract of brain and urine resisted CNBr treatment, as did leu- enkephalin, while met-enkephalin and β-endorphin showed marked diminutions of their biological activity. In further experiments, samples were incubated with nitrous acid according to the method described by Karrer (1959). Under these conditions, primary and secondary amino groups will be altered, so that the pharmacological potency disappears if they are essential for the opiate receptor interaction. As indicated in table 54.1, the extracts of brain and urine were not affected with respect to their potency to inhibit the twitch tension of the GPI, whereas the opioid peptides completely lost their biological activity, as did controls conducted with normorphine.

Additional characterization was conducted using paper electrophoresis in a buffer of pH 2.0 (acetic acid, 120 ml; formic acid, 20 ml; propyleneglycol, 100 ml; distilled water to 1000 ml). The materials were subjected to electrophoresis (10 V/cm) for 6–8 hours at room temperature. Thereafter, biological activity was located by placing small sections of the developed paper into the Krebs–Ringer solution bathing the strips. The electrophoretic separation of an amount comprising twice the ED_{50} revealed the following mobility of the substances towards the cathode. Ornithine was used as reference compound (R_{or})

opiate-like activity, urine extract	R_{or}	= 0.42
opiate-like activity, brain extract	R_{or}	= 0.30
met-enkephalin	R_{or}	= 0.33
leu-enkephalin	R_{or}	= 0.33
β-endorphin	R_{or}	= 0.40

The R_{or} values indicate cationic properties of the extracts from urine, as has been reported by Goldstein and Cox (1977), and brain. However, the urine extract appeared to possess a stronger basic property compared to the brain material. Attempts to visualize the opiate-like acting urine or brain material by ninhydrin were unsuccessful, but provided clear reactions in the case of met-enkephalin or β-endorphin. However, increasing the amount of opiate-like activity of urine or brain extract to 10 times the ED_{50} resulted in a slightly visible spot in the areas where opioid-like activity was detected. Despite this ninhydrin treatment opioid-like activity was still observed. When brain and urine extracts were examined for behavior on paper electrophoresis at alkaline conditions (pH 8.6), no migration towards the anode was observed.

DISCUSSION

The data presented here extend former investigations with opiate-like acting substances from brain and urine, which display properties unlike those of the opioid peptides (Schulz *et al.*, 1977*a*; Schulz and Wüster, 1977). It appears that the heptane/chloroform extracts from both sources lack a S-methyl group of methionine, which is essential for binding to the opiate receptor. Such a group is known to be present on endorphins derived from β-LPH. Another criterion important for the characterization of these materials is their resistance to nitrous acid exposure, indicating a lack of primary or secondary amino groups, which might be essential for the interaction with opiate receptors. In support of this finding is the failure of ninhydrin to destroy the opiate-like activity of the materials. Although there are some similarities between extracts from brain and urine, differences are apparent in their onset of inhibitory action on the GPI as well as on their migration in an electrical field. Substances extracted from urine are less lipophilic than the brain material, as indicated by its faster onset of action, and displays stronger cationic properties.

So far, the results presented here taken together with others, for example, resistance to Pronase P, a high lipophilicity, and a high resistance to acid hydrolysis (Wüster *et al.*, 1978), are in conflict with the concept that peptides represent the only endogenous ligands for the opiate receptors. Materials investigated here do not bind to morphine antibodies and their biological activity is antagonized by naloxone, which is unlike the properties of a 'non-peptide, morphine-like compound' extracted from the CNS (Gintzler *et al.*, 1978; Blume *et al.*, 1977).

Supported by Deutsche Forschungsgemeinschaft.

REFERENCES

Blume, A., Shorr, J., Finberg, J. and Spector, S. (1977). *Proc. natn. Acad. Sci. U.S.A.*, **74**, 4927–31
Gintzler, A. R., Levy, A. and Spector, S. (1976). *Proc. natn. Acad. Sci. U.S.A.*, **73**, 2132–6
Gintzler, A. R., Gershon, M. D. and Spector, S. (1978). *Science*, **199**, 447–8
Goldstein, A. and Cox, B. M. (1977). *Fedn. Proc.*, **36**, 3895
Gross, E. (1967). In *Methods of Enzymology*, (ed. C. H. W. Hirs) **11**, Academic Press, New York, pp. 238–55
Henderson, G., Hughes, J. and Kosterlitz, H. W. (1972). *Brit. J. Pharmac.*, **46**, 764–6
Karrer, P. (1959). In *Lehrbuch der organischen Chemie*, Georg Thieme, Stuttgart, pp. 142–52
Schulz, R. and Goldstein, A. (1972). *J. Pharmac. exp. Ther.*, **183**, 404–10
Schulz, R. and Wüster, M. (1977). *Eur. J. Pharmac.*, **43**, 383–4
Schulz, R., Wüster, M. and Herz, A. (1977*a*). *Life Sci.*, **21**, 105–16
Schulz, R., Wüster, M., Simantov, R., Snyder, S. and Herz, A. (1977*b*). *Eur. J. Pharmac.*, **41**, 347–8
Wüster, M., Loth, P. and Schulz, R. (1978). *Advances in Biochemical Psychopharmacology*, (eds. E. Costa and M. Trabucchi) Raven Press, New York, in press

55
Characterization of a peptide from the serum of psychotic patients

Roberta M. Palmour*, Frank R. Ervin†, Herbert Wagemaker‡ and Robert Cade∮
(*Department of Genetics, University of California, Berkeley,
†Neuropsychiatric Institute, University of California, Los Angeles,
‡Department of Psychiatry, University of Louisville Medical School, Louisville,
∮Department of Medicine, University of Miami, Miami, Florida, U.S.A.)

The group of psychotic disorders collectively known as schizophrenia continues to be a critical problem for modern psychiatry, accounting for a large proportion of mental hospital bed use, large expenditures for community care and tragedy for many families. Although the work of Kety and Rosenthal (1968) clearly indicates a major genetic contribution to the etiology of such diseases, the biochemical concomitants of these severe disruptions of brain function have remained obscure. The heterogeneity of the patient population suggests underlying biochemical and genetic heterogeneity. While some investigators have studied possible neuronal excess of, or hyper-sensitivity to, neurotransmitters, others have attempted to find a neurotoxic component in the brain or physiological fluids of schizophrenic patients. The embarrassing fate of some of these hypotheses (and of the studies investigating them) has produced a widespread reluctance to pursue other similar suggestions. Nonetheless, the report of Wagemaker and Cade (1977), describing the remission of psychotic symptoms in a group of drug-resistant schizophrenic patients after hemodialysis, suggested an experimental approach. If improvement following dialysis is not a general effect of physiological stress, then some neurochemically active material which either causes psychiatric symptomatology or reflects the underlying neurochemical pathology might be found in the dialysate. Earlier reports of clinical improvement with peritoneal or hemodialysis lend credence to the attempt (Tholen *et al.*, 1960; Opolon *et al.*, 1976). Because dialysis primarily removes low molecular weight components (less than 5000 daltons) it seemed reasonable to look for amines, amino acids and peptides known to have CNS activity. This chapter summarized clinical data on 14 patients treated by Wagemaker and Cade, and reports preliminary biochemical studies of the hemodialysate and serum from six of these patients.

EXPERIMENTAL

Patients and treatment

Fourteen young, chronic process schizophrenics who had manifested psychotic symptomatology, including Schneiderian first-rank symptoms, for more than 3 but less than 15 years, were chosen for the study (table 55.1). All had good premorbid adjustment and had been treated with antipsychotic medications in

Table 55.1 Patient summary

Patient	Drug history	Removed from drugs	BPRS	Treatment outcome
Ct	Navane, Elavil	Night before	43–22	Good
Me	Chlorpromazine, Stelazine	Night before	61–2	Good
Ry	Chlorpromazine, Prolixin	9 Months before	54–0	Good
Pa	Stelazine	Night before	46–0	Good
Eg	Navane, Haldol	Night before	53–0	Good
To	Mellaril	Night before	49–7	Good
Hy	Navane	Night before	43–6	Good
Ch	Mellaril	Night before	41–5	Good
Ho	Chlorpromazine	7 Months before	55–3	Good
Br	Mellaril, Stelazine	Night before	65–31	Moderate
Be	Stelazine	Night before	57–31	Moderate
Ha	Prolixin	Night before	62–22–48	Poor
Sc	Prolixin	Night before	42–69	Poor
Wo	Chlorpromazine	Night before	67–34–62	Poor

adequate doses before entering the dialysis program. Each patient manifested abnormalities of thought and behavior, including inability to work or go to school, and inability to participate in meaningful personal relationships. Renal function was clinically normal in all cases. Informed consent was obtained from each patient before implantation of an arteriovenous shunt and initiation of a series of 14 to 16 consecutive weekly dialyses. Aliquots of dialysate were removed from the first, eighth and sixteenth dialysates and were stored frozen before analysis. Venous blood samples (heparin as anticoagulant) were drawn before dialysis in some instances, and plasma was separated by centrifugation (3000 *g*) and stored at –20 °C.

Amino acid and peptide analysis

Dialysates were concentrated to a standard amino acid concentration by lyophilization and the amino acid and peptide composition was evaluated by microcolumn lithium hydroxide physiological fluids analysis on a Beckman Model 121 M Amino Acid Analyzer, using a five-buffer (pH 2.85, 3.60, 4.17, 5.28, 6.50), two-temperature (64 °C, 41 °C) system. Each peak was quantitated planimetrically. Semi-quantitative estimation of the amount of specific peptides present has been calculated using approximate C values derived from the amino acid content of the peptide determined following purification and/or from C values calculated following analysis of standard synthetic peptides of similar sequence and composition.

Peptides and amino acids were also evaluated by high voltage paper electrophoresis (Whatman No. 1 paper; pH 1.9 pyridine: AcOH:HOH, 2:98:900; 3000 V; 45-90 min), followed by staining with cadmium acetate, ninhydrin or 1-nitroso-2-naphthol.

Purification of peptides

Peptides were purified from a 50-fold concentration of dialysate fluid, using standard techniques of ion exchange chromatography and gel filtration. Aliquots of dialysate fluid (4.1) were lyophilized and reconstituted in a commercially-available physiological salts solution (Dianeal, Travenol Labs) containing 0.1 M formic acid. Peptides and amino acids were desalted on a Sephadex G-50 column (0.9 × 75 cm) equilibrated and eluted with 1 M formic acid; fractions containing amino acids and peptides were identified following high-voltage paper electrophoresis and ninhydrin-staining of aliquots from each fraction. Ninhydrin-positive fractions were concentrated by lyophilization, and reconstituted in the starting buffer for the next chromatographic step. Frequently the desalting operation was repeated, following washing of the column with at least 5 1 1 M formic acid. Desalted peptides were then fractionated by ion exchange chromatography on Aminex A-4 resin (0.9 × 30 cm, 37 °C) using a linear *N*-ethylmorpholine-pyridine-AcOH gradient system (0.5-2.0 M pyridine, pH 2.5-5.0). Fractions containing 1 ml were collected and analyzed by high voltage electrophoresis. Appropriate pools were prepared, lyophilized and reconstituted for final purification by high voltage electrophoresis (Whatman No. 3MM paper, pH 1.9 or 6.0 pyridine: AcOH: HOH buffer, 2500-3500 V, 30-120 min). The positions of peptides were identified by staining guide strips; peptides were cut out and eluted in 0.1 M formic acid.

Analysis of peptides

The molecular weights of purified peptides were estimated by gel filtration using insulin, bacitracin and synthetic peptides of known molecular weights as calibration standards. Relative elution positions ($V_e - V_0$) of known peptides were plotted against the logarithm of the molecular weights. The amino acid content of the peptides was determined on the Model 121 M following acid hydrolysis (6 N HCl, 110 °C) in sealed, evacuated tubes for 18, 48 and 72 hours; following initial experiments, a crystal of phenol was added to protect tyrosine residues. The sulphophenylisothiocyanate derivatives (Inman *et al.*, 1972) of peptides from patients Eg and Ry have been partly sequenced using manual Edman degradation (Gray, 1967) or automatic Edman degradation on the Beckman Model 890 Sequenator (Niall, 1975). Residues have been identified directly following HI hydrolysis (Smithies *et al.*, 1971).

Behavioral and neurophysiological experiments

Adult cats were implanted with electrodes in the frontal cortex, the reticular formation and both amygdalae as well as with i.v.t cannulae for the administration of peptides directly into the CNS. At least 10 days was allowed for recovery from surgery. Peptide purified from patient Ry (100 μg per injection) was introduced into the ventricles of two separate cats, following baseline recording.

Recording was initiated 2 min after the administration of peptide and continued uninterrupted for 1 hour. Gross behavioral observations were performed simultaneously. Electroencephalograms were obtained on each cat for at least 1 hour at 12 hour intervals until electrophysiological and behavioral effects subsided. Synthetic β-endorphin (100 μg per injection), and [D-Ala^2, Met^5]-enkephalinamide and [D-Ala^2, Leu^5]-enkephalinamide (30 μg per injection) were administered as reference compounds; behavioral and electrophysiological observations were collected as described above.

RESULTS

Clinical outcome

At the end of the research protocol period, nine of the fourteen patients showed good improvement, as measured by the Brief Psychiatric Rating Scale (BPRS) and by a renewed ability to work, go to school and lead a productive existence (table 55.1). This was in stark contrast to their pre-dialysis condition when most were either in psychiatric hospitals or in a state of severe personality deterioration. Two patients showed moderate improvement, BPRS scores dropping from 65 and 57 to 31; these two patients exhibited increased function and improved personal relationships. Three patients did not respond favorably to dialysis. Two of these individuals required hospitalization and treatment with neuroleptics following acute psychotic episodes, while the third patient showed initial improvement, but has remained only mildly improved during many weeks of dialysis. Both psychotic patients experienced uncontrollable sleep deprivation during the period of the protocol.

All 14 patients were removed from antipsychotic medication before initiation of the protocol, and remained without antipsychotic medications throughout the dialysis period. Two patients (Ry, Ho) had terminated antipsychotic medication 9 and 6 months before dialysis. Some patients required sleep medication during the dialysis protocol; they were given Dalmane or chloral hydrate.

Dialysate screening

Partial biochemical analysis on dialysate from six patients (1-5 and 10 on table 55.1) is presented here. We reasoned that if a characteristic molecule were being removed by dialysis, then its concentration in dialysate 1 should be substantially greater than its concentration in dialysate 16. Thus, in screening the dialysate samples, samples from dialysates 1 and 16 from each patient were compared with one another, so that each patient served as his own control. The superimposition of the eluate from amino acid analysis of dialysis 1 (solid) and dialysis 16 (dashed) from a single patient is depicted in figure 55.1. Two fractions appear to be more plentiful in dialysate 1. The more prominent peak (A) elutes in the region of asparagine while the other peak of interest (B) coelutes with tryptophan. Similar elution patterns are seen for other individual samples. Following acid hydrolysis of an aliquot of dialysate 1, peak A disappears, suggesting that it is a peptide.

Peptides and amino acids were also evaluated by high voltage paper electrophoresis. When the electrophoretic patterns from paired dialysates 1 and 16 are compared (figure 55.2), a single ninhydrin-positive, tyrosine-positive peptide is

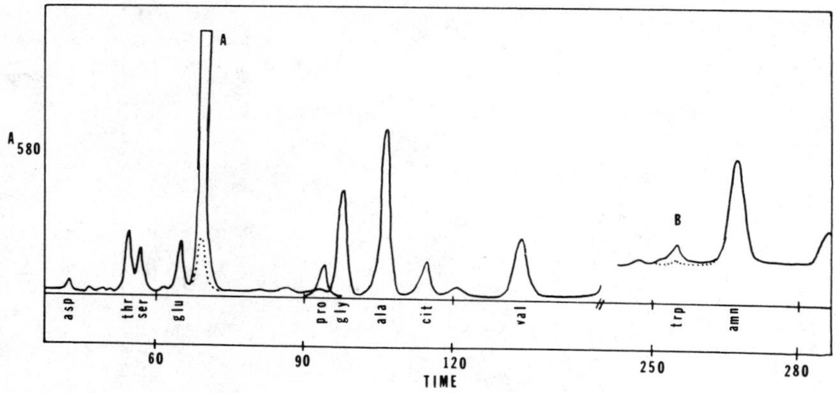

Figure 55.1 Analysis of ninhydrin-positive components of 1st (solid) and 16th (dotted) dialysates from a typical patient (Ct), following approximately five-fold concentration of dialysate to a standard amino acid content. Absorbance at 580 nm is plotted against elution time on a LiOH physiological fluids program on a Beckman Model 121 M Amino Acid Analyzer (details in text). Elution times of some of the common amino acids found in serum and urine are indicated; the portions of the chromatogram before 30 min, between 150 and 240 min and after 290 min are omitted. The two peaks found to be more plentiful in dialysate 1 are labeled A and B; A elutes at approximately the same times as asparagine, while B coelutes with tryptophan. Both A and B disappear following acid hydrolysis; there is no large increase in any single amino acid (including aspartic) following hydrolysis, suggesting that peak A is a peptide.

found to be greatly enriched in dialysate 1 from five of six patients, although the intensity of staining varies from patient to patient. This material coelutes with the peak of high concentration seen previously by amino acid analysis. Furthermore, the electrophoretic mobility of the ninhydrin-positive, tyrosine-positive spot is consistent from patient to patient.

Using the semi-quantitative method described above for estimating the concentration of peptide in peak A, we have approximated the amount of material present. Figure 55.3 shows that in five of six patients there is at least a hundred-fold excess of material in dialysate 1 as compared to that in dialysate 16. Furthermore, the quantity of material present in dialysate 8 from two of the patients suggests that metabolic stores are being gradually diminished. BPRS scores are plotted in figure 55.3B. In one patient (figure 55.3C) there continues to be a considerable quantity of material present in dialysate 16. Although there was an improvement in the BPRS for this patient, post-dialysis social adjustment was ambiguous. In another patient (figure 55.3D) levels of material in the first, ninth and sixteenth dialysates, in post-dialysis relapse serum, relapse dialysate and serum after dialysis were examined. Although there are some methodological problems with the identification of material in the serum, our present methodology suggests that there is a high concentration of material in the serum before relapse dialysis and a much lower concentration after relapse dialysis. Furthermore, although the concentration of peptide in this patient's sixteenth dialysate was very low, the concentration in the relapse dialysate was quite high.

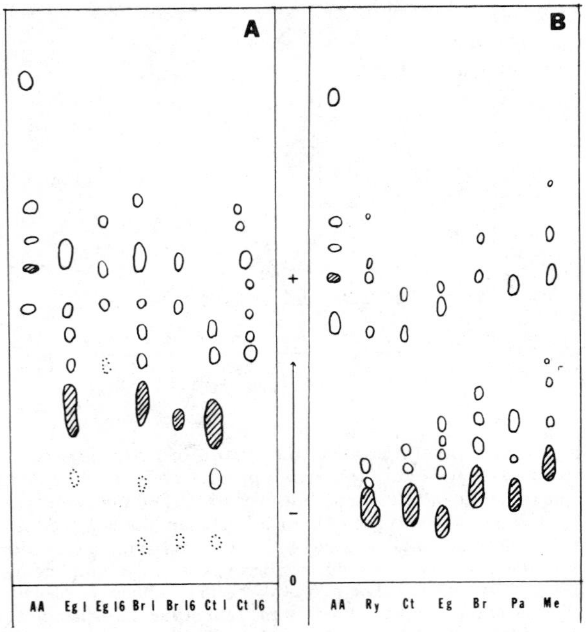

Figure 55.2 Tracing of high-voltage electrophoretograms of dialysate peptides and amino acids, pH 1.9 pyridine acetate buffer, stained with cadmium acetate ninhydrin (circled) or 1-nitroso-2-naphthol (cross-hatched). A, Concentrates (50-fold) of 1st and 16th dialysates from three separate patients were run at 3 kV, 60 min, then stained for ninhydrin-positive and tryosine-positive material. Amino acid standards (Channel 1) include tyrosine. B, Concentrates (50-fold) of 1st dialysates from all six patients studied were run at 3 kV for 50 min and stained as above.

Purification and properties of peptide

Peptide from four patients (Ct, Eg, Pa, Ry) has been purified to electrophoretic homogeneity, using the protocol described in the experimental section of this paper. A single N-terminal amino acid, tyrosine, was obtained following reaction of an aliquot of each peptide with phenylisothiocyanate, conversion to the PTH derivative and identification by g.l.c. and t.l.c. (Palmour and Ervin, unpublished results). The molecular weight of each peptide is approximately 3000 daltons, as determined by gel filtration on a calibrated column (figure 55.4). The amino acid composition of peptide derived from each of these patients is presented in table 55.2, both as molar fractions and as residues of amino acid present. The compositions are quite similar to one another and are generally consistent with published compositions of β-endorphin. The sulphophenylisothiocyanate derivatives of peptides from patients Eg and Ry have been partly sequenced using both manual and automatic procedures. Quantitative data from the first eight degradations of peptide Eg are presented in table 55.3. The complete amino acid sequence of peptide from patient Eg is

Tyr-Gly-Gly-Phe-Leu-Thr-Ser-Glx-Lys-Ser-Glx-Thr-Pro-Leu-
Val-Thr-Leu-Phe-Lys-Asx-Ala-Ile-Ile-Lys-Asx-Ala- ? -Lys-(Lys, Gly, Glx).

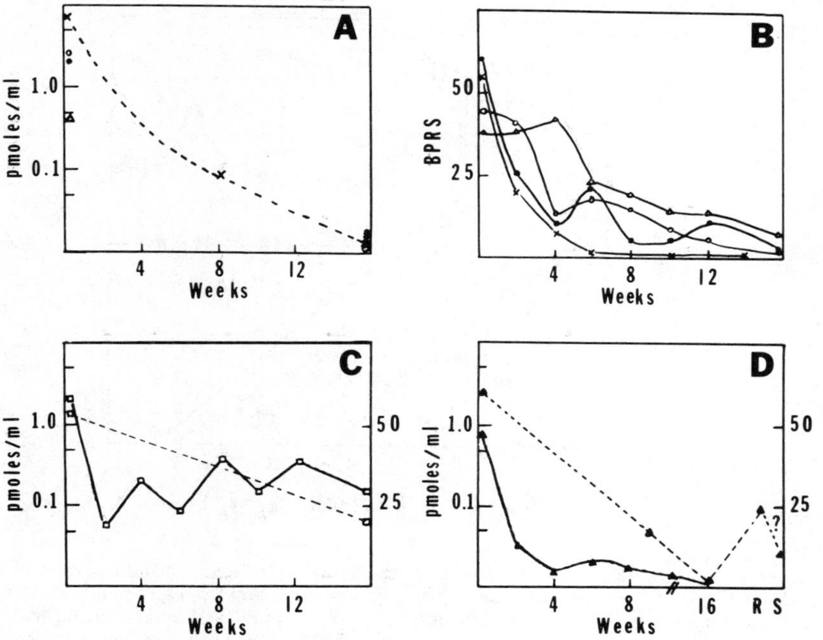

Figure 55.3 A graphic representation of the decline in peptide concentration from dialysates 1 to 16 and its reappearance in relapse in one patient. A, A semi-quantitative estimate (details in text) of the concentration of peptide in four patients (X, Eg; ○, Pa; •, Me; △, Ct) is plotted on a logarithmic scale as a function of number of weeks of dialysis. A curve is traced only for the patient for whom data on the level of peptide at 8 weeks of dialysis are available. B, Brief Psychiatric Rating Scale (BPRS) scores are plotted for the same four patients as a function of number of weeks of dialysis. C, Levels of peptide (dashed line) and BPRS scores (solid line) are plotted for a patient (□, Br) whose progress was ambiguous. D, Levels of peptide (dashed line) and BPRS scores (solid line) are plotted for a patient (▲, Ry) whose relapse dialysate (R) and serum after dialysis (S) were analyzed for levels of peptide. The methodology for examination of this peptide is not yet sufficiently sensitive to permit absolute quantification.

Although amide residues remain to be assigned, and although there are still some ambiguities near the C-terminus of the molecule, the present sequence appears to be identical to that of normal human β-endorphin with one exception: in position 5 there is a Leu residue rather than a Met residue. Analysis of the N-terminal portion of material from patient Ry demonstrates that the leu-enkephalin pentapeptide is present in that peptide as well. Analysis of material from other patients is in progress; it seems likely that peptides Ct and Pa contain both leucine and methionine in position 5.

We have compared the chromatographic and electrophoretic properties of peptides from patient Eg with those of synthetic β-endorphin. Although the elution pattern on preparative and analytical ion exchange chromatography and the migration pattern on t.l.c. in some solvent systems is extremely similar for β-endorphin and the molecule we report here, on high voltage electrophoresis β-endorphin has a faster mobility than does the dialysate peptide. Although both

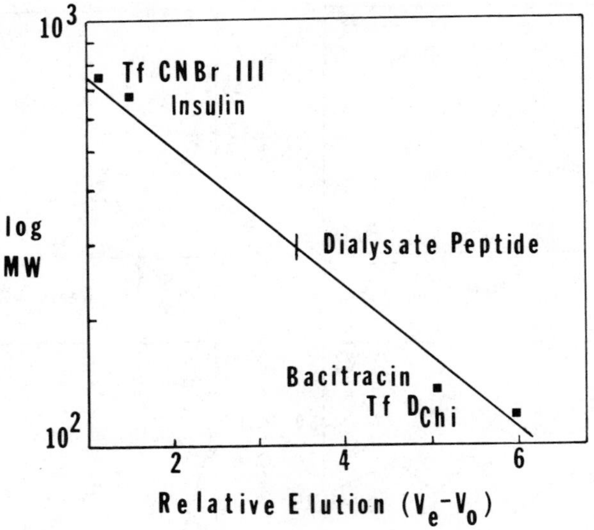

Figure 55.4 Molecular weight estimation of the peptide purified from 1st dialysate of four patients. Gel filtration was performed on a calibrated Sephadex column as described in the text, and relative elution positions of marker peptides were plotted against the logarithms of the appropriate molecular weights. The elution position of dialysate peptides corresponds to a molecular weight of approximately 3000. Tf peptides were purified and sequenced previously from human transferrin.

Table 55.2 Composition of purified peptides*

	Eg	Pa	Ry	Ct
Lys	0.1826 (6.0)	0.1550 (5.4)	0.1568 (5.2)	0.1831 (5.9)
Asp	0.0725 (2.4)	0.0669 (2.3)	0.0750 (2.6)	0.0690 (2.1)
Thr	0.1018 (3.3)	0.1117 (3.9)	0.0810 (2.7)	0.0920 (2.9)
Ser	0.0594 (1.7)	0.0544 (1.0)	0.0626 (2.1)	0.0646 (2.0)
Glu	0.0887 (2.9)	0.0900 (3.2)	0.0992 (3.3)	0.1057 (3.3)
Pro	0.0306 (1.0)	0.0255 (0.9)	0.0289 (1.0)	0.0394 (1.2)
Gly	0.1154 (3.8)	0.1289 (4.5)	0.0976 (3.2)	0.0944 (2.9)
Ala	0.0690 (2.3)	0.0703 (2.5)	0.0925 (3.1)	0.0520 (1.6)
Val	0.0324 (1.1)	0.0279 (1.0)	0.0352 (1.1)	0.0306 (1.0)
Met	0.0101 (0.3)	0.0184 (0.6)	0.0198 (0.7)	0.0209 (0.6)
Ile	0.0611 (2.0)	0.0641 (2.2)	0.0683 (2.3)	0.0682 (2.1)
Leu	0.0946 (3.1)	0.0918 (2.7)	0.0952 (2.7)	0.0660 (2.1)
Tyr	0.0261 (0.9)	0.0297 (1.0)	0.0259 (0.9)	0.0381 (1.2)
Phe	0.0620 (2.0)	0.0627 (2.1)	0.0596 (2.0)	0.0741 (2.3)
	32.8	34.3	32.9	31.2

*Expressed as molar fractions (number of residues)

Table 55.3 Sequence of dialysate peptide*

	1	2	3	4	5	6	7	8
Lys†	tr		0.0177	0.0043	tr	tr	0.0073	0.0179
Asp			0.0076					
Thr					0.0045	*0.0975*	tr	
Ser	tr	tr				0.0084	*0.0095*	0.0307
Glu							0.0086	*0.1775*
Gly	0.0278	*0.2640*	*0.4019*	0.1103	0.0049	0.0021	tr	0.0056
Ala	0.0131	0.0078	tr	tr		0.1763‡	0.0716§	0.0120
Leu				0.0170	*0.2446*	0.0995	0.0314	tr
Tyr	*0.0531*	0.0098	tr					
Phe			0.0123	*0.3120*	0.0549	tr		

*Peptide from patient Eg; manual Edman degradation with direct identification of residues by amino acid analysis following HI hydrolysis.
†Residues expressed as μmol amino acid.
‡Hydrolysis of threonine with HI yields both Thr and α-aminobutyric acid.
§Hydrolysis of serine with HI primarily yields alanine

leu and met-enkephalin have been reported in the brains and pituitaries of various animals, and although the generation of met-enkephalin from β-LPH by way of β-endorphin has been reasonably proposed (Hughes *et al.*, 1975; Lazarus *et al.*, 1976), a similar precursor molecule for leu-enkephalin has not yet been described. Whether the leu-endorphin we report here is a normal brain constituent or whether it is an atypical molecule generated by the substitution of a leucyl for a methionyl codon in the structural gene encoding β-LPH is not clear. A single nucleotide substitution would account for a methionine to leucine shift.

Behavioral and neurophysiological observations

Intraventricular administration of leu-endorphin and of [D-Ala^2, Leu^5]-enkephalinamide elicit paroxysmal hypersynchronous firing from amygdala (figure 55.5), as has previously been reported by Henriksen *et al.* (1977). By contrast to their observations with β-endorphin, we have observed very long lasting activity (greater than 36 hours) and alterations of the synchrony of firing of the reticular formation as well. Control administration of synthetic β-endorphin, but not of [D-Ala^2, Met^5]-enkephalinamide, resulted in paroxysmal hypersynchronous amygdala firing of much shorter duration than that observed with leu-endorphin. Behavioral alterations observed during the duration of pharmacological action included ataxia, motor stereotypies, inability to orient to new surroundings and epileptic 'absences'. Again the duration of behavioral alterations was much longer with leu-endorphin than with synthetic β-endorphin.

DISCUSSION

These findings suggest many questions and many further studies. We would like to comment on two of these areas. First, the relationship between circulating leu-endorphin, psychotic disorder and/or hemodialysis remains an enigma. For example, is the high concentration of this molecule due to the stress of dialysis?

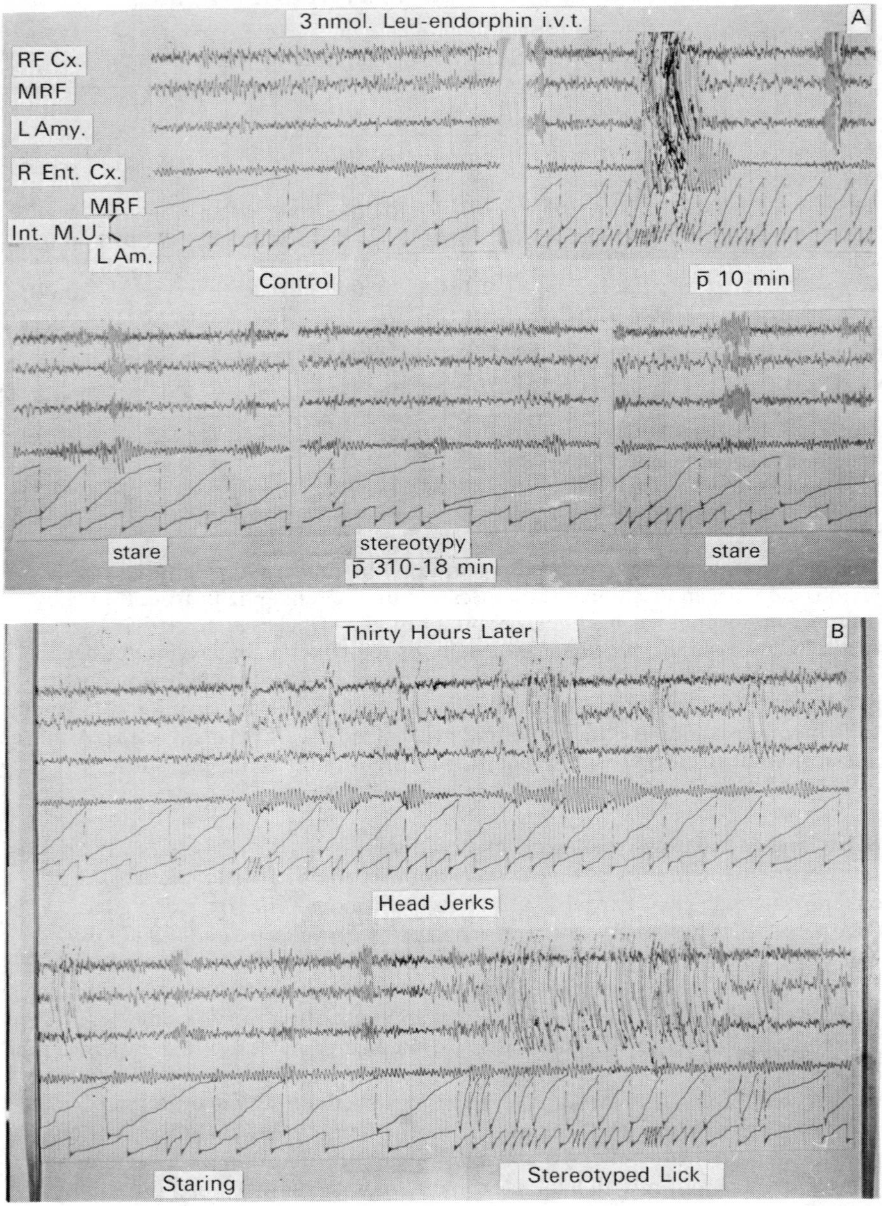

Figure 55.5 Electrophysiological effects of i.v.t. injection of leu-endorphin. Three nanomol of [Leu[5]]-endorphin purified from patient Ry (sequence analysis presented in text) was injected into a 2 kg cat through an i.v.t. cannula at time 0. Recordings were taken at 25 mm/s on a Grass polygraph from semimicroelectrodes implanted in the right frontal cortex (RFC), Mesencephalic reticular formation (MRF), left amygdala (LAm) and entorhinneal cortex (ERC). The two lower tracings represent the integrated multiunit activity from the MRF and

We are familiar with animal studies suggesting the secretion of opioid peptides in response to stress (Madden *et al.*, 1977) and with the recent elegant demonstration that β-endorphin and ACTH are concomitantly secreted in stressed animals (Guillemin *et al.*, 1977*a*). In some of these studies it appears that levels of opiate peptides decline in chronically stressed animals. In man, renal dialysis has been reported to increase serum levels of β-MSH (another hormone cleaved from β-LPH) which were positively correlated with the duration of dialysis. ACTH levels, though high, were not abnormal (Gilles *et al.*, 1975). In contrast, we have found a negative correlation between endorphin levels and duration of dialysis. One might still argue that psychotic, in contrast to renal patients, show a high endocrine stress response, and later, an habituation to the experience of dialysis. Were this the case, one might not expect to see the increased endorphin levels in the 17th dialysate of relapsed patients, as we see in this study. Furthermore, preliminary data from the examination of dialysate from renal patients suggests that high levels of endorphins are not characteristic of those dialysates. We are currently evaluating the endocrinological profile of renal and psychotic patients being treated with hemodialysis.

Another possibility is that the high endorphin levels are a consequence of long-term treatment with neuroleptic drugs. Again we have not yet studied this possibility thoroughly. However, two separate laboratories have failed to find increased levels of β-MSH in phenothiazine-treated patients, although MSH levels are increased in experimental animals receiving phenothiazines (Plummer *et al.*, 1975). In one patient reported in this study, phenothiazines had been discontinued

---

the LAm, respectively. The slope of the integrator ramp is directly proportional to the rate of firing for these units. A, The earliest electrographic changes were noted 3.5 min after injection. From left to right, and top to bottom: (1) baseline recording, animal alert and relaxed, grooming or resting, before any injection; (2) after injection, there was a marked increase in grooming, particularly in the perineal area and a tendency to posture; episodes of fixed stare lasted 10–30 s and episodes of stereotyped licking of the forepaw and/or the cage occurred. By day 2, motor awkwardness, loss of placing reaction and mild cataleptic rigidity were increased. Stereotyped licking was more marked and urine drinking occurred. Electrographically, the record is dominated by hypersynchronous spindle bursts appearing through the MRF, left amygdala (LAm) and Cortex (Cx). There is some indication that these bursts originate in the reticular formation (RF), but note their similarity to activity induced by hallucinogens such as quipazine. In records 3 and 5, isolated spindle bursts are illustrated, recorded concomitantly with episodes of fixed stare. Between episodes (4), the record looks quite normal for periods of several minutes, during which the animal was in a bizarre posture and manifested stereotyped grooming of the forelimb. B, Thirty hours later, both the recordings and the behaviors continued to be at least as strongly modified as they were during the first few hours post-injection; there were, however, longer periods of apparently normal sleep. Throughout the record, there were periods of abrupt spindling (top) accompanied by myoclonic jerks of the head and neck. Such an episode was characteristically accompanied by an increase in unit firing in the RF and often in the LAm as well; it was not infrequently terminated by a protracted bout of stereotypic grooming. Bursts of hypersynchronous spindles continued to appear during this period, but much of the record is dominated by less well-organized episodes of spiking or irregular fast activity, especially in the RF (bottom). These late effects are suggestive of the effects seen after the administration of [D-Ala^2, Leu^5]-enkephalinamide (Ervin, Palmour and Guzman, unpublished results). During this later period, the animal was fearful of handling, and when placed in an unfamiliar cage, vocalized and showed poorly organized threat responses to observers and to other cats.

9 months before dialysis. Moreover, the appearance of endorphins in relapse dialysates mitigates against the notion that this is simply a chronic drug effect.

Finally, the behavioral and neurochemical properties of this molecule are of extreme interest. In addition to the studies reported here, we have tested crude preparations of this material in chickens, rabbits, rats and monkeys and have found a continuum of behavioral effects ranging from drowsiness, ataxia and stereotypies to limbic seizures, convulsions and death. Carefully controlled dose response and drug interaction studies are now under way. Studies of the metabolism and breakdown of the molecule in animal preparations using radiolabelled endorphins have also been initiated. It is interesting to note that Guillemin *et al.* (1977) have recently reported that synthetic leu-endorphin binds more avidly to brain receptors than does met-endorphin. Although the neurophysiological mechanisms of endorphin function are still unclear, the alterations of neuroendocrine regulation and dopaminergic transmission which could be engendered by prolonged binding of this neuroactive molecule to specific receptor sites bears investigation.

In summary, we report the presence of a new biological material, leu-endorphin. Its presence in high concentrations in a group of drug-resistant, psychotic patients and its positive correlation with states of remission or relapse suggests it to be an important key to understanding the pathophysiology of this small subset of the psychoses. Because it has not been identified in normal brain or pituitary, we cannot at this time distinguish between the abnormal production or impaired degradation of a normally occurring molecule and the presence of a genetically variant molecule.

Further studies of the electrophysiological effects of [Met^5]-β-endorphin revealed that high doses (100 μg) elicit long-lasting (> 36 h) alterations.

REFERENCES

Gilles, J. J. H., Eady, R. A. J., Rees, L. H., Munro H. H. and Moorhead, J. F. (1975).*Br. Med. J.*, **1**, 656–8

Gray, W. R. (1967). *Meth. Enzymol.*, **XI**, 469–71

Guillemin, R., Vargo, T., Rossier, J., Minick, S., Ling, N., Rivier, C., Vale, W. and Bloom, F. (1977*a*). *Science*, **197**, 1367–9

Guillemin, R., Ling, N., Burgus, R., Bloom, F. and Segal, D. (1977*b*). *Psychoneuroendocrinology*, **2**, 59–62

Henriksen, S. J., Bloom, F. E., Ling, N. and Guillemin, R. (1977). *Soc. Neurosci.*, 933

Hughes, J., Smith, T. W., Kosterlitz, H. W., Fothergill, L. A., Morgan, B. A. and Morris, H. R. (1975). *Nature*, **258**, 577–9

Inman, J. K., Hannon, J. E. and Appela, E. (1972). *Biochem. biophys. Res. Commun.*, **46**, 2075

Kety, S., Rosenthal, D., Schulsinger, F. and Wender, P. (1968). In *The Transmission of Schizophrenia*, (eds. S. Kety and D. Rosenthal). Oxford University Press, Oxford

Lazarus, L. H., Ling, N. and Guillemin, L. (1976). *Proc. natn. Acad. Sci. U.S.A.*, **73**, 2156–9

Madden, J., Akil, H., Patrick, R. L. and Barchas, J. (1977). *Nature*, **265**, 358–60

Niall, H. D. (1975). In *Protein Sequence Determination*, (ed. S. B. Needleman). 2nd ed. Springer, New York

Opolon, P., Rapin, J. R., Huguet, C., Granger, A., Delorme, M. L., Boschat, M. and Sausse, A. (1976). *Trans. Am. Soc. Artif. Int. Organs*, **22**, 701–8

Plummer, N. A., Thody, A. J., Burton, J. L., Goolamali, S. K., Shuster, S., Cole, E. N. and Boyns, A. R. (1975). *J. clin. endocr. Med.*, **41**, 380–2

Smithies, O., Gibson, D., Fanning, E. M., Goodfliesh, R. M., Gilman, J. G. and Balentyne, D. L. (1971). *Biochemistry,* **10**, 4912–21

Tholen, H., Stricker, E., Feer, H., Massini, M. A. and Straub, H. (1960). *Deutsch. Med. Wochenschrift,* **85**, 1012–3

Wagemaker, H. and Cade, R. (1977). *Am. J. Psychiat.,* **134**, 684–5

Summary of basic research

Candace B. Pert and Agu Pert (Section on Biochemistry and Pharmacology, Biological Psychiatry Branch, National Institute of Mental Health, Bethesda, Maryland, U.S.A.)

The study of endorphins and opiate receptors continues to expand wildly in all directions as it captures the imaginations of scientists in virtually every field. Only 6 months elapsed between the last meeting of the International Narcotics Research Conference held in New Hampshire and the symposium on Endorphins in Mental Health Research reported in this volume. It is a credit to the ingenuity of the investigators at this meeting that they were able to make so many new discoveries in such a short time. In this brief summary, we have tried to touch on most of them, but we cannot claim to have covered everything of importance.

Little light was shed at this meeting on the synthetic pathways for enkephalin or β-endorphin production in central nervous tissue. In a mouse pituitary tumor cell line, however, the beautiful agreement between two elegant studies (Mains and Eipper; Herbert *et al.*) left little doubt that a very large (31K) protein is the gene product precursor for the manufacture of pituitary β-endorphin. This protein, appropriately dubbed 'pro-opiocortin' by Udenfriend's group, contains β-lipotropin (β-LPH) at the C-terminal, ACTH in the middle and a very large hunk of an, as yet unidentified sequence, at the N-terminal. While pro-opiocortin is the major component of both rat and camel pituitary (Udenfriend *et al.*), its presence in brain at this time can only be surmised from the close association between β-LPH, β-endorphin and ACTH radioimmunoassayable material within the same neurons (Watson *et al.*).

Evidence that ACTH and β-LPH pituitary release are closely coupled continues to mount following the original report by Guillemin *et al.* (1977) that ACTH and β-endorphin levels rise concurrently following the sudden fracture of the tibia or adrenalectomy. Krieger *et al.* reported a highly significant correlation of elevated plasma ACTH and β-LPH concentrations in patients with Cushing's disease, Nelson's syndrome, or the ectopic ACTH syndrome. Plasma concentrations of ACTH and β-LPH in her patients also rose together after insulin-induced hypoglycemic stress or vasopressin administration. Herbert *et al.* reported that ACTH and β-endorphin release from pituitary cultures were concurrently stimulated by hypothalamic extract (CRF) and blocked by dexamethasone. In Herbert's study, ACTH and β-endorphin were released virtually mol for mol, while Krieger reported an ACTH/LPH ratio which ranged from 2.4–3.7, possibly due to differences in distribution volume or rate of degradation between the two hormones. The exciting discovery by Smyth and Lakarian that both brain and pituitary contain a substantial quantity of N-terminal acylated C-fragment (β-endorphin) and β-LPH suggests one possible mechanism for the uncoupling of ACTH and opioid activity, since N-acylation of the critical terminal tyrosine residue would destroy affinity for opiate receptors.

While Graf *et al.* demonstrated that pituitary homogenates are capable of liberating β-endorphin from the opiate-inert β-LPH, almost nothing is really known of the enzymatic steps in endorphin synthesis and destruction. The degradation scheme of Smyth and Zakarian for β-endorphin [(LPH_{61-91}) → C^1-fragment (LPH_{61-87}) and then to α or γ-endorphin and met-enkephalin with cleavage of the terminal tyrosine] is not in agreement with that of Graf *et al*. who believe cleavage of Leu^{77}-Phe^{78} is the rate limiting step of β-endorphin destruction, which is then followed by removal of the now susceptible N-terminal tyrosine.

While endorphin is a hormone itself, there is no doubt that enkephalin or endorphin acting as a neurotransmitter in the hypothalamus regulates the release of other hormones from the anterior pituitary (see Guidotti and Grandison, LaBrie *et al.*, Miller *et al.* and Fredrickson *et al.*). Potent enkephalin analogues, morphine and β-endorphin all produce dramatic increases in serum levels of growth hormone (GH) and prolactin (PRL). Naloxone can not only antagonize opiate-induced GH and PRL release, but also produces a decrease in basal PRL (Guidotti and Grandison, Fredrickson *et al.*,) and GH (Fredrickson *et al.*,) levels, suggesting that ongoing enkephalinergic tone modulates the basal levels of these hormones. All the data, including particularly the intrahypothalamic microinjection by Guidotti and Grandison, are consistent with a hypothalamic locus of modulation. Stress-induced release of PRL (Guidotti and Grandison) can be blocked by naloxone as well, suggesting that enkephalinergic activity has a role in this phenomenon.

Several other substances, not yet chemically characterized, were reported to possess opiate-like activity by some criteria—the smoke has definitely not yet cleared in this area! Wüster *et al.* report a non-peptide substance found in brain with naloxone-reversible activity in the guinea pig ileum and mouse vas deferens. Teschemacher *et al*. find their Pronase-resistant substance in blood, urine and milk, as well as pituitary. The material is naloxone-reversible in the guinea pig ileum, but neither of the above materials is recognized by morphine antisera. Spector *et al.* report on the morphine-like compound (MLC) originally identified by its reactivity to antisera prepared against morphine. MLC, which is not a peptide, produces opiate receptor inhibition, marked inhibition in the smooth muscle-plexus preparations, as well as a striking behavioral effect after i.v.t. injection. None of the pharmacological effects of MLC is naloxone reversible, but an endogenous opiate of such high affinity that reversal by an antagonist is impossible is certainly not unimaginable. Also relevant is the report by Musacchio *et al.* that the naloxone-reversible, calcium-dependent release of what was previously thought to by endorphin, by strong stimulation of the guinea pig ileum, has a dissociation rate far too slow to be either β-endorphin or enkephalin. Klee *et al.* demonstrated that pepsin digests of wheat gluten generate an 'exorphin' (exogenous morphine) which produces naloxone reversible opiate-like effects in both the vas deferens and adenylate cyclase assay. This finding could breathe new life into the theory that wheat gluten in food is a factor in the pathology of schizophrenia.

With regard to schizophrenia, Terenius *et al*. continue to report on their radioreceptor assay for opiate-like substances in cerebrospinal fluid with which elevated levels of certain chromatographic fractions are detected in the CSF of some mentally ill patients. Terenius's claim that the material detected in his radioreceptor assay is a peptide is based on its destruction by pronase and trypsin, although it is not recognized by antibodies prepared against β-endorphin or met-enkephalin. In direct contradiction, Udenfriend *et al.* report that human CSF is devoid of any peptide endorphin activity and contains only MLC. The astounding revelation of Palmour *et al.* that first dialysates of schizophrenic blood contain such high levels of the peptide Leu^{64}-β-endorphin that complete biochemical identification is possible was met with considerable skepticism. To obtain one milligram of pure peptide (the quantity required for peptide identification) from the approximately 7 l of blood which undergoes dialysis in one individual would require blood levels of about 5×10^{-5} M, an extraordinarily high value, about four orders of magnitude above those in stressed rats. Udenfriend *et al.*, moreover, emphasized that they had failed to detect any leu-enkephalin or leu-β-endorphin in rat or camel pituitary.

Determination of brain levels of neurotransmitters generally gives only very insensitive or ambiguous assessments of neurotransmitter usage. Yang *et al.* have made a good start at developing a method for assessing enkephalin turnover by measuring the incorporation of i.v.t. administered [^{3}H] amino acids into met-enkephalin purified by an antibody affinity column. The experiments of Childers and Snyder suggested that enkephalin is rarely utilized and its release is uncommon. After sufficient cyclohexamide administration to block 90 per cent of protein synthesis, enkephalin levels fell so very slowly that 12 hours were required in order to observe a significant reduction. Pert and Bowie described a novel method for assessing the very small but functionally important pool of endorphin which is associated with opiate receptors. They found changes in opiate receptor occupancy with cold-induced stress, sleep deprivation, and strenuous exercise. Enkephalin levels, on the other hand, are quite resistant to alteration by opiate administration or environmental stimuli, but chronic administration of neuroleptics (Hong *et al.*; Wise and Stein) were shown markedly to increase enkephalin levels—whether by increasing or decreasing turnover is unknown.

The important question of the possibility and organization of multiple opiate receptors received little attention at this meeting. Creese *et al.* pointed out that opiates fall into two groups: (a) those with great sensitivity to sodium and reduced ability to displace [^{3}H] met-enkephalin; and (b) those with low 'sodium shifts' and more equivalent ability to displace [^{3}H] met-enkephalin and [^{3}H] dihydromorphine binding. They postulate that enkephalin and other group (b) opiates possess an extra lipophilic binding site for receptor attachment. Watson *et al.* described experiments in which several brain regions appear to contain more met-enkephalin than leu-enkephalin binding sites. Pert and Bowie emphasized that opiate receptors can be classed as 'occupied' or 'unoccupied'. The ways to categorize and divide opiate receptors continue to multiply with no one as yet offering a parsimonious categorization which simultaneously explains all of the binding data, the differential pharmacological sensitivity of the guinea pig ileum compared with the vas deferens (Lord *et al.*, 1977) and the subtle differences in the pharmacological profiles of morphine and some benzomorphans in the dog (Martin *et al.* 1976).

The number of potent enkephalin analogues containing the D-Ala^2 substitution first reported by Pert *et al.* (1976) continues to multiply. This modification preserves opiate receptor affinity and bestows resistance to degradative enzymes (see Marks and Lajtha). Of particular interest are the Sandoz analogue, FK33-824 (Tyr-D-Ala-Gly-MePhe-Met(O)-ol), which is four times as active as morphine even after s.c. injection in mice (see Extein *et al.*) and the Lilly analogue, Tyr-D-Ala-Gly-Phe-N(CH_3)-Met-$CONH_2$, which is also so potent that it is active by a peripheral route (see Fredrickson and Smithwick). Of potential therapeutic importance is the discovery that the Lilly analogue is unable to produce naloxone-precipitated withdrawal jumping even after 2 weeks of very high dose chronic administration. Miller *et al.* report on the structures and sometimes surprising pharmacological profiles of the most extensive series of metabolically stable enkephalin analogues synthesized to date. Li has prepared a number of β-endorphin analogues whose immunological reactivity, not surprisingly, bears no relation to their receptor potency. D-Ala^2 substitution retains β-endorphin's pharmacological potency but does not improve it as would be expected, since β-endorphin itself is already much more resistant to degradation than enkephalin. Interestingly, the substitution Phe^{27}, Gly^{31} in the only positions where human and camel β-endorphin differ, results in an analogue slightly more potent than the natural form.

There were some very hearty discussions of the accuracy of various determinations of enkephalin levels. Converting all data to pmol/mg protein with the assumption that 1 mg protein = 10 mg wet weight and that one rat striatum weighs 50 mg, it can be calculated that Bloom, Miller and Costa are in very close agreement with mean met-enkephalin values of about 2.5 pmol/mg hypothalamus protein and 2.0 pmol/mg striatal protein. Udenfriend reported the richest striatum, containing a full order of magnitude more met-enkephalin. Watson's values for hypothalamus were about four times higher. The cause of the discrepancies are unknown but presumably must relate to differences in conservation during extraction or cross-reactivity with interfering substances.

Studies using radioimmunoassays and immunocytochemical techniques have revealed endorphins in brain as well as the pituitary. These two endorphin systems appear to be independent since hypophysectomy does not alter the levels of brain endorphins (Miller *et al.*, Goldstein and Cox). There also appear to be two independent endorphin systems in brain—one encoded by β-endorphin and the other by met or leu-enkephalin. Bloom *et al.* and Watson *et al.* reported the presence of two groups of β-endorphin neurons in brain using immunocytochemical techniques. One group has their perikarya located in and dorso-lateral to the arcuate nucleus of the hypothalamus; the other group is located more anterior and lateral in the basal hypothalamus. Varicosities from these neurons have been followed to a number of midline structures near the ventricles, including various hypothalamic nuclei, midline thalamus, pontine periaqueductal grey matter, dorsal raphe and locus coeruleus. Forebrain structures that appear to be innervated by β-endorphin-containing neurons include the lateral septum and the nucleus accumbens.

While the β-endorphin encoded neuronal pathways seem to be rather restricted in origin and distribution, the enkephalin-coded systems are much more ubiquitous in brain. Uhl *et al.* reported immunofluorescent enkephalinergic fibers and terminals in the substantia gelatinosa of dorsal horn of the spinal cord, as well as the substantia gelatinosa of the spinal trigeminal nucleus in the medulla. The presence of enkephalins in these regions may serve to modulate pain transmission at a rather early level of integration. Lower levels of fluorescence were found in the ventral and dorsal portions of the pontine reticular formation. Enkephalinergic cell bodies were also observed in a number of hindbrain regions including the raphe magnus, medial vestibular nucleus and the dorsal cochlear nucleus. At the level of the locus coeruleus, the densest fiber terminals, as well as cell body fluorescence, was found in the medial aspect of the dorsal tegmental nucleus of Gudden. In the mesencephalon, fibers and cell bodies were found in the medial aspect of the interpeduncular nucleus. The periaqueductal grey matter contained enkephalinergic cell bodies but only modest densities of fibers and terminals which appeared to extend into the lateral midbrain. Miller *et al.* and Jacobowitz *et al.* described more rostral enkephalinergic perikarya and projections. Positive staining cell bodies and nerve terminals were found in the lateral septum, amygdala, hippocampus, globus pallidus, caudate nucleus and nucleus accumbens. Apparently, not all enkephalinergic cells are interneurons as has been previously suggested. Uhl *et al.* presented evidence for at least two enkephalinergic pathways. Lesions of the central nucleus of the amygdala (one region high in enkephalinergic cell bodies) resulted in the loss of fluorescence in the ventrolateral stria terminals, suggesting the presence of an amygdalo-fugal enkephalinergic pathway. In addition, some enkephalinergic neurons appear to project from the caudate nucleus to the globus pallidus since injections of kainic acid (a neurotoxin that destroys cell bodies) into the head of the caudate/putamen resulted in a substantial depletion of enkephalinergic fluorescence in portions of the globus pallidus. Jacobowitz *et al.* postulated the existence of an enkephalinergic pathway that may have its origin in the globus pallidus and which projects through the medial forebrain bundle toward the olfactory tubercle and the septal region. Future mapping studies will undoubtedly reveal whether there are other long enkephalinergic pathways or whether enkephalin is generally contained within interneurons.

A number of groups also reported on the brain distribution of enkephalin using RIA. In general, it seems that the highest enkephalin levels are associated with areas that have the densest enkephalinergic terminal and cell body concentrations (Miller *et al.*, Bloom *et al.*). The presence of enkephalinergic terminals, cell bodies and endogenous enkephalin in limbic forebrain and hindbrain regions, the diencephalon and extrapyramidal structures suggests an important modulatory role of enkephalins in affective states, pain perception, autonomic functions, as well as motor behavior.

If endorphins are indeed novel neurotransmitters or neuromodulators, they appear to be predominantly inhibitory in nature. Bloom *et al.* found that most cells in the CNS were inhibited by the iontophoretic application of opiate alkaloids, as well as peptides. Exceptions to this were the pyramidal cells in the hippocampus and the Pukinje cells in the cerebellum. Enkephalin also appears to be inhibitory in the spinal cord. Zieglgänsberger and Tulloch found that iontophoretically applied enkephalin inhibited spontaneous, as well as glutamate and substance P-induced, excitation of cells in the dorsal horn. Enkephalin, however, was not found to produce changes in membrane potential or resistance like hyperpolarizing inhibitory neurotransmitters. Instead, enkephalin seems to depress the rate of rise of the postsynaptic excitatory potential by altering sodium influx into the cell. These findings strongly suggest a postsynaptic action for enkephalin at least in the spinal cord.

Mudge *et al.*, on the other hand, presented evidence that [D-Ala^2, Met^5] enkephalin inhibits potassium-evoked release of substance P from sensory neuron cultures. They suggested that enkephalin may instead decrease the entry of calcium into nerve cells thereby decreasing the release of substance P or other excitatory neurotransmitters. These findings, in turn, suggest a presynaptic site of action of enkephalins and opiate alkaloids in the spinal cord. It is possible, of course, that enkephalin acts through both mechanisms to inhibit the transmission of nociceptive information at the level of the spinal cord.

The wide spectrum of pharmacological effects exhibited by opioid alkaloids presumably reflects the normal involvement of endogenous opioids in a variety of physiological processes.

For example, low doses of opiates have been shown to increase core temperatures while high doses have been shown to decrease it. Herz and Bläsig also found similar effects following administration of the systemically active potent opioid peptide FK233-824. The same investigators also found that naloxone inhibited emotionally-induced hyperthermia. The role of endorphins in temperature regulation was also substantiated by Goldstein and Cox, who indicated that naloxone induced a slight but significant hyperthermic response, and by Holaday *et al.* It seems likely that one of the physiological roles of enkephalins, at least in mammals, is to modulate body temperature.

The potent analgesic profile of opiates and opioid peptides and the presence of endorphins in brain regions known to process pain information suggests the existence of an endogenous pain suppression system. If this system is tonically active, then it should be possible to produce hyperalgesia by blocking the effects of endorphin with appropriate opiate antagonists. Although results from studies using this approach have been rather equivocal (Goldstein and Cox) Fredrickson *et al.* were able to demonstrate consistent hyperalgesia in the hot-plate paradigm following systemic naloxone. Interestingly, the same investigators also observed a diurnal rhythm in control nociceptive reactions as well as in the hyperalgesic effects of naloxone and the analgesic effects of morphine. These findings presumably reflect the natural rhythmic oscillations in the activity of endorphins.

Low dosages of opiates produce hyperactivity in rats while high doses produce a depression of motor behavior and catatonia which is often followed by motor excitation. Intraventricular injections of β-endorphin, enkephalin, as well as morphine, were also found to produce similar biphasic effects on spontaneous locomotor behavior in rats (A. Pert *et al.*, Segal *et al.*). The excitatory and inhibitory opiate effects appear to be mediated through distinct and different neuroanatomical systems. Injections of morphine and [D-Ala^2, Met^5]-enkephalin into the nucleus accumbens produced only increases in locomotor activity while injections of morphine into the periaqueductal grey matter, ventral thalamus and dorsal hippocampus produced only inhibition of activity.

If endogenous endorphin systems in brain are active in modulating motor behaviors then opiate antagonists should be effective in modifying motor activity. Depression of motor activity in rats was, in fact, reported by both A. Pert *et al.*

and Segal *et al.* following the systemic administration of naloxone. Kelleher and Goldberg also found naloxone produced dose-dependent decreases in operant responding in monkeys. The ability of naloxone to produce only depression of motor activity suggests either that the enkephalinergic systems which increase motor output are the only ones that are tonically active or that these are the more dominant.

Herz and Bläsig also compared the catatonic potencies of various opiate alkaloids and opioid peptides. All produce catatonia which was qualitatively similar. Morphine, however, appeared to have a catatonic potency that was lower than that of the peptides. One reason for this may be the confounding nonspecific excitatory effects exhibited by morphine (Jacquet) which are not seen with other opiates or opioid peptides.

The catatonic actions of opiates have often been ascribed to their inhibitory actions on striatal dopamine neurons. Perez-Cruet *et al.* did in fact, report that apomorphine blocked β-endorphin-induced catatonia and that β-endorphin increased homovanillic acid (HVA) in the striatum. These findings seem to support the notion that β-endorphin blocks dopamine neurons. Extein *et al.*, on the other hand, found that HVA levels in the CSF of monkeys were not modified by FK33-824. While there appear to be some similarities between dopaminergic blocking agents and opiates and opioid peptides, the mechanisms underlying the catatonic effects of opiates and the cataleptic effects of neuroleptics cannot be the same. A. Pert *et al.* suggest that morphine and phenothiazines induce immobility through entirely different neural substrates.

Opiates also have the ability to initiate and maintain self-administration behavior in laboratory animals. Presumably, their euphorigenic actions underlie this property. Stein and Belluzzi found that rats will also self-administer enkephalins into the ventricular space, thereby suggesting a euphorigenic property for enkephalins. The same authors also proposed that electrical self-stimulation of certain brain regions depends in part on the release of enkephalin. On the basis of the ability of naloxone to antagonize electrical self-stimulation from the periaqueductal grey matter, as well as other enkephalin-rich brain regions, these investigators have suggested that endogenous opioid peptides may actually mediate the 'drive-reducing' reward function which corresponds to the state of satisfaction or well-being associated with goal attainment. Alternatively, the rewarding effects of enkephalins and opiate alkaloids may be determined by a direct or indirect activation of ascending catecholamine pathways which have also been implicated in mediating hedonistic behavior (Stein and Belluzzi).

Many issues still remain unresolved—they will require clarification by further experiments. However, we dare not list the important questions toward which future research 'should' be directed. Breakthroughs have a way of coming from unpredictable directions, and this field will surely continue to have its share of surprises.

Summary of clinical research

Glenn C. Davis and William J. Bunney Jr. (National Institute of Mental Health, Bethesda, Maryland, U.S.A.)

Isolation of the opiate receptor and subsequent elucidation of a family of opiate-like peptides has dramatically opened a new era in our understanding of brain biology. Because of the extensive effects of opiates on behavior and mood, there has been a rapid introduction of these basic biochemical and pharmacological findings into clinical studies. The physiological roles of the various endorphins as neurotransmitters and endocrine effectors have yet to be clearly defined, but the dramatic implications for clinical medicine are such that basic and clinical studies have proceeded in parallel. This volume contains clinical studies of the effects of narcotic antagonists, the clinical and pharmacological effects of the endogenous opiate β-endorphin, studies examining the pharmacology of these substances in animals, and basic papers (reviewed by Pert and Pert, pp. 594–600) that appear to have clinical relevance.

Kline and Lehmann, and Angst *et al.*, report the effects of β-endorphin administered in single doses of up to 10 mg in patients suffering from a variety of psychiatric illnesses. Kline and Lehmann report improvement in the symptoms of schizophrenia in 1 to 5 days after the administration of β-endorphin and, in case-study format, report improvement in a variety of other psychiatric illnesses. Angst *et al.* report a marked and persistent improvement in two of six depressed patients administered β-endorphin in an open trial. These investigators found that three of six depressed patients switched into mania or hypomania after injection.

Catlin *et al.* found relief of cancer pain in two of three patients given β-endorphin i.v. while Hosobuchi and Li report prolonged analgesia after i.v.t. administration.

Because of the enormous interest in the pharmacology and possible therapeutic efficacy of these drugs, Tocus and Brown reviewed the procedures for obtaining investigational drug status for new peptides such as β-endorphin.

A number of investigators (Perez-Cruet *et al.*; Davis *et al.*; Janowsky *et al.*; Gunne *et al.*; Berger *et al.*; Emrich *et al.*) report their experience with the narcotic antagonists, naloxone and naltrexone, in schizophrenia, affective illness and catatonia. Perez-Cruet *et al.*, Davis *et al.*, Janowsky *et al.*, and Gunne *et al.* failed to find naloxone effective in reducing the psychotic symptoms of schizophrenia. Emrich *et al.* and Berger *et al.* report that naloxone reduced or eliminated auditory hallucinations in most of their schizophrenics. Emrich *et al.* also found that the delusions of their patients were reduced.

Janowsky *et al.* found general anti-manic effects of naloxone in mood, motor and speech parameters, while Davis *et al.* found the rate and amount of speech reduced in a dose-dependent fashion in one patient using a placebo-controlled, repeated-dose design. Emrich *et al.*, on the other hand, did not find anti-manic effects in two patients administered naloxone.

Davis *et al.*, Gunne *et al.*, and Emrich *et al.* did not observe any anti-depressant effects of naloxone in a small number of depressed patients tested. Davis *et al.* and Emrich *et al.* found naloxone without effect in a small number of patients with catatonic features.

Thus no conclusion can yet be drawn as to the therapeutic effects of narcotic antagonists in schizophrenia, mania, depression and catatonia. Methodological issues of dose, duration of patient evaluation, patient selection criteria, and rating measures are discussed by the authors.

Physiological, pharmacological, and subjective effects of naloxone in volunteer groups may be found in the papers of Jones; Davis *et al.*; and Goldstein and Cox.

Thus a functional role for endorphins in mental illness remains speculative but the studies found within this volume should serve as an excellent guide for subsequent investigations.

Contributors index

Subject index